Human Experimentation and Research

The International Library of Medicine, Ethics and Law

Series Editor: Michael D. Freeman

Titles in the Series

Human Experimentation and Research

Edited by

George F. Tomossy and David N. Weisstub

University of Sydney, Australia and Université de Montréal, Canada

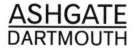

ASHGATE
DARTMOUTH

Published by
Dartmouth Publishing Company
Ashgate Publishing Limited
Gower House
Croft Road
Aldershot
Hants GU11 3HR
England

Ashgate Publishing Company
Suite 420
101 Cherry Street
Burlington, VT 05401-4405
USA

Ashgate website: http://www.ashgate.com

British Library Cataloguing in Publication Data
Human experimentation and research. – (The international
   library of medicine, ethics and law)
   1. Human experimentation in medicine – Moral and ethical
   aspects 2. Human experimentation in medicine – Law and
   legislation
   I. Tomossy, George F. II. Weisstub, David N., 1944–
   174.2'8

Library of Congress Cataloging-in-Publication Data
Human experimentation and research / edited by George F. Tomossy and David N. Weisstub.
        p. cm. — (International library of medicine, ethics, and law)
   Includes bibliographical references.
   ISBN 0-7546-2226-6 (alk. paper)
      1. Human experimentation in medicine—Law and legislation. 2. Human experimentation
in medicine—Moral and ethical aspects. I. Tomossy, George F. II. Weisstub, David N.,
1944– III. Series.

   K3611.H86H86 2003
   174'28—dc21

                                                                          2003045351

ISBN 0 7546 2226 6

Printed in Great Britain by The Cromwell Press, Trowbridge, Wiltshire

Contents

PART II   PROTECTING HUMAN SUBJECTS

PART III   RISK AND RESPONSIBILITY

PART IV   GLOBALIZATION AND CORPORATION – TRUST AND PARTICIPATION

Acknowledgements

The editors and publishers wish to thank the following for permission to use copyright material.

George J. Annas (1996), 'Questing for Grails: Duplicity, Betrayal and Self-Deception in Postmodern Medical Research', *Journal of Contemporary Health Law and Policy*, **12**, pp. 297–324. Copyright © George J. Annas.

Ashgate Publishing Limited for the essay: David J. Rothman (1998), 'The Nuremberg Code in Light of Previous Principles and Practices in Human Experimentation', in Ulrich Tröhler and Stella Reiter-Theil in cooperation with Eckhard Herych (eds), *Ethics Codes in Medicine: Foundations and Achievements of Codification Since 1947*, Ashgate: Aldershot, pp. 50–59.

Association of American Medical Colleges for the essay: Mark Yarborough and Richard R. Sharp (2002), 'Restoring and Preserving Trust in Biomedical Research', *Academic Medicine*, **77**, pp. 8–14. Copyright © 2002 Association of American Medical Colleges.

American Society of Law, Medicine and Ethics for the essays: Jesse A. Goldner (2000), 'Dealing with Conflicts of Interest in Biomedical Research: IRB Oversight as the Next Best Solution to the Abolitionist Approach', *Journal of Law, Medicine and Ethics*, **28**, pp. 379–404. Copyright © 2000 American Society of Law, Medicine and Ethics; Charles Weijer (2000), 'The Ethical Analysis of Risk', *Journal of Law, Medicine and Ethics*, **28**, pp. 344–61. Copyright © 2000 Charles Weijer; Nancy M.P. King (2000), 'Defining and Describing Benefit Appropriately in Clinical Trials', *Journal of Law, Medicine and Ethics*, **28**, pp. 332–43. Copyright © 2000 American Society of Law, Medicine and Ethics; Robert J. Levine (1988), 'Uncertainty in Clinical Research', *Law, Medicine and Health Care*, **16**, pp. 174–82. Copyright © 1998 American Society of Law, Medicine and Ethics. Reprinted with the permission of the American Society of Law, Medicine and Ethics. All rights reserved.

Arnold Journals & Reference for the essay: S. Senn (2002), 'Ethical Considerations Concerning Treatment Allocation in Drug Development Trials', *Statistical Methods in Medical Research*, **11**, pp. 403–11. Copyright © 2002 Arnold.

Blackwell Publishing Ltd for the essays: Eric M. Meslin, Heather J. Sutherland, James V. Lavery and James E. Till (1995), 'Principlism and the Ethical Appraisal of Clinical Trials', *Bioethics*, **9**, pp. 399–418. Copyright © 1995 Blackwell Publishers Ltd; Richard Ashcroft (1999), 'Equipoise, Knowledge and Ethics in Clinical Research and Practice', *Bioethics*, **13**, pp. 314–26. Copyright © 1999 Blackwell Publishers Ltd; David Wendler (2002), 'What Research with Stored Samples Teaches us about Research with Human Subjects', *Bioethics*, **16**, pp. 33–54. Copyright © 2002 Blackwell Publishers Ltd; Trudo Lemmens and Benjamin Freedman (2000), 'Ethics Review for Sale? Conflict of Interest and Commercial Research Review Boards', *Milbank Quarterly Review*, **78**, pp. 547–84.

Series Preface

Few academic disciplines have developed with such pace in recent years as bioethics. And because the subject crosses so many disciplines important writing is to be found in a range of books and journals, access to the whole of which is likely to elude all but the most committed of scholars. The International Library of Medicine, Ethics and Law is designed to assist the scholarly endeavour by providing in accessible volumes a compendium of basic materials drawn from the most significant periodical literature. Each volume contains essays of central theoretical importance in its subject area, and each throws light on important bioethical questions in the world today. The series as a whole – there will be fifteen volumes – makes available an extensive range of valuable material (the standard 'classics' and the not-so-standard) and should prove of inestimable value to those involved in the research, teaching and study of medicine, ethics and law. The fifteen volumes together – each with introductions and bibliographies – are a library in themselves – an indispensable resource in a world in which even the best-stocked library is unlikely to cover the range of materials contained within these volumes.

It remains for me to thank the editors who have pursued their task with commitment, insight and enthusiasm, to thank also the hard-working staff at Ashgate – theirs is a mammoth enterprise – and to thank my secretary, Anita Garfoot for the enormous assistance she has given me in bringing the series from idea to reality.

MICHAEL FREEMAN
Series Editor
Faculty of Laws
University College London

Introduction: Human Research Ethics

Human experimentation is essential for advancing scientific knowledge and thereby for improving the longevity and quality of human lives. Yet the pursuit of this laudable ambition may come into conflict with moral values to which we might be equally committed, such as the sanctity of life and personal autonomy. The twentieth century has produced an unprecedented number of technological and medical advances; but this history is also littered with tragic revelations of professional scandals and the exploitation of vulnerable persons. What are the boundaries of ethically permissible experimentation with human subjects? Or, as posed by Katz (1993, p. 34), 'When, if ever, is it justified to use human beings as subjects for research, considering that they also serve as means for the ends of others?' the answer to this question, however phrased, is by no means straightforward. While there is a general consensus that the sacrifice of individuals for the benefit of society should be minimized, if not avoided altogether, this tension between society and the individual pervades philosophical and policy discussions in research ethics.

Decision-making concerning the use of human beings in experiments must reconcile a range of interests, as well as balance potential risks and benefits. With mounting international pressure for improved healthcare in the face of constrained resources and ageing populations, the challenge *not* to use persons 'as means for the ends of others' is becoming all the more difficult. Moreover, the concomitant phenomena of globalization and corporatization of science in recent decades are forcing the rethinking of traditional paradigms in research ethics. A complex web of interests, including substantial economic considerations, has replaced the classic 'society–individual' dialectic. While the ethical precepts of *justice, beneficence* and *respect for persons*, articulated over 25 years ago in the historic US *Belmont Report* (1978), continue to anchor existing research ethics policies, it nevertheless behoves us to reconsider their continued relevance (or perhaps force) in a modern corporatized research culture. Risks and the consequences of unethical experiments are not necessarily confined to isolated subjects and can impact whole communities or future generations. Incidents of ethical wrongdoing can have even broader implications by undermining public trust in the research enterprise. Furthermore, inequities in the distribution of the benefits of research, which are easily exported from one jurisdiction to another, present new dilemmas for regulators and investigators alike. The topic of the ethics of human experimentation at the start of the new millennium continues to remain, therefore, a fluid domain of inquiry, demanding self-reflection, responsive criticism and perhaps novel solutions.

The scholarly literature on human research ethics is as rich as it is at times controversial. A full exploration of the legal, technical, ethical and moral problems raised by human experimentation, which are of ongoing importance in bioethics discourse and public health policy decision-making, would amount to a vast undertaking. This volume is intended to canvass only some of the issues.[1] An attempt has been made to select a number of scholarly works that review the historical and philosophical foundations of research ethics (Part I), legal and regulatory dilemmas in protecting human subjects (Part II), notions of risk and responsibility (Part III), and some future challenges inspired by a global research industry (Part IV). The central theme that permeates the essays in this volume – and the field of research ethics generally, for that matter – is recognition of the need for vigilance in protecting individuals against the barrage of external interests that might threaten their dignity and bodily integrity.

The Historical and Philosophical Foundations

An appropriate place to begin any exploration of the issues raised by the conduct of research involving human subjects in the post-war era is the oft-cited 'courageous article' (Katz, 1993, p. 31) in the *New England Journal of Medicine* by Henry Knowles Beecher (1966).[2] Foremost amongst his concerns was the dramatic upward trend of available funds and demand for research over the prior two decades that could foreseeably exceed 'the supply of available responsible investigators'. He described the increasing dominance of medical academia by investigators, how this also created pressures on 'ambitious young physicians', and noted that the societal value of human experimentation, coupled with the growth of clinical research as a distinct profession, could lead to an 'unfortunate separation between the interests of science and the interests of the patient'. Beecher correctly attributes a pivotal role to the investigator, noting that the most reliable safeguard for ethical research is 'an intelligent, informed, conscientious, compassionate, responsible investigator' (see also Beecher, 1970, p. 79).

Yet, as Katz (1993, p. 34) notes, Beecher's ethical investigator 'could only come into being . . . after the value conflicts inherent in research are clarified and choices are made about the priorities to be given to competing values'. But what are these 'competing values'? Exploring this question is relevant not only for establishing a value framework for decision-making by investigators, but also in rationalizing the practice of human experimentation itself. A credible moral foundation is needed in order to construct an ethically sound system wherein persons can be exposed to risks for the benefit of others, either by being called upon to submit to these risks willingly, perhaps in response to a social duty to do so, or as in some cases by actually being conscripted into service through benevolent deception, coercion or surrogate consent.

The traditional framework for philosophical reflection on human experimentation is summarized in Chapter 1 by Hans Jonas in what has become a classic essay in research ethics:[3]

> The setting for the conflict most consistently invoked in the literature is the polarity of individual versus society – the possible tension between the individual good and the common good, between private and public welfare. (p. 4)

This conflict of values is echoed throughout the research ethics literature and official policies, but is invariably resolved in favour of the individual. The consensus conveyed by both the Declaration of Helsinki and European Convention on Human Rights and Biomedicine, for example, is that human experimentation is both necessary and acceptable,[4] provided that appropriate safeguards to protect human subjects are in place.[5] Indeed, a review of official research ethics policies will reveal this to be the case across most jurisdictions (for example, Brody, 1998, pp. 31–54, 119–38).

In the quest for values in research, different philosophical ideologies will yield different results. In Chapter 2, Ruth Macklin and Susan Sherwin assess both deontological and utilitarian approaches. In the case of persons unable to provide consent, they find a Kantian response to be too restrictive, while a utilitarian calculus can too easily contribute to exploitation of their vulnerability. Instead, they favour a model based on the conception of justice put forward by Rawls (1971). But irrespective of whether even this approach provides the best solution, Macklin and Sherwin's analysis reveals the limits of applying any singular philosophical standpoint to found a value base in research ethics. One must, in the end, arrive at some sort of compromise between ideological poles. As Weisstub (1998, p. 2) noted:

> ... we are prepared nonetheless to assert that between the Western Judeo-Christian ethic and a popular consciousness achieved in this century with respect to what can be understood as a liberal ethic, we can balance the individualistic-modernist morality of which we have become a part, and the public interest and communitarian ethic upon which we justify some curtailments of absolute freedom in the nature of a broader good.

A good example of compromise is the historic *Belmont Report* (1978), authored by the National Commission for the Protection of Human Subjects of Biomedical and Behavioral Research (US), which eschewed any single ethical theory (Levine, 1986, pp. 11–12). Instead, it enunciated the principles of *respect for persons*, *beneficence* and *justice*[6] to guide ethics committees in their deliberations. These principles remain the cornerstone of research regulations in the United States, having also been adopted as the basis for policies in other jurisdictions, such as Canada (Tri-Council, 1998).

A principle-based approach, although having notable supporters (for example, Veatch, 1981; Engelhardt, jr, 1996) and widespread application, is not without detractors (see, in particular, Gert *et al.*, 1997; Toulmin, 1981).[7] The central objection to 'principlism'[8] is that it does not embody 'an articulated, established, and unified moral system capable of providing guidance' (Gert *et al.*, 1997, p. 75). In response to this line of criticism, in Chapter 3 Eric Meslin *et al.* assess the principles offered by Beauchamp and Childress against standard meta-criteria used to assess normative theories. They argue that principles, while not being wholly adequate to serve as a foundation for ethical decision-making, need only to be supplemented by 'sensitivity to context'[9] in the evaluation of clinical trials:

> ... principles should function as heuristics that can be specified in the context of clinical trials, acting not as formal rules for decision making, but rather as cognitive prompts for thinking about the types of considerations that research involving human subjects ought to accommodate. (p. 90)

A statement of ethical principles or standards is relevant not only to guide decision-makers, but also to assist in judging their actions and thereby provide a basis for moral accountability. Regrettably, reviewing professional conduct, including when it was officially sanctioned, has been a necessary exercise on numerous occasions.[10] The promulgation of the Nuremberg Code[11] in response to the Nazi experiments is the most significant such event in the history of research ethics. David Rothman concludes in Chapter 4 that the importance of this ruling is not so much its role in formulating ethical principles, since these were all known and established previously, but in entrenching them in a formal code under legal sanction. As Childress notes in Chapter 5, its greatest legacy is a 'fundamental and absolute commitment to the rights and welfare of research subjects, whatever the prospect of scientific advancement' (p. 113). But when judgements are made in relation to events that occurred many years in the past, it raises a profound controversy concerning the universality of ethical principles. In Chapter 6 Allen

Buchanan relates how the question of retrospective moral judgement troubled the members of the Advisory Commission on Human Radiation Experiments (ACHRE) throughout their deliberations (ACHRE, 1996, ch. 4). The heart of the Committee's framework is a distinction between the wrongness of actions and culpability of agents. Various principles were deemed to be universal and not time-bound, thus making retrospective judgement possible; while factors such as a lack of evidence, cultural variables and conflicting obligations, could serve to mitigate culpability even where the underlying act was found to be 'wrong'. A determination of the wrongness of a past act would not necessarily imply that the person who committed it is blameworthy. Tom Beauchamp (Chapter 7)[12] while praising the ACHRE for being 'decisive beyond what might reasonably have been anticipated in light of its broad and diverse mission' (p. 141) found the Committee's treatment of the matters of culpability and possible exculpation to be lacking, thus compromising the essential objectives of the process to achieve future deterrence and provide justice for wronged individuals.[13]

Despite the difficulties associated with retrospective judgement, revelations of scandals in human research have been instrumental in stimulating regulatory reforms. But to say that transformative moments in the history of research ethics and regulation occur only as a result of scandal, while partly true, is an oversimplification. Official policies emerge due to a number of other reasons including concern about new technologies or their application, and broader social movements (Brody, 1998, pp. 197–99). Indeed, as Jay Katz notes in Chapter 13, the response of codification and regulation in research was a response to the revelation that 'reliance on the ethical conscience, inculcated in physician-investigators during their medical education, provided insufficient protection to the human rights of subjects of medical research' (p. 227). The recurring *prescriptive* response by *external* forces to govern the research universe is significant. As Rothman (1998, p. 42) observed,

> . . . the history of human experimentation makes clear that left to itself, medicine in its collective capacity does not necessarily generate change, even when a sizeable gap separates professed ideals from actual practice. The impetus must come from outside, whether from a court, as with Nuremberg, or from federal regulation, as with the [institutional review board].

Rothman rightly reinforces the need for accountability – for external oversight to judge and ascribe blame to those who commit unethical acts.

Unethical research, however, raises concerns beyond those of its direct consequence to subjects. In Chapter 8, Arthur Caplan discusses the scientific validity of unethical research[14] by examining the incorporation of the results of the Tuskegee Syphilis Study into the scientific literature. He critiques two components of the argument that good science is incompatible with bad ethics: useful or valid scientific findings cannot be generated from obviously immoral conduct, and the body of scientific knowledge should not accept any findings thus obtained.[15] He concludes that '[t]he acceptance of the Tuskegee study findings as valid refutes the argument that bad ethics is always incompatible with valid science' (p. 145) but that further use of the data should be accompanied by discussion of its ethical deficiencies.[16]

Ethical violations have, of course, a broader implication: destruction of 'trust' in the research enterprise. This theme is explored by Sissela Bok (Chapter 9) whose essay was written in response to a growing prevalence of the use of deception in psychological and behavioural studies. Bok emphasizes the importance of truth-telling, cautioning against undermining the traditional protections of subjects on the basis of risk–benefit calculations and arguing that a failure to do so could have broader ramifications in terms of damaging trust in professionals and their institutions. Loss of trust can result not only from failings in truthful disclosure, but from more general exchanges and relationships. In Chapter 10, Nancy Kass *et al.* draw upon extensive subject interviews conducted by the ACHRE and find that patients participated in research for a number of reasons along the scale between self-interest to altruism. They also found that interviewees placed substantial trust in the integrity and benevolence of investigators and their institutions, so much so that it might ultimately hinder the fulfilment of the informed consent process. Kass *et al.* echo, in a fashion, the concerns raised by Bok:

> The stories these patient-subjects told about why they decided to participate in research suggest that the current emphasis in research on analyses of benefits and risks and on subjects' autonomous decisionmaking is insufficient. The paradigm must be enriched with a sensitivity to the profound trust participants place in researchers and the research enterprise. (pp. 166–67)

A further challenge to Beecher's 'responsible investigator' arises when the roles of healer and scientist coincide. In Chapter 11, George Annas is highly critical of such 'double lives', stating that '[d]oubling and duplicity in both language and action have become the hallmark of experimentation in the United States and most of the developed world (p. 172). He lays part of the blame on the dominance of market ideology, which places profit-making as the highest priority. He is particularly critical of terms such as 'therapeutic research', which he views as infecting and obfuscating the true nature of the exchange between subject and researcher (see also Verdun-Jones and Weisstub, 1998). Annas rightly concludes that:

> To confront not only our mortality, but also our morality, we must use language to clarify rather than obscure what we do to one another. Minimally, we must correctly identify and describe roles and responsibilities in human experimentation. In our postmodern world, it may not be realistic to think we can always distinguish research from therapy, physicians from scientists, or subjects from patients. Nonetheless, it is morally imperative to use language to clarify differences because ignoring these differences undermines the integrity of scientific research, the integrity of the medical profession, and the rights and welfare of patients and subjects. (p. 196)

The problem, however, as Katz argues in Chapter 13, goes beyond obfuscatory language, a lack of clarity in professional roles and blind trust in the legitimacy of the invitation to participate in research. It also arises from the ideology of medical professionalism when applied to research. By this, Katz refers to the traditional argument put forward by medical professionals for non-disclosure based on paternalistic justifications in the guise of beneficence. He is justly critical of arguments that endorse a therapeutic privilege in the doctor–patient relationship, and particularly so in research.

The difficulty in deriving a satisfactory solution from any single philosophical ideology to moral problems in research ethics highlights their complexity. Sometimes, as David Weisstub explores in Chapter 12, these questions 'have led us quite naturally to make, arguably in good faith, a set of both moral and legal fictions in order that our social needs have respectable "justificatory" ethics' (p. 203). He does not suggest that these are mere rationalizations, but rather sincere attempts to balance different goals that may be in either explicit or implicit conflict. He warns, however, to guard against unquestioning reliance on such solutions, as they 'cannot only be misleading, but also a contributing factor to the kind of dependency where moral failures can be most pronounced' (p. 203). Protecting human subjects requires, therefore, not only a staunch commitment to fundamental ethical principles, but also sensitivity to the ways in which moral and legal fictions, deliberate or unintended obfuscations in professional roles and outright violations of subjects' rights can damage an implicit trust in the integrity of science and its officers. While Beecher's 'conscientious investigator' is an invaluable agent in this endeavour, history has judged sole reliance on this frontline defence to be insufficient. Without a means of enforcing or holding accountable those charged with this responsibility, philosophical inquiry into the rights of subjects and interests of science becomes a merely academic pursuit.

Protecting Human Subjects

Part II of this volume explores some of the ethical, legal and regulatory responses to the dilemmas of subject protection and balancing of values in research.

It is appropriate to frame the task of protecting human research participants as a societal responsibility. Indeed, ensuring the fair treatment and safety of the subjects from whom societal gains derive should be viewed as an implied public duty. As Jonas admonishes in Chapter 1, 'Let us not forget that progress is an optional goal, not an uncompromising commitment' (p. 29). Thus, despite an insatiable demand for social advances, the evolution of research ethics policies has rightly supported, at least in principle, limits on the sacrifices that can be demanded of citizens in the name of progress and restraints on the activities of those involved in its pursuit. A range of alternative approaches for the best method of achieving this objective, however, continues to be debated.

The most pronounced trend in research ethics governance over recent decades has been towards increasingly formal external oversight. This has involved a process of codification, development of the ethics committee review system, promulgation of official regulations and enactment of statutes (see, generally, McNeill, 1993, chs 1–6).[17] As Paul Benson explains in his review of social controls in human biomedical research (Chapter 14), the move in the United States towards 'externally developed, bureaucratically administered, and formally sanctioned rules' (p. 280) was largely a result of dissatisfaction with the success of internal controls, including both informal procedures and codes. Benson also notes the limited influence of the courts on developing legal controls (see also Roth *et al.*, 1987, pp. 427–29), with judicial rulings on conduct in research being generally sparse throughout common-law jurisdictions.[18] Continuing in this trend, Jonathan Moreno (Chapter 15) presages the next era in research regulation in the United States as one of 'strong protectionism'. He designates the peer or committee review process as a transitionary phase and describes the past twenty-odd years as 'a compromise that combined substantial researcher discretion with rules enforced by a minimal bureaucracy' (p. 286). Moreno views this trend as a historical inevitability that is motivated by recognition of a duty owed to protect those who participate in research, and is sceptical of efforts to combat this trend, including the suggestion that education or improved cooperation between review boards and investigators could be an alternative to expanding external control mechanisms (for example, Koski, 1999).

Moreno's criticism should not be viewed as belittling the importance of researcher integrity, but instead perhaps as resignation to the persistence of forces promoting external controls. Indeed, Moreno appears to be wary of strong protectionism insofar as it might 'inadvertently result in undermining physician investigators' sense of personal moral responsibility' (p. 293). If such an alienation of responsibility were to occur, it would arguably undermine the legitimacy of any governance structure that must depend, at least in part, on the sound judgement and ethical conduct of its agents, which will always include the investigator as the pivotal point of contact with the subject. As Barber *et al.* (1973, pp. 186–89) observed in their classic study, both internal and external social controls are inevitable for a profession to become and remain socially responsible, which they view as the desirable and essential feature of any 'profession'. An ideal environment which, in their view, best serves the interests of a profession would rely solely on internal controls (self-regulation). However, they concluded that, even in cases where such mechanisms are nearly perfect, external controls are unavoidable. At the very least, society will have an expectation of effective internal governance but also demand some level of accountability. The demand for external controls will rise whenever confidence in self-regulation wanes, which at its highest level can include recourse to law. Unsurprisingly, Katz's critique in Chapter 13 relates to both internal and external controls, the former at the level of clarifying the investigator–subject relationship in the consent dialogue, and the latter in recommending a national regulatory policy-making authority.[19] Indeed, recent scholarship clearly supports recognition of the 'need for responsibility and accountability at every level of the research enterprise' (Mastroianni, this volume, p. 306).

In Chapter 16, Alexander Capron, a former Commissioner of the National Bioethics Advisory Commission, also argues strongly in favour of national, independent oversight for the effective protection of human subjects. He notes that the regulatory framework in the United States has remained more or less unchanged for the past 35 years, identifying five constant features of this model: diffused authority, delegated responsibility, individualized decision-making, a 'peer review' format and limitation of federal rules. One could broadly describe these points as characterizing a system that lacks any cohesive authoritative force for policy formulation or regulatory control. Capron identifies delegation of responsibility as particularly problematic, despite being well-intended in deferring to the ethical character of the research professions. He argues that:

> . . . the time has come for a paradigm shift, not simply evolutionary adjustments of the details of the regulations but a new way of developing, promulgating, monitoring, and revising the regulations. To effect a new paradigm, we need to consolidate authority in this field in a new, independent federal office, linked to but not controlled by research-sponsors. (p. 297)

Anna Mastroianni (Chapter 17) fully supporting Capron's call for a national oversight body, further emphasizes the importance of accountability in instilling public trust. She recommends that any such body should be charged not only with identifying and providing guidance on issues of concern, but also with providing adequate monitoring and follow-up. Within such a framework, external controls could be calibrated according to specific needs. In other words, in some cases guidelines might suffice, but if after following up on their effectiveness these were found to be inadequate, more formal steps, such as promulgating regulations, should be within the ambit of such a body's authority. To date, this next step in the development of external controls – creation of a national oversight body – has been avoided in the United States – and in many other jurisdictions for that matter (for example, Law Reform Commission of Canada, 1989).[20]

The matter of legal and regulatory protections is especially relevant for research involving vulnerable populations. These traditionally include children (Ramsey, 1976; 1977; McCormick, 1976; Nicholson, 1986; McLean, 1992; Grodin and Glantz, 1994; Kopelman, 2000), the elderly (Glass, 1993; High and Doole, 1995; Keyserlingk *et al.*, 1995; Dresser, 2001a; Tomossy *et al.*, 2001), persons with cognitive disabilities or disorders (see below), and prisoners (Lasagna, 1969; Arboleda-Florez, 1991; Verdun-Jones *et al.*, 1998; Hornblum, 1998), but have also included women and minorities (Charo, 1993; McCarthy, 1994), military personnel (Annas, 1998), patients requiring emergency care (Karlawish and Hall, 1996; Fost, 1998), the terminally ill (Gray *et al.*, 1995; Addicott, 1999) and communities, particularly indigenous groups (Weijer, 1999). Infamous incidents involving these populations include unethical studies of hepatitis on children (Rothman and Rothman, 1984; Lederer and Grodin, 1994), cancer cells in both terminally ill elderly patients and prisoners (Langer, 1964; Cassel, 1985; Hornblum, 1997), and radioisotopes on developmentally disabled children (West, 1998). Unfortunately, such occurrences cannot be simply relegated to the past. Only recently, the Maryland Court of Appeals criticized a leading US research institution harshly for the ethics of a lead abatement study conducted on economically disadvantaged children, and found that a duty of care *was* owed by investigators to their subjects which could form the basis of an action of negligence.[21]

As Schuklenk (2000, p. 969) noted, 'Research ethics are essentially about ways to ensure that vulnerable people are protected from exploitation and other forms of harm.' The key criterion for 'vulnerability' in the context of research is an inability to protect oneself from exploitation or exposure to unreasonable risks of harm (see, for example, Weisstub *et al.*, 1996). Arguably, all subjects are potentially vulnerable owing to their dependence on investigators to assess and communicate risks properly, and to make at least some decisions on their behalf. Only investigators possess the specialized knowledge required to understand the full extent of possible risks – at least as far as they can be reasonably predicted – and how these might impact on a given subject. Indiscriminately treating a group as 'vulnerable' might, of course, raise concerns about paternalism or outright discrimination. Yet a protectionist approach is not only warranted, but is also consistent with the ongoing trend in research ethics portrayed thus far: growing recognition of the need for increasing external controls of research activities. Vulnerable persons require, by definition, at least some level of assistance, whether by enhancing their ability to make decisions or by actively protecting them from harm. While autonomy-based arguments rejecting external regulatory interference in research might have some appeal in the case of 'non-vulnerable' persons, they fall short in the case of individuals whose autonomy is compromised even to the slightest degree. A fully competent adult, when aggrieved, can normally litigate. Children or cognitively impaired adults, however, cannot as readily avail themselves of the same judicial remedies. They must rely on external forces to defend their interests.

As Capron (1997, p. 25) observed, 'No type of research raises more problems than research with the mentally impaired, particularly those who are institutionalised for treatment.' Regrettably, effective legal governance is lacking in many jurisdictions. In Chapter 18, Marshall Kapp describes the regulation of research involving decisionally impaired adults in the United States as being in a 'dynamic state'. By this, he points to the high level of uncertainty concerning actual legal duties. Kapp's advice to mental health professionals, who can often become directly or indirectly involved in research protocols, is to be 'thoroughly conversant with existing, as well as credible proposed, statutes, administrative rules, and judicial decisions pertaining to research involving mentally impaired human subjects' (p. 326). His exposition of the evolution of regulatory controls and reactions to these efforts illustrates the difficulties faced in the attempt to regulate this area in a manner that balances the goals of subject protection, allows much-needed research to proceed, and avoids stigmatization of a population that has historically suffered extensive prejudice and exploitation.

Some have been highly critical of recommendations to increase regulatory controls governing research with 'persons with mental disorders that might affect decision-making capacity' such as those put forward by the National Bioethics Advisory Commission (1998). For example, in Chapter 19, Robert Michels is sceptical about whether singling out this area for regulatory reform would in fact enhance public confidence in research. He further remarks that an 'absence of special regulations . . . does not necessarily define a vacuum [which the NBAC 'rushed' to fill], and providing additional regulations is not the best solution to all problems (p. 333). His greatest concern, also flagged by Moreno in Chapter 15, is that regulations might 'undermine researchers' sense of moral responsibility as their attention shifts from their obligation to research subjects to their compliance with the regulations' (p. 333). The views represented by Michels reflect what might appear to be professional distaste for external legalistic interference. This may be justified. Poorly conceived, inflexible or cumbersome regulation might indeed curb research freedom, inhibit medical innovation, and interfere with the rights of individuals belonging to 'vulnerable populations' to participate in research and enjoy the prospect of an improved quality of life. However, the alternative of a non-regulated environment justifiably encounters resistance not only from proponents of regulation who mistrust market controls in general, but also from those responding to specific deficiencies in legal systems that the market cannot solve. Such legal gaps can compromise subject protection *as well as* the pursuit of vital health research.

To illustrate, George Tomossy and David Weisstub discuss, in Chapter 20, why research involving cognitively impaired adults has generally been found to stand on shaky legal ground in common-law jurisdictions. Courts have rightly resisted allowing surrogate decision-makers to submit their wards to procedures that do not accord with their best interests or which cannot be rationalized on the basis of a substituted judgement test.[22] Experimentation, which is, by definition, a non-benefit-producing intervention, is unlikely to be endorsed by a court, except perhaps in cases of nil or negligible risk (see also Queensland Law Reform Commission, QLRC, 1996, p. 393; Law Commission (UK), 1995, paras 6.33, 6.37; Dickens, 1998). To resolve this dilemma, Tomossy and Weisstub recommend guardianship law, including the provision of explicit statutory authority for advance and proxy consent on behalf of decisionally impaired persons (see also Backlar, 1998).[23] They argue that, in the absence of statutory clarification, researchers may be exposed unnecessarily to liability and possibly criminal sanction (Law Reform Commission of Canada, 1989), even where proxy consent has been obtained. Since neither alternative – proceeding in the absence of legal clarity or ceasing research altogether – is acceptable, legislative reform becomes not only desirable, but necessary.

Formulating research ethics policies must occur in a manner that is supportive of our devotion to principles of autonomy and personal inviolability. The protection of 'vulnerable' persons would be an especially important measure of success in this regard. The regulation debate discloses that ethical proscriptions or legal rules will fail if they are ignored, inconsistent, ineffective or not enforced. The challenge of research ethics regulation, then, is to create a governance framework that prioritizes subject protection by stimulating ethical conduct rather than merely proscribing it. Law need not be perceived as being in conflict with either science or research professionals. Although law must prove its legitimacy as a source of oversight by actually being followed *as well as* enforced, it equally serves as a force to legitimate practices that are inherently controversial (for example, Roach Anleu, 2001). Both internal (professional) and external (legal/regulatory) controls are therefore necessary in order to achieve the desired dynamic relationship between legal controls and actual practice.

Risk and Responsibility

The modern trend towards stronger protectionism described in Part II should not be perceived as diminishing the importance of the research professional. Indeed, given the rising complexity and continued social relevance of health research, the call for Beecher's 'responsible investigator' has never been greater. As Part IV of this volume conveys, the pressures now assailing investigators have increased dramatically. The very character of research has changed, most likely irreversibly, from the pursuit of purportedly philanthropic ambitions in quiet academic settings to the modern blending of economic and societal interests within a global corporate setting. The traditional individual–societal dialectic described in Part I is therefore no longer valid, having been replaced by a web of conflicting interests. But before discussing these issues, it is necessary to address some of the core concepts that underpin the ethical justification of clinical trials and ethical requirements for exchanges with subjects: risk of harm, benefit and uncertainty.

Managing risks of harm and benefits – minimizing the former and maximizing the latter – is a vital component of ethical research design and a core feature of research ethics review. Yet, as Charles Weijer notes in Chapter 21, ethics committees may be placing too much emphasis on the consent process and not enough on the risk–benefit calculus. This is troubling considering that the validity of an 'informed' consent hinges on the quality of disclosure of risks. An inadequate risk assessment, either by the investigator or the ethics committee, can undermine even the most carefully thought-out consent form. Subjects do not generally possess the expertise necessary to assess risks themselves and must rely on the investigator and safeguards of ethics reviews. This inherent vulnerability mandates a special duty owed to the subject that includes the effective evaluation, minimization and communication of risks.

The problem with 'risk' and 'benefit' is not only that they are amorphous concepts, but that these terms are often used incorrectly. Levine (1986, p. 37) describes risk 'in terms of probability that a certain harm will occur' and benefit as denoting 'something of value that can be supplied upon demand'. His preferred antonym for 'benefit' is 'injury'. Weijer reaffirms Levine's model, with respect to his categories of risk (physical, psychological, social and economic), and analyses the work of the Belmont Commission, whose recommendations continue to provide the foundations of risk–benefit analysis in research in the United States. Weijer is critical of inconsistencies in the existing US system and favours a 'comprehensive approach' that involves the systematic assessment of individual components of a study. Each component is to be distinguished on the basis of whether it has a 'therapeutic' or 'non-therapeutic' outcome for the subject and must be justified in its own right. Deconstructing a protocol in this manner is important in order to avoid classifying it as 'therapeutic' solely on the basis of some, or a few, therapeutic procedures.[24]

Characterizing 'risk' is not the only potential source of confusion; 'benefit' is equally troublesome and often misrepresented. This is unfortunate, as the two concepts are inextricably linked. In Chapter 22, Nancy King identifies the description of 'benefits' as an area to which investigators and ethics review committees should pay greater attention. She notes that a 'therapeutic misconception'[25] continues to prejudice patient-subject perceptions of the purpose and expected outcome of research involvement. King distinguishes three types of possible benefits from research: direct, collateral and aspirational. With patient-subjects generally being concerned with direct benefits, conflation with either of the other two categories, whether deliberate or inadvertent, is problematic.

The risk–benefit equation also needs to be conceived more broadly than merely as a balancing process of immediate harms and gains. In Chapter 23, David Wendler presents three models of subject involvement:

> The subject model traces to the claim that individuals' primary interests relevant to research are their interests in avoiding harm. . . . The experiential model recognizes a broader range of interests as relevant to individuals' research involvement, requiring that one consider whether the research might affect the individuals in any way, not simply whether it might harm them. . . . The contribution model recognizes that individuals' interests extend beyond their own experiences. In particular, individuals have interests in the projects to which they contribute. (p. 400 & p. 414)

Most existing regulatory frameworks operate under an experiential model which promotes informed consent as a means of enabling individuals (or their substitute decision-makers) to have adequate control over their lives. Yet, as Wendler argues, the experiential model falls short in areas where a person isn't directly affected by the research – such as research involving anonymous tissue samples – and informed consent may be seen to be unnecessary. A 'contribution model', on the other hand, where a subject might have an interest in the outcome of the study, provides a rational basis for requiring informed consent despite the absence of personal risk or gain. The growing influence of research advocates (see generally Dresser, 2001b), both in promoting subjects' rights and setting funding priorities, may further legitimate a contribution model of research involvement as subjects may increasingly elect to participate only in research that is ethically sound or which pursues goals they support.

A fundamental aspect of risks of harm and benefits is the existence of uncertainty. Acknowledging this fact is vital in establishing a healthy (and ethical) dialogue between doctor and patient (Katz, 1984), as 'every time a physician administers a drug to a patient, he is in a sense performing an experiment' (Blumgart, 1969, p. 44). The ethically significant distinction between research and therapy, however, is their respective *degree* of uncertainty. Research, a process of inquiry intended to 'contribute to generalizable knowledge' (Levine, 1986, p. 3), is, by definition, rooted more firmly in the unknown rather than in therapy. The purpose of the clinical trial – and the modern emphasis on evidence-based medicine, for that matter – is to manage or alleviate uncertainty. Yet it must be remembered that, as noted by Robert Levine in Chapter 24, while the randomized clinical trial (RCT) – the standard method for evaluating treatments – does contribute towards this objective, it by no means replaces uncertainties with certainties:

> We must continue to be skeptical about our 'certainties' and persistent in our pursuit of better intellectual tools to distinguish between knowledge and ignorance. In the foreseeable future it will be necessary

for us to continue to grapple with the problem of uncertainty, to learn how best to deal with it and to communicate about it with subjects and prospective subjects of research. (p. 424; see also Levine, 1986, pp. 207–10)

A recurring and related theme in the conduct of randomized clinical trials is the notion of 'equipoise'. Introduced by Fried (1974, pp. 51–56) in his classic treatment of the subject of human experimentation, 'equipoise' can be explained as 'a state of genuine uncertainty on the part of the clinical investigator regarding the comparative therapeutic merits of each arm in a trial' (Freedman, this volume, p. 427). Refinement of this principle has been tackled from several vantage points in the literature. In Chapter 25, Freedman distinguishes between *theoretical* equipoise – 'when, overall, the evidence on behalf of two alternative treatment regimens is exactly balanced' (p. 429) – and *clinical* equipoise, which exists when 'there is no consensus within the expert clinical community about the comparative merits of the alternatives to be tested' (p. 430). Levine, in Chapter 24, also supports Freedman's model, which has also been adopted in Canadian (Tri-Council, 1998, p. 7.1) and US guidelines (Office for Human Research Protections, 2001). Yet although this variation helps transcend the vagaries of individual clinical perception, it remains open to criticism concerning the composition of the 'community' from which this 'consensus' should be derived (for example, Gifford, 1995, 2001; Alderson, 1996). Others advocate further expansion of the concept in the form of 'community equipoise', which incorporates the preferences of both patients and clinicians (Karlawish and Lantos, 1997; Karlawish and Whitehouse, 1998). Both Levine and Freedman do respond to the needs of subjects by advocating that equipoise be incorporated into the informed consent process, but, as with informed consent generally, problems can arise with patients with diminished capacity. Kahn (1999, p. 279) is therefore amply justified in asking, 'given the difficulty in achieving equipoise with professionals, how can we possibly hope for anything approaching equipoise at work in the motivations of research subjects?'.

The question that follows is whether 'equipoise', even if expanded to include the perceptions of patients and researchers, is an adequate construct for managing uncertainty in clinical trials. Ultimately, a conceptual foundation for equipoise should perhaps be sought in epistemology. As Richard Ashcroft discusses in Chapter 26, 'equipoise is a situation involving beliefs, rather than knowledge' (p. 439). Various methodological solutions have also been proposed, including employing alternatives to the RCT, such as unbalanced randomization (Avins, 1998) or adaptive clinical trials (Pullman and Wang, 2001), which place less of a burden on clinicians to superimpose collective perceptions of uncertainty on their own decision-making. Or, rather than seek a precise point at which competing uncertainties are in equilibrium, one could embrace a modified concept such as 'equiphase', which describes 'a range of probabilities over which a patient is risk indifferent . . . and a range of "prior" probability estimates which the doctor's mind . . . cannot distinguish' (Chard and Lilford, 1998, p. 898). Instead of broadening the region of equipoise, S. Senn, in Chapter 27, proposes that the decision to enrol a patient in a clinical trial should be based not on relative uncertainty about equivalent therapeutic value, but rather on a certainty that no treatment option is *inferior* to the other. He resolves the clinician's dilemma by regarding society as 'defining through the regulatory process the standard of care (potentially) available' (p. 448) according to which clinicians are expected to base their decisions. In so doing, the question of equipoise (or uncertainty), in effect, becomes socially managed.[26]

The use of the placebo in clinical trials raises a distinct set of ethical dilemmas. As Baruch Brody notes in Chapter 28, placebo controls represent 'scientific advantages rather than absolute needs for scientific validity', which means that 'they might be outweighed in at least some cases by other concerns such as ethical concerns' (p. 458).[27] The general response has been to deem the use of a placebo unethical when a known therapeutic treatment exists (for example, De Deyn and D'Hooge, 1996).[28] However, as Senn argues, a blanket prohibition of this sort is incorrect. The issue is examined in detail by Brody in his critique of the development of thrombolytic therapy for myocardial infarction (see also Brody, 1995). Brody concludes that those particular trials – where, as part of the clinical trial design, known therapeutic interventions were denied to patients receiving emergency treatment – were indeed unethical. He proposes a normative standard to assess the validity of such trials: first, the subjects' valid consent to being randomized, if they are able to provide it; and, second, a normative assessment by the ethics review process that 'a reasonable person of an average degree of altruism and risk-aversiveness' (p. 464) might consent to being randomized. Brody's approach is appealing as it aims to reconcile scientific needs with the moral duty to protect subjects. His standard serves to provide the starting point for determining the ethical validity of a trial, qualified by the requirement of subject consent wherever possible, thus stopping short of ascribing a duty to participate.[29]

The tension between individual and collective ethics is apparent in debates about risks of harm, benefits, uncertainty, and the ethics of clinical trials generally. Fertile ground for debate remains, particularly with regard to the notion of equipoise – although a number of important themes emerge from these exchanges that are consistent with those canvassed earlier in this volume. While duly acknowledging societal goals, deference continues to be paid overall to the rights of subjects. It is held to be reasonable that individuals can be asked to submit to some level of risk for the greater good, but this risk has to be reasonable and not disproportionate to the expected benefits. The call for proper disclosure of possible risks of harm, benefits, as well as uncertainty, serves to reassure subjects of the scientific validity and social need for undertaking a risk. Closely related to this duty is the need to avoid a therapeutic misconception from developing in the mind of the patient-subject. Recognizing enhanced means for subject participation, such as through the contribution model, as well as attempts to expand the notion of equipoise to include subject perceptions, further support the principle of respect for persons and the right to self-determination. Yet, as with the doctrine of informed consent, owing to the complexity of the factors involved in the decision-making process, one must inevitably rely on the integrity of the investigator and enrolling clinician, as well as on social controls such as the ethics review system, to set boundaries and protect subjects' interests. As will be shown in Part IV, the globalization and corporatization of the research endeavour has introduced a number of factors that make the proper discharge of this obligation more difficult. With the growing recognition of conflicts of interest in the corporate research environment, as well as blurred lines of accountability across jurisdictions, social regulation of research – including of core concepts such as risk, benefit and uncertainty – is becoming increasingly important.

Globalization and Corporatization – Trust and Participation

The modern era of human experimentation is faced with many challenges for regulators, sponsors, subjects and investigators alike. Four themes have been selected: globalization, corporatization, trust and public participation.[30] As with most themes in research ethics, they are closely linked. The effects of globalization would not be as extensive without the transnational expansion of the pharmaceutical and biotechnology industries; and the demand by health consumers and research participants to participate in policy decisions concerning research agendas and subject protection would not be as insistent in a climate of complete public trust in regulatory authorities, research professions, their institutions and sponsors. Likewise, health consumer and subject activism is largely responsible for the outcry against global inequities in healthcare and the distribution of the benefits of research, which are themselves problems that stem, in part, from the market orientation of health research and commodification of science. These interrelationships create a difficult environment for policy formulation as regulators must look to both national and international solutions to ethical dilemmas, and may also have to rethink the wisdom of allowing market forces to reign free in areas so deeply affecting human well-being.

Biomedical research has been significantly transformed by the forces of globalization. The amount of international research has increased dramatically over recent decades and will continue to do so as a consequence of a number of factors, including ongoing efforts to harmonize drug regulation and promote mutual acceptance of clinical trial data (Dominguez-Urban, 1997).[31] Globalization imposes additional burdens on regulatory authorities, not only to ensure that efficacy and safety data for new drugs submitted from foreign clinical trials are indeed translatable to local populations, but also to verify that standards of good clinical practice and ethical conduct are consistent with those of the home jurisdiction (for example, Office of Inspector General, 2001).[32] There is also the related concern of trial sponsors 'shopping around' for the least onerous (and possibly most favourably inclined) regulatory environment, as well as for the purpose of avoiding potential litigation in the event of adverse effects (for example, Lurie *et al.*, 1994). The liability and accountability of multinational corporations conducting international research, which, if privately funded, also happens to fall between the cracks of most regulatory regimes that are grounded in government funding agencies, presents a complex dilemma, both for national authorities as well as subjects.[33]

In Chapter 29, Ruth Macklin relates some of the principal ethical issues raised by international research and examines the ongoing debate between cultural relativists and universalists concerning the validity of transplanting ethical principles derived from Western ethical and legal traditions to other cultures (see also Macklin, 1999). For example, the consent requirement that is the cornerstone of 'Western' research ethics policies is viewed differently in cultures where community-based, rather than individual, decision-making is the norm. In such cases, is it 'ethical imperialism' to force such requirements on other cultures? Or should one adopt a position of 'ethical pluralism', which holds that rules governing research practices might vary according to the country where they are carried out? It is commonly argued that if research is unethical in one jurisdiction – for example, due to a lack of individual informed consent – it should still not be conducted in another jurisdiction where the requirement is different. Does it not, as Macklin asks, constitute a contradiction to try to have it both ways? A further example involves the use of placebo-controlled trials where a known treatment exists but is otherwise unavailable in the country where the trial is taking place, most likely owing to its prohibitive cost. The ethics of these trials, such as for drugs to prevent mother-to-child transmission of HIV/AIDS, have been intensely debated in recent years.[34] In 2000, after Macklin wrote her essay, the Declaration of Helsinki was revised to reflect a universal standard whereby such trials would be unethical (Bland and Kerr, 2002). This clarification, however, occurred only as a consequence of strong criticism of the language of an earlier proposed revision that would have permitted such trials to take place (Levine, 1999; Lurie and Wolfe, 1999).[35]

The broader question that Macklin and others raise, however, is that of justice – the equitable distribution of risks *and* benefits arising from research. The debate about placebo-controlled trials in developing countries has served to heighten awareness about gross inequities in healthcare resources between developing and affluent countries (de Zulueta, 2001, p. 91). Revision of the Declaration of Helsinki will be insufficient 'without some means of strengthening capacity to promote and implement such standards' (Singer and Benatar, 2001, p. 747). Both national and international regulatory intervention, including binding international agreements, have been called for to address these issues (Bassiouni *et al.*, 1981; Dominguez-Urban, 1997). But desirable as the latter might be, if the extensive delays and controversy surrounding the ratification of the Council of Europe's Convention on Human Rights and Biomedicine[36] (for example, De Wachter, 1997) are to serve as any indication, a global convention on the protection of subjects is unlikely to occur in the near future. Benatar (2001, p. 338) is justified, therefore, in stating that the best hope for long-term results lies in recognizing the adverse impact of globalization, which will require 'a paradigm shift in thinking and action – towards reciprocal relationships between individuals, society, and the notion of rational self-interest and long term interdependence'. Hopefully, this theme will be allowed to run its course over the years to come.

The second major theme relates to the impact of commercial forces.[37] As funding models continue to rely more heavily on industry sources, classic relationships, such as in academic and clinical settings, are rapidly being eclipsed by commercial exchanges. This transformation has raised alarms from a number of health professionals, academics and journal editors alike. In Chapter 30, Marcia Angell, who was until recently editor of the *New England Journal of Medicine*, asks a provocative question: 'Is academic medicine for sale?'. Besides the possibility of business ties biasing research outcomes, her greatest concern is the influence of business goals on the educational mission of medical schools. Angell recognizes the value of cooperation between academia and industry (see also Gelijns and Thier, 2002), but cautions that '[t]he incentives of the marketplace should not become woven into the fabric of academic medicine' (p. 449). James Rule and Adil Shamoo, in Chapter 31, explore the ethical issues in university– industry relationships in greater detail, succinctly contrasting both negative and positive perspectives. They rightly identify conflicts of interest as the central issue.[38] And likewise, in Chapter 32, Thomas Bodenheimer expresses his concerns about the influence of the pharmaceutical industry on the research community. Trial design, data analysis, control over publication and authorship – all are areas cited by Bodenheimer as presenting challenges for researchers to remain independent of pressures exerted by corporate sponsors. In particular, he worries about increasingly prevalent networks of for-profit contract research organizations (CROs), which he describes as being 'heavily tipped toward industry interests' (p. 517). In Chapter 33, Trudo Lemmens and Benjamin Freedman echo this concern. The research ethics committee review has become the cornerstone of subject protection over recent decades. The rising volume of research conducted by CROs has logically led to the birth of the *commercial* ethics review, which is competitive by reducing the time typically taken for ethics review and corresponding opportunity cost associated with this delay. A conflict of interest arises from this client relationship (see also Office of Inspector General, 1998).[39] Lemmens and Freedman are particularly sensitive to the fact that it is an activity that has largely escaped public scrutiny, arguing that a fiduciary relationship should extend to bodies that are supposedly established to protect research participants. They recommend that ethics review committees should be 'situated on a continuum somewhere between administrative tribunals and administrative licensing boards' (p. 528), thereby benefiting from the experience of dealing with conflicts of interest in administrative law.

Conflicts of interest have received significant attention in recent years for good reason. As Jesse Goldner relates in Chapter 34, undisclosed pecuniary interests of researchers have occasionally clouded the judgement of clinician-investigators who enrolled unsuitable subjects in research with tragic results, including serious injury and death. A range of individual and institutional conflicts can come into play, such as subject recruitment fees to clinicians (see also Caulfield and Griener, 2002), gifts from sponsors and stock options, as well as institutional dependence on industry funding owing to decreasing levels of public support. As with conflicts of interest in other professions, they need not be blatant, as the mere *appearance* of a conflict can be sufficient to raise the ire of the media, government entities or increasingly active subjects' rights coalitions. Indeed, in recent years, public media scandals have significantly damaged the reputation of various institutional icons, well-known for research excellence. Such revelations, while regrettably historically necessary to stimulate a regulatory response, can have a marked impact on public trust in science, government and researchers. Goldner, while agreeing in principle with Angell that sources of conflict of interest should ideally be removed from the research exchange altogether, quite reasonably does not advocate a complete prohibition. The political will to achieve such a solution does not exist, given the strong inherent links between sponsors and their clinical or academic counterparts. He emphasizes the role that should be played by ethics review committees and of mandatory disclosure as part of the informed consent process, but rightly notes that both regulatory and procedural measures must be adopted in order to empower committees to effectively discharge these additional burdens.

The importance of preserving public trust in the research endeavour cannot be understated. It is increasingly being argued that a loss of trust will markedly reduce the availability of willing subjects, as well as lead to even stronger procedural intervention by regulatory bodies. In Chapter 35, Mark Yarborough and Richard Sharp relate how, as a result of recent media coverage of tragic deaths in biomedical research, public confidence in research institutions has indeed been placed in jeopardy. The relationship between the public, government and the media is aptly described by Thomas (1997) as a triangle with media at its apex, where disturbances at any point can disrupt public trust in research. This conceptualization might be further enhanced by visualizing the trust dynamic rather as a diamond, with industry and government occupying the lateral points, media at the pinnacle and the public (which includes the subject) at its base. Recognizing these relationships is important because, as Chalmers and Pettit (1998) described, political reactions to scandals serve only to fuel the 'controversy machine', which is an inefficient engine to drive regulatory reform.[40] A proactive approach is eminently preferable.

A holistic approach to research regulation is equally essential. Each participant in the research endeavour must contribute to this effort. Yarborough and Sharp argue that institutions must take proactive measures beyond mere compliance with existing regulatory requirements. This would include collaboration with the public, 'robust institutional oversight', and training programmes to build professional character. The importance of instilling a 'culture of conscience and responsibility' is likewise emphasized by Goldner in Chapter 34 in addressing the threat of conflicts of interest. A responsibility for preserving public trust would also logically lie both with government and industry, being the most powerful forces to effect change. However, as mentioned earlier, research participants have become empowered in recent years, largely as a result of increased awareness through the media of the secret world (and scandals) of human experimentation. The public's role is not limited to activism demanding enhanced regulatory protections and transparency in oversight. Research advocates are also vying for better involvement in the processes of ethics review and policy formulation, such as in setting research funding priorities (Dresser, 1999, 2001b; Resnik, 2001; Zucker, 2001, p. 244). Consulting the public in debates governing controversial issues is likewise urged by David Resnik in Chapter 36. Using the area of stem cell research as a case study, he warns against the tendency of governments to use legislation as a blunt instrument to curtail controversial activities. He shows how a ban in federally funded research on stem cells and cloning has resulted in forcing such experiments into the private sphere or to migrate to less restrictive jurisdictions. The proper solution, he argues, must be applied with discretion and care, and derive from meaningful discussion with scientists, industry and the public.

Given that human subjects are indispensable participants in research and also its ultimate beneficiaries, it is appropriate, thus, to end on the theme of public participation. Resnik's call for 'serious, informed, and sincere debate about the social, ethical, cultural, and scientific issues associated with biomedicine and biotechnology before enacting more rules and regulations' (p. 602) is well worth heeding. Enhanced regulatory controls are indeed necessary, as evidenced by the historical record of abuses; but as discussed earlier, their legitimacy will depend most strongly on the degree to which they are *accepted*. Effective dialogue can only contribute to this objective. As Katz eloquently noted in his individual statement as a member of ACHRE (1996, p. 856),

> ... the problems inherent in research with human subjects – advancing science and protecting subjects of research – are complex. Society can no longer afford to leave the balancing of individual rights against scientific progress to the low-visibility decision-making of IRBs with regulations that are porous and invite abuse. The important work that our Committee has done in its evaluation of the radiation experiments conducted by governmental agencies and the medical profession during the Cold War once again confronts us with the human and societal costs of too relentless a pursuit of knowledge. If this is a price worth paying, society should be forced to make these difficult moral choices in bright sunlight and through a regulatory process that constantly strives to articulate, confront, and delimit those costs.

Acknowledgements

We are grateful to Professor Terry Carney of the Faculty of Law, University of Sydney, for his comments on drafts of this text. The opinions expressed in this chapter remain those of the authors.

Notes

1   The topic of genetic research, for example, although of rapidly increasing significance in this area, has been deliberately omitted in deference to another volume in this series.

2   Beecher's landmark article is reprinted as Chapter 1 in another volume in this series, *Ethics and Medical Decision-Making*, edited by Professor Michael D. Freeman.

3   This essay was part of a special issue of *Dædalus – Journal of the American Academy of Arts and Science*, edited by Paul A. Freund. The essays in that issue were subsequently reprinted in Freund (1983). See also Schafer (1983, 2001) and Fethe (1993) for scholarly critiques of Jonas' classic essay. Jonas' essay was also the topic of discussion at a recent meeting of the President's Council on Bioethics (US) (transcript available at: http://www.bioethics.gov/200209/session1.html).

4   An interesting corollary to the question of whether individuals *can* be used as experimental subjects is whether individuals have a *duty to volunteer*. In Chapter 1, Jonas argues this question in the negative. Caplan (1988), however, argues in favour of such a duty.

5   See Article 5 of the revised Declaration of Helsinki (2000): 'In medical research on human subjects, considerations related to the well-being of the human subject should take precedence over the interests of science and society'; and also article 2 of the European Convention on Human Rights and Biomedicine (1997): 'The interests and welfare of the human being shall prevail over the sole interest of society or science.'

6   These three core principles were later expanded to four by Beauchamp and Childress (2001, 5th edn) to also include *non-maleficence*.

7   See chapters 7–11 in another volume in this series, *Ethics and Medical Decision-Making*, edited by Professor Michael D. Freeman, for critiques of the principle-based approach, including the mentioned essay by Toulmin.

8   For the source of this term, see Clouser and Gert (1990), reprinted as Chapter 11 of the aforementioned volume (see note 7).

9   By 'sensitivity to context', Meslin *et al.* refer to the 'facts, situations, relationships and circumstances that arise for given individuals at given points in time' (p. 80).

10   The history of human experimentation is replete with post-war abuses of human rights, including the Cameron 'depatterning' studies at the Royal Victoria Hospital in Montreal in the late 1950s (Cooper, 1986), the cervical cancer study at the National Women's Hospital in Auckland, in the 1960s (Coney, 1988; New Zealand Committee *et al.*, 1988), and the chemical warfare experiments conducted during the Second World War in Australia (Goodwin, 1998) and up to the 1980s in the United Kingdom at Porton Down (see the series of essays reported by the BBC between 1999 and 2001, including 'Porton Down probe launched' (30 July 2001), available at: http://news.bbc.co.uk/1/hi/uk/1463993.stm). Of course, all of these events collectively pale in comparison with the atrocities committed during the Second World War (see generally Mitscherlich, 1949; Müller-Hill, 1988; Proctor, 1988; Caplan, 1992; Brackman, 1988; Williams and Wallace, 1989).

11   The Nuremberg Code constituted part of the judgment resulting from *U.S.* v. *Karl Brandt et al., Trials of War Criminals Before the Nuremberg Military Tribunal Under Control Council Law No. 10*, Vol. 2, Nuremberg, October 1946–April 1949 (Washington, DC: US Government Printing Office, 1949), pp. 181–82.

12   Chapters 6 and 7 in this volume were part of a special issue of the *Kennedy Institute of Ethics Journal* that examined the work of the ACHRE.

13   The Committee did make findings of blameworthiness in a general sense, even to the level of stating that 'government officials and investigators are blameworthy for not having had policies and practices in place to protect the rights and interests of human subjects' (ACHRE, 1996, pp. 788–89, finding 11c), but it failed to do so in the case of individuals even where, as Beauchamp shows, the violation of basic principles could not but lead to a determination of inexcusable culpability.

14   In this context, 'unethical research' refers to otherwise scientifically valid results that were obtained through the unethical use of human subjects. Cases of fraudulent or misrepresented results in the literature raise an entirely different set of issues and worries for journal editors and the scientific community (for example, Farthing *et al.*, 2001).

15   With regard to the latter, the Declaration of Helsinki (article 27) holds that reports of experiments that were not conducted in accordance with its principles should not be published. Angell (1992, p. 282), a recent editor of the *New England Journal of Medicine*, described three justifications for non-publication in such instances: to deter unethical work; to preserve the primacy of subjects' rights; and to emphasize that scientific knowledge is not the ultimate good in society. Luna (1997),

strongly in favour of editors not publishing obviously unethical results, argued further that, in dubious cases, a critique of ethical problems should accompany the publication of results, allowing investigators the opportunity for a rebuttal.

16 It should be noted that the Tuskegee Study is by no means the only known example of unethical research finding its way into the scientific literature or of unethical results (and their originators) being cultivated in some other way. Prominent examples include the reintegration of Nazi scientists into military and industry hierarchies after the war and non-prosecution of Japanese doctors for their crimes against prisoners of war in China during the Second World War in exchange for disclosure of the results of their experiments (Bower, 1987; Brackman, 1988; Williams and Wallace, 1989).

17 At present, explicit legislation governing human experimentation exists in many jurisdictions: France (Byk, 1998), the Canadian Province of Quebec (Verdun-Jones and Weisstub, 1995), Denmark (Riis, 1998), the Netherlands (van Leeuwen 2001) and various states of the United States (Benson and Roth, 1988).

18 Although on the rise in recent years, De Ville (2002) argues that litigation will probably not be an effective means of ensuring retrospective accountability in human experimentation, although it may serve a key role in driving prospective accountability.

19 See also Goldner (1993, pp. 104–34) in which he responds to Katz's criticisms.

20 While the principal US federal inspectorate (Office for Protection of Research Risks) was recently upgraded (now Office for Human Research Protections) and, as a result, made more independent (Shalala, 2000), a true national oversight body as described has yet to be created.

21 *Grimes* v. *Kennedy Krieger Institute, Inc.*, 782 A.2d 807 (Md. 2001). See also Kopelman (2002), Ross (2002), Glantz (2002), and Mastroianni and Kahn (2002).

22 In the absence of guiding legislation, courts in common-law systems have historically acted through their supervisory *parens patriae* jurisdiction to make decisions on behalf of those who cannot care for themselves, such as children or adults with diminished mental capacity.

23 The mechanism provided by the Civil Code of the Canadian province of Quebec currently requires that protocols involving 'a group of children or incapable persons of full age' must be approved by the Minister of Health and Social Services (Civil Code of Quebec, art. 20). In the Australian states of New South Wales and Queensland, this approval must be obtained from the state Guardianship Tribunal (Adult Guardianship Act 1987, ss. 45AA-AB; Guardianship and Administration Act 2000, s. 72).

24 Such an approach, it might be noted, is also consistent with the concerns expressed by Annas in Chapter 11 about the ambiguity created by blending antonymous constructs such as 'therapeutic research'.

25 A 'therapeutic misconception' can occur when the patient-subject incorrectly ascribes a therapeutic character to an intervention that is essentially experimental in nature (Appelbaum *et al.*, 1982; Berg *et al.*, 2001, pp. 288–90; Fried, 2001).

26 The dominance of individual versus consensus opinion to determine the ethical validity of enrolling patients in clinical trials continues to be the focus of intense debate as illustrated by recent exchanges in the *British Medical Journal* (Enkin, 2000; Weijer *et al.*, 2000) and the *Canadian Medical Association Journal* (Sackett, 2000; Shapiro and Glass, 2000). As portrayed in the *British Medical Journal*, the debate has been couched in terms of competing principles: the uncertainty principle versus clinical equipoise. However, as Lilford and Djulbegovic (2001) note in their response, the two concepts should not be viewed as mutually exclusive. They suggest that the question should instead be: 'How much uncertainty can we accept before entering a patient into a trial and by whom (patients, physicians, and the community)?'.

27 Senn, in Chapter 27, disposes of the argument that placebos can be ethically justified as effective treatments in their own right.

28 For a contrary view, see Miller and Brody (2002), as well as the excellent series of peer commentaries to their position in that issue of the *American Journal of Bioethics*.

29 See also note 4. Brody's standard is compatible with Senn's application of Rawls' notion of justice in which Senn views the decision to enrol a subject from the 'original position' of a healthy individual.

30 Genetic research, as already mentioned, has been deliberately left out to be covered in another volume in this series. On the commercialization of genetic research, see also Caulfield and Williams-Jones (1999).

31 Whether such projects as the International Conference on Harmonization will succeed as envisaged, however, has yet to be seen, particularly since individual countries will probably wish to retain their vetos with regard to the approval of drug products (Eakin, 1999). Moreover, it must be remembered that the ICH Guidelines for Good Clinical Practice govern only procedural aspects of research; substantive measures, such as the enactment of enforceable legislation, are also required (Hirtle *et al.*, 2000). The European Union, however, in light of EU Directive 2001/20/EC ('Directive of the European Parliament and of the Council on the approximation of the laws, regulations and administrative provisions of the Member States relating to implementation of good clinical practice in the conduct of clinical trials on medicinal products for human use'), is well on the way to harmonizing regulatory standards between its member states. The Directive also requires member states to legislate appropriate protections for vulnerable populations.

32 In the United States, for example, the National Bioethics Advisory Commission (2001) recommended that clinical trials be approved by ethics committees in *both* the foreign jurisdiction where the study is taking place *as well as* an American institutional review board.

33 Ethical and regulatory concerns associated with international research in developing countries were covered in a detailed series of investigative reports in *The Washington Post*, entitled 'The Body Hunters', accessible at: http://www.washingtonpost.com/wp-dyn/world/issues/bodyhunters/ (last accessed December 2002).

34 See also the chapters on clinical research in developed countries in another volume in this series, *AIDS: Society, Ethics and Law*, edited by Professor Udo Schüklenk (2001).

35 The language of an earlier proposed revision to the Declaration of Helsinki – not the text that was ultimately endorsed – adopted the double standard of the 'highest attainable' and 'highest sustainable' in the host country (Luna, 2001).

36 Convention for the Protection of Human Rights and Dignity of the Human Being with Regard to the Application of Biology and Medicine: Convention on Human Rights and Biomedicine. European Treaty Series No. 164. It is worth mentioning that (as of 12 January 2003) although the Convention has come into force, only 15 states have ratified it in addition to 16 signatories. There are a number of notable absences: Germany, the United Kingdom, Russia and each of the non-European states that had participated in its elaboration, including Canada, the United States, Australia and Japan. An additional protocol under the Convention specifically on biomedical research, however, is currently under preparation.

37 The effects of corporatization on medicine more broadly will be canvassed in a forthcoming volume in this series, *Medicine and Industry*.

38 See also the excellent exchange on conflict of interest in university-industry in *Academic Medicine* (Kodish *et al.*, 1996; Blumenthal, 1996; Frankel, 1996; Pritchard, 1996); Walsh, Graber and Wolfe (1997); Kevles (2001); and Resnik and Shamoo (2002).

39 Similar arguments concerning the need for independent ethics review (that is, detached from stakeholders or beneficiaries of the research) have also been made in the context of the appointment of non-institutional members to ethics committees, as well as placing ethics review outside the purview of funding authorities (see note 20).

40 The US experience of patchy regulations for research involving adults with impaired decision-making capacity is demonstrative of the 'controversy machine' in action. See Kapp's discussion in Chapter 18.

References

ACHRE (US Advisory Committee on Human Radiation Experiments) (1996), *Final Report of the Advisory Committee on Human Radiation Experiments*, New York: Oxford University Press.

Addicott, D.C. (1999), 'Regulating Research on the Terminally Ill: A Proposal for Heightened Safeguards', *Journal of Contemporary Health Law and Policy*, **15**(2), pp. 479–524.

Alderson, P. (1996), 'Equipoise as a Means of Managing Uncertainty: Personal, Communal and Proxy', *Journal of Medical Ethics*, **22**(3), pp. 135–39.

Angell, M. (1992), 'Editorial Responsibility: Protecting Human Rights by Restricting Publication of Unethical Research', in G.J. Annas and M.A. Grodin (eds), *The Nazi Doctors and the Nuremberg Code: Human Rights in Human Experimentation*, New York: Oxford University Press, pp. 276–85.

Annas, G.J. (1998), 'Protecting Soldiers from Friendly Fire: The Consent Requirement for Using Investigational Drugs and Vaccines in Combat', *American Journal of Law & Medicine*, **24**(2–3), pp. 245–60.

Appelbaum, P.S., Roth, L.H. and Lidz, C. (1982), 'The Therapeutic Misconception: Informed Consent in Psychiatric Research', *International Journal of Law and Psychiatry*, **5**(3–4), pp. 319–29.

Arboleda-Florez, J. (1991), 'Ethical Issues Regarding Research on Prisoners', *International Journal of Offender Therapy and Comparative Criminology*, **35**(1), pp. 1–5.

Avins, A.L. (1998), 'Can Unequal Be More Fair? Ethics, Subject Allocation, and Randomised Clinical Trials', *Journal of Medical Ethics*, **24**(6), pp. 401–408.

Backlar, P. (1998), 'Advance Directives for Subjects of Research who have Fluctuating Cognitive Impairments due to Psychotic Disorders (such as Schizophrenia)', *Community Mental Health Journal*, **34**(3), pp. 229–40.

Barber, B., Lally, J.J., Makarushka, J.L. and Sullivan, D. (1973), *Research on Human Subjects: Problems of Social Control in Medical Experimentation*, New York: Russell Sage Foundation.

Bassiouni, M.C., Baffes, T.G. and Evrard, J.T. (1981), 'An Appraisal of Human Experimentation in International Law and Practice: The Need for International Regulation of Human Experimentation', *Journal of Criminal Law and Criminology*, **72**(4), pp. 1597–666.

Beauchamp, T.L. and Childress, J.F. (2001), *Principles of Biomedical Ethics*, 5th edn, New York: Oxford University Press.

Beecher, H.K. (1966), 'Ethics and Clinical Research', *New England Journal of Medicine*, **274**(24), pp. 1354–60.

Beecher, H.K. (1970), *Research and the Individual: Human Studies*, Boston, MA: Little, Brown.

Benatar, S.R. (2001), 'Commentary: Justice and Medical Research: A Global Perspective', *Bioethics*, **15**(4), pp. 333–40.

Benson, P.R. and Roth, L.H. (1988), 'Trends in the Social Control of Medical and Psychiatric Research', *Law & Mental Health*, **4**, pp. 1–47.

Berg, J.W., Appelbaum, P.S., Lidz, C.W. and Parker, L.S. (2001), *Informed Consent: Legal Theory and Clinical Practice*, 2nd edn, Oxford: Oxford University Press.

Bland, J.M. and Kerr, D. (2002), 'Fifth Revision of Declaration of Helsinki. Clause 29 Forbids Trials from Using Placebos When Effective Treatment Exists', *British Medical Journal*, **324**(7343), p. 975.

Blumenthal, D. (1996), 'Ethics Issues in Academic–Industry Relationships in the Life Sciences: The Continuing Debate', *Academic Medicine*, **71**(12), pp. 1291–96.

Blumgart, H.L. (1969), 'The Medical Framework for Viewing the Problem of Human Experimentation', in P.A. Freund (ed.), *Experimentation with Human Subjects*, London: George Allen and Unwin, pp. 39–65.

Bower, T. (1987), *The Paperclip Conspiracy: The Battle for the Spoils and Secrets of Nazi Germany*, London: M. Joseph.

Brackman, A.C. (1988), *The Other Nuremberg: The Untold Story of the Tokyo War Crimes Trials*, New York: Quill.

Brody, B.A. (1995), *Ethical Issues in Drug Testing, Approval, and Pricing: The Clot-Dissolving Drugs*, New York: Oxford University Press.

Brody, B.A. (1998), *The Ethics of Biomedical Research: An International Perspective*, New York: Oxford University Press.

Byk, C. (1998), 'French Law and Biomedical Research: A Practical Experiment', in D.N.Weisstub (ed.), *Research on Human Subjects: Ethics, Law, and Social Policy*, 1st edn, Oxford: Pergamon Press, pp. 158–74.

Caplan, A. (1988), 'Is There an Obligation to Participate in Biomedical Research?', in S.F. Spicker (ed.), *The Use of Human Beings in Research: With Special Reference to Clinical Trials*, Dordrecht: Kluwer Academic Publishers, pp. 229–48.

Caplan, A.L. (1992), *When Medicine Went Mad: Bioethics and the Holocaust*, Totowa, NJ: Humana Press.

Capron, A.M. (1997), 'Incapacitated Research', *Hastings Center Report*, **27**(2), pp. 25–27.

Cassel, C.K. (1985), 'Research in Nursing Homes. Ethical Issues', *Journal of the American Geriatric Society*, **33**(11), pp. 795–99.

Caulfield, T. and Griener, G. (2002), 'Conflicts of Interest in Clinical Research: Addressing the Issue of Physician Remuneration', *Journal of Law, Medicine and Ethics*, **30**(2), pp. 305–308.

Caulfield, T. and Williams-Jones, B. (1999), *The Commercialization of Genetic Research: Ethical, Legal, and Policy Issues*, New York: Kluwer Academic/Plenum Publishers.

Chalmers, D. and Pettit, P. (1998), 'Towards a Consensual Culture in the Ethical Review of Research. Australian Health Ethics Committee', *Medical Journal of Australia*, **168**(2), pp. 79–82.

Chard, J.A. and Lilford, R.J. (1998), 'The Use of Equipoise in Clinical Trials', *Social Science and Medicine*, **47**(7), pp. 891–98.

Charo, R.A. (1993), 'Protecting Us to Death: Women, Pregnancy, and Clinical Research Trials', *Saint Louis University Law Journal*, **38**(1), pp. 135–87.

Clouser, K.D. and Gert, B. (1990), 'A Critique of Principalism', *Journal of Medicine and Philosophy*, **15**(2), pp. 219–36.

Coney, S. (1988), *The Unfortunate Experiment*, Auckland, NZ: Penguin.

Cooper, G. (1986), *Opinion of George Cooper, Q.C., Regarding Canadian Government Funding of the Allan Memorial Institute in the 1950s and 1960s*, Ottawa: Supply and Services, Canada.

De Deyn, P.P. and D'Hooge, R. (1996), 'Placebos in Clinical Practice and Research', *Journal of Medical Ethics*, **22**(3), pp. 140–46.

De Ville, K. (2002), 'The Role of Litigation in Human Research Accountability', *Accountability in Research*, **9**(1), pp. 17–43.

De Wachter, M.A. (1997), 'The European Convention on Bioethics', *Hastings Center Report*, **27**(1), pp. 13–23.

de Zulueta, P. (2001), 'Randomised Placebo-Controlled Trials and HIV-Infected Pregnant Women in Developing Countries. Ethical Imperialism or Unethical Exploitation?', *Bioethics*, **15**(4), pp. 289–311.

Dickens, B.M. (1998), 'The Legal Challenge of Health Research Involving Children', *Health Law Journal*, **6**, special edition, pp. 131–48.

Dominguez-Urban, I. (1997), 'Harmonization in the Regulation of Pharmaceutical Research and Human Rights: The Need to Think Globally', *Cornell International Law Journal*, **30**, pp. 245–86.

Dresser, R. (1999), 'Public Advocacy and Allocation of Federal Funds for Biomedical Research', *Milbank Quarterly*, **77**(2), pp. 257–74, 175.

Dresser, R. (2001a), 'Dementia Research: Ethics and Policy for the Twenty-first Century', *Georgia Law Review*, **35**(2), pp. 661–90.

Dresser, R. (2001b), *When Science Offers Salvation: Patient Advocacy and Research Ethics*, Oxford: Oxford University Press.

Eakin, D.V. (1999), 'The International Conference on Harmonization of Pharmaceutical Regulations: Progress or Stagnation?', *Tulsa Journal of Comparative and International Law*, **6**, pp. 221–45.

Engelhardt, H.T., jr (1996), *The Foundations of Bioethics*, 2nd edn, New York: Oxford University Press.

Enkin, M.W. (2000), 'Clinical Equipoise and not the Uncertainty Principle is the Moral Underpinning of the Randomised Controlled Trial: Against', *British Medical Journal*, **321**(7263), pp. 757–58.

Farthing, M.J.G., Lock, S. and Wells, F.O. (2001), *Fraud and Misconduct in Biomedical Research*, 3rd edn, London: BMJ Books.

Fethe, C. (1993), 'Beyond Voluntary Consent: Hans Jonas on the Moral Requirements of Human Experimentation', *Journal of Medical Ethics*, **19**(2), pp. 99–103.

Fost, N. (1998), 'Waived Consent for Emergency Research', *American Journal of Law and Medicine*, **24**(2–3), pp. 163–83.

Frankel, M.S. (1996), 'Perception, Reality, and the Political Context of Conflict of Interest in University–Industry Relationships', *Academic Medicine*, **71**(12), pp. 1297–304.

Freeman, M.D. (2001), *Ethics and Medical Decision-Making*, Aldershot: Ashgate.

Freund, P.A. (ed.) (1970), *Experimentation and Human Subjects*, New York: G. Brazilier.

Fried, C. (1974), *Medical Experimentation: Personal Integrity and Social Policy*, Amsterdam: North-Holland Publishing Co.

Fried, E. (2001), 'The Therapeutic Misconception, Beneficence, and Respect', *Accountability in Research*, **8**(4), pp. 331–48.

Gelijns, A.C. and Thier, S.O. (2002), 'Medical Innovation and Institutional Interdependence: Rethinking University–Industry Connections', *Journal of the American Medical Association*, **287**(1), pp. 72–77.

Gert, B., Culver, C.M. and Clouser, K.D. (1997), *Bioethics: A Return to Fundamentals*, New York: Oxford University Press.

Gifford, F. (1995), 'Community-Equipoise and the Ethics of Randomized Clinical Trials', *Bioethics*, **9**(2), pp. 127–48.

Gifford, F. (2001), 'Uncertainty about Clinical Equipoise. Clinical Equipoise and the Uncertainty Principles Both Require Further Scrutiny', *British Medical Journal*, **322**(7289), p. 795.

Glantz, L.H. (2002), 'Nontherapeutic Research with Children: *Grimes* v *Kennedy Krieger Institute*', *American Journal of Public Health*, **92**(7), pp. 1070–73.

Glass, K.C. (1993), 'Informed Decision-making and Vulnerable Persons: Meeting the Needs of the Competent Elderly Patient or Research Subject', *Queen's Law Journal*, **18**, pp. 191–238.

Goldner, J.A. (1993), 'An Overview of Legal Controls on Human Experimentation and the Regulatory Implications of Taking Professor Katz Seriously', *Saint Louis University Law Journal*, **38**(1), pp. 63–134.

Goodwin, B. (1998), *Keen as Mustard: Britain's Horrific Chemical Warfare Experiments in Australia*, St Lucia, Qd: University of Queensland Press.

Gray, J.N., Lyons, P.M. and Melton, G.B. (1995), *Ethical and Legal Issues in AIDS Research*, Baltimore, MD: Johns Hopkins University Press.

Grodin, M.A. and Glantz, L.H. (1994), *Children as Research Subjects: Science, Ethics, and Law*, New York: Oxford University Press.

High, D.M. and Doole, M.M. (1995), 'Ethical and Legal Issues in Conducting Research Involving Elderly Subjects', *Behavioral Sciences and the Law*, **13**(3), pp. 319–35.

Hirtle, M., Lemmens, T. and Sprumont, D. (2000), 'A Comparative Analysis of Research Ethics Review Mechanisms and the ICH Good Clinical Practice Guideline', *European Journal of Health Law*, **7**, pp. 265–92.

Hornblum, A.M. (1997), 'They were Cheap and Available: Prisoners as Research Subjects in Twentieth Century America', *British Medical Journal*, **315**(7120), pp. 1437–41.

Hornblum, A.M. (1998), *Acres of Skin: Human Experiments at Holmesburg Prison*, New York: Routledge.

Kahn, J. (1999), 'Equipoise and the Problem of Research Subjects with Diminished Capacity', *Accountability in Research*, **7**(2–4), pp. 277–82.

Karlawish, J.H. and Hall, J.B. (1996), 'The Controversy over Emergency Research. A Review of the Issues and Suggestions for a Resolution', *American Journal of Respiratory and Critical Care Medicine*, **153**(2), pp. 499–506.

Karlawish, J.H. and Lantos, J. (1997), 'Community Equipoise and the Architecture of Clinical Research', *Cambridge Quarterly of Healthcare Ethics*, **6**(4), pp. 385–96.

Karlawish, J.H. and Whitehouse, P.J. (1998), 'Is the Placebo Control Obsolete in a World after Donepezil and Vitamin E?', *Archives of Neurology*, **55**(11), pp. 1420–24.

Katz, J. (1984), *The Silent World of Doctor and Patient*, New York: Free Press.

Katz, J. (1993), '"Ethics and Clinical Research" Revisited. A Tribute to Henry K. Beecher', *Hastings Center Report*, **23**(5), pp. 31–39.

Kevles, D.J. (2001), 'Principles, Property Rights, and Profits: Historical Reflections on University/Industry Relations', *Accountability in Research*, **8**(4), pp. 293–307.

Keyserlingk, E.W., Glass, K., Kogan, S. and Gauthier, S. (1995), 'Proposed Guidelines for the Participation of Persons with Dementia as Research Subjects', *Perspectives in Biology and Medicine*, **38**(2), pp. 319–61.

Kodish, E., Murray, T. and Whitehouse, P. (1996), 'Conflict of Interest in University–Industry Research Relationships: Realities, Politics, and Values', *Academic Medicine*, **71**(12), pp. 1287–90.

Kopelman, L.M. (2000), 'Children as Research Subjects: A Dilemma', *Journal of Medicine and Philosophy*, **25**(6), pp. 745–64.

Kopelman, L.M. (2002), 'Pediatric Research Regulations under Legal Scrutiny: Grimes Narrows their Interpretation', *Journal of Law, Medicine and Ethics*, **30**(1), pp. 38–49.

Koski, E.G. (1999), 'Resolving Beecher's Paradox: Getting Beyond IRB Reform', *Accountability in Research*, **7**(2–4), pp. 213–25.

Langer, E. (1964), 'Human Experimentation: Cancer Studies at Sloan Kettering Stir Public Debate on Medical Ethics', *Science*, **143**, p. 551.

Lasagna, L. (1969), 'Special Subjects in Human Experimentation', in P.A. Freund (ed.), *Experimentation with Human Subjects*, London: George Allen and Unwin, pp. 262–75.

Law Commission (UK) (1995), *Mental Incapacity*, Report No. 231, London: The Law Commission.

Law Reform Commission of Canada (1989), *Biomedical Experimentation Involving Human Subjects (Working Paper 61)*, Ottawa: Law Reform Commission of Canada.

Lederer, S.E. and Grodin, M.A. (1994), 'Historical Overview: Pediatric Experimentation', in M.A.Grodin and L.H. Glantz (eds), *Children as Research Subjects: Science, Ethics, and Law*, New York: Oxford University Press, pp. 3–28.

Levine, R.J. (1986), *Ethics and Regulation of Clinical Research*, 2nd edn, Baltimore, MD: Urban & Schwarzenberg.

Levine, R.J. (1999), 'The Need to Revise the Declaration of Helsinki', *New England Journal of Medicine*, **341**(7), pp. 531–34.

Lilford, R.J. and Djulbegovic, B. (2001), 'Uncertainty about Clinical Equipoise. Equipose and Uncertainty Principle are not Mutually Exclusive', *British Medical Journal*, **322**(7289), p. 795.

Luna, F. (1997), 'Vulnerable Populations and Morally Tainted Experiments', *Bioethics*, **11**(3–4), pp. 256–64.

Luna, F. (2001), 'Is "Best Proven" a Useless Criterion?', *Bioethics*, **15**(4), pp. 273–88.

Lurie, P., Bishaw, M., Chesney, M.A., Cooke, M., Fernandes, M.E., Hearst, N. *et al.* (1994), 'Ethical, Behavioral, and Social Aspects of HIV Vaccine Trials in Developing Countries', *Journal of the American Medical Association*, **271**(4), pp. 295–301.

Lurie, P. and Wolfe, S.M. (1999), 'Proposed Revisions to the Declaration of Helsinki. Paving the Way for Globalization in Research', *Western Journal of Medicine*, **171**(1), p. 6.

McCarthy, C.R. (1994), 'Historical Background of Clinical Trials Involving Women and Minorities', *Academic Medicine*, **69**(9), pp. 695–98.

McCormick, R.A. (1976), 'Experimentation in Children: Sharing in Sociality', *Hastings Center Report*, **6**(6), pp. 41–46.

Macklin, R. (1999), *Against Relativism: Cultural Diversity and the Search for Ethical Universals in Medicine*, New York: Oxford University Press.

McLean, S. (1992), 'Medical Experimentation with Children', *International Journal of Law and the Family*, **6**(1), pp. 173–91.

McNeill, P.M. (1993), *The Ethics and Politics of Human Experimentation*, Cambridge: Cambridge University Press.

Mastroianni, A.C. and Kahn, J.P. (2002), 'Risk and Responsibility: Ethics, Grimes v Kennedy Krieger, and Public Health Research Involving Children', *American Journal of Public Health*, **92**(7), pp. 1073–76.

Miller, F.G. and Brody, H. (2002), 'What Makes Placebo-Controlled Trials Unethical?', *American Journal of Bioethics*, **2**(2), pp. 3–9.

Mitscherlich, A. (1949), *Doctors of Infamy: The Story of Nazi Medical Crimes*, New York: Henry Schuman.

Müller-Hill, B. (1988), *Murderous Science: Elimination by Scientific Selection of Jews, Gypsies, and Others, Germany 1933–1945*, Oxford: Oxford University Press.

National Bioethics Advisory Commission (US) (1998), *Research Involving Persons with Mental Disorders That May Affect Decisionmaking Capacity. Volume I: Report and Recommendations of the National Bioethics Advisory Commission*, Washington, DC: Government Printing Office.

National Bioethics Advisory Commission (US) (2001), *Ethical and Policy Issues in International Research: Clinical Trials in Developing Countries. Volume 1: Report and Recommendations*, Washington, DC: Government Printing Office.

National Commission for the Protection of Human Subjects and Biomedical and Behavioral Research (USA) (1978), *The Belmont Report: Ethical Principles and Guidelines for the Conduct of Research Involving Human Subjects*, Washington, DC: DHEW.

New Zealand Committee of Inquiry into Allegations Concerning the Treatment of Cervical Cancer at a

National Women's Hospital and into Other Related Matters and Cartwright, S.R. (1988), *The Report of the Committee of Inquiry into Allegations Concerning the Treatment of Cervical Cancer at National Women's Hospital and into Other Related Matters*, Auckland, NZ: The Committee.

Nicholson, R.H. (1986), *Medical Research with Children – Ethics, Law, and Practice*, Oxford: Oxford University Press.

Office for Human Research Protections (2001), *Institutional Review Board Guidebook*, 2nd edn, http://ohrp.osophs.dhhs.gov/irb/irb-guidebook.htm

Office of Inspector General (1998), *Report of Institutional Review Boards: The Emergence of Independent Boards*, Report No. OEI-01-97-00192; 6/98, London: HMSO.

Office of Inspector General (2001), *The Globalization of Clinical Trials: A Growing Challenge in Protecting Human Subjects*, Report No. OEI-01-00-00190, London: HMSO.

Pritchard, M.S. (1996), 'Conflicts of Interest: Conceptual and Normative Issues', *Academic Medicine*, **71**(12), pp. 1305–13.

Proctor, R. (1988), *Racial Hygiene: Medicine Under the Nazis*, Cambridge, MA: Harvard University Press.

Pullman, D. and Wang, X. (2001), 'Adaptive Designs, Informed Consent, and the Ethics of Research', *Controlled Clinical Trials*, **22**(3), pp. 203–10.

Queensland Law Reform Commission (1996), *Assisted and Substituted Decisions: Decision-Making by and for People with a Decision-Making Disability. Vol. 1*, Brisbane: QLRC.

Ramsey, P. (1976), 'The Enforcement of Morals: Nontherapeutic Research on Children', *Hastings Center Report*, **6**(4), pp. 21–30.

Ramsey, P. (1977), 'Children as Research Subjects: A Reply', *Hastings Center Report*, **7**(2), pp. 40–42.

Rawls, J. (1971), *A Theory of Justice*, Cambridge, MA: Belknap Press of Harvard University Press.

Resnik, D.B. (2001), 'Setting Biomedical Research Priorities: Justice, Science, and Public Participation', *Kennedy Institute of Ethics Journal*, **11**(2), pp. 181–204.

Resnik, D.B. and Shamoo, A.E. (2002), 'Conflict of Interest and the University', *Accountability in Research*, **9**(1), pp. 45–64.

Riis, P. (1998), 'Ethical Guidelines for Epidemiological Research', in D.N. Weisstub (ed.), *Research on Human Subjects: Ethics, Law, and Social Policy*, 1st edn, Oxford: Pergamon Press, pp. 588–98.

Roach Anleu, S.L. (2001), 'The Legal Regulation of Medical Science', *Law and Policy*, **23**(4), pp. 417–40.

Ross, L.F. (2002), 'In Defense of the Hopkins Lead Abatement Studies', *Journal of Law, Medicine and Ethics*, **30**(1), pp. 50–57.

Roth, L.H., Appelbaum, P.S., Lidz, C.W., Benson, P. and Winslade, W.J. (1987), 'Informed Consent in Psychiatric Research', *Rutgers Law Review*, **39**(2–3), pp. 425–41.

Rothman, D.J. (1998), 'Bringing Ethics to Human Experimentation: The American Experience', in D.N. Weisstub (ed.), *Research on Human Subjects: Ethics, Law, and Social Policy*, 1st edn, Oxford: Pergamon Press, pp. 35–43.

Rothman, D.J. and Rothman, S.M. (1984), *The Willowbrook Wars*, 1st edn, New York: Harper & Row.

Sackett, D.L. (2000), 'Equipoise, a Term Whose Time (If It Ever Came) Has Surely Gone', *Canadian Medical Association Journal*, **163**(7), pp. 835–36.

Schafer, A. (1983), 'Experimentation with Human Subjects: A Critique of the Views of Hans Jonas', *Journal of Medical Ethics*, **9**(2), pp. 76–79.

Schafer, A. (2001), 'Research on Elderly Subjects', in D.N. Weisstub, D.C. Thomasma, S. Gauthier and G.F. Tomossy (eds), *Aging: Decisions at the End of Life*, Dordrecht: Kluwer Academic Publishers, pp. 171–205.

Schüklenk, U. (2000), 'Protecting the Vulnerable: Testing Times for Clinical Research Ethics', *Social Science and Medicine*, **51**(6), pp. 969–77.

Shalala, D. (2000), 'Protecting Research Subjects – What Must be Done', *New England Journal of Medicine*, **343**(11), pp. 808–10.

Shapiro, S.H. and Glass, K.C. (2000), 'Why Sackett's Analysis of Randomized Controlled Trials Fails, But Needn't', *Canadian Medical Association Journal*, **163**(7), pp. 834–35.

Singer, P.A. and Benatar, S.R. (2001), 'Beyond Helsinki: A Vision for Global Health Ethics', *British Medical Journal*, **322**(7289), pp. 747–48.

Thomas, R.A. (1997), 'The Government's Role in Public Trust of Biomedical Science', *Accountability in Research*, **5**, pp. 205–23.

Tomossy, G.F., Weisstub, D.N. and Gauthier, S. (2001), 'Regulating Ethical Research Involving Cognitively Impaired Elderly Subjects: Canada as a Case Study', in D.N. Weisstub, D.C. Thomasma, S. Gauthier and G.F. Tomossy (eds), *Aging: Decisions at the End of Life*, Dordrecht: Kluwer Academic Publishers, pp. 227–54.

Toulmin, S. (1981), 'The Tyranny of Principles', *Hastings Center Report*, **11**(6), pp. 31–39.

Tri-Council (1998), *Tri-Council Policy Statement: Ethical Conduct for Research Involving Humans*, Ottawa: Ministry of Supply and Services.

van Leeuwen, E. (2001), 'Dutch Law and Ethics Concerning the Experimental Treatment of Early Psychosis', *Schizophrenia Research*, **51**(1), pp. 63–67.

Veatch, R.M. (1981), *A Theory of Medical Ethics*, New York: Basic Books.

Verdun-Jones, S. and Weisstub, D.N. (1995), 'Consent to Human Experimentation in Quebec: The Application of the Civil Law Principle of Personal Inviolability to Protect Special Populations', *International Journal of Law and Psychiatry*, **18**(2), pp. 163–82.

Verdun-Jones, S.N. and Weisstub, D.N. (1998), 'Drawing the Distinction Between Therapeutic Research and Non-therapeutic Experimentation: Clearing a Way Through the Definitional Thicket', in D.N. Weisstub (ed.), *Research on Human Subjects: Ethics, Law, and Social Policy*, 1st edn, Oxford: Pergamon Press, pp. 88–110.

Verdun-Jones, S.N., Weisstub, D.N. and Arboleda-Florez, J. (1998), 'Prisoners as Subjects of Biomedical Experimentation: Examining the Arguments For and Against a Total Ban', in D.N. Weisstub (ed.), *Research on Human Subjects: Ethics, Law, and Social Policy*, 1st edn, Oxford: Pergamon Press, pp. 503–30.

Walsh, M.E., Graber, G.C. and Wolfe, A.K. (1997), 'University–Industry Relationships in Genetic Research: Potential Opportunities and Pitfalls', *Accountability in Research*, **5**(4), pp. 265–82.

Weijer, C. (1999), 'Protecting Communities in Research: Philosophical and Pragmatic Challenges', *Cambridge Quarterly of Healthcare Ethics*, **8**(4), pp. 501–13.

Weijer, C., Shapiro, S.H. and Glass, K.C. (2000), 'Clinical Equipoise and Not the Uncertainty Principle is the Moral Underpinning of the Randomised Controlled Trial', *British Medical Journal*, **321**(7263), pp. 756–57.

Weisstub, D.N. (1998), 'The Ethical Parameters of Experimentation', in D.N. Weisstub (ed.), *Research on Human Subjects: Ethics, Law, and Social Policy*, 1st edn, Oxford: Pergamon Press, pp. 1–34.

Weisstub, D.N., Arboleda-Florez, J. and Tomossy, G.F. (1996), 'Establishing the Boundaries of Ethically Permissible Research with Special Populations', *Health Law in Canada*, **17**(2), pp. 45–63.

West, D. (1998), 'Radiation Experiments on Children at the Fernald and Wrentham Schools: Lessons for Protocols in Human Subject Research', *Accountability in Research*, **6**(1–2), pp. 103–25.

Williams, P. and Wallace, D. (1989), *Unit 731: Japan's Secret Biological Warfare in World War II*, 1st edn, New York: Free Press.

Zucker, C. (2001), 'Are New Laws Needed to Protect Human Subjects?', *Accountability in Research*, **8**(3), pp. 235–44.

Part I
The Historical and Philosophical Foundations

[1]

HANS JONAS

Philosophical Reflections on Experimenting with Human Subjects

WHEN I was first asked to comment "philosophically" on the subject of human experimentation, I had all the hesitation natural to a layman in the face of matters on which experts of the highest competence have had their say and still carry on their dialogue. As I familiarized myself with the material,[1] any initial feeling of moral rectitude that might have facilitated my task quickly dissipated before the awesome complexity of the problem, and a state of great humility took its place. Nevertheless, because the subject is obscure by its nature and involves fundamental, transtechnical issues, any attempt at clarification can be of use, even without novelty. Even if the philosophical reflection should in the end achieve no more than the realization that in the dialectics of this area we must sin and fall into guilt, this insight may not be without its own gains.

The Peculiarity of Human Experimentation

Experimentation was originally sanctioned by natural science. There it is performed on inanimate objects, and this raises no moral problems. But as soon as animate, feeling beings become the subjects of experiment, as they do in the life sciences and especially in medical research, this innocence of the search for knowledge is lost and questions of conscience arise. The depth to which moral and religious sensibilities can become aroused is shown by the vivisection issue. Human experimentation must sharpen the issue as it involves ultimate questions of personal dignity and sacrosanctity. One difference between the human experiments and the physical is this: The physical experiment employs small-scale, artificially devised substitutes for that about which knowledge is to be obtained, and the experimenter extrapolates from these models and simulated conditions to nature at large. Something deputizes for the "real thing"—balls rolling down an inclined plane for sun and planets, electric discharges from a condenser for real lightning, and so on. For the most part, no such substitution is possible in the biological sphere. We must operate on the original itself, the real thing in the fullest sense, and perhaps affect it irreversibly. No simulacrum can take its place. Especially in the human sphere, experimentation loses entirely the advantage of the clear division between vicarious model and true object. Up to a point, animals may fulfill the proxy role of the classical physical experiment. But in the end man himself must furnish knowledge about himself, and the comfortable separation of noncommittal experiment and definitive action vanishes. An experiment in education affects the lives of its subjects, perhaps a whole generation of schoolchildren. Human experimentation for whatever purpose is always *also* a responsible, nonexperimental, definitive dealing with the subject himself. And not even the noblest purpose abrogates the obligations this involves.

Can both that purpose and this obligation be satisfied? If not, what would be a just compromise? Which side should give way to the other? The question is inherently philosophical as it concerns not merely pragmatic difficulties and their arbitration, but a genuine conflict of values involving principles of a high order. On principle, it is felt, human beings *ought not* to be dealt with in that way (the "guinea pig" protest); on the other hand, such dealings are increasingly urged on us by considerations, in turn appealing to principle, that claim to override those objections. Such a claim must be carefully assessed, especially when it is swept along by a mighty tide. Putting the matter thus, we have already made one important assumption rooted in our "Western" cultural tradition: The prohibitive rule is, to that way of thinking, the primary and axiomatic one; the permissive counter-rule, as qualifying the first, is secondary and stands in need of justification. We must justify the infringement of a primary inviolability, which needs no justification itself; and the justification of its infringement must be by values and needs of a dignity commensurate with those to be sacrificed.

"Individual Versus Society" as the Conceptual Framework

The setting for the conflict most consistently invoked in the literature is the polarity of individual versus society—the possible tension between the individual good and the common good, be-

Philosophical Reflections on Human Experimentation

tween private and public welfare. Thus, W. Wolfensberger speaks of "the tension between the long-range interests of society, science, and progress, on one hand, and the rights of the individual on the other."[2] Walsh McDermott says: "In essence, this is a problem of the rights of the individual versus the rights of society."[3] Somewhere I found the "social contract" invoked in support of claims that science may make on individuals in the matter of experimentation. I have grave doubts about the adequacy of this frame of reference, but I will go along with it part of the way. It does apply to some extent, and it has the advantage of being familiar. We concede, as a matter of course, to the common good some pragmatically determined measure of precedence over the individual good. In terms of rights, we let some of the basic rights of the individual be overruled by the acknowledged rights of society—as a matter of right and moral justness and not of mere force or dire necessity (much as such necessity may be adduced in defense of that right). But in making that concession, we require a careful clarification of what the needs, interests, and rights of society are, for society—as distinct from any plurality of individuals—is an abstract and as such is subject to our definition, while the individual is the primary concrete, prior to all definition, and his basic good is more or less known. Thus, the unknown in our problem is the so-called common or public good and its potentially superior claims, to which the individual good must or might sometimes be sacrificed, in circumstances that in turn must also be counted among the unknowns of our question. Note that in putting the matter in this way—that is, in asking about the right of society to individual sacrifice—the consent of the sacrificial subject is no necessary part of the *basic* question.

"Consent," however, is the other most consistently emphasized and examined concept in discussions of this issue. This attention betrays a feeling that the "social" angle is not fully satisfactory. If society has a right, its exercise is not contingent on volunteering. On the other hand, if volunteering is fully genuine, no public right to the volunteered act need be construed. There is a difference between the moral or emotional appeal of a cause that elicits volunteering and a right that demands compliance—for example, with particular reference to the social sphere, between the *moral claim* of a common good and society's *right* to that good and to the means of its realization. A moral claim cannot be met without consent; a right can do without it. Where consent is present anyway,

221

the distinction may become immaterial. But the awareness of the many ambiguities besetting the "consent" actually available and used in medical research prompts recourse to the idea of a public right conceived independently of (and valid prior to) consent; and, vice versa, the awareness of the problematic nature of such a right makes even its advocates still insist on the idea of consent with all its ambiguities: An uneasy situation exists for both sides.

Nor does it help much to replace the language of "rights" by that of "interests" and then argue the sheer cumulative weight of the interests of the many over against those of the few or the single individual. "Interests" range all the way from the most marginal and optional to the most vital and imperative, and only those sanctioned by particular importance and merit will be admitted to count in such a calculus—which simply brings us back to the question of right or moral claim. Moreover, the appeal to numbers is dangerous. Is the number of those afflicted with a particular disease great enough to warrant violating the interests of the non-afflicted? Since the number of the latter is usually so much greater, the argument can actually turn around to the contention that the cumulative weight of interest is on *their* side. Finally, it may well be the case that the individual's interest in his own inviolability is itself a public interest such that its publicly condoned violation, irrespective of numbers, violates the interest of all. In that case, its protection in *each* instance would be a paramount interest, and the comparison of numbers will not avail.

These are some of the difficulties hidden in the conceptual framework indicated by the terms "society-individual," "interest," and "rights." But we also spoke of a moral call, and this points to another dimension—not indeed divorced from the societal sphere, but transcending it. And there is something even beyond that: true sacrifice from highest devotion, for which there are no laws or rules except that it must be absolutely free. "No one has the right to choose martyrs for science" was a statement repeatedly quoted in the November, 1967, *Dædalus* conference. But no scientist can be prevented from making himself a martyr for his science. At all times, dedicated explorers, thinkers, and artists have immolated themselves on the altar of their vocation, and creative genius most often pays the price of happiness, health, and life for its own consummation. But no one, not even society, has the shred of a right to expect and ask these things. They come to the rest of us as a *gratia gratis data.*

Philosophical Reflections on Human Experimentation

The Sacrificial Theme

Yet we must face the somber truth that the *ultima ratio* of communal life is and has always been the compulsory, vicarious sacrifice of individual lives. The primordial sacrificial situation is that of outright human sacrifices in early communities. These were not acts of blood-lust or gleeful savagery; they were the solemn execution of a supreme, sacral necessity. One of the fellowship of men had to die so that all could live, the earth be fertile, the cycle of nature renewed. The victim often was not a captured enemy, but a select member of the group: "The king must die." If there was cruelty here, it was not that of men, but that of the gods, or rather of the stern order of things, which was believed to exact that price for the bounty of life. To assure it for the community, and to assure it ever again, the awesome *quid pro quo* had to be paid ever again.

Far be it from me, and far should it be from us, to belittle from the height of our enlightened knowledge the majesty of the underlying conception. The particular *causal* views that prompted our ancestors have long since been relegated to the realm of superstition. But in moments of national danger we still send the flower of our young manhood to offer their lives for the continued life of the community, and if it is a just war, we see them go forth as consecrated and strangely ennobled by a sacrificial role. Nor do we make their going forth depend on their own will and consent, much as we may desire and foster these: We conscript them according to law. We conscript the best and feel morally disturbed if the draft, either by design or in effect, works so that mainly the disadvantaged, socially less useful, more expendable, make up those whose lives are to buy ours. No rational persuasion of the pragmatic necessity here at work can do away with the feeling, mixed of gratitude and guilt, that the sphere of the sacred is touched with the vicarious offering of life for life. Quite apart from these dramatic occasions, there is, it appears, a persistent and constitutive aspect of human immolation to the very being and prospering of human society—an immolation in terms of life and happiness, imposed or voluntary, of few for many. What Goethe has said of the rise of Christianity may well apply to the nature of civilization in general: "*Opfer fallen hier, / Weder Lamm noch Stier, / Aber Menschenopfer unerhoert.*"[4] We can never rest comfortably in the belief that the soil from which our satisfactions sprout is not wa-

223

tered with the blood of martyrs. But a troubled conscience compels
us, the undeserving beneficiaries, to ask: Who is to be martyred?
in the service of what cause? and by whose choice?

Not for a moment do I wish to suggest that medical experimentation on human subjects, sick or healthy, is to be likened to pri-
meval human sacrifices. Yet something sacrificial is involved in the
selective abrogation of personal inviolability and the ritualized exposure to gratuitous risk of health and life, justified by a presumed
greater, social good. My examples from the sphere of stark sacrifice
were intended to sharpen the issues implied in that context and to
set them off clearly from the kinds of obligations and constraints
imposed on the citizen in the normal course of things or generally
demanded of the individual in exchange for the advantages of civil
society.

The "Social Contract" Theme

The first thing to say in such a setting-off is that the sacrificial
area is not covered by what is called the "social contract." This
fiction of political theory, premised on the primacy of the individual, was designed to supply a rationale for the *limitation* of individual freedom and power required for the existence of the body
politic, whose existence in turn is for the benefit of the individuals.
The principle of these limitations is that their *general* observance
profits all, and that therefore the individual observer, assuring this
general observance for his part, profits by it himself. I observe
property rights because their general observance assures my own;
I observe traffic rules because their general observance assures my
own safety; and so on. The obligations here are mutual and general;
no one is singled out for special sacrifice. For the most part, *qua* limitations of my liberty, the laws thus deducible from the hypothetical "social contract" enjoin me from certain actions rather than
obligate me to positive actions (as did the laws of feudal society).
Even where the latter is the case, as in the duty to pay taxes, the
rationale is that I am myself a beneficiary of the services financed
through these payments. Even the contributions levied by the welfare state, though not originally contemplated in the liberal version
of the social contract theory, can be interpreted as a personal insurance policy of one sort or another—be it against the contingency
of my own indigence, the dangers of disaffection from the laws in
consequence of widespread unrelieved destitution, or the disadvan-

Philosophical Reflections on Human Experimentation

tages of a diminished consumer market. Thus, by some stretch, such contributions can still be subsumed under the principle of enlightened self-interest. But no complete abrogation of self-interest at any time is in the terms of the social contract, and so pure sacrifice falls outside it. Under the putative terms of the contract alone, I cannot be required to die for the public good. (Thomas Hobbes made this forcibly clear.) Even short of this extreme, we like to think that nobody is entirely and one-sidedly the victim in any of the renunciations exacted under normal circumstances by society "in the general interest"—that is, for the benefit of others. "Under normal circumstances," as we shall see, is a necessary qualification. Moreover, the "contract" can legitimize claims only on our overt public actions and not on our invisible private being. Our powers, not our persons, are beholden to the commonweal. In one important respect, it is true, public interest and control do extend to the private sphere by general consent: in the compulsory education of our children. Even there, the assumption is that the learning and what is learned, apart from all future social usefulness, are also for the benefit of the individual in his own being. We would not tolerate education to degenerate into the conditioning of useful robots for the social machine.

Both restrictions of public claim in behalf of the "common good"—that concerning one-sided sacrifice and that concerning the private sphere—are valid only, let us remember, on the premise of the primacy of the individual, upon which the whole idea of the "social contract" rests. This primacy is itself a metaphysical axiom or option peculiar to our Western tradition, and the whittling away of this axiom would threaten the tradition's whole foundation. In passing, I may remark that systems adopting the alternative primacy of the community as their axiom are naturally less bound by the restrictions we postulate. Whereas we reject the idea of "expendables" and regard those not useful or even recalcitrant to the social purpose as a burden that society must carry (since their individual claim to existence is as absolute as that of the most useful), a truly totalitarian regime, Communist or other, may deem it right for the collective to rid itself of such encumbrances or to make them forcibly serve some social end by conscripting their persons (and there are effective combinations of both). We do not normally—that is, in nonemergency conditions—give the state the right to conscript labor, while we do give it the right to "conscript" money, for money is detachable from the person as labor is not.

225

Even less than forced labor do we countenance forced risk, injury, and indignity.

But in time of war our society itself supersedes the nice balance of the social contract with an almost absolute precedence of public necessities over individual rights. In this and similar emergencies, the sacrosanctity of the individual is abrogated, and what for all practical purposes amounts to a near-totalitarian, quasi-Communist state of affairs is *temporarily* permitted to prevail. In such situations, the community is conceded the right to make calls on its members, or certain of its members, entirely different in magnitude and kind from the calls normally allowed. It is deemed right that a part of the population bears a disproportionate burden of risk of a disproportionate gravity; and it is deemed right that the rest of the community accepts this sacrifice, whether voluntary or enforced, and reaps its benefits—difficult as we find it to justify this acceptance and this benefit by any normal ethical categories. We justify it transethically, as it were, by the supreme collective emergency, formalized, for example, by the declaration of a state of war.

Medical experimentation on human subjects falls somewhere between this overpowering case and the normal transactions of the social contract. On the one hand, no comparable extreme issue of social survival is (by and large) at stake. And no comparable extreme sacrifice or foreseeable risk is (by and large) asked. On the other hand, what is asked goes decidedly beyond, even runs counter to, what it is otherwise deemed fair to let the individual sign over of his person to the benefit of the "common good." Indeed, our sensitivity to the kind of intrusion and use involved is such that only an end of transcendent value or overriding urgency can make it arguable and possibly acceptable in our eyes.

Health as a Public Good

The cause invoked is health and, in its more critical aspect, life itself—clearly superlative goods that the physician serves directly by curing and the researcher indirectly by the knowledge gained through his experiments. There is no question about the good served nor about the evil fought—disease and premature death. But a good to whom and an evil to whom? Here the issue tends to become somewhat clouded. In the attempt to give experimentation the proper dignity (on the problematic view that a value be-

Philosophical Reflections on Human Experimentation

comes greater by being "social" instead of merely individual), the health in question or the disease in question is somehow predicated of the social whole, as if it were society that, in the persons of its members, enjoyed the one and suffered the other. For the purposes of our problem, public interest can then be pitted against private interest, the common good against the individual good. Indeed, I have found health called a national resource, which of course it is, but surely not in the first place.

In trying to resolve some of the complexities and ambiguities lurking in these conceptualizations, I have pondered a particular statement, made in the form of a question, which I found in the *Proceedings* of the November *Dædalus* conference: "Can society afford to discard the tissues and organs of the hopelessly unconscious patient when they could be used to restore the otherwise hopelessly ill, but still salvageable individual?" And somewhat later: "A strong case can be made that society can ill afford to discard the tissues and organs of the hopelessly unconscious patient; they are greatly needed for study and experimental trial to help those who can be salvaged."[5] I hasten to add that any suspicion of callousness that the "commodity" language of these statements may suggest is immediately dispelled by the name of the speaker, Dr. Henry K. Beecher, for whose humanity and moral sensibility there can be nothing but admiration. But the use, in all innocence, of this language gives food for thought. Let me, for a moment, take the question literally. "Discarding" implies proprietary rights—nobody can discard what does not belong to him in the first place. Does society then own my body? "Salvaging" implies the same and, moreover, a use-value to the owner. Is the life-extension of certain individuals then a public interest? "Affording" implies a critically vital level of such an interest—that is, of the loss or gain involved. And "society" itself—what is it? When does a need, an aim, an obligation become social? Let us reflect on some of these terms.

What Society Can Afford

"Can Society afford. . . ?" Afford what? To let people die intact, thereby withholding something from other people who desperately need it, who in consequence will have to die too? These other, unfortunate people indeed cannot afford not to have a kidney, heart, or other organ of the dying patient, on which they depend for an extension of their lease on life; but does that give them a right to it? Does it oblige society to procure it for them? What is it that *society* can or cannot afford—leaving aside for the moment the question of what it has a *right* to? It surely can afford to lose members through death; more than that, it is built on the balance of death and birth decreed by the order of life. This is too general, of course, for our question, but perhaps it is well to remember. The specific question seems to be whether society can afford to let some people die whose death might be deferred by particular means if these were authorized by society. Again, if it is merely a question of what society can or cannot afford, rather than of what it ought or ought not to do, the answer must be: Of course, it can. If cancer, heart disease, and other organic, noncontagious ills, especially those tending to strike the old more than the young, continue to exact their toll at the normal rate of incidence (including the toll of private anguish and misery), society can go on flourishing in every way.

Here, by contrast, are some examples of what, in sober truth, society cannot afford. It cannot afford to let an epidemic rage unchecked; a persistent excess of deaths over births, but neither too great an excess of births over deaths; too low an average life-expectancy even if demographically balanced by fertility, but neither too great a longevity with the necessitated correlative dearth of youth in the social body; a debilitating state of general health; and things of this kind. These are plain cases where the whole condition of society is critically affected, and the public interest can make its imperative claims. The Black Death of the Middle Ages was a *public* calamity of the acute kind; the life-sapping ravages of endemic malaria or sleeping sickness in certain areas are a public calamity of the chronic kind. A society as a whole can truly not "afford" such situations, and they may call for extraordinary remedies, including, perhaps, the invasion of private sacrosanctities.

This is not entirely a matter of numbers and numerical ratios. Society, in a subtler sense, cannot "afford" a single miscarriage of justice, a single inequity in the dispensation of its laws, the violation of the rights of even the tiniest minority, because these undermine the moral basis on which society's existence rests. Nor can it, for a similar reason, afford the absence or atrophy in its midst of compassion and of the effort to alleviate suffering—be it widespread or rare—one form of which is the effort to conquer disease of any kind, whether "socially" significant (by reason of number)

Philosophical Reflections on Human Experimentation

or not. And in short, society cannot afford the absence among its members of *virtue* with its readiness to sacrifice beyond defined duty. Since its presence—that is to say, that of personal idealism—is a matter of grace and not of decree, we have the paradox that society depends for its existence on intangibles of nothing less than a religious order, for which it can hope, but which it cannot enforce. All the more must it protect this most precious capital from abuse.

For what objectives connected with the medico-biological sphere should this reserve be drawn upon—for example, in the form of accepting, soliciting, perhaps even imposing the submission of human subjects to experimentation? We postulate that this must be not just a worthy cause, as any promotion of the health of anybody doubtlessly is, but a cause qualifying for transcendent social sanction. Here one thinks first of those cases critically affecting the whole condition, present and future, of the community. Something equivalent to what in the political sphere is called "clear and present danger" may be invoked and a state of emergency proclaimed, thereby suspending certain otherwise inviolable prohibitions and taboos. We may observe that averting a disaster always carries greater weight than promoting a good. Extraordinary danger excuses extraordinary means. This covers human experimentation, which we would like to count, as far as possible, among the extraordinary rather than the ordinary means of serving the common good under public auspices. Naturally, since foresight and responsibility for the future are of the essence of institutional society, averting disaster extends into long-term prevention, although the lesser urgency will warrant less sweeping licenses.

Society and the Cause of Progress

Much weaker is the case where it is a matter not of saving but of improving society. Much of medical research falls into this category. A permanent death rate from heart failure or cancer does not threaten society. So long as certain statistical ratios are maintained, the incidence of disease and of disease-induced mortality is not (in the strict sense) a "social" misfortune. I hasten to add that it is not therefore less of a human misfortune, and the call for relief issuing with silent eloquence from each victim and all potential victims is of no lesser dignity. But it is misleading to equate the fundamentally human response to it with what is owed to society: It is

229

owed by man to man—and it is thereby owed by society to the individuals as soon as the adequate ministering to these concerns outgrows (as it progressively does) the scope of private spontaneity and is made a public mandate. It is thus that society assumes responsibility for medical care, research, old age, and innumerable other things not originally of the public realm (in the original "social contract"), and they become duties toward "society" (rather than directly toward one's fellow man) by the fact that they are socially operated.

Indeed, we expect from organized society no longer mere protection against harm and the securing of the conditions of our preservation, but active and constant improvement in all the domains of life: the waging of the battle against nature, the enhancement of the human estate—in short, the promotion of progress. This is an expansive goal, one far surpassing the disaster norm of our previous reflections. It lacks the urgency of the latter, but has the nobility of the free, forward thrust. It surely is worth sacrifices. It is not at all a question of what society can afford, but of what it is committed to, beyond all necessity, by our mandate. Its trusteeship has become an established, ongoing, institutionalized business of the body politic. As eager beneficiaries of its gains, we now owe to "society," as its chief agent, our individual contribution toward its *continued pursuit*. Maintaining the existing level requires no more than the orthodox means of taxation and enforcement of professional standards that raise no problems. The more optional goal of pushing forward is also more exacting. We have this syndrome: Progress is by our choosing an acknowledged interest of society, in which we have a stake in various degrees; science is a necessary instrument of progress; research is a necessary instrument of science; and in medical science experimentation on human subjects is a necessary instrument of research: Therefore, human experimentation has come to be a societal interest.

The destination of research is essentially melioristic. It does not serve the preservation of the existing good from which I profit myself and to which I am obligated. Unless the present state is intolerable, the melioristic goal is in a sense gratuitous, and not only from the vantage point of the present. Our descendants have a right to be left an unplundered planet; they do not have a right to new miracle cures. We have sinned against them if by our doing we have destroyed their inheritance—which we are doing at full blast; we have not sinned against them if by the time they come

Philosophical Reflections on Human Experimentation

around arthritis has not yet been conquered (unless by sheer neglect). And generally, in the matter of progress, as humanity had no claim on a Newton, a Michelangelo, or a St. Francis to appear, and no right to the blessings of their unscheduled deeds, so progress, with all our methodical labor for it, cannot be budgeted in advance and its fruits received as a due. Its coming-about at all and its turning out for good (of which we can never be sure) must rather be regarded as something akin to grace.

The Melioristic Goal, Medical Research, and Individual Duty

Nowhere is the melioristic goal more inherent than in medicine. To the physician, it is not gratuitous. He is committed to curing and thus to improving the power to cure. Gratuitous we called it (outside disaster conditions) as a *social* goal, but noble at the same time. Both the nobility and the gratuitousness must influence the manner in which self-sacrifice for it is elicited and even its free offer accepted. Freedom is certainly the first condition to be observed here. The surrender of one's body to medical experimentation is entirely outside the enforceable "social contract."

Or can it be construed to fall within its terms—namely, as repayment for benefits from past experimentation that I have enjoyed myself? But I am indebted for these benefits not to society, but to the past "martyrs," to whom society is indebted itself, and society has no right to call in my personal debt by way of adding new to its own. Moreover, gratitude is not an enforceable social obligation; it anyway does not mean that I must emulate the deed. Most of all, if it was wrong to exact such sacrifice in the first place, it does not become right to exact it again with the plea of the profit it has brought me. If, however, it was not exacted, but entirely free, as it ought to have been, then it should remain so, and its precedence must not be used as a social pressure on others for doing the same under the sign of duty.

Indeed, we must look outside the sphere of the social contract, outside the whole realm of public rights and duties, for the motivations and norms by which we can expect ever again the upwelling of a will to give what nobody—neither society, nor fellow man, nor posterity—is entitled to. There are such dimensions in man with trans-social wellsprings of conduct, and I have already pointed

231

to the paradox, or mystery, that society cannot prosper without them, that it must draw on them, but cannot command them.

What about the moral law as such a transcendent motivation of conduct? It goes considerably beyond the public law of the social contract. The latter, we saw, is founded on the rule of enlightened self-interest: *Do ut des*—I give so that I be given to. The law of individual conscience asks more. Under the Golden Rule, for example, I am required to give as I wish to be given to under like circumstances, but not in order that I be given to and not in expectation of return. Reciprocity, essential to the social law, is not a condition of the moral law. One subtle "expectation" and "self-interest," but of the moral order itself, may even then be in my mind: I prefer the environment of a moral society and can expect to contribute to the general morality by my own example. But even if I should always be the dupe, the Golden Rule holds. (If the social law breaks faith with me, I am released from its claim.)

Moral Law and Transmoral Dedication

Can I, then, be called upon to offer myself for medical experimentation in the name of the moral law? *Prima facie,* the Golden Rule seems to apply. I should wish, were I dying of a disease, that enough volunteers in the past had provided enough knowledge through the gift of their bodies that I could now be saved. I should wish, were I desperately in need of a transplant, that the dying patient next door had agreed to a definition of death by which his organs would become available to me in the freshest possible condition. I surely should also wish, were I drowning, that somebody would risk his life, even sacrifice his life, for mine.

But the last example reminds us that only the negative form of the Golden Rule ("Do not do unto others what you do not want done unto yourself") is fully prescriptive. The positive form ("Do unto others as you would wish them to do unto you"), in whose compass our issue falls, points into an infinite, open horizon where prescriptive force soon ceases. We may well say of somebody that he ought to have come to the succor of B, to have shared with him in his need, and the like. But we may not say that he ought to have given his life for him. To have done so would be praiseworthy; not to have done so is not blameworthy. It cannot be asked of him; if he fails to do so, he reneges on no duty. But *he* may say of himself, and only he, that he ought to have given his life. *This*

Philosophical Reflections on Human Experimentation

"ought" is strictly between him and himself, or between him and God; no outside party—fellow man or society—can appropriate its voice. It can humbly receive the supererogatory gifts from the free enactment of it.

We must, in other words, distinguish between moral obligation and the much larger sphere of moral value. (This, incidentally, shows up the error in the widely held view of value theory that the higher a value, the stronger its claim and the greater the duty to realize it. The highest are in a region beyond duty and claim.) The ethical dimension far exceeds that of the moral law and reaches into the sublime solitude of dedication and ultimate commitment, away from all reckoning and rule—in short, into the sphere of the *holy*. From there alone can the offer of self-sacrifice genuinely spring, and this—its source—must be honored religiously. How? The first duty here falling on the research community, when it enlists and uses this source, is the safeguarding of true authenticity and spontaneity.

The "Conscription" of Consent

But here we must realize that the mere issuing of the appeal, the calling for volunteers, with the moral and social pressures it inevitably generates, amounts even under the most meticulous rules of consent to a sort of *conscripting*. And some soliciting is necessarily involved. This was in part meant by the earlier remark that in this area sin and guilt can perhaps not be wholly avoided. And this is why "consent," surely a non-negotiable minimum requirement, is not the full answer to the problem. Granting then that soliciting and therefore some degree of conscripting are part of the situation, who may conscript and who may be conscripted? Or less harshly expressed: Who should issue appeals and to whom?

The naturally qualified issuer of the appeal is the research scientist himself, collectively the main carrier of the impulse and the only one with the technical competence to judge. But his being very much an interested party (with vested interests, indeed, not purely in the public good, but in the scientific enterprise as such, in "his" project, and even in his career) makes him also suspect. The ineradicable dialectic of this situation—a delicate incompatibility problem—calls for particular controls by the research community and by public authority that we need not discuss. They can mitigate, but not eliminate the problem. We have to live with the ambiguity, the treacherous impurity of everything human.

Self-Recruitment of the Research Community

To whom should the appeal be addressed? The natural issuer of the call is also the first natural addressee: the physician-researcher himself and the scientific confraternity at large. With such a coincidence—indeed, the noble tradition with which the whole business of human experimentation started—almost all of the associated legal, ethical, and metaphysical problems vanish. If it is full, autonomous identification of the subject with the purpose that is required for the dignifying of his serving as a subject—here it is; if strongest motivation—here it is; if fullest understanding— here it is; if freest decision—here it is; if greatest integration with the person's total, chosen pursuit—here it is. With self-solicitation, the issue of consent in all its insoluble equivocality is bypassed *per se*. Not even the condition that the particular purpose be truly important and the project reasonably promising, which must hold in any solicitation of others, need be satisfied here. By himself, the scientist is free to obey his obsession, to play his hunch, to wager on chance, to follow the lure of ambition. It is all part of the "divine madness" that somehow animates the ceaseless pressing against frontiers. For the rest of society, which has a deep-seated disposition to look with reverence and awe upon the guardians of the mysteries of life, the profession assumes with this proof of its devotion the role of a self-chosen, consecrated fraternity, not unlike the monastic orders of the past; and this would come nearest to the actual, religious origins of the art of healing.

It would be the ideal, but not a real solution to keep the issue of human experimentation within the research community itself. Neither in numbers nor in variety of material would its potential suffice for the many-pronged, systematic, continual attack on disease into which the lonely exploits of the early investigators have grown. Statistical requirements alone make their voracious demands; were it not for what I have called the essentially "gratuitous" nature of the whole enterprise of progress, as against the mandatory respect for invasion-proof selfhood, the simplest answer would be to keep the whole population enrolled, and let the lot, or an equivalent of draft boards, decide which of each category will at any one time be called up for "service." It is not difficult to picture societies with whose philosophy this would be consonant. We are agreed that ours is not one such and should not become one. The specter of it is indeed among the threatening utopias on

Philosophical Reflections on Human Experimentation

our own horizon from which we should recoil, and of whose advent by imperceptible steps we must beware. How then can our mandatory faith be honored when the recruitment for experimentation goes outside the scientific community, as it must in honoring another commitment of no mean dignity? We simply repeat the former question: To whom should the call be addressed?

"Identification" as the Principle of Recruitment in General

If the properties we adduced as the particular qualifications of the members of the scientific fraternity itself are taken as general criteria of selection, then one should look for additional subjects where a maximum of identification, understanding, and spontaneity can be expected—that is, among the most highly motivated, the most highly educated, and the least "captive" members of the community. From this naturally scarce resource, a descending order of permissibility leads to greater abundance and ease of supply, whose use should become proportionately more hesitant as the exculpating criteria are relaxed. An inversion of normal "market" behavior is demanded here—namely, to accept the lowest quotation last (and excused only by the greatest pressure of need), to pay the highest price first.

As such a rule of selection is bound to be rather hard on the number-hungry research industry, it will be asked: Why all the fuss? At this point we had better spell out some of the things we have been tacitly presupposing all the time. What is wrong with making a person an experimental subject is not so much that we make him thereby a means (which happens in social contexts of all kinds), as that we make him a thing—a passive thing merely to be acted on, and passive not even for real action, but for token action whose token object he is. His being is reduced to that of a mere token or "sample." This is different from even the most exploitative situations of social life; there the business is real, not fictitious. The subject, however much abused, remains an agent and thus a "subject" in the other sense of the word. The soldier's case, referred to earlier, is instructive: Subject to most unilateral discipline, forced to risk mutilation and death, conscripted without, perhaps against, his will—he is still conscripted with his capacities to act, to hold his own or fail in situations, to meet real challenges for real stakes. Though a mere "number" to the High Command, he is not a token and not a thing. (Imagine what he

235

would say if it turned out that the war was a game staged to sample observations on his endurance, courage, or cowardice.)

These compensations of personhood are denied to the subject of experimentation, who is acted upon for an extraneous end without being engaged in a real relation where he would be the counterpoint to the other or to circumstance. Mere "consent" (mostly amounting to no more than permission) does not right this reification. The "wrong" of it can only be made "right" by such authentic identification with the cause that it is the subject's as well as the researcher's cause—whereby his role in its service is not just permitted by him, but *willed.* That sovereign will of his which embraces the end as his own restores his personhood to the otherwise depersonalizing context. To be valid it must be autonomous and informed. The latter condition can, outside the research community, only be fulfilled by degrees; but the higher the degree of the understanding regarding the purpose and the technique, the more valid becomes the endorsement of the will. A margin of mere trust inevitably remains. Ultimately, the appeal for volunteers should seek this free and generous endorsement, the appropriation of the research purpose into the person's own scheme of ends. Thus, the appeal is in truth addressed to the one, mysterious, and sacred source of any such generosity of the will—"devotion," whose forms and objects of commitment are various and may invest different motivations in different individuals. The following, for instance, may be responsive to the "call" we are discussing: compassion with human suffering, zeal for humanity, reverence for the Golden Rule, enthusiasm for progress, homage to the cause of knowledge, even longing for sacrificial justification (do not call that "masochism," please). On all these, I say, it is defensible and right to draw when the research objective is worthy enough; and it is a prime duty of the research community (especially in view of what we called the "margin of trust") to see that this sacred source is never abused for frivolous ends. For a less than adequate cause, not even the freest, unsolicited offer should be accepted.

The Rule of the "Descending Order" and
Its Counter-Utility Sense

We have laid down what must seem to be a forbidding rule. Having faith in the transcendent potential of man, I do not fear that the "source" will ever fail a society that does not destroy it—

Philosophical Reflections on Human Experimentation

and only such a one is worthy of the blessings of progress. But "elitistic" the rule is (as is the enterprise of progress itself), and elites are by nature small. The combined attribute of motivation and information, plus the absence of external pressures, tends to be socially so circumscribed that strict adherence to the rule might numerically starve the research process. This is why I spoke of a descending order of permissibility, which is itself permissive, but where the realization that it is a *descending* order is not without pragmatic import. Departing from the august norm, the appeal must needs shift from idealism to docility, from high-mindedness to compliance, from judgment to trust. Consent spreads over the whole spectrum. I will not go into the casuistics of this penumbral area. I merely indicate the principle of the order of preference: The poorer in knowledge, motivation, and freedom of decision (and that, alas, means the more readily available in terms of numbers and possible manipulation), the more sparingly and indeed reluctantly should the reservoir be used, and the more compelling must therefore become the countervailing justification.

Let us note that this is the opposite of a social utility standard, the reverse of the order by "availability and expendability": The most valuable and scarcest, the least expendable elements of the social organism, are to be the first candidates for risk and sacrifice. It is the standard of *noblesse oblige;* and with all its counter-utility and seeming "wastefulness," we feel a rightness about it and perhaps even a higher "utility," for the soul of the community lives by this spirit.[6] It is also the opposite of what the day-to-day interests of research clamor for, and for the scientific community to honor it will mean that it will have to fight a strong temptation to go by routine to the readiest sources of supply—the suggestible, the ignorant, the dependent, the "captive" in various senses.[7] I do not believe that heightened resistance here must cripple research, which cannot be permitted; but it may slow it down by the smaller numbers fed into experimentation in consequence. This price—a possibly slower rate of progress—may have to be paid for the preservation of the most precious capital of higher communal life.

Experimentation on Patients

So far we have been speaking on the tacit assumption that the subjects of experimentation are recruited from among the healthy. To the question "Who is conscriptable?" the spontaneous answer is:

237

Least and last of all the sick—the most available source as they are under treatment and observation anyway. That the afflicted should not be called upon to bear additional burden and risk, that they are society's special trust and the physician's particular trust— these are elementary responses of our moral sense. Yet the very destination of medical research, the conquest of disease, requires at the crucial stage trial and verification on precisely the sufferers from the disease, and their total exemption would defeat the purpose itself. In acknowledging this inescapable necessity, we enter the most sensitive area of the whole complex, the one most keenly felt and most searchingly discussed by the practitioners themselves. This issue touches the heart of the doctor-patient relation, putting its most solemn obligations to the test. Some of the oldest verities of this area should be recalled.

The Fundamental Privilege of the Sick

In the course of treatment, the physician is obligated to the patient and to no one else. He is not the agent of society, nor of the interests of medical science, the patient's family, the patient's co-sufferers, or future sufferers from the same disease. The patient alone counts when he is under the physician's care. By the simple law of bilateral contract (analogous, for example, to the relation of lawyer to client and its "conflict of interest" rule), he is bound not to let any other interest interfere with that of the patient in being cured. But manifestly more sublime norms than contractual ones are involved. We may speak of a sacred trust; strictly by its terms, the doctor is, as it were, alone with his patient and God.

There is one normal exception to this—that is, to the doctor's not being the agent of society vis-à-vis the patient, but the trustee of his interests alone—the quarantining of the contagious sick. This is plainly not for the patient's interest, but for that of others threatened by him. (In vaccination, we have a combination of both: protection of the individual and others.) But preventing the patient from causing harm to others is not the same as exploiting him for the advantage of others. And there is, of course, the abnormal exception of collective catastrophe, the analogue to a state of war. The physician who desperately battles a raging epidemic is under a unique dispensation that suspends in a nonspecifiable way some of the strictures of normal practice, including possibly those against experimental liberties with his patients. No rules can be devised

Philosophical Reflections on Human Experimentation

for the waiving of rules in extremities. And as with the famous shipwreck examples of ethical theory, the less said about it the better. But what is allowable there and may later be passed over in forgiving silence cannot serve as a precedent. We are concerned with non-extreme, non-emergency conditions where the voice of principle can be heard and claims can be adjudicated free from duress. We have conceded that there are such claims, and that if there is to be medical advance at all, not even the superlative privilege of the suffering and the sick can be kept wholly intact from the intrusion of its needs. About this least palatable, most disquieting part of our subject, I have to offer only groping, inconclusive remarks.

The Principle of "Identification" Applied to Patients

On the whole, the same principles would seem to hold here as are found to hold with "normal subjects": motivation, identification, understanding on the part of the subject. But it is clear that these conditions are peculiarly difficult to satisfy with regard to a patient. His physical state, psychic preoccupation, dependent relation to the doctor, the submissive attitude induced by treatment—everything connected with his condition and situation makes the sick person inherently less of a sovereign person than the healthy one. Spontaneity of self-offering has almost to be ruled out; consent is marred by lower resistance or captive circumstance, and so on. In fact, all the factors that make the patient, as a category, particularly accessible and welcome for experimentation at the same time compromise the quality of the responding affirmation that must morally redeem the making use of them. This, in addition to the primacy of the physician's duty, puts a heightened onus on the physician-researcher to limit his undue power to the most important and defensible research objectives and, of course, to keep persuasion at a minimum.

Still, with all the disabilities noted, there is scope among patients for observing the rule of the "descending order of permissibility" that we have laid down for normal subjects, in vexing inversion of the utility order of quantitative abundance and qualitative "expendability." By the principle of this order, those patients who most identify with and are cognizant of the cause of research—members of the medical profession (who after all are sometimes patients themselves)—come first; the highly motivated and educated, also

239

least dependent, among the lay patients come next; and so on down the line. An added consideration here is seriousness of condition, which again operates in inverse proportion. Here the profession must fight the tempting sophistry that the hopeless case is expendable (because in prospect already expended) and therefore especially usable; and generally the attitude that the poorer the chances of the patient the more justifiable his recruitment for experimentation (other than for his own benefit). The opposite is true.

Nondisclosure as a Borderline Case

Then there is the case where ignorance of the subject, sometimes even of the experimenter, is of the essence of the experiment (the "double blind"-control group-placebo syndrome). It is said to be a necessary element of the scientific process. Whatever may be said about its ethics in regard to normal subjects, especially volunteers, it is an outright betrayal of trust in regard to the patient who believes that he is receiving treatment. Only supreme importance of the objective can exonerate it, without making it less of a transgression. The patient is definitely wronged even when not harmed. And ethics apart, the practice of such deception holds the danger of undermining the faith in the *bona fides* of treatment, the beneficial intent of the physician—the very basis of the doctor-patient relationship. In every respect, it follows that concealed experiment on patients—that is, experiment under the guise of treatment— should be the rarest exception, at best, if it cannot be wholly avoided.

This has still the merit of a borderline problem. This is not true of the other case of necessary ignorance of the subject—that of the unconscious patient. Drafting him for nontherapeutic experiments is simply and unqualifiedly impermissible; progress or not, he must never be used, on the inflexible principle that utter helplessness demands utter protection.

When preparing this paper, I filled pages with a casuistics of this harrowing field, but then scratched out most of it, realizing my dilettante status. The shadings are endless, and only the physician-researcher can discern them properly as the cases arise. Into his lap the decision is thrown. The philosophical rule, once it has admitted into itself the idea of a sliding scale, cannot really specify its own application. It can only impress on the practitioner a general maxim or attitude for the exercise of his judgment and consci-

Philosophical Reflections on Human Experimentation

ence in the concrete occasions of his work. In our case, I am afraid, it means making life more difficult for him.

It will also be noted that, somewhat at variance with the emphasis in the literature, I have not dwelt on the element of "risk" and very little on that of "consent." Discussion of the first is beyond the layman's competence; the emphasis on the second has been lessened because of its equivocal character. It is a truism to say that one should strive to minimize the risk and to maximize the consent. The more demanding concept of "identification," which I have used, includes "consent" in its maximal or authentic form, and the assumption of risk is its privilege.

No Experiments on Patients Unrelated to Their Own Disease

Although my ponderings have, on the whole, yielded points of view rather than definite prescriptions, premises rather than conclusions, they have led me to a few unequivocal yeses and noes. The first is the emphatic rule that patients should be experimented upon, if at all, *only* with reference to *their* disease. Never should there be added to the gratuitousness of the experiment as such the gratuitousness of service to an unrelated cause. This follows simply from what we have found to be the *only* excuse for infracting the special exemption of the sick at all—namely, that the scientific war on disease cannot accomplish its goal without drawing the sufferers from disease into the investigative process. If under this excuse they become subjects of experiment, they do so *because*, and only because, of *their* disease.

This is the fundamental and self-sufficient consideration. That the patient cannot possibly benefit from the unrelated experiment therapeutically, while he might from experiment related to his condition, is also true, but lies beyond the problem area of pure experiment. Anyway, I am discussing nontherapeutic experimentation only, where *ex hypothesi* the patient does not benefit. Experiment as part of therapy—that is, directed toward helping the subject himself —is a different matter altogether and raises its own problems, but hardly philosophical ones. As long as a doctor can say, even if only in his own thought: "There is no known cure for your condition (or: You have responded to none); but there is promise in a new treatment still under investigation, not quite tested yet as to effectiveness and safety; you will be taking a chance, but all things considered, I

241

judge it in your best interest to let me try it on you"—as long as
he can speak thus, he speaks as the patient's physician and may err,
but does not transform the patient into a subject of experimenta-
tión. Introduction of an untried therapy into the treatment where
the tried ones have failed is not "experimentation on the patient."

Generally, there is something "experimental" (because tentative) about every individual treatment, beginning with the diagnosis itself; and he would be a poor doctor who would not learn
from every case for the benefit of future cases, and a poor member
of the profession who would not make any new insights gained
from his treatments available to the profession at large. Thus,
knowledge may be advanced in the treatment of any patient, and
the interest of the medical art and all sufferers from the same
affliction as well as the patient may be served if something happens to be learned from his case. But this gain to knowledge and
future therapy is incidental to the *bona fide* service to the present
patient. He has the right to expect that the doctor does nothing
to him just in order to learn.

In that case, the doctor's imaginary speech would run, for instance, like this: "There is nothing more I can do for you. But you
can do something for me. Speaking no longer as your physician
but on behalf of medical science, we could learn a great deal about
future cases of this kind if you would permit me to perform certain experiments on you. It is understood that you yourself would
not benefit from any knowledge we might gain; but future patients
would." This statement would express the purely experimental
situation, assumedly here with the subject's concurrence and with
all cards on the table. In Alexander Bickel's words: "It is a different
situation when the doctor is no longer trying to make [the patient]
well, but is trying to find out how to make others well in the
future."[8]

But even in the second case of the nontherapeutic experiment
where the patient does not benefit, the patient's own disease is
enlisted in the cause of fighting that disease, even if only in others.
It is yet another thing to say or think: "Since you are here—in
the hospital with its facilities—under our care and observation,
away from your job (or, perhaps, doomed), we wish to profit
from your being available for some other research of great interest
we are presently engaged in." From the standpoint of merely
medical ethics, which has only to consider risk, consent, and the
worth of the objective, there may be no cardinal difference be-

Philosophical Reflections on Human Experimentation

tween this case and the last one. I hope that my medical audience will not think I am making too fine a point when I say that from the standpoint of the subject and his dignity there is a cardinal difference that crosses the line between the permissible and the impermissible, and this by the same principle of "identification" I have been invoking all along. Whatever the rights and wrongs of any experimentation on any patient—in the one case, at least that residue of identification is left him that it is his own affliction by which he can contribute to the conquest of that affliction, his own kind of suffering which he helps to alleviate in others; and so in a sense it is his own cause. It is totally indefensible to rob the unfortunate of this intimacy with the purpose and make his misfortune a convenience for the furtherance of alien concerns. The observance of this rule is essential, I think, to attenuate at least the wrong that nontherapeutic experimenting on patients commits in any case.

On the Redefinition of Death

My other emphatic verdict concerns the question of the redefinition of death—acknowledging "irreversible coma as a new definition for death."[9] I wish not to be misunderstood. As long as it is merely a question of when it is permitted to cease the artificial prolongation of certain functions (like heartbeat) traditionally regarded as signs of life, I do not see anything ominous in the notion of "brain death." Indeed, a new definition of death is not even necessary to legitimize the same result if one adopts the position of the Roman Catholic Church, which here for once is eminently reasonable—namely that "when deep unconsciousness is judged to be permanent, extraordinary means to maintain life are not obligatory. They can be terminated and the patient allowed to die."[10] Given a clearly defined negative condition of the brain, the physician is allowed to allow the patient to die his own death by *any* definition, which of itself will lead through the gamut of all possible definitions. But a disquietingly contradictory purpose is combined with this purpose in the quest for a new definition of death, in the will to *advance* the moment of declaring him dead: Permission not to turn off the respirator, but, on the contrary, to keep it on and thereby maintain the body in a state of what would have been "life" by the older definition (but is only a "simulacrum" of life by the new)—so as to get at his organs and tissues under the ideal conditions of what would previously have been "vivisection."[11]

Now this, whether done for research or transplant purposes, seems to me to overstep what the definition can warrant. Surely it is one thing when to cease delaying death, but another when to start doing violence to the body; one thing when to desist from protracting the process of dying, but another when to regard that process as complete and thereby the body as a cadaver free for inflicting on it what would be torture and death to any living body. For the first purpose, we need not know the exact borderline with absolute certainty between life and death—we leave it to nature to cross it wherever it is, or to traverse the whole spectrum if there is not just one line. All we need to know is that coma is irreversible. For the second purpose we must know the borderline; and to use any definition short of the maximal for perpetrating on a *possibly* penultimate state what only the ultimate state can permit is to arrogate a knowledge which, I think, we cannot possibly have. *Since we do not know the exact borderline between life and death,* nothing less than the maximum definition of death will do—brain death plus heart death plus any other indication that may be pertinent—before final violence is allowed to be done.

It would follow then, for this layman at least, that the use of the definition should itself be defined, and this in a restrictive sense. When only permanent coma can be gained with the artificial sustaining of functions, by all means turn off the respirator, the stimulator, any sustaining artifice, and let the patient die; but let him die all the way. Do not, instead, arrest the process and start using him as a mine while, with your own help and cunning, he is still kept this side of what may in truth be the final line. Who is to say that a shock, a final trauma, is not administered to a sensitivity diffusely situated elsewhere than in the brain and still vulnerable to suffering? a sensitivity that we ourselves have been keeping alive? No fiat of definition can settle this question.[12] But I wish to emphasize that the question of possible suffering (easily brushed aside by a sufficient show of reassuring expert consensus) is merely a subsidiary and not the real point of my argument; this, to reiterate, turns on the indeterminacy of the boundaries between *life and death,* not between sensitivity and insensitivity, and bids us to lean toward a maximal rather than a minimal determination of death in an area of basic uncertainty.

Philosophical Reflections on Human Experimentation

There is also this to consider: The patient must be absolutely sure that his doctor does not become his executioner, and that no definition authorizes him ever to become one. His right to this certainty is absolute, and so is his right to his own body with all its organs. Absolute respect for these rights violates no one else's rights, for no one has a right to another's body. Speaking in still another, religious vein: The expiring moments should be watched over with piety and be safe from exploitation.

I strongly feel, therefore, that it should be made quite clear that the proposed new definition of death is to authorize *only* the one and *not* the other of the two opposing things: only to break off a sustaining intervention and let things take their course, not to keep up the sustaining intervention for a final intervention of the most destructive kind.

There would now have to be said something about nonmedical experiments on human subjects, notably psychological and genetic, of which I have not lost sight. But having overextended my limits of space by the most generous interpretation, I must leave this for another occasion. Let me only say in conclusion that if some of the practical implications of my reasonings are felt to work out toward a slower rate of progress, this should not cause too great dismay. Let us not forget that progress is an optional goal, not an unconditional commitment, and that its tempo in particular, compulsive as it may become, has nothing sacred about it. Let us also remember that a slower progress in the conquest of disease would not threaten society, grievous as it is to those who have to deplore that their particular disease be not yet conquered, but that society would indeed be threatened by the erosion of those moral values whose loss, possibly caused by too ruthless a pursuit of scientific progress, would make its most dazzling triumphs not worth having. Let us finally remember that it cannot be the aim of progress to abolish the lot of mortality. Of some ill or other, each of us will die. Our mortal condition is upon us with its harshness but also its wisdom—because without it there would not be the eternally renewed promise of the freshness, immediacy, and eagerness of youth; nor, without it, would there be for any of us the incentive to number our days and make them count. With all our striving to wrest from our mortality what we can, we should bear its burden with patience and dignity.

DÆDALUS

REFERENCES

1. G. E. W. Wolstenholme and Maeve O'Connor (eds.), *CIBA Foundation Symposium, Ethics in Medical Progress: With Special Reference to Transplantation* (Boston, 1966); "The Changing Mores of Biomedical Research," *Annals of Internal Medicine* (Supplement 7), Vol. 67, No. 3 (Philadelphia, September, 1967); *Proceedings of the Conference on the Ethical Aspects of Experimentation on Human Subjects*, November 3-4, 1967 (Boston, Massachusetts; hereafter called *Proceedings*); H. K. Beecher, "Some Guiding Principles for Clinical Investigation," *Journal of the American Medical Association*, Vol. 195 (March 28, 1966), pp. 1135-36; H. K. Beecher, "Consent in Clinical Experimentation: Myth and Reality," *Journal of the American Medical Association*, Vol. 195 (January 3, 1966), pp. 34-35; P. A. Freund, "Ethical Problems in Human Experimentation," *New England Journal of Medicine*, Vol. 273 (September 23, 1965), pp. 687-92; P. A. Freund, "Is the Law Ready for Human Experimentation?", *American Psychologist*, Vol. 22 (1967), pp. 394-99; W. Wolfensberger, "Ethical Issues in Research with Human Subjects," *World Science*, Vol. 155 (January 6, 1967), pp. 47-51; See also a series of five articles by Drs. Schoen, McGrath, and Kennedy, "Principles of Medical Ethics," which appeared from August to December in Volume 23 of *Arizona Medicine*. The most recent entry in the growing literature is E. Fuller Torrey (ed.), *Ethical Issues in Medicine* (New York, 1968), in which the chapter "Ethical Problems in Human Experimentation" by Otto E. Guttentag should be especially noted.

2. Wolfensberger, "Ethical Issues in Research with Human Subjects," p. 48.

3. *Proceedings*, p. 29.

4. *Die Braut von Korinth:* "Victims do fall here, /Neither lamb nor steer, / Nay, but human offerings untold."

5. *Proceedings*, pp. 50-51.

6. Socially, everyone is expendable relatively—that is, in different degrees; religiously, no one is expendable absolutely: The "image of God" is in all. If it can be enhanced, then not by any one being expended, but by someone expending himself.

7. This refers to captives of circumstance, not of justice. Prison inmates are with respect to our problem in a special class. If we hold to some idea of guilt, and to the supposition that our judicial system is not entirely at fault, they may be held to stand in a special debt to society, and their offer to serve—from whatever motive—may be accepted with a minimum of qualms as a means of reparation.

8. *Proceedings*, p. 33. To spell out the difference between the two cases: In the first case, the patient himself is meant to be the beneficiary of the experiment, and directly so; the "subject" of the experiment is at the same time its object, its end. It is performed not for gaining knowledge, but for helping him—and helping him in the *act* of performing it, even if

Philosophical Reflections on Human Experimentation

by its results it also contributes to a broader testing process currently under way. It is in fact part of the treatment itself and an "experiment" only in the loose sense of being untried and highly tentative. But whatever the degree of uncertainty, the motivating anticipation (the wager, if you like) is for success, and success here means the subject's own good. To a pure experiment, by contrast, undertaken to gain knowledge, the difference of success and failure is not germane, only that of conclusiveness and inconclusiveness. The "negative" result has as much to teach as the "positive." Also, the true experiment is an act distinct from the uses later made of the findings. And, most important, the subject experimented on is distinct from the eventual beneficiaries of those findings: He lets himself be used as a means toward an end external to himself (even if he should at some later time happen to be among the beneficiaries himself). With respect to his own present needs and his own good, the act is gratuitous.

9. "A Definition of Irreversible Coma," Report of the *Ad Hoc* Committee of Harvard Medical School to Examine the Definition of Brain Death, *Journal of the American Medical Association,* Vol. 205, No. 6 (August 5, 1968), pp. 337-40.

10. As rendered by Dr. Beecher in *Proceedings,* p. 50.

11. The Report of the *Ad Hoc* Committee no more than indicates this possibility with the second of the "two reasons why there is need for a definition": "(2) Obsolete criteria for the definition of death can lead to controversy in obtaining organs for transplantation." The first reason is relief from the burden of indefinitely drawn out coma. The report wisely confines its recommendations on application to what falls under this first reason—namely, turning off the respirator—and remains silent on the possible use of the definition under the second reason. But when "the patient is declared dead on the basis of these criteria," the road to the other use has theoretically been opened and will be taken (if I remember rightly, it has even been taken once, in a much debated case in England), unless it is blocked by a special barrier in good time. The above is my feeble attempt to help doing so.

12. Only a Cartesian view of the "animal machine," which I somehow see lingering here, could set the mind at rest, as in historical fact it did at its time in the matter of vivisection: But its truth is surely not established by definition.

[2]

Experimenting on Human Subjects: Philosophical Perspectives *

Ruth Macklin†

and

Susan Sherwin‡

The ethical problems that attend the use of human subjects present difficult questions both for researchers and for society. The authors investigate these issues from various philosophical points of view, focusing on the theories of Immanuel Kant and John Stuart Mill. After exploring the shortcomings of these theories as guides for resolving the ethical questions inherent in human experimentation, the authors suggest John Rawls' theory of social justice as a model for making ethical judgments.

I. INTRODUCTION

THE USE OF human beings in scientific research raises fundamental issues that lie at the heart of philosophical inquiry. The first question that arises concerning experimentation on human subjects is: Why are we disturbed at all by such experimentation? Put more precisely, why do questions arise about experimentation on human beings when there are no similar questions concerning experimentation on inanimate objects? This general question is the basis for the more specific questions to which the analysis in this paper will be addressed.

There is, of course, an obvious and, indeed, trivial answer to the broader question: Human beings are persons, and persons should be treated differently from things, or inanimate objects. This obvious answer is one that we all accept and that we presuppose in

* Supported in part by the National Endowment for the Humanities under Grant No. EH-6028-111, and under the auspices of the Moral Problems in Medicine Project at Case Western Reserve University. The contents of this article do not necessarily represent the view of the Endowment.

† Associate Professor of Philosophy, Case Western Reserve University. B.A., Cornell University, 1958; M.A., Case Western Reserve University, 1966; Ph.D., 1968.

‡ Assistant Professor of Philosophy, Dalhousie University (Halifax, Nova Scotia). B.A., York University (Toronto), 1969; Ph.D., Stanford University, 1974.

our worries about experimenting on human subjects. However, the deeper, philosophical answer to the basic question constitutes an explication and justification of the claim asserted in the trivial response. We want to know the nature of persons, the centrally important characteristics[1] of human beings, which make them different from inanimate objects in a way that is relevant to how human beings ought to be treated. The answer to this question requires that we explore some territory that lies at the intersection of the two following philosophical areas: philosophy of mind and ethics.

Before turning to a brief look at the cluster of general questions in philosophy of mind and ethics which relate to the nature of persons and how human beings ought to be treated, it would be well to identify the two specific questions on which this paper will focus: (1) What kinds of experiments on human beings can be morally justified? and (2) Under what constraints should experimental subjects be selected or allowed to participate? In a philosophical examination of these questions, it is necessary to note several specific concepts that are prominent in the area in which ethics and philosophy of mind intersect and that bear crucially on the sorts of values we must identify and explore. These concepts include the presumed rationality and autonomy of persons as well as the notions of voluntariness, coercion, and paternalism. All of the concepts bear on the central moral values in our view of human beings: that since persons have an intrinsic worth and an inherent dignity, they ought to be treated with respect. Not surprisingly, these concepts and values cluster around the debates and dilemmas relating to "informed consent," a preeminent concern in human experimentation.[2] The discussion in this paper will focus on the specific application of these concepts to the problems surrounding human experimentation and look briefly at some of the philosophical underpinnings.

---

1. Sometimes what we refer to here as "centrally important characteristics" are termed "essential properties" or the "essence" of human beings. In such accounts, notably those of Plato and Aristotle, all things—including persons—are assumed to have an essence, or that which makes them the kind of thing they are. Many modern accounts, especially those of existentialist philosophers, deny that man has an essence. We want to be neutral concerning these essentialist or antiessentialist metaphysical positions, and so we hope that our terminology is acceptable to anyone who has any views whatever on this subject. All we intend in referring to "centrally important characteristics" is that set of attributes or properties, possessed by humans, which leads to our having moral rules, ethical beliefs, systems of reward and punishment, or anything else presupposing human responsibility for human actions.

2. *See* Cowan, *Human Experimentation: The Review Process in Practice,* 25 CASE W. RES. L. REV. 533, 536-37 (1974).

II. THE PHILOSOPHICAL BACKGROUND

Among other things, philosophy of mind is an inquiry into the nature of persons. What, if anything, is unique or special about persons? How do their characteristics, abilities, structure, and function differ from those of other entities that we categorize as things, machines, or instruments? Unless we can begin to formulate an answer to this type of question, we cannot move to the basic ethical questions which this paper addresses. In attempting to spell out the answer to the inquiry in philosophy of mind, we will construct a framework for an ethical theory that offers moral principles for how we ought to treat people or what sorts of actions are morally permissible. It is not sufficient for an ethical theory merely to assert such principles, but it also must offer a justification for them. Moral philosophy is not casuistry, a study of cases of conscience in an attempt to give specific solutions to problematic ethical dilemmas. Instead, philosophical ethics seeks to offer general moral principles and a thorough justification for their adoption and application in a wide variety of situations in which any person might find himself. This presupposes at least a provisional account of the nature of persons.

A further word about moral philosophy is in order. Unlike specific ethical codes of behavior or even ethical prescriptions or commandments that derive from religious sources, philosophical ethical theories generally avoid dogmatic principles or rigid, exceptionless commands. One purpose of a sound philosophical ethics is to mediate between an unjustified dogmatism, on the one hand, and an unwarranted moral skepticism on the other. Hence, philosophical ethics places a premium on the giving of reasons, both in support of the moral principles themselves and against the competing claims of dogmatic ethics and moral skepticism. Moreover, as we shall try to show in the account that follows, the fundamental moral principles of the most prominent ethical theories can serve as a basis for addressing the specific issues that arise in connection with experimentation on human subjects.

We return now to a closer look at the general question posed at the outset: What are the centrally important characteristics of human beings, which render them different from inanimate objects in a way that is relevant to how human beings ought to be treated? After laying the groundwork through inquiry into this question—including a brief look at two prominent ethical theories—we shall be prepared to discuss the ethically relevant criteria for answering the two specific questions pertinent to human experimentation: (1) What kinds of experiments can be justified? and (2) Under what constraints should subjects be selected or allowed to participate?

The first human characteristic relevant to our concerns here is that of sentience. Human beings, like other higher forms of animal life, are sentient creatures; that is, they are capable of feeling pleasure and pain under a wide range of predictable circumstances. What is more, people pursue pleasure and seek to avoid pain. Some philosophers and psychologists have gone so far as to claim that pursuit of pleasure and avoidance of pain are the sole factors motivating human behavior.[3] We need not go this far, however, in order to acknowledge the primacy of pain and pleasure as determinants of human action. It is this basic fact of sentience, conjoined with the teleological principle that people seek pleasurable ends and avoid actions with painful or unpleasant consequences, that has led to the widespread acceptance of one prominent ethical theory, utilitarianism.

One of the leading utilitarians, the 19th century English philosopher, John Stuart Mill, argued that pleasure is the sole thing that is good as an end. Since each person takes his own pleasure or happiness to be his ultimate aim or goal, toward which all particular activities are a means, Mill claimed that the value that should be maximized in the community as a whole is the greatest happiness of all. For the most part, Mill followed his utilitarian predecessor, Jeremy Bentham, in adopting the "Greatest Happiness Principle" as the fundamental moral principle of his ethical theory.[4]

---

3. Such a view may be found in the words of Jeremy Bentham:

Nature has placed mankind under the governance of two sovereign masters, *pain* and *pleasure*. It is for them alone to point out what we ought to do, as well as to determine what we shall do. On the one hand the standard of right and wrong, on the other the chain of causes and effects, are fastened to their throne.

Bentham, *An Introduction to the Principles of Morals and Legislation,* in PROBLEMS OF MORAL PHILOSOPHY 151 (2d ed. P. Taylor 1972).

Freud expressed a similar view:

The sovereign tendency obeyed by these primary processes is easy of recognition; it is called the pleasure-pain (Lust-Unlust) principle, or more shortly the pleasure-principle. These processes strive towards gaining pleasure; from any operation which might arouse unpleasantness ("pain") mental activity draws back (repression).

S. FREUD, *Formulation Regarding the Two Principles in Mental Functioning,* in GENERAL PSYCHOLOGICAL THEORY 22 (reissued 1963).

4. Mill writes, "the principle of utility, or, as Bentham latterly called it, the greatest happiness principle, has had a large share in forming the moral doctrines even of those who most scornfully reject its authority." J.S. MILL, UTILITARIANISM 6 (Bobbs-Merrill 1957).

As Mill himself stated, under the principle of utility, "actions are right in proportion as they tend to promote happiness; wrong as they tend to produce the reverse of happiness. By happiness is intended pleasure and the absence of pain; by unhappiness, pain and the privation of pleasure."[5] In order to prevent any misunderstanding of this influential theory, a bit more needs to be said by way of explication and interpretation of the utilitarian moral principle.

First, it should be emphasized that Mill explicitly disavows the interpretation of his theory as a "gross form" of hedonism.[6] While he clearly identifies happiness and pleasure, as shown in the above-quoted statement of the utilitarian principle, Mill nevertheless argues for a qualitative distinction among pleasures in addition to the usual distinction in terms of quantity or amount—the view held by Bentham and others. Mill writes:

> It is quite compatible with the principle of utility to recognize the fact that some kinds of pleasure are more desirable and more valuable than others. It would be absurd that, while in estimating all other things quality is considered as well as quantity, the estimation of pleasure should be supposed to depend on quantity alone.[7]

Thus, although Mill does identify happiness and pleasure, he argues against the mistake of confounding "the two very different ideas of happiness and content."[8] These so-called "higher pleasures" include the pleasures of the intellect, of the feelings and imagination, and of the moral sentiments—all of which are to be accorded a higher value as pleasures than those of "mere sensation."

A second, related point should also be stressed in explicating Mill's view. Utilitarianism might be criticized as being a crass, majority-rule doctrine, in which a preference for any action or state of affairs whatsoever of 51 percent of the population renders that action or state of affairs morally acceptable. This criticism rests on a misinterpretation of the intent of the utilitarian moral position. Throughout his essay, and especially in the lengthy final chapter entitled "On the Connection Between Justice and Utility," Mill expresses concern for minority rights and, indeed, the basic rights of persons. The claimed weakness of the utilitarian position lies in Mill's response to an objector who asks why society ought to defend

---

5. *Id.* at 10.
6. *Id.* at 9.
7. *Id.* at 12.
8. *Id.* at 13.

a person in the possession of his rights; Mill replies: "I can give him no other reason than general utility."[9]   Although nonutilitarians such as Immanuel Kant and John Rawls[10] have found Mill's answer unsatisfactory, a careful reading of Mill's writings reveals a pervasive humane and humanitarian thread woven throughout.   A serious problem remains, however, in that the principle of utility alone —as a fundamental moral principle—does not seem able to account for a variety of ethical duties and precepts of justice without the additional corollaries and interpretive remarks offered by Mill and other defenders of utilitarianism.

In summary, we should emphasize again that utilitarians claim that their ethical theory is derivable from certain indisputable facts about human beings—sentience and the tendency of persons to seek pleasure or happiness and avoid pain or unhappiness.   It is clear that the utilitarian principle often provides the basis for how people actually make judgments about the rightness and wrongness of actions.   As we shall see below, this ethical principle is frequently the operative criterion that guides many decisions in specific cases of experimentation on humans.   In particular, it seems that utility is the underlying moral principle in the notion of the "risk-benefit" equation, about which more will be said later.[11]

We now turn to the second basic characteristic of human beings, with which another prominent ethical theory is closely associated.   This attribute of the human species is rationality, and one major ethical theory that arises largely out of this human characteristic is the doctrine of the 18th century German philosopher, Immanuel Kant.   Closely linked with the concept of rationality is that of personal autonomy, to which ethical values are attached. Kant's ethical system begins by presupposing rationality and autonomy as fundamental characteristics of persons.   He then constructs a moral theory that is applicable to all rational beings, who possess what he describes as an autonomous, self-legislating will.   The inherent autonomy of each person, which is produced by his rationality, requires that each person be treated as a creature having dignity and, therefore, worthy of respect.   In Kant's view, rationality and autonomy are the essential humanity-conferring properties and give rise to the moral principle that persons should be accorded dignity and treated with respect.

---

9. *Id.* at 66.

10. *See* Kant, *Fundamental Principles of the Metaphysics of Morals,* in PROBLEMS OF MORAL PHILOSOPHY 236-37 (2d ed. P. Taylor 1972); J. RAWLS, A THEORY OF JUSTICE 209-11 (1971).

11. Text accompanying note 37 *infra.*

Kant used the term rationality to apply to an attribute of the human species rather than to an attribute of individual persons. As a result, the Kantian framework does not give us a criterion for distinguishing between rational individuals and irrational or nonrational individuals. Instead, it treats the human species (or any other "higher" beings) as having the capacity to reason and form concepts and, hence, as possessing the attribute of rationality. Some further distinctions and an explication of several specifiable senses of rational will be offered in section III, below. We hope to show that each of these different senses of rational is a key concept in problems relating to informed consent in special groups of experimental subjects: young children and the aged, the mentally retarded, the so-called "mentally ill," and prisoners. What is required at this point is a brief account of the way in which the concept of rationality and that of autonomy are linked in Kant's theory. We may then see how the human characteristic of rationality gives rise to some fundamental ethical values and moral principles.

Kant's notion of morality is that "its law must be valid, not merely for men, but for all *rational creatures generally*, not merely under certain contingent conditions or with exceptions, but with *absolute necessity* . . . ."[12] This passage makes explicit Kant's concept of morality as one that is applicable to all rational beings rather than one whose application is designed specifically for humans; it also exhibits the tone of his moral philosophy, which has led many to object that it is an implausibly rigid ethical system, since its law commands "with absolute necessity." On the basis of this notion of the nature and scope of morality, Kant formulates his account of the derivation of the commands of ethics:

> [S]ince moral laws ought to hold good for every rational creature, we must derive them from the general concept of a rational being. . . .
>
> . . . .
>
> Everything in nature works according to laws. Rational beings alone have the faculty of acting according *to the conception* of laws, that is according to principles, *i.e.* have a *will*. Since the deduction of actions from principles requires *reason*, the will is nothing but practical reason.[13]

Kant terms the fundamental moral principle or law of morality "the categorical imperative,"[14] since the moral law commands ab-

---

12. *Id.* at 222.
13. *Id.* at 223-24.
14. *Id.* at 228.

solutely (categorically) rather than conditionally (hypothetically).

In the archaic language in which Kant himself expresses it, the categorical imperative states: *"Act only on that maxim whereby thou canst at the same time will that it should become a universal law."*[15] Kant argues that all imperatives of duty can be deduced from this one fundamental principle, since persons can always formulate a maxim for each act they consider performing and then test the maxim for conformity to the fundamental principle, or categorical imperative. If the maxim passes the test, that is, if it can consistently be willed by the agent as a universal law, applicable to all rational creatures, then the contemplated action is morally permissible or morally right. We should emphasize here that this is a purely formal requirement for Kant, a necessary condition for an imperative to count as a moral law. The test Kant postulates is generally referred to, in an alternative formulation, as the requirement of generalization, or universalizability, in ethics. The core idea in all these views is that a moral law is one that holds for all persons similar in relevant respects in all like circumstances. Thus, what is right for one would be right for all similar persons in similar circumstances. Moreover, for a maxim to pass the test of the categorical imperative, it is not a matter of whether or not the agent can will the maxim to be a universal law as a matter of psychological fact. It is, rather, a question of logical consistency: maxims that cannot be willed to be universal laws, as prescribed by the categorical imperative, fail either because they lead to a logical contradiction or because such a will would contradict itself. A good will formulates and acts only on those maxims that prescribe our duties; morally right acts are those done for the sake of duty. So, for example, if a person contemplated breaking a promise when it was inconvenient for him to keep it, he would have to formulate a maxim of the following form: it is morally permissible to break promises when it is inconvenient to keep them. This maxim cannot (consistently) be universalized, since if everyone acted in accordance with it, the social institution of promising would soon break down, and there would no longer be a meaningful concept of a promise.

There is but one categorical imperative according to Kant, and yet he offers what he terms a second formulation of this fundamental principle: *"So act as to treat humanity, whether in thine own person or in that of any other, in every case as an end withal, never*

---

15. *Id.* at 229.

as means only."[16]   It is not our concern here to debate the question whether or not this statement is another formulation of the same principle or a new principle based on additional assumptions; we leave that debate to Kantian scholars.   The second formulation succeeds in capturing a common moral sentiment: we ought to treat our fellow human beings as ends in themselves and not as mere means or instruments for our own purposes, even to serve so-called "noble" aims.   It is this second formulation of Kant's categorical imperative that seems especially appropriate as a moral principle applicable in cases of human experimentation, for we can always test proposed actions using human subjects against the principle that persons should be treated as ends, never as mere means. Kant claims that "[t]he foundation of this principle is: *rational nature exists as an end in itself.*"[17]

Finally, Kant offers what he considers the third formulation of the categorical imperative, from which the notion of autonomy emerges.   The "third practical principle of the will, which is the ultimate condition of its harmony with the universal practical reason [is] the idea *of the will of every rational being as a universally legislative will.*"[18]   This capacity of every human will to be a universally legislating will is what constitutes the principle of autonomy of the will, which, according to Kant, is claimed to be "the basis of the dignity of human and of every rational nature."[19]   We can see, then, how the fundamental characteristic of rationality and the derivative concept of autonomy form the foundation for those values most central to our humane moral beliefs.   From Kant's moral philosophy we obtain the important value conception of the intrinsic worth or dignity of human beings.   In arguing for the central importance of duty in a conception of morality, Kant sums up these interrelationships as follows:

> The practical necessity of acting on this principle, *i.e.* duty, does not rest at all on feelings, impulses, or inclinations, but solely on the relation of rational beings to one another, a relation in which the will of a rational being must always be regarded as *legislative*, since it otherwise could not be conceived as *an end in itself*.   Reason then refers every maxim of the will, regarding it as legislating universally, to every other will and also to every action towards oneself; and this not on account of any other practical motive or

16. *Id.* at 234-35.
17. *Id.* at 234.
18. *Id.* at 236.
19. *Id.* at 239.

any future advantage, but from the idea of the *dignity* of a rational being, obeying no law but that which he himself also gives.[20]

The ethical theories of Kant and Mill each propose a basic general principle, according to which any moral agent can test his contemplated actions to ascertain their moral rightness or wrongness. In Kant's system, the central moral notion is that of duty, and the intrinsic human values are autonomy and dignity, both derived from the essential human attribute of rationality. Mill bases his theory on the empirically ascertained attribute of sentience in persons along with the observable goal-directed behavior of human beings in their pursuit of pleasure or happiness and avoidance of pain and suffering. The basic conceptions of morality found in both Kant and Mill seem to be required for a full account of our common moral sentiments and beliefs. In addition, they both provide a general principle under which we can subsume particular actions or subordinate moral rules in order to test their moral acceptability or validity. One need not consider himself a hedonist in order to accept the utilitarian principle, nor need one adhere, in general, to a duty-oriented conception of ethics in order to acknowledge the importance of the categorical imperative (in any of the formulations Kant suggests).

III. Ethical Concepts

Having laid the groundwork through a brief examination of two major normative theories in philosophical ethics, we turn next to an exploration of several subordinate concepts in ethics—concepts that relate directly to the moral problems surrounding human experimentation. Arising out of the facts of man's sentience and pursuit of his own happiness or welfare, and also out of the fundamental human attribute of rationality and the derived notions of autonomy and dignity, the subordinate ethical concepts relevant to experimenting on humans include coercion and paternalism, autonomy and dependency.

The concepts we are about to examine all converge on the central concern in human experimentation: the need to obtain the informed consent of the experimental subject. It is evident that only by obtaining informed consent can we be sure we are treating the experimental subject as an end, and not as mere means; neglecting to seek informed consent would indicate a deeper failure to recognize the autonomy and, hence, the humanity of the subject. All

---

20. *Id.* at 238.

three formulations of Kant's categorical imperative are relevant
to our understanding of why we deem informed consent an important prerequisite for any experimentation on human beings.

It is appropriate, however, to begin our inquiry with a further
look at the concept of rationality, since that notion lies at the roots
of Kant's ethical system and is also the recurrent issue in problems
relating to special groups of experimental subjects (*e.g.*, children,
the retarded, the mentally ill). The concept of rationality is problematic, partly because it is not a purely descriptive concept but is
itself a normative notion, and, more importantly, because the term
rational has several related yet distinct senses. Perhaps the most
fundamental sense is that in which the concept of rationality pur-
ports to distinguish one class of beings or entities from all other entities or creatures. In this way, man is defined as "the rational animal," and so rationality is seen as a distinctive or essential property
of the human species. It is this sense of rationality that appears to
be Kant's conception, providing the basis for his ethical system. It is
not clear, however, whether this sense of the term applies only to
the human species (and, if they exist, "higher" beings such as God
and angels), although it is intended to apply to all persons, *qua*
members of the human species. The scope of this sense of rational
remains open, with conceptual arguments offered on behalf of considering highly advanced computers, robots of the future, and, perhaps, dolphins as rational entities. It is worth speculating about
whether we would become gravely concerned about experimenting on dolphins (in a way different from our ordinary concerns about
animals) if, as a result of empirical inquiry, conceptual decision, or
both, we determined that dolphins were rational creatures. It appears that both the attributes of sentience and rationality are required to generate what we consider moral concern for existing entities, in the sense that requires our treating them with dignity and
respect. Computers and present-day robots lack the property of sentience, so even if we were to ascribe rationality to them, this alone
would not require that we treat them in accordance with moral
principles (although we may nonetheless decide that they should be
kept in good repair). There is an asymmetry, then, between the
possession of rationality alone and the possession of sentience alone,
in respect to our treatment of non-human entities. The possession of sentience alone is a criterion for our treating creatures with
some moral concern, as shown by our behavior towards higher forms
of animal life and by the laws and regulations governing the use of

animals in experimental contexts.[21] We propose to bypass a discussion of experimenting on animals here, noting simply that sentience alone introduces the propriety of moral attitudes and behavior. It remains an open question whether the existence of rationality alone would similarly entitle its possessor to moral treatment at the hands of human beings.

The sense of rationality as necessarily applying to all human creatures is not a helpful notion when we want to distinguish among human beings in respect of their rationality, for special purposes. These purposes may include a perceived need to interfere with the behavior of those persons who are deemed irrational, whether on their own behalf (*i.e.*, paternalistically), or for the good of society (*i.e.*, coercively). Whether persons lacking in rationality in a qualitative sense, may be treated in ways that are morally impermissible when performed on fully rational humans is a central question arising in the context of experimentation on human subjects. The so-called mentally ill, the retarded, young children, the senile aged—all these persons have been considered, at the very least, as lacking full-scale rationality, if not as wholly irrational.

We turn next to two related yet distinct senses of rational, which appear to constitute the usual criteria for distinguishing persons generally considered rational from those deemed irrational or non-rational. In one of its common meanings, the term rational denotes the capacity of humans to use their reason (rationality) to maximize their chosen or accepted ends. This is the sense in which a rational person can defer the temptation of short range gain or pleasure for the sake of a longer term goal that he holds to be more important. Such a sense of rationality also encompasses the conception of a rational person as one who is good at calculation and inductive as well as deductive reasoning, since these are necessary attributes for consistently being able to choose the best means to one's ends. The other closely related sense of rational refers to the chosen ends themselves. In this sense of the term, the chosen means, if any, are not a criterion for ascribing rationality to the agent; it is, rather, the ends themselves that confer rationality. Self-destructive ends, painful or unprofitable goals, apparently pointless acts—all these are characteristic of the irrational, as the correlative notion. Thus, persons who attempt suicide are considered irrational by psychiatrists and others, and, as a result, are subjected to coercive measures

---

21. *E.g.*, Laboratory Animal Welfare Act, 7 U.S.C. §§ 2131-55 (1970); 9 C.F.R. §§ 3.1-.114 (1973).

such as involuntary hospitalization. It is evident that the foregoing senses of the term irrational are different, since a person may be rational in one of these senses and irrational according to the other.[22] Nevertheless, these two senses of rational and irrational enter prominently into ethical considerations in experimenting on humans.

One major concern in human experimentation is the question of the competence of persons to give their consent. The relevant meaning of competence here encompasses both of the senses of rational discussed immediately above. While it is patently clear that infants, the severely retarded, and wholly uncommunicative emotionally disturbed persons are not competent to give consent in any of the requisite senses of rational, the concepts in question fall along a continuum and may be difficult to apply in borderline cases.[23] In approaching such problems, we should view the senses of rational and irrational either as enduring attributes of the persons to whom they apply or else as temporary attributes that cut across a wide range of abilities or capacities of a person. It is evident that infants, the severely retarded, or the emotionally disturbed lack the functional capacity, in general, for making intelligent decisions or rational choices, engaging in careful deliberations, or adopting prudent long-range ends or goals. Whether the class of persons lacks full-scale rationality or competence as an enduring attribute (*e.g.*, the mentally retarded), or whether the irrational or non-rational status is temporary but pervades the whole personality (*e.g.*, infants and "curable" mental patients), the above-noted concepts of rationality cut across most or all of a person's cognitive and deliberative abilities and capacities. There is, however, another use of the term irrational in which it applies only to a temporary and localized attribute of persons. Two sorts of examples serve to illustrate this use. First, there are cases in which a person might have temporary mood disturbances (*e.g.*, depression) during which time he is not fully rational and may even contemplate suicide; most of the time, however, he can function adequately and well, even as a highly compe-

22. An example might be the person who "successfully" commits suicide—with efficiency and with the least financial and emotional cost to others.
23. It is generally held that lack of competence or rationality in a person warrants interference with his autonomy by others, in the belief that such interference is justified if it is necessary to the person's health or welfare. This sort of interference is central to the meaning of the concept of paternalism—a concept that plays a key role in human experimentation when the experimental subjects themselves are unable to give informed consent.

tent professional or academic.   Secondly, there are cases in which a
person might be suffering from temporary shock (*e.g.*, after an accident) or profound grief (*e.g.*, following the death of a loved one)
or even extreme fear and anxiety (*e.g.*, prior to difficult surgery on
oneself or one's child).   In both categories the competence
of such persons may be called into question, even if the lack
of rationality exhibited is temporary or confined to a small area of
their total activities.   Such an application of the notion of rationality
enters prominently into judgments concerning informed consent:
Under what circumstances can consent be considered fully informed, and who besides the experimental subject himself ought to
be allowed to grant consent?

A word should be said about some of the epistemological issues
pertaining to informed consent.   While our primary focus in this article is on the ethical issues in experimentation on human subjects,
philosophical problems of knowledge are relevant as well.   The
chief epistemological concern arises because the notion of "being
informed" is none too clear.   It is obvious that there are vastly different amounts of information that a person may possess, and, as a
result, varying degrees of one's being informed.   The question in the
present connection is, how much information, and what specific sorts
of information, ought a person have before his consent can properly
be said to be informed?[24]   Some persons—usually, but not always,
physicians[25]—claim that a patient, or lay persons in general, can
never be fully informed.   In order for them to be, the argument
runs, they would have to know as much as the physician knows
about diseases, risks, complications, statistics about similar cases,
and perhaps a range of other facts.   If people had to know all these
facts, theories, and statistics in order to be truly informed, consent
could rarely be given even for most therapeutic procedures, much
less for a variety of experiments employing human subjects.[26]   So,
it is reasonable to look for some standard other than "full and com-

---

24. *See* Cowan, *supra* note 2, at 552-53, for a listing of the Department of
Health, Education, and Welfare's criteria for informed consent.

25. *E.g.*, Letter to the Editor from Nicholas J. Demy, M.D., 217 J.A.M.A.
696-97 (1971); Ingelfinger, *Informed (But Uneducated) Consent*, 287 NEW
ENG. J. MED. 465-66 (1972).

26. As Dr. Cowan notes, much the same problem exists on institutional
review committees as a result of the medical ignorance of nonphysician members. *See* Cowan, *supra* note 2, at 558. Ironically, it would seem that the nonphysician reviewer's ignorance might be the very factor that would best qualify
him to appreciate just how informed the consent given by an equally ignorant
subject is.

plete information" on which to base consent. Just what such a standard should be remains a problem to be solved, but it is not insurmountable. Focus should probably be in the area of ascertaining what information is relevant for an experimental subject's consent to be sufficiently informed. While judgments about relevance are also subject to dispute, at least the problem becomes more manageable. An additional epistemological issue is the difficulty that the physician or experimenter faces in determining whether the experimental subject has the requisite understanding of the relevant information to grant his informed consent.[27] Evidence is sometimes brought forth to show that even when patients or experimental subjects are given the necessary information, for a variety of possible reasons they may not adequately process or comprehend that information. So even when experimental subjects have been properly informed (told) by others about a proposed experiment, the subjects may nonetheless remain uninformed (lacking in understanding) in important ways.

Aside from these epistemological issues concerning what it is to be informed and how we can tell when a person really is informed in a particular case, there are the primary ethical difficulties relating to autonomy and dependency, paternalism and coercion. An analysis of the manner in which consent is obtained reveals how such ethical questions arise. Such an analysis requires an explication of the notion of voluntariness, in the sense that means "uncoerced actions."[28] In addition to being informed, consent must also be voluntary, or uncoerced, in order not to violate our moral principles prohibiting interference with other autonomous persons. It is precisely at this point that most of the moral problems are found concerning the use of prisoners as experimental subjects, and some of these same issues arise with other institutionalized populations,

---

27. This difficulty has prompted some institutional review committees to require that a family member witness the giving of consent in order to further insure that the subject actually understood the full impact of his consent. *Id.* at 553-54.

28. There are other related meanings of the term "voluntary" besides the sense rendered here as "uncoerced." Especially in legal contexts, the notion of voluntariness may have a somewhat different application than the sense explicated in this article. Voluntariness is a somewhat problematic concept, and we do not intend to stipulate a definition; nor do we imply that the sense of the term that means "uncoerced" is the only or even the primary sense. Rather, we hope to capture the meaning that is central to the notion of a genuine volunteer: one who (voluntarily) offers himself for some purpose without being coerced.

such as the aged or the terminally ill.[29]　Consent for research, therefore, must be voluntary and granted by mentally competent, rational agents who are properly informed.

For present purposes, we may identify several special classes of "dependent persons." These categories include children,[30] mentally retarded persons, the aged, prisoners, and the mentally ill—especially those emotionally disturbed persons who are institutionalized. The individuals comprising these classes of persons are functionally incapacitated or undeveloped in some way, and, therefore, tend to be viewed as less capable of autonomous actions and decisions than are normal adults. While some of these individuals are dependent because of less-than-normal capacity to think or reason or make judgments (*e.g.*, young children and mentally retarded persons), others, such as prisoners, are rendered dependent in special ways by the actions of society. The constraints placed on institutionalized persons constitute limitations on their freedom in ways that raise serious questions about their ability to grant fully voluntary consent to serve as experimental subjects. The ethical problems come to focus on the element of coercion that seems to be present on many occasions when informed consent is sought.

How can we tell when voluntariness is present? There are paradigm cases of coerced actions—those that are performed under threat of violence or some other negative sanction. If I am accosted by someone with a gun who demands, "Your money or your life!" and I hand over my purse, do I do so voluntarily? In one sense, I do it voluntarily since I choose this alternative rather than the other, less desirable one. So, I voluntarily hand over my purse rather than risk death at the hands of the gunman. In another sense, this action does not seem wholly voluntary when compared with other cases in which I act not under threat of violence but willingly or "out of my own volition" or "of my own free will," as it is commonly put. In one perfectly ordinary way of speaking, I

---

29. An example of ethically suspect research on old persons who were hospitalized and terminally ill is the cancer study performed at the Jewish Chronic Disease Hospital in Brooklyn, New York. In this experiment, cancer cells were implanted in these patients, and it was charged that some of the experiments in this study were performed without the informed consent of the participants. For a full discussion, see EXPERIMENTATION WITH HUMAN BEINGS 9-66 (J. Katz ed. 1972).

30. For a discussion of some special problems associated with experimentation on children in connection with the development and testing of drugs, *see* Cowan, *supra* note 2, at 556-57.

hand over my purse to the gunman "against my will." There is, it appears, a problematic conceptual issue that needs to be addressed if we are to be able to assess when a person's decisions and actions are truly voluntary, in the sense of not coerced. We still have a problem of deciding what criteria to employ in judging when informed consent is truly voluntary and when a competent adult experimental subject is performing actions or making decisions under some form of coercion, however subtle. Critics of the use of prisoners (as well as other institutionalized persons) in research contend that the very role of prisoner precludes fully voluntary decision and action on the part of such individuals.[31] This contention maintains that an element of coercion always exists in the very nature of the prisoner's role and in the constraints inherent in an institutionalized setting. We should be aware that debate on these issues rests only partly on moral considerations; much of the disagreement often lies in conceptual and factual matters, as well. For example, if the parties to a dispute about the morality of using prisoners in research could agree on whether prisoners can, in principle, ever volunteer in an uncoerced manner, or whether, on the contrary, their being prisoners entails an element of coercion in all behavior that involves prison officials and outsiders, they would come closer to settling the moral dilemma that lies at the heart of this issue.

Unlike prisoners, who are rendered dependent by the actions of society, other types of persons suffer reduced autonomy because of a natural dependence. The aged may suffer from impaired mental capacity, like retarded persons, and young children are not yet capable of autonomous decision and action. It is natural, and perhaps even necessary in many cases, to assume a protective attitude toward persons who are functionally incapacitated in some way. This attitude is exhibited, for example, in the phenomenon of "maternal instinct" in humans and other mammals. Dependent status makes the elderly and the retarded especially vulnerable to a variety of experimental treatments, only some of which might benefit them.[32]

31. *See* Lasagna, *Special Subjects in Human Experimentation*, 98 DAEDA-LUS 449-55 (1969); Mitford, *Experiments Behind Bars*, ATLANTIC MONTHLY, Jan. 1973, at 64, 73.

32. In the cancer study cited in note 29 *supra*, the researchers made no claims about possible benefits to the experimental subjects themselves. In contrast, the researchers who deliberately exposed retarded children at the Willow-brook State School to viral hepatitis defended their research on the grounds that these children would have contracted hepatitis even without this artificial

When research is viewed as possibly or probably beneficial to the experimental subjects, it is justified on paternalistic grounds, namely: Interference is warranted because it will promote the welfare of the subjects themselves. Where no perceived benefit is possible or likely for the subjects themselves, an attempt to justify the interference cannot be based on paternalistic grounds. Rather, the experimenter must seek some other justification for treating persons as having less than full autonomy, that is, treating them in a coercive manner. People in institutions of any sort might be viewed as ideal subjects for experimentation because of the ease of observing them, the ability of researchers to select control groups, the opportunity for repetitive or long-term research using the same subjects, and so on. Unfortunately, however, these same institutionalized persons are often ideal subjects for another reason: their dependency and diminished human capacities render them easy prey to coercive measures of all sorts, including use in medical experiments by well-intentioned as well as unscrupulous researchers.

All of the moral issues in this broad area might be phrased in terms of the ethical notion of the rights of persons: What are the rights of children, retarded persons, and the mentally ill? In general, how ought persons who are functionally incapacitated be viewed with respect to the presence or absence of their human rights? What sorts of attributes must a person have—or lack—in order to retain basic human rights such as the right not to be interfered with or the right to be granted full-fledged freedom and autonomy? Who, if anyone, has the right to grant consent for experimentation on minor children, retarded persons, or the mentally ill? Conceiving the moral issues in terms of rights and duties is, however, only one way of placing them in an ethical perspective. Questions of the sort under discussion here do not seem to be made clearer or easier to answer by formulating them in terms of rights. Indeed, the ethical waters are often muddied by a variety of claims about people's rights that are difficult to substantiate. This is partly because of a range of problems associated with the notion of rights: Where do they come from? How do we know when they exist or in whom they reside? How do we settle conflicts of rights or disagreements about their existence or nonexistence in particular

---

exposure, but in the experimental setting the children would be "better off" since they would be under careful observation by the researchers and the hepatitis could be kept under control. The Willowbrook research is described by Saul Krugman and Joan P. Giles in *Viral Hepatitis: New Light on an Old Disease,* 212 J.A.M.A. 1019-29 (1970).

cases?   These difficulties are much less pronounced when we are dealing with legal rights, rather than with moral rights, which are not embodied in written laws.   Moral philosophy addresses itself to such problems and issues, but has produced no universally applicable answer in all the years of debate.   We believe, therefore, that knotty moral problems are not simplified by being couched in terms of people's rights, though it does not follow that talk about rights or appeals to rights ought to be eliminated entirely from our moral discourse.   Since a good deal of ethical philosophy and many of our ordinary moral sensibilities and convictions are concerned with the basic rights of persons, we may still recognize the legitimacy of the notion of rights even if that notion is hard to understand fully and difficult to apply.

It is important to provide a clear analysis and explication of all of the ethical concepts we have discussed in this section, so that we can develop criteria that are useful and applicable in practice when informed consent must be obtained.   It may be that some paternalistic acts are justifiable in experimental contexts, while others are not.   We may decide that our fundamental ethical principles preclude the introduction of any coercive elements into the selection of experimental subjects or the attempt to gain their consent. Without careful analysis, we risk making our practical criteria too weak or too strong, too vague or too ambiguous, and therefore, inappropriate or difficult to apply.

IV.   THEORY AND PRACTICE

Let us turn now to the specific ethical questions arising from the practice of experimenting on human subjects: (1) What experiments can be morally justified? and (2) Under what constraints should subjects be selected?   In the account that follows, we shall show how one might obtain reasoned answers to these questions by using the philosophical theories and conceptual analyses sketched above.

In answering these questions, it makes a great deal of difference which ethical theory we choose to adopt.   The theories of Kant and Mill are substantively different, and in some cases they yield different answers to moral questions.   We must, therefore, weigh the options carefully and examine the consequences of adopting either theory.   Once committed to a theory, we should try to be consistent and avoid appealing to our chosen theory only when its directives suit us, while choosing some alternative conception when they do not.

At first glance, it would seem that the acceptance of Kant's account requires that we consider all experiments using human subjects as wrong: experimenters necessarily use their subjects as means, since the subjects are, in a sense, instruments in the experiment. A closer look, however, shows that Kant's imperative is to treat persons as ends and not as means merely. It is permissible to treat persons as means, provided that we also consider them as ends.

Unfortunately, the language of "means" and "ends" is very con-confusing, and Kant does little to illuminate the matter. It is clear, though, that he cannot be enjoining us from ever using other persons to further our own ends. We treat persons as means when we hire them to move our furniture, cut our hair, treat our illnesses, and draw up contracts for us. It is a fact of life in any social environment that we treat people as means; in fact, it is generally believed that the chief purpose of societies is for people to band together to meet each other's needs in the most efficient way.[33] Kant's injunction, therefore, cannot be construed as prohibiting any use whatsoever of another person for our own purpose. Rather, it prescribes that we not treat a person exclusively as a means. We must also attend to the individual's chosen ends and avoid using the person to meet our ends, unless by doing so we are contributing to the attainment of his own chosen ends.

With respect to experimentation, Kant would surely approve of those experiments in which an intended or hoped-for aim is some benefit to the subjects themselves. If an experiment is conducted both as a therapeutic attempt and to help others or to further knowledge, it is acceptable by this standard. Even if the subjects do not themselves need this treatment but merely have an interest in the success of the research for some other reason (for example, if the research is investigating an illness from which a relative suffers, or the subjects have a scientific curiosity about the matter, or, simply, are acting altruistically), the experiment would still be acceptable.

Nonetheless, Kant would find even these experiments unjustifiable if they could result in a reduction of an individual's ability to function as an independent, autonomous, rational agent. Rationality and autonomy are the most important human characteristics,

33. One of the earliest statements of this view appears in PLATO, THE REPUBLIC, Book II, 367e-372a (F. Cornford transl. Oxford Univ. 1945).

454 *CASE WESTERN RESERVE LAW REVIEW* [Vol. 25:434

and, as we noted earlier, they form the basis of our moral framework. Any act that might reduce these capacities would violate an important standard of human dignity and would be inconsistent with the third formulation of the categorical imperative.[34] By this standard, all forms of novel exploratory experimentation on ways of effecting behavior change in humans would be suspect, be they behavior modification techniques, psychosurgery, or new chemical or electrical stimuli to the brain. The notorious syphilis experiment done at the Tuskegee Institute,[35] in which unwitting subjects suffering from syphilis were left untreated for more than thirty years, was immoral according to Kant's criterion because it was known that many subjects would become mad in the stage of tertiary syphilis, and it is morally wrong to bring about or promote irrationality.

Kant also argues that being alive must be a fundamental value for everyone. Most people naturally choose life over death. For those who do not, Kant offers arguments to show that everyone who is able to choose has an obligation not to terminate his own life. It follows that others must respect this universally binding human end and that any experiment involving the death (or even a serious likelihood of death) of its subjects is wrong. Hence, even if the subjects are willing to risk their lives for the sake of the experiment, they are mistaken, for they ought to value their lives above most other considerations. It is wrong for anyone to violate this fundamental end. The only possible exceptions to the presumption against experiments involving death would be those cases in which death is imminent without the experiment, or where life is otherwise seriously threatened, say, by a high probability of contracting some fatal disease; but even then it would be right for subjects only to agree to a risk of death, while still refusing to allow certain death in the cause of science.

There is another whole set of experiments that Kant would object to: those involving deception. His ethical theory requires persons to act only in accordance with maxims that they could consistently will to be universal law. It appears to be clear to Kant that truth-telling fulfills this criterion while lying does not; thus it is always wrong to lie. Hence, any experiment that involves deliberate lying could not be justified in spite of its potential benefits. This is-

---

34. *See* note 18 *supra* and accompanying text.

35. *See Hearings on S. 2071, S. 2072, and H.R. 7724 Before the Subcomm. on Health of the Senate Comm. on Labor and Public Welfare*, 93d Cong., 1st Sess., pt. 4, at 1187-1253 (1973).

sue is especially pertinent in the social sciences, where a great deal of research is conducted by means of deceptive experiments. The most famous of the genre is one run by Stanley Milgram in the mid-1960's, in which he investigated the degree to which persons will respond to authority.[36] The procedure involved telling subjects that they were to administer painful and even fatal electric shocks to other volunteers on direction from an experimenter. The supposed recipient of the shock was actually a stooge, who cried out and made other appropriate responses on signal, but suffered no ill effects. Since it was important to the study that the subjects believed themselves to be actually adminstering shocks, and since 65 percent of the subjects administered what would have been fatal shocks, it was obviously ethically preferable to use deception. The only alternative (except not experimenting at all) would have been to administer killing dosages of shock. Nevertheless, a Kantian would not approve of this procedure, but would claim that lying in itself is wrong and cannot be made right by the goodness of its consequences. If the only way that this sort of experiment could have been conducted without lying would have been by killing people, then the experiment was unjustifiable in any form and should not have been conducted.

The utilitarian answer to the question of what experiments are morally justifiable is much easier to formulate, though surely no easier to apply. The utilitarian principle requires us to act in the way that produces the greatest general balance of happiness over unhappiness. In order to determine whether an experiment is justified, a utilitarian must calculate the "expected utility," that is, the good or happiness or welfare likely to come of it. The calculation proceeds by estimating the amount of happiness and multiplying that amount by the probability of its coming about as a result of this experiment, thereby obtaining a measure of the benefit at stake. The utilitarian must then weigh that benefit against the anticipated risk, determined by multiplying the amount of harm by the probability of its occurrence. The measure is complex, for it must include all the possible good and bad effects of the experiment—including feelings engendered in the general population, feelings of satisfaction or guilt on the part of participants, and consequences of actions done as a direct result of the experiment. However complex the utilitarian calculation may be, something very much like it ap-

---

36. *See* Milgram, *Behavioral Study of Obedience*, 67 J. ABNORMAL SOCIAL PSYCHOLOGY 371-78 (1963).

pears to be the underlying moral principle in the notion of the risk-benefit equation, as mentioned earlier.[37]

There is an obvious problem here for both Kantians and utilitarians. By the very nature of experimentation, research contexts often make possible studies for which the results are as yet unknown. Kant's principle refuses to permit experiments that will result in decreased autonomy on the part of the subject; Mill's principle allows only experiments that produce the greatest balance of good over evil in terms of pleasurable or painful consequences. The problem that confronts the prospective experimenter, then, lies in the fact that we cannot accurately predict the results. Inability to predict results does not, however, grant a license to act in total disregard of consequences (as, for example, in radically innovative experimental attempts). Instead, this unfortunate feature demands a strong responsibility on the part of researchers to study as best they can the possible or likely results and requires them to engage only in those tests with human subjects in which the experimenters are assured that there is little chance of significant harm to the subjects. Mistakes might still be made, just as mistakes are made in all other areas of human activity, but if researchers have sincerely tried to reduce the likelihood of risk and have not attempted an experiment when they have reason to believe serious harm may result, then they are justified in performing it.

Utilitarianism permits a wide range of experiments that Kantians would never consider. For instance, utilitarians would probably approve an experiment expected to provide a cure for cancer, even though it was expected to cause its early subjects to develop untreatable cancer; Kantians would surely object. Utilitarians as well as Kantians would object to the Tuskegee syphilis experiments, but on different grounds: Whereas Kantians would object to the loss of the subjects' autonomy as a result of illness and possible insanity, the utilitarians would object because the experiments did little good. If the experiments had been better designed and were likely to succeed in producing some significant, useful knowledge leading to beneficial results for humanity, utilitarians might be willing to approve, despite the resulting illness and insanity generated by the tests.

Still, utilitarians do not operate with a simple risk-benefit table that approves any experiment whatsoever where benefit measures highest. They are obliged to choose the option with the best ratio

---

37. Text accompanying note 11 *supra*.

of benefit to risk, and so they have a strong responsibility to minimize risks. It is important to investigate alternative courses of action that might further improve the ratio, even if the benefit already
outweighs the risk. In practice, this requirement would prevent
Mill and most utilitarians from engaging in many experiments that
are threatening to life or that interfere with the basic rights of persons.[38] If a great risk is present, utilitarians would generally assume that the experimenter should wait before performing this particular test and seek a safer means of obtaining the result. However,
if no safe alternative can be devised, and if the expected benefit
clearly outweighs the risk, in terms of happiness or well-being and
pain or suffering, then utilitarians are obliged to permit experiments
that Kantians would unconditionally oppose.

According to either conception of ethics, we can identify some
types of experiments that are morally wrong; even if it were possible to obtain willing volunteers for such experiments, it would be
wrong to perform them according to the fundamental moral principles of these theories. However, this analysis does not completely
resolve our ethical questions because there are further moral conditions to be met even within the range of experiments that are unjustifiable in principle. In general, these further considerations have
to do with some conception of the individuals involved as experimental subjects. In the Kantian framework, human beings are thought
to be autonomous creatures having dignity, and, hence, deserving
respect. According to Mill, human beings are happier if they are
treated with dignity and respect and if their personal freedom is
made as extensive as is socially feasible.[39] The difference between
these two views in this regard lies in the ultimate end each theory
posits. For Mill, pleasure or happiness is the ultimate end for
man, so all actions must promote that end; for Kant, the only thing
good in itself is a good will—a will whose motive for actions is that
they be done for the sake of duty. In any case, it follows from either
theory that we have a prima facie obligation to treat other persons

38. Mill claims that the moral agent must assure himself that in benefiting some persons by his actions "he is not violating the rights, that is, the legitimate and authorized expectations, of anyone else." J.S. MILL, *supra* note 4,
at 25.

39. Mill refers to "the love of liberty and personal independence" in man,
and to "a sense of dignity, which all human beings possess in one form or
other, and in some, though by no means in exact, proportion to their higher
faculties, and which is so essential a part of the happiness of those in whom
it is strong that nothing which conflicts with it could be otherwise than momentarily an object of desire to them." *Id.* at 13.

honestly, to seek their consent in matters affecting them, and to be sensitive to their interests. The most effective way to attain these goals when dealing with subjects of experimentation is by obtaining their informed consent for all that we do with them.

In practice, such obligations are more easily fulfilled with certain groups of subjects than with others, thus it may be that while an experiment is permissible if done with one set of subjects, it is impermissible if done with some other group of subjects. As we have stressed, the ideal situation is one in which the experimental subjects are fully rational persons who have offered genuinely informed, voluntary consent. Under such conditions, there is considerable assurance that the researchers are not using the subjects solely as means. We cannot justify using persons as subjects of experiments against their will. If they actively resist participation, using them would violate Kant's prescription not to treat persons as mere means; Mill, too, would consider this an unjustified interference with the basic rights of persons. Thus, it is wrong to coerce people into serving as subjects when they have decided otherwise. It follows, then, that any coercive use of prisoners in experimentation is wrong.

The need for informed consent is a most difficult requirement, since it is common for research to deal exclusively with a condition only experienced by "dependent persons"—those not clearly capable or clearly incapable of providing informed consent. Medical researchers cannot investigate all the problems of prenatal injury without experimenting on fetuses, nor can medical or social scientists gain an understanding of the workings of Down's syndrome (mongolism) without experimenting on some of its victims. Psycho-pharmacologists must surely use psychotic patients to develop effective antipsychotic drugs, and gerontologists can only understand senility by conducting research on the senile. Obviously, the list could be extended to cover every class of persons limited by some medical or psychological condition.[40] The potential benefits are great; the risks may be small. In so many cases the only hope of reducing suffering involves using persons who are unable to provide informed consent. Our problem is to decide when, if ever, we are justified in conducting an experiment without obtaining informed consent.

---

40. One class which has posed great difficulty for drug researchers is children. Because of the controversy over whether or not a child can give informed consent, "investigators are becoming progressively more reluctant to test new drugs in children." Cowan, *supra* note 2, at 557.

Utilitarians have no serious problem in these cases. There is a genuine disutility in allowing the practice of treating people as experimental subjects without their consent. Consider, as an extreme example, the wide-scale discomfort and anxiety experienced even to this day as a result of experiments performed by the Nazis. As a mere practical consideration the full cooperation of subjects, which can be expected after their consent has been obtained, should result in the greater success of many experiments. Still, there are times when we would be scientifically better off without worrying about informed consent.[41] In such cases if we instituted some special experimental constraints with the aim of reducing anxiety about the possibility of Nazi-like atrocities, such experiments would be in accord with the utilitarian principle; hence, it would be justifiable on that theory to use subjects without their consent. In fact, utilitarianism seems to mandate the use of subjects with limited abilities whenever possible. Since such subjects are less likely to benefit society in other ways than are normal persons, it is in the social interest to take risks with their lives rather than with the lives of those fully rational persons who may make some other sort of contribution. Moreover, there is reason to believe that at least some of these individuals actually suffer less than others, or have less potential for happiness (*e.g.*, fetuses, the severely retarded, the dying who are already suffering). If this is so, and if the general aim is to maximize the balance of happiness over pain in society, then there are further grounds for using these sorts of persons as experimental subjects.

It appears that we are now caught between extremes on the problem of experimentation: Kant's position is so rigid it seems implausibly strong, while the utilitarian solution seems almost heartless and inadequate to account for all our moral sensibilities. As a way out of this impasse, we shall introduce a line of reasoning developed by John Rawls and spelled out in detail in his book, *A Theory of Justice*.[42] Rawls works out an alternative conception of morality, which appeals to the insights of both of his predecessors.

Rawls is dissatisfied with the utilitarian approach, for it fails to account adequately for that element of justice commonly conceived as fairness. Two examples, one hypothetical and the other histori-

---

41. Dr. Cowan cites as one example of such a situation the "double blind trial" in drug studies, wherein it is crucial to keep the subjects ignorant of the nature of the drug being tested on them. Such ignorance would, of course, preclude the giving of fully informed consent. Cowan, *supra* note 2, at 554-55.

42. J. RAWLS, *supra* note 10.

cal, serve to illustrate this failure: If it would help in understanding and eventually curing depression to stimulate a person's brain with electrodes in order to produce in him a permanent, incapacitating state of depression that could be carefully studied and recorded until death, utilitarians would consent to the study. If they were convinced that the experiments would be useful, utilitarians would also be likely to allow the cancer study Southam and Levin performed on the unaware, aged inmates of the Jewish Chronic Disease Hospital, in which cancer cells were injected under their skin.[43] In objecting to these features of the utilitarian moral theory, Rawls observes that "there is no reason in principle why the greater good of some should not compensate for the lesser losses of others; or more importantly, why the violation of the liberty of a few might not be made right by greater good shared by many."[44] Rawls believes however that many people would charge such measures with being unfair, and justifiably so; unlike the utilitarians, he believes this would be a morally relevant objection.[45] He agrees that our ethical considerations ought to account for the general welfare, but he argues that they must also be concerned with justice, as well.[46] It is not sufficient to worry only about maximizing happiness and minimizing pain.

In order to convey what is involved in determining a just solution, Rawls uses a thought experiment commonly appealed to in the literature of social and political philosophy. He asks us to imagine what a group of persons in a carefully defined original position would agree to if they were deciding amongst themselves on their social organization.[47] Such a thought experiment is key to all social contract theories;[48] the important feature of any social contract is that everyone enter it willingly, that it be the sort of commitment all could agree to. Rawls uses this technique because he believes that a just procedure is one that does not take advantage of anyone but

---

43. *See* note 29 *supra.*
44. J. RAWLS, *supra* note 10, at 26.
45. *Id. passim* (especially at 3-4).
46. *Id.* at 4-5.
47. *Id.* at 11-22.
48. The most prominent examples of such theories are, of course, those of Hobbes, Locke, and Rousseau. The terms of the contracts envisioned by these theories are not all the same; they arise out of the details of whichever original position the particular social contract theorist assumes. *See* T. HOBBES, LEVIATHAN; J. LOCKE, OF CIVIL GOVERNMENT; J. ROUSSEAU, THE SOCIAL CONTRACT.

rather, allows everyone equality—a truly fair arrangement.[49] Such equality does not exist in real life, for actual social contracts are entered into by parties who are most concerned with fostering their own interests. Those with power are able to influence others and ensure a contract which, instead of being fair, unjustly supports the interests of the powerful at the expense of the weak. So the need arises for a thought experiment, and Rawls asks us to imagine a situation in which we have to agree on a standard of justice to apply to all future arrangements, without being able to account for our particular interests.

To construct this hypothetical situation Rawls directs us to imagine ourselves under a "veil of ignorance,"[50] whereby we do not know any specific facts about ourselves: neither our wealth, social position, talents, preferences, age, nor race. We would know only the general facts of human nature on which Mill based his notion of a person's rights: that humans are sentient, that they are concerned with their own well-being, that they function in a society, and that their happiness depends upon fulfilling a certain life plan. Rawls argues that anyone making a decision under this constraint would have to act fairly, and deliberately avoid exploiting anyone, because it is possible that the decisionmaker might turn out to be the one exploited. The decisionmaker under the veil of ignorance will be most concerned with protecting himself from the worst fate. As a result, not knowing precisely who he himself is prior to the lifting of the veil of ignorance, he will have to act so as to protect everyone from such a fate. Hence, no one will be exploited or taken advantage of by using such a procedure. Everyone commits himself in advance to the system that is most fair.

While this is clearly an impractical suggestion since no one can block out all particular knowledge about himself, it is a valuable exercise nonetheless. Rawls does not expect us to experience literally the veil of ignorance. The situation is described in an attempt to capture our intuitions of what it would be like to act genuinely fairly, to be in a fully equal position where we would treat all alike and not favor ourselves.[51] In doing so, we can secure the aim Kant had in mind in the first formulation of the categorical imperative, where he requires us to question whether the maxim of our action could consistently be adopted as a universal law.[52]

49. J. RAWLS, *supra* note 10, at 12.
50. *Id*. at 12, 136-42.
51. *See id*. at 18-19.
52. *See* note 15 *supra* and accompanying text.

Rawls uses the above-described conception to help formulate the principles of justice that he believes appropriate for evaluating the major institutions of society.[53] He argues that if persons were constrained in such a manner that rendered them all equal, they would adopt two principles of justice, which can be roughly stated as follows: (1) Everyone is entitled to the greatest equal liberty compatible with a like liberty for all; and (2) Inequalities are to be arranged so that they benefit the least advantaged and that positions associated with such inequalities are open to all. Further, these principles are ordered, so that no consideration—not even the satisfaction of the second principle—can justify depriving someone of a liberty open to others.

Rawls' theory provides us with a standard of justice by which to evaluate social institutions. There are other criteria that a society must also fulfill in order to be considered good. It should, for example, be efficient, productive, and conducive to happiness. But the criterion of justice is primary and inviolable; it cannot be overridden by utilitarian considerations.

Applying these precepts in the context of experimentation, we may note first that Rawls' theory, like Kant's, rejects some experiments in principle no matter what benefit might be gained from them. In particular, Rawls would judge impermissible all experiments that violate a liberty to which a person is entitled. Any experiment that might deprive its subjects of freedom of thought, freedom of the person, civil liberties, and political liberty, would be wrong under his conception. No experiment likely to render its subjects unable to act as autonomous, independent beings could be approved. Going even beyond Kant, Rawls would protect purely social or political liberties—those that are not natural products of an autonomous will but, rather, arise out of particular social constitutions that define and legitimize such rights.

As an example of experimentation that would call into play Rawls' concepts, consider some possible uses of electric shock. Aversion therapy with electric shocks has been used to control "compulsive gambling, homosexuality, compulsive eating, . . . writer's cramp, . . . habitual blushing, . . . and marital infidelity."[54] Presumably, some social scientists are curious to know whether such techniques might enable us to destroy motivation to vote, to form social bonds, or even to speak, in order that they

---

53. J. RAWLS, *supra* note 10, at 302-03.
54. J. KATZ, *supra* note 29, at 445.

may discover how essential and ingrained these needs are in the human makeup. According to the Rawlsian conception of ethics, however, it would be wrong to conduct all such experiments.

The second principle of justice would prohibit taking advantage of the sick for the sake of others' well-being. An unequal distribution of risks, like other unequal distributions, can be justified only if it benefits those who are currently disadvantaged. Experiments that are therapeutic and may benefit their subjects, as well as help protect the medically well-off, would meet this requirement. However, experiments that are designed to help persons other than their subjects, and may in fact harm the subjects, are not permissible if the subjects are already worse off than the beneficiaries. Hence, Rawls would not approve of the Southam and Levin cancer study at the Jewish Chronic Disease Hospital, nor would he approve of any study using dying persons for the interests of others where the research did not also benefit its subjects. Similarly, he would disapprove of the use of retarded persons as subjects in experiments that were not directly related to their condition. If the Willowbrook study done by Saul Krugman were conceived of as an attempt to infect inmates of an institution with hepatitis virus in order to develop a vaccine useful to others, it too would fail the test. However, Krugman argues that the participants in this experiment were certain to contract the disease anyway, and so they were not made worse off but rather were benefited by the careful attention the experiment provided.[55] If this assessment is correct, the experiment seems to satisfy this condition of justice. However, it could be argued that the fully competent, rational staff members at Willowbrook were in the same position with respect to contracting hepatitis and could just as well have been used as experimental subjects. If there were another option of choosing subjects who could also be selected without inflicting undue harm, it would have been preferable to use those who could provide informed consent. Experiments without informed consent are always to be viewed as a last resort. In general, however, the second principle of Rawls' theory of justice appears to preclude the use of institutionalized persons in experiments that threaten their well-being, since all such persons are appropriately viewed as disadvantaged.

According to Rawls then, it is unjust to use dependent persons as subjects for experiments unrelated to their condition. It is wrong to take advantage of their limited rationality and diminished ca-

55. Krugman & Giles, *supra* note 32, at 1018-29.

pacities in order to serve the ends of others. However, there is still the problem of experimental research that investigates the very conditions with which such persons are afflicted. For example, since the effects of drugs may differ considerably in infants and in adults, how could the effects of new drugs on infants ever be established, if experiments on infants are prohibited?[56]

Rawls' principles do not give us clear guidance on this issue, but by following his line of reasoning as a model we can gain a more specific understanding of our responsibilities toward dependent persons, as well as some direction concerning how they ought to be treated with regard to experimentation. Rawls claims that the just solution is always one to which everyone could agree in advance.[57] Some medical conditions even provide a realistic framework for using the assumption of the relevant veil of ignorance, since we do not know in advance which of us will be victims of many diseases. Thus it is reasonable to assume that a fair procedure for selecting subjects for medical and psychological research in such cases is one upon which we can now agree without knowing our personal connection to the disease. It is, for instance, in the interest of all potential sufferers of heart disease to agree to undergo some discomfort for the sake of a study that might help eradicate the disease. Even without assuming any altruistic motives in people, it is reasonable to expect them to be willing to agree to such a procedure simply because they wish to protect themselves from developing untreatable heart disease. By the same token, people might also be expected to agree to participate in certain studies aimed at reducing the ill effects of the disease in those who are victimized by it. Since it is rational for all concerned to agree to experiments without undue risk, we can conclude that persons should all be willing to provide informed consent when called upon to participate. Relying on the sense of justice of those whose participation is needed, however, it is appropriate to insist upon informed consent in such cases,

---

56. Stated simply:

> [O]ne cannot use new drugs in children unless they have been certified for use in children. But one cannot get new drugs certified for use in children because it is nonbeneficial research and one cannot do nonbeneficial research in children. Hence, either the pediatricians practice illegally or the children become therapeutic orphans.

Cowan, *supra* note 2 at 557.

57. This view is implicit in *A Theory of Justice* and is stated explicitly in Rawls, *Justice as Fairness*, 67 THE PHILOSOPHICAL REV. 164, 171 (1958): "The idea is that everyone should be required to make *in advance* a firm commitment, which others also may reasonably be expected to make . . . ."

and to reserve the right of refusal in keeping with the spirit of Rawls' first principle—the greatest liberty principle.

In experimenting on persons with Down's syndrome we cannot employ directly analogous reasoning because the veil of ignorance is no longer real (though many can assume it in contemplating bearing such a child). Still, using Rawls' model we can try to determine what we would agree to if we took seriously the possibility that we might be affected by the condition. What research on both healthy and afflicted children would we agree to, in the interest of curing or treating Down's syndrome, if we seriously expected to be subjects of such research ourselves? What risks or suffering would we agree to in the interest of minimizing the severity and incidence of this condition? We need not actually experience the condition in order to address this question, any more than we have to be the worst off member of society to recognize the rightness of Rawls' principles of justice. We must simply try, so far as we are able, to determine what it would be like to have Down's syndrome.

Such an approach is significantly different from Kant's proposed method of accounting for everyone. Kant recommended that we treat every human being the same, *qua* member of the human species.[58] All persons were assumed to be entitled to the same treatment by virtue of belonging to a rational species. In contrast, Rawls' procedure licenses treating people differently according to their special interests. Kant takes the Golden Rule literally, advising us to do to others as we would want them to do to us. Rawls modifies it by recommending that we do to others as we would want them to do to us if we were they.[59] While we might not want to have brain surgery done on us now, we might be willing and eager to have it done if we were suffering violent headaches that might be alleviated by surgery; we might even decide now that we want it done in the event we were ever to suffer such headaches, even if at that later point we were too irrational to agree to it. Similarly, although we would not want to be institutionalized during a present state of full mental capacity, if we were so severely retarded that we could not care for our own needs, we might well want to be institutionalized if we were capable of choosing.

In following Rawls' method, we must imagine what we would choose in various circumstances, knowing full well that if such conditions obtained, we would be incapable of rational choice. This

---

58. *See* discussion of Kant in text following notes 11 and 21 *supra*.
59. J. RAWLS, *supra* note 10, *passim* (especially at 95-108).

reasoning justifies paternalism in cases involving persons who are not fully rational, for rational agents would want to insure themselves against any situation in which they might lack the power to pursue their own interest. In the original position, "the parties adopt principles stipulating when others are authorized to act in their behalf and to override their present wishes if necessary; and this they do recognizing that sometimes their capacity to act rationally for their good may fail, or be lacking altogether."[60]

Hence, while justice requires us to extend liberty as far as possible, it also provides for a cautious use of paternalism when an individual is not rational enough to care for his own interests. Such paternalism is justified by the fact that it is rational to choose to have someone behave paternalistically towards us should we become incapable of looking out for ourselves. Thus, all persons are likely to agree to such a practice, provided it includes carefully designed constraints prohibiting paternalism when persons are rational enough to decide for themselves.

If someone were called upon to make a paternalistic decision on our behalf, that person would be required "to do what we would do for ourselves if we were rational . . . ."[61] For ourselves, when contemplating a paternalistic action, "[a]s we know less and less about a person, we act for him as we would act for ourselves from the standpoint of the original position."[62]

If the preceding account provides an acceptable model for morally justified paternalism, it follows that when a decision needs to be made on behalf of a dependent person whether or not he should participate in an experiment, the task is to determine whether it would be rational for anyone to agree from the position of the relevant veil of ignorance. Experiments with high risk or poor risk-benefit ratios would not pass this test, since it can be assumed that no rational agent in the original position would agree to be a participant. In other words, experiments must at least meet rigid utilitarian standards to be approved by this method; but they must not bear too high a cost for any particular individual.

According to Rawls' theory, the researcher is always in a better moral position when he has obtained genuinely informed consent; having gained consent, the experimenter is most assured of acting in accordance with what the experimental subject himself could

---

60. *Id.* at 249.
61. *Id.*
62. *Id.*

agree to. Further, the second principle of justice urges that hardships be distributed in a manner that serves the interests of the disadvantaged. Since it is reasonable to hold that persons who are not fully rational are disadvantaged by virtue of their diminished capacities, it seems clear that they should not be made to suffer any further for the sake of people who are more advantaged.

If, therefore, the use of human beings as experimental subjects can be justified at all, it is best to choose those who have provided informed consent rather than those who have not. An example of a wholly unjustifiable experiment is one performed in 1949 to investigate the possibility of toxic effects from agene, a substance used in the manufacture of flour.[63] There had previously been many reports of its toxic effects on animals and there was a desire to know if it was also toxic for humans. Thus, eighty boys, whose ages ranged from 10 to 15 years, were chosen from a residential school, and all were fed agenized flour for 6 months. When no ill effects developed, two adults were put on agenized flour for 6 weeks. Surely, if the experiment had to be conducted at all, it could have begun with adult volunteers—perhaps, the experimenters themselves.

If there is no alternative but to use subjects who cannot provide informed consent, and if the experiment is warranted in terms of its risk-benefit ratio, then a third party has a right to consent on behalf of the subject only if (1) the decisionmaker has good reason to believe it is a decision the person would in fact make if he were rational, or (2) lacking such information, it is in accordance with a decision any rational person would make knowing he might be in the subject's place. On this model, the paternalistic decisionmaker must ask: "Would it be rational for me to agree if I were he?"

In concluding this section, we turn to a distinctive range of moral problems arising in connection with a special class of persons whose use in experimentation has occasioned much debate. We refer, of course, to prisoners, whose circumstances give rise to a unique sort of dilemma. Prison conditions are such that the freedom of prisoners is severely restricted in ways that render them susceptible to various forms of coercion. Moreover, some members of our society clearly seem to value the lives of prisoners less than the lives of others; in Kantian terminology, prisoners are sometimes perceived as possessing less dignity and, as a result, are viewed as

---

63. *See* Elithorn, Johnson & Crosskey, *Effects of Agenised Flour on Man,* THE LANCET, Jan. 22, 1949, at 143.

less deserving of respect. Such an attitude requires justification before it can be incorporated into any moral arguments, and it surely cannot be justified within the scope of Kant's theory. It is, nevertheless, an attitude that some people have and are prepared to act on. Because of these circumstances it is important to guarantee the prohibition of any coercive use of prisoners in experiments.

However, there is a further problem with using prisoners as ex-experimental subjects—a problem that is related to the unusual circumstances inherent in a prisoner's situation. It is sometimes argued that the prison environment actually distorts the needs and desires of its inmates to a point where prisoners are no longer fully capable of accurately identifying their own interests.[64] For instance, in prison a dollar assumes a value very much out of proportion to its normal worth, for the ability to purchase cigarettes or chocolates becomes a matter of paramount importance to those allowed little opportunity to make choices.[65] Even this small sum may appear to be of such importance that the prisoner will sacrifice what others perceive to be his genuine well-being in pursuit of it. Under these circumstances, it is quite easy for someone who does not so value that dollar to get prisoners to take risks to which a rational agent in a natural social setting would never agree. Experimenters are in a position to take advantage of this unfortunate situation and any resultant nonrational preferences of prisoners.

If the judgment is correct that prisoners are responding inappropriately to options presented—that they are neglecting their overall well-being for the sake of lesser ends—then there is reason to believe that we cannot consider their consent to participate in experiments as legitimate, even if they have been fully informed about the details of the experiment. It would seem that prisoners themselves may mistakenly identify their own ends; they may act in ways that bring about a reduction in their own well-being. Now, it is true that we all do this to some extent, but the point is that an identifiable pattern seems to exist according to which many persons appear to lose perspective on their interests in similar ways under prison conditions.[66] Such uniformity allows us to specify the particular areas in which their surroundings decrease the ability of prisoners to make rational decisions.

Nevertheless, it may be the case that inmates' interests are genu-

---

64. *See* Mitford, *supra* note 31, at 64-73.
65. *Id.*
66. *Cf.* M. PAPPWORTH, HUMAN GUINEA PIGS 63-68 (1967).

inely changed in the prison environment and, as a result, such prisoners are not misperceiving their ends or acting irrationally. A proper evaluation of this issue will require a complex, well-confirmed theory of human ends of a sort not currently provided by psychology or the social sciences generally. But if we suspect that prisoners' preferences have become inappropriately distorted, and, further, if in applying Rawls' test we decide that we would not want to be in circumstances leading us to reorder our current values if we were to find ourselves in prison, then we are obliged to protect prisoners from making agreements we fear might be irrational. For example, the current practice of using prisoners in the first phase of drug-testing on humans[67] seems to reflect an assumption that no free, rational person would agree to be among the first human beings subjected to the drug. If this assumption is true, Rawls' model yields the conclusion that this use of prisoners is unwarranted.

Kant insists that we respect a person's ends if ever we use him as a means. If prison renders some persons incapable of accurately perceiving their ends, an experimenter who responds to their mistakenly identified ends would fail to satisfy Kant's imperative. Experimenters who obtain subjects by meeting prisoners' mistakenly chosen ends—who actively take advantage of this confusion—are treating these persons as means and not as ends. However, there are some experiments that do address the prisoner-subjects' legitimate ends, be they a sense of altruism, a chance of parole, or even minimal monetary reward. Such experiments could then be justified, provided they also meet the requirements for informed consent as discussed above: the prisoner-subject's decision to participate must be a rational choice for him to make under the circumstances, and, further, the options open to him should be such that his consent can be considered wholly voluntary in the relevant respect; that is, it must be uncoerced.

V. Conclusion

In providing a theoretical framework for analyzing the moral dilemmas that arise in human experimentation,[68] we have exam-

---

67. *See id.* at 62, 65, 67; Experimentation with Human Beings, *supra* note 29, at 1041-49.

68. There are some areas of concern that have been barely mentioned in this article. One large area is significant in much social scientific research: the use of deception. This technique causes special problems because it appears necessary to deceive the subjects in some experiments (especially in psychology) in order to investigate the topic under inquiry. But subjects who are deceived are not, by definition, informed, and so informed consent can never

ined the issues involved in experimenting on human subjects from a number of philosophical perspectives. We began by looking at the fundamental questions concerning human experimentation as an acceptable moral practice: Why is there an ethical issue at all surrounding the use of humans in research? What characteristics do human beings have that set up presumptions against using people in experiments as we use inanimate objects or lower forms of life?[69] We found that the characteristics of sentience and rationality in the human species are the properties that give rise to the need for ethical principles of a general sort, from which particular moral judgments flow, assessing the rightness or wrongness of any action.

The two major ethical traditions in modern Western philosophy, represented in turn by John Stuart Mill and Immanuel Kant, both have at their base a moral principle that emphasizes the intrinsic value or inherent worth of one or both of these fundamental attributes of humans. Sentience, conjoined with the related capacity for purposive or goal-directed behavior, and rationality, along with its derivative concepts of autonomy and the inherent dignity of humans, together comprise a framework for ethical judgments or moral decisionmaking in virtually any human context. As we saw,

---

be obtained in principle. When confronted with objections to deception in psychological experiments, some researchers known to these writers dismiss them as arising out of too rigid an adherence to ethical rules that prescribe truthtelling. If, however, we are justified in attaching significant moral value to the practice of obtaining fully informed, voluntary consent, then the simple reply based on truth-telling will not satisfy the serious objector to deception in social scientific research. Here, it would seem, the risk-benefit ratio assumes some importance since the experimenter is obliged to seek ways of conducting research without deception, so that the informed consent of his subjects can be obtained. Moreover, if he can find no experimental design compatible with obtaining genuinely informed consent, then the potential benefits of the experiment (or the research in general) must be objectively assessed in light of the fact that human beings are being used without their informed consent by a researcher as a means to his scientific ends.

There are other special problems of an ethical nature in social scientific research (*e.g.*, maintaining confidentiality), and in still other areas of medicine there exist a variety of related issues, such as the use of untreated control groups in experimentation with new drugs or therapeutic procedures, and the widespread use of placebos in experimental therapeutic contexts. The sort of analysis offered in this paper can easily be extended to cover these related issues, and once equipped with one or more basic moral principles, which lie at the heart of a well-founded ethical theory, we can approach almost all special cases and new situations in which moral dilemmas occur.

69. The use of higher animals is, of course, the subject of much debate because such creatures more closely resemble humans in particular, relevant respects.

the contemporary theory of justice propounded by John Rawls draws on elements from these and other philosophical traditions (*e.g.*, the social contract theories) and proposes a pair of principles for evaluating institutions and social arrangements where justice is a concern. While it seems to us that Rawls' theory is superior in a a number of ways to those of Mill and Kant in its application to ethical issues in human experimentation, ultimately the choice of a basic moral principle is left to each individual. Rawls' account might provide a means of settling ethical disputes between, say, a utilitarian and a Kantian over what kind of research on human subjects is morally justifiable. As we have seen, actions that are morally permissible according to the utilitarian theory may be impermissible according to Kant. Rawls' conjectural method enables us to bypass dilemmas of this sort in seeking a just, fair solution to moral problems. His account is not problem-free, but it does seem significantly applicable to ethical issues in human experimentation.

Of course, the application of ethical theories to everyday, practical matters is not an easy task. In addition, conflicts of legitimate interest among persons and conflicts of fundamental principles will always arise, in the nature of human contingencies. The consistent, conscientious practice of morally justifiable behavior is difficult, as most people know by experience and observation. It is our hope that the philosophical perspectives presented in this paper will, at least, clarify and illuminate our thinking on a range of moral concerns we all share about experimentation on human subjects.

[3]

PRINCIPLISM AND THE ETHICAL APPRAISAL OF CLINICAL TRIALS

ERIC M. MESLIN, HEATHER J. SUTHERLAND, JAMES V. LAVERY, JAMES E. TILL

ABSTRACT

For nearly two decades, the process of reviewing the ethical merit of research involving human subjects has been based on the application of principles initially described in the U.S. National Commission's Belmont Report, *and later articulated more fully by Beauchamp and Childress in their* Principles of Biomedical Ethics. *Recently, the use of ethical principles for deliberating about moral problems in medicine and research, referred to in the pejorative sense as "principlism", has come under scrutiny. In this paper we argue that these principles can provide a foundation for the source of ethical appraisal of human research, but are not themselves wholly adequate for this purpose. Therefore, we further propose that (1) principles should be understood as heuristics that can be "specified" as described by DeGrazia (1992), and (2) that the principle-based approach should be supplemented by formally incorporating "sensitivity to context" into the evaluation of clinical trials.*

A. INTRODUCTION

The determination of the ethical acceptability of clinical trials involving human subjects is a bi-level ethical exercise requiring assessment criteria and procedures on the one hand, and a sound theoretical basis for adopting these standards on the other. For Research Ethics Boards (REBs)[1] charged with reviewing the ethical acceptability of specific scientific protocols, the first-level task is an eminently practical one. Individual protocols are analyzed for

---

[1] Committees to review human subjects research are known by various names. In the U.S. they are known as Institutional review Boards (IRBs), in the U.K. and Europe as Research Ethics Committees (RECs), and in Canada as Research Ethics Boards (REBs).

400   ERIC M. MESLIN ET AL

relevant ethical features, or lack thereof, and judged ethically acceptable or unacceptable accordingly.

The second and more fundamental level of ethical consideration in research involving human subjects is the justification for the criteria used by REBs in their evaluations of ethical acceptability. The normative foundation that underlies these criteria is ultimately what determines whether or not their use is defensible. In this paper we examine the philosophical justification for adopting one particular method of appraising the ethical acceptability of clinical research involving human subjects — the use of certain ethical principles — and provide an argument for supplementing it.

Little has been written on the justification for the enterprise of medical research,[2] and even less attention has been directed towards the justification for evaluating the ethical criteria for assessing clinical trials. The purpose of research ethics review has been generally understood to involve the protection of the rights and welfare of human subjects.[3] More recently, however, evidence of a broadened mandate for research ethics review which includes the assessment of scientific merit has been found in several guidelines, such as the Medical Research Council of Canada *Guidelines*,[4] the "Good Clinical Practice" guidelines of the European Economic Community,[5] and in the CIOMS *International Ethical Guidelines for Biomedical Research Involving Human Subjects*.[6]

These guidelines suggest that the assessment of ethical and scientific merit is now widely accepted to be jointly necessary and sufficient conditions for the activation of a clinical trial. Moreover,

---

[2] The best arguments are still those of Claude Bernard in his *Introduction to the Study of Experimental Medicine*, 1865, trans. Henry C. Greene, New York: Owen Publications, 1957; Hans Jonas' "Philosophical reflections on experimentation with human subjects", in Paul A. Freund, ed. *Experimentation with Human Subjects*, New York: American Academy of Sciences, 1969; and Leon Eisenberg, "The social imperatives of medical research" *Science*: 1977; 198: 1105—1110. For a commentary on this relative silence in arguments regarding justification, see LeRoy Walters, "Research with human and animal subjects", in Tom L. Beauchamp and LeRoy Walters. eds. *Contemporary Issues in Bioethics*. 3rd. ed. Belmont, CA: Wadsworth, 1989.

[3] Henry K. Beecher, "Ethics and clinical research", *New England Journal of Medicine* 1966, 74: 1354—60.

[4] Medical Research Council of Canada. *Guidelines on Research Involving Human Subjects*. Ottawa: Ministry of Supply and Services, 1987, p. 15.

[5] CPMP Working Party on Efficiency of Medicinal Products. *Good Clinical Practice for Trials on Medicinal Products in the European Community*. Brussels: Commission of European Communities, 1988.

[6] Council of International Organizations of Medical Sciences. *International Ethical Guidelines for Biomedical Research Involving Human Subjects*. Geneva: CIOMS, 1993.

PRINCIPLISM AND THE ETHICAL APPRAISAL   401

they clearly take this assessment to be the task of REBs. But even if the purpose of research ethics review and the mandate of REBs were defined more restrictively to include only subject protection, two central problems remain: first, which criteria best satisfy this objective at the conceptual level; and second, do these criteria, when applied to protocols by REBs, adequately protect subjects? The first problem is an issue in justification of the principle-based approach criteria; and the second is an empirical question concerning the effectiveness of the criteria at realizing the stated objective.

The paper has three objectives: (1) to propose a set of meta-criteria that can be used to assess the principle-based source of ethical appraisal that currently provides the foundation for the specific criteria used for ethical review of clinical trials; (2) to assess, in relation to the meta-criteria, the principle-based approach described by the U.S. National Commission for the Protection of Human Subjects in the *Belmont Report*,[7] and developed more rigorously by Beauchamp and Childress in *Principles of Biomedical Ethics*;[8] and (3) to recommend incorporating the concept of "sensitivity to context" into the evaluation of clinical research using the strategy of "specification" suggested by David DeGrazia.[9] In particular, we will argue that this latter strategy, in effect, makes the principle-based approach more relevant to ethics review, and in so doing reveals and emphasizes the role of principles as heuristics. We argue that rather than obviating the role of principles, "sensitivity to context" clarifies and thereby improves their practical role in research ethics review.

B.   DETERMINING THE APPROPRIATE META-CRITERIA

The task of identifying meta-criteria that will be used to assess sub-criteria is not new, having been developed for both normative ethical theories and empirical theories. For example, in his book *Morality: A New Justification for the Moral Rules*, Bernard Gert defends his theory of morality using the following meta-criteria:

> I believe that I have presented a moral theory that yields a **clear, coherent, and comprehensive** description of the moral system

[7] U.S. National Commission for the Protection of Human Subjects of Biomedical and Behavioral Research. *The Belmont Report: Ethical Principles and Guidelines for the Conduct of Research Involving Human Subjects*. Washington, D.C.: DHEW, 1978.

[8] Tom L. Beauchamp and James F. Childress, *Principles of Biomedical Ethics*. 4th. ed. New York: Oxford University Press, 1994.

[9] David DeGrazia, "Moving Forward in Bioethical Theory: Theories, Cases, and Specified Principlism", *Journal of Medicine and Philosophy* 1992, 17: 511–539.

that thoughtful **people actually use** when deciding how to act or in making moral judgments.[10]

Other moral philosophers have suggested similar criteria. For example, Mappes and Zembaty suggest that one ought to assess competing theories on the basis of internal consistency, completeness, simplicity, reconcilability with the moral life, and usefulness (or effective guidance), the latter two being of particular relevance to ethical theories.[11] Frankena suggests that a normative theory, and particularly a normative theory of obligation, should "guide us in the making of decisions and judgments about actions in particular situations".[12] Beauchamp and Childress suggest eight general conditions to determine the adequacy of ethical theories: clarity, internal consistency (coherence), completeness, simplicity, explanatory power, justificatory power, output power, and practicability."[13]

Given that the purpose of research ethics review is to make a decision about the *ethical* acceptability of human research, then it seems reasonable to refer to the criteria that have been suggested for assessing normative theory. It is evident that several criteria are common to these five lists (three of which are proposed to appraise ethical theories in general, and two of which are offered by the theorists themselves as criteria for judging their own and other theories). Taken together, the criteria of effective guidance, coherence, completeness, simplicity and reconcilability, provide a starting point for an assessment of the criteria that might be used to appraise the ethical acceptability of clinical trials. We think it reasonable, however, to assume that at the very least, the meta-criterion of usefulness or *effective guidance* ought to serve as the basis for assessing general ethical appraisal sources that will be used to assess clinical trials. We say "the basis", since other criteria will be necessary to prevent implausible or incoherent actions from being recommended.[14] An ethical appraisal source that provides better guidance for assessing research protocols than alternative sources would be considered superior. Its ultimate

[10] Bernard Gert. *Morality: A New Justification for the Moral Rules.* New York: Oxford University Press, 1988, pp. viii, emphasis added.

[11] Thomas A. Mappes and Jane S. Zembaty, "Biomedical ethics and ethical theory". In *Biomedical Ethics.* 3rd ed., eds. Thomas Mappes and Jane S. Zembaty. New York: McGraw-Hill, 1992.

[12] William K. Frankena, *Ethics.* Engelwood Cliffs: Prentice Hall, 1973.

[13] Beauchamp and Childress, *op cit.* pp. 45–47.

[14] David DeGrazia (personal communication, March 1993), suggested to us that an action guide can be very clear and specific, but not meet with universal acceptance (e.g. "don't allow any non-therapeutic research").

PRINCIPLISM AND THE ETHICAL APPRAISAL   403

value, however, would be determined by the number of meta-criteria it satisfied in addition to effective guidance.

We now consider the "four principles"[15] of bioethics attributed to Beauchamp and Childress's *Principles of Biomedical Ethics*, because it is the most rigorous presentation of the principles initially described in the *Belmont Report*. This latter document is now a widely-accepted ethical appraisal standard for human subjects research.[16] We first consider how these principles match up against the meta-criteria suggested above and what problems still remain.

C.   THE MATCH-UP OF PRINCIPLES WITH META-CRITERIA

Any ethics appraisal source that is useful, coherent, complete, clear and reconcilable is likely to be considered valuable by REBs. Do these principles satisfy these meta-criteria? In particular, do these principles offer a sufficiently secure basis as an appraisal source to warrant supplementation by contextual criteria in research ethics review? It would only be necessary for the principles to satisfy meta-criteria if they were being proposed as a moral theory. Given that they are not intended to be a moral theory, why subject them to such an evaluation? There are two reasons. First, we believe that the meta-criteria are important indicators for judging the rigour of a way of thinking that has normative force. That is, even though the four principles do not constitute a moral theory *per se*, they have been afforded a prominent role as action guides in bioethics.

Second, the process of considering the appropriateness of the four principles as a standard for grounding the criteria for research ethics review requires a justification. We are adopting a pragmatic approach to justification, as described initially by Feigl.[17] Feigl has argued that the process of *external* justification (which attempts to provide rational explanations for entire institutions of thought, in contrast with *internal* justification, which provides explanations for propositions within an established system of rules) is a pragmatic activity requiring two components: first, the identification of the practical purposes, goals, or objectives of an institution; and second,

[15] The "four principles" term is used in Raanan Gillon (ed.), *Principles of Health Care Ethics*. Wiley: West Sussex, England, 1994.

[16] By "widely-accepted" we mean simply that these principles have been adopted either verbatim or in part by research ethics regulations, guidelines and other instruments in North America. Increasingly, though, international organizations, such as the CIOMS have incorporated these principles.

[17] Herbert Feigl, "De principiis non disputatum . . . ?" In *Philosophical Analysis*. ed. Max Black, Ithaca NY: Cornell University Press, 1950.

404   ERIC M. MESLIN ET AL

the identification of the standards or criteria that are best able to satisfy these objectives.[18] We believe this approach both explains why we ought to subject the four principles to the meta-criteria, and suggests how well they satisfy these meta-criteria.

Effective Guidance

Principlism is not simply a theoretical construct; it is well entrenched in the bioethics literature, and specifically entrenched in guidelines and regulations for research involving human subjects. This widespread adoption of the principle-based approach can be traced to the mandate of the U.S. National Commission:

> to identify the basic ethical principles that should underlie the conduct of biomedical and behavioral research and to develop guidelines which should be followed to assure that research is conducted in accordance with these principles.[19]

The Commission recommended that three principles or "general prescriptive judgments" be used in the context of protocol review: respect for persons, beneficence and justice. These principles provide the foundation for the specific criteria of ethics appraisal of human research:

> *Informed Consent.* Respect for persons requires that subjects, to the degree that they are capable, be given the opportunity to choose what shall or shall not happen to them. This opportunity is provided when adequate standards for informed consent are satisfied.

> *Assessment of Risks and Benefits.* The requirement that research be justified on the basis of a favourable risk/benefit assessment bears a close relation to the principle of beneficence, just as the moral requirement that informed consent be obtained is derived primarily from the principle of respect for persons.

> *Selection of Subjects.* The principle of justice gives rise to moral requirements that there be fair procedures and outcomes in the selection of research subjects.

What is not clear, however, is whether these specific criteria are necessarily derived from the ethical principles of respect for persons, beneficence, and justice, or even whether it is necessary to accept these principles, and not others. There is no agreement about the number of

---

[18] Ibid. See also Wesley Salmon. *The Foundations of Scientific Inference*. Pittsburgh: University of Pittsburgh Press, 1960.

[19] National Commission, *Belmont Report*, p. 2.

PRINCIPLISM AND THE ETHICAL APPRAISAL   405

ethical principles or their content. Frankena identifies only beneficence and justice as important ethical principles, letting beneficence include the obligations to do good and to avoid harm. Beauchamp and Childress use four (distinguishing between non-maleficence and beneficence). Robert Veatch, in *A Theory of Medical Ethics* (New York: Basic Books, 1981), includes under a general principle of beneficence two further principles: the Hippocratic Principle of benefitting patients according to the judgment and ability of a physician, and a principle of utility (in contrast with Frankena who argues that utility is a principle derivative from beneficence). Moreover, in addition to autonomy and justice, Veatch includes other principles in his list: contract keeping, avoiding killing, and honesty.

The difficulty, then, in linking the meta-criterion of effective guidance to the ethical principles is one that confronts all methods or frameworks in bioethics: how is it that one takes a necessarily general or abstract theory (or principle) and *applies* it to a concrete case, such as deciding whether a particular clinical trial is ethically acceptable? Clouser and Gert suggested that the application of principles to cases is problematic because (at least in Beauchamp and Childress' version) the explanation of a principle involves a "description of several ways in which the authors think beneficence or autonomy or justice is a relevant moral consideration; we do not get a specific directive for action".[20]

We will suggest below that principles are useful in research ethics review in that they function as heuristic devices that provide REB members with cognitive strategies for thinking about important ethical considerations, and for interpreting the ethical relevance of contextual details, in the review of a protocol.

Internal Consistency

Principle-based ethics appraisal can be traced to more than one moral theory, and as many introductory bioethics texts illustrate, these monistic theories tend to occupy much of the moral terrain in discussions of the theoretical foundations of bioethics. Indeed, one of the conveniences of embracing both deontological and utilitarian reasoning in bioethics is that the critiques that each have of the other can be accommodated. The *Belmont Report* is a particularly apt example of this combining. In this respect principlism can be said to be consistent with the theories from which it is derived. The principle of respect for autonomy, for example, can be derived from

[20]   K. Danner Clouser and Bernard Gert, "A critique of principlism", *Journal of Medicine and Philosophy* 1990, 15: 220.

406   ERIC M. MESLIN ET AL

both deontology and utilitarianism; beneficence and non-maleficence can plausibly emerge from utilitarian theory. The principle of
justice is somewhat more elusive to attribute to one theory, in part
because as stated it has almost no content, and because so many
theories include a principle of justice.

If principlism is interpreted — as Clouser and Gert have done —
as an attempt to replace moral theory, then certain charges of
inconsistency will be difficult to defend against. For example, one
can easily imagine situations in which it is acceptable to justify
giving priority to respect for autonomy (e.g., where competent adult
subjects are given the opportunity to consent to participate in a
clinical trial of a new drug), and yet in another situation which looks
remarkably similar, priority is given to another of the ethical
principles, such as beneficence (e.g., where competent adult subjects
are required to remain in one arm of a trial until it is completed in
order to maximize the potential for acquiring valuable knowledge).

But principlism need not be interpreted this rigidly. Internal
consistency may be considered in a more pragmatic manner. Put
very simply, if principles function as heuristics they can avoid
intractable conflicts (and the charges of inconsistency that accompany them) by framing and encouraging a dialectical review
process. This process, initially described by Richardson[21] and more
particularly for bioethics by DeGrazia,[22] involves the constant
specification of moral norms in a manner suggestive of reflective
equilibrium. Therefore, principles may be seen to be internally
consistent insofar as they facilitate this dialectical process and avoid
the dead-end conflicts that can occur when principlism is understood
simply as an inflexible deductive framework.

We suggest that, despite specific instances of conflict between
principles, they do, in fact, facilitate practical decision-making by
REBs, and that they are able to do so because REBs do not subscribe
to them as features of a rigid deductive model of moral justification.

Completeness

The National Commission understood the principles of respect for
persons, beneficence, and justice to be both relevant and comprehensive to research involving human subjects. Nothing in the
current U.S. regulatory mechanism for overseeing the protection of
human subjects, specifically the U.S. Federal Policy for the

---

[21] Henry F. Richardson, "Specifying norms as a way to resolve concrete ethical
problems", *Philosophy and Public Affairs* 1990; 19: 279–310.
[22] DeGrazia, *op. cit.*

PRINCIPLISM AND THE ETHICAL APPRAISAL   407

Protection of Human Subjects, suggests anything to the contrary. By explaining how principles are derived from two standard moral theories, giving preference to neither, little room is left for alternative theories or approaches. This may have led to the conclusion that the principles derived from those theories were, likewise, exhaustive of those possible for use.

In our narrower interpretation of principlism described above, we are not so much concerned with the completeness of the principles *per se*, but rather that they adequately delineate the field of moral considerations relevant to research ethics review. Other principles, for example truth telling, bodily integrity, freedom of choice, could be regarded as "fundamental" to research ethics review, but these do not necessarily challenge the comprehensiveness of the principles in the more general role that we have ascribed to them.

Clarity

One of the commendable features of the principle-based approach is that the principles are simple to define with clarity for use by non-philosophers, although the philosophical foundations of the principles themselves are not simple. The *Belmont Report* provides definitions of the three ethical principles as follows:

1. *Respect for Persons*. Respect for persons incorporates at least two ethical convictions: first, that individuals should be treated as autonomous agents, and second, that persons with diminished autonomy are entitled to protection. The principle of respect for persons thus divides into two separate moral requirements: the requirement to acknowledge autonomy and the requirement to protect those with diminished autonomy.

2. *Beneficence*. "Beneficence" is often understood to cover acts of kindness or charity that go beyond strict obligation. In this document, beneficence is understood in a stronger sense, as an obligation. Two general rules have been formulated as complementary expressions of beneficent actions in this sense: (1) do not harm and (2) maximize possible benefits and minimize possible harm.

3. *Justice*. Who ought to receive the benefits of research and bear its burdens? This is a question of justice, in the sense of "fairness in distribution" or "what is deserved". An injustice occurs when some benefit to which a person is entitled is denied without good reason or when some burden is imposed unduly.

Defined in this way, several conceptual concerns are apparent, some of which were evident to Beauchamp and Childress. For

408   ERIC M. MESLIN ET AL

example, the principle of respect for persons seems to blur the distinction between respect for autonomous choice, and respect for the moral agent. Similarly, the principle of beneficence blends uncritically the positive injunction to do good and promote well being with the directive to avoid or prevent harm from occurring (nonmaleficence).[23] It was for these reasons that Beauchamp and Childress began the project that resulted in the *Principles*. Clouser and Gert have argued, however, that little progress has been made in making the principles clear — or at least clear enough to function as action guides — since the definitions of these principles are vaguely described in the *Principles*, functioning instead as "chapter headings". Still, our interpretation of principlism requires, not that the principles provide a clear and simple *solution* to each and every moral issue that surfaces in research ethics review, but rather that they provide a reasonable account of the moral topography of research ethics review in language and concepts that are familiar and readily understandable to REB members.

Reconcilability with experience

If a general principle-based ethics necessarily stems from general classes of moral theory such as consequentialism and deontology, it is unlikely to adequately reflect a general moral point of view. However, if reconcilability refers to the degree to which a source of ethical appraisal sufficiently accounts for the practical experience of REBs within society, then it is more likely to enjoy acceptance.

Little is known about the "moral point of view" of REBs, apart from the studies of attitudes about, and decisions by, these committees.[24] We are unaware of any assessment of the degree to which principlism reflects any committee's philosophic point of

---

[23] Beauchamp, Tom L. 1993. "The principles approach", *Hastings Center Report*. Spec. Supp. 23 (November/December): S9.

[24] Bradford Gray, "An assessment of institutional review committees in human experimentation". *Med. Care*. 1975; 13: 318; Robert A. Cooke, and Alan S. Tannenbaum, "A survey of institutional review boards and research involving human subjects", in: National Commission for the Protection of Human Subjects of Biomedical and Behavioral Research, *Report and Recommendations: Institutional Review Boards, Appendix*. Washington DC: USGPO, 1977, 1.1 – 1.303; Jerry L. Mashaw, "Thinking About Institutional Review Boards", in: President's Commission for the Study of Ethical Problems in Medicine and Biomedical and Behavioral Research, *Whistleblowing In Biomedical Research*, Washington D.C., 1981, 3 – 23; Pauline Allen, and W.E. Watters, "Attitudes to research ethical committees", *Journal of Medical Ethics*, 1983; 9, 61 – 65; Michael A. Grodin, Beth E. Zaharoff, Paula V. Kaminow, "A 12-year audit of IRB decisions", *QRB*. 1986; 82 – 86 Claire Gilbert, KWM Fulford, C. Parker, "Diversity in the practice of district

PRINCIPLISM AND THE ETHICAL APPRAISAL 409

view. This is perhaps not surprising since it is difficult to conceive of a moral theory that would deny these mid-level principles. The adoption of a principle-based approach in guidelines and regulations, however, is an indication of the general acceptance of principlism. This point of view may be what Bankowski was referring to, in suggesting that it is desirable to pursue a set of global ethical norms to guide research, when he observed that "[t]he ethical principles of research involving human subjects are identical everywhere".[25]

If principlism can be defended on the grounds that it represents a type of distillation of our general shared values as applied in practice to health care ethics, it would seem to be reconcilable with our common experience, and therefore of value in the review of research protocols. It is important to reiterate, however, that in our interpretation the principles themselves play only a guiding role in determining what are either shared or acceptable *instantiations* of these values. The advantage offered by the principles is that they do, in fact, provide a generally accepted framework of values within which individual contextual considerations may be evaluated. As described above, this very process is also of great importance to the continuous reassessment of the framework itself.

The degree to which the principles "match up" against the meta-criteria gives only a rough approximation of the success of this source of ethics appraisal. Indeed, if principlism is not perceived to be relevant from the perspective of individuals or REBs who review research, its utility is questionable, since it is equally likely that the specific criteria described in *The Belmont Report*, namely informed consent, assessment of risk and benefit, and selection of subjects, will be identified as principles themselves. We believe that the weaknesses of principlism do not render useless the application of ethical principles to research ethics review. On the contrary, we see many of the criticisms of principlism to be relevant specifically to principlism as a substitute for moral theory, a claim we have not

ethics committee", *British Medical Journal*, 1989; 299: 1437–1439; Jerry Goldman and Martin D. Katz, "Inconsistency and Institutional Review Boards", *Journal of the American Medical Association* 1989; 248: 197–202; Judith N. Miller, "Ethics review in Canada: highlights from a national workshop: Part 1", *Annals of the Royal College of Physicians and Surgeons of Canada* 22 (November, 1989): 515–523. For a more comprehensive discussion of many of these issues, see Paul M. McNeill, *The Ethics and Politics of Human Experimentation*, Cambridge: Cambridge University Press, 1993.

[25] Zbigniew Bankowski, J.F. Dunne, Sev S. Fluss, "Ethics standards for research across nations and cultures", in: Medical Research Council of Canada [Documents] *Towards an International Ethic for Research with Human Beings*. Ottawa: MRC, 1987.

410   ERIC M. MESLIN ET AL

made. Rather, we will suggest that some of the key elements of principlism described above may in fact offer tenable grounds on which to supplement principlism so that it can provide more effective guidance for REBs. Next we suggest how principles can be specified as the source for ethical assessment of clinical trials.

D.   SPECIFICATION OF PRINCIPLES AS HEURISTICS FOR ETHICS APPRAISAL

REBs assess the ethics of protocols using guidelines and criteria that can be traced to a series of policies and proposals established by the U.S. Public Health Service in the late 1960s and early 1970s.[26] Yet there has been no formal assessment of the philosophic justification for adopting this set of criteria, and little attention has focused on the justification for the widespread adoption of these principles as the standard from which specific review criteria can be derived.

The practice of applying these principles to cases is now commonly referred to as "principlism". Criticisms of principlism have generally involved concerns about the adequacy of its theoretical basis. For example, Clouser and Gert have defined principlism as:

> the practice of using principles to replace both moral theory and particular moral rules and ideals in dealing with the moral problems that arise in medical practice.[27]

The more restricted form of principlism is intended to provide a framework to facilitate and direct deliberations about practical issues — specifically the evaluation of clinical trials — rather than about general moral questions. Several authors have described various types of principlism.[28] All of these descriptions see the ethical principles as being derived from a cluster of moral theories, for example those of Mill, Hume, Kant, and Rawls. Frankena refers to his theory as a mixed deontological theory.[29] While Veatch's theory is decidedly deontological, it admits that utilitarian considerations are relevant.[30] Beauchamp and Childress, while admitting that they "present only some elements of a comprehensive *general* theory"[31] refer to it as a "common-morality" theory.[32]

---

[26] Ruth R. Faden, and Tom L. Beauchamp, *A History and Theory of Informed Consent*. New York: Oxford University Press, 1986, pp. 200–232.

[27] Clouser and Gert, *op. cit.*, p. 219.

[28] See for example, Frankena, Beauchamp and Childress, and Veatch.

[29] Frankena, *op. cit.* p. 43.

[30] Veatch, *op. cit.* Ch. 4.

[31] Beauchamp and Childress, *op. cit.*, p. 45.

[32] *Ibid.*, pp. 100–106.

PRINCIPLISM AND THE ETHICAL APPRAISAL   411

The mixed or composite nature of the theory that underlies principlism, although seen as a failing by some critics, has recently been identified as a potentially fruitful point of departure in the pursuit of a model for bioethical theory. DeGrazia, building on previous work by Richardson, has identified three features of principlism that, he argues, make it particularly appropriate for modification or supplementation by what he refers to as "specification". We believe that these features provide a useful grounding for our objective of incorporating contextual considerations into the framework of bioethical principlism:

(1) It (principlism) acknowledges the lack of a rationalist foundation for morality, thereby vindicating the use of intuition at some level; (2) It acknowledges the lack of a supreme moral principle or set of explicitly-related principles from which all correct moral judgements can be *derived*; and (3) It acknowledges the need for a justification procedure that can (at least generally) distinguish correct intuitive judgements from incorrect ones, so that the whole theory is not reducible to intuitionism.[33]

As Richardson, DeGrazia and others[34] have argued, these considerations suggest that the process whereby principles are applied or "specified" in deliberations about real moral issues (in this case the ethics review of research protocols) is a dialectical and discursive one. It is clear that this argument has had an effect. Beauchamp and Childress now acknowledge the role that specification plays in modifying their principle-based approach:

Abstract principles, then, must be developed conceptually and shaped normatively to connect with concrete action guides and practical judgements . . . In light of the indeterminacy in general norms, we accept Henry Richardson's argument that the specification of our principles is essential to determining what counts as an instance of that principle and to overcome some moral conflicts.[35]

In clinical research, a number of general norms may be specified that we expect are well known to clinicians, investigators, REBs, and (hopefully) patients. These include: research is an activity designed to produce generalizable knowledge; research involving human subjects must be scientifically and ethically acceptable;

[33] DeGrazia, *op. cit.* pp. 523–524.
[34] See for example, B. Andrew Lustig, "The Method of Principlism: A Critique of the Critique", *Journal of Medicine and Philosophy* 1992; 17: 490; Ronald M. Green, "Method in Bioethics: A Troubled Assessment", *Journal of Medicine and Philosophy*, 1990; 15: 179–97.
[35] Beauchamp and Childress, *Principles*, pp. 28–29.

412   ERIC M. MESLIN ET AL

patients participating in clinical trials must be made aware of the
nature of the study, what it will involve, the potential harms and
benefits to them from participating; information about individual
patients/subjects should not be part of published reports of
research.[36] Depending on the individual study, however, additional
particular norms may be specified. For example, in a study aimed at
assessing the efficacy of treating breast cancer using various surgical or
medical methods (e.g., mastectomy, lumpectomy, chemotherapy,
radiotherapy), additional norms may be specified for different
individuals: for some women, retaining their identity requires that
mutilating surgery always be rejected; for some investigators,
maintaining strict randomization procedures (where subjects to agree
to participate would not know in advance which intervention they
would receive) is essential for completion of a scientifically valid study.

What then is the relationship between the specification of norms
in a clinical trial and the role of principles in research ethics review?
Considering the nature of the dynamic relationship between the *tools*
(principles) and the *work* (research ethics review) has led us to
propose a model in which principles function as heuristics,
delineating the general scope of ethical acceptability and thereby
providing a conceptual and moral framework within which the
contextual details of a given protocol may be examined. Tversky
and Kahneman have described a heuristic as a strategy that helps
individuals simplify complex sets of information.[37] We believe that
principles might function in a similar way for REB members. This
relationship is a dialectical one since certain features of a protocol,
when considered as elements of the broader context of the proposed
clinical trial, may challenge the general boundaries as defined by the
principles, and vice-versa. This process is a more modest version of
the kind of reflective equilibrium that DeGrazia believes grounds his
proposal of specified principlism, and is clearly more modest than
the kind of reflective equilibrium proposed by Rawls[38] and
extended by Daniels.[39]

---

[36] These norms are part of a more detailed account of the ethical foundations of
science, human research, publication and dissemination discussed in Meslin, EM.
"Toward an ethic in dissemination of new knowledge in primary care research", in
EV Dunn, et al. *Disseminating Research/Changing Practice: Research Methods in Primary
Care Research*, Vol 6. Thousand Oaks, CA: Sage Publications, 1994, pp. 32–44.

[37] Amos Tversky and Daniel Kahneman, "Judgment under uncertainty:
heuristics and biases", *Science* 1974, 1985: 1124–1131.

[38] John A. Rawls, *A Theory of Justice*. Cambridge, MA: Harvard University
Press, 1971.

[39] Norman Daniels, "Wide Reflective equilibrium and Theory Acceptance in
Ethics", *Journal of Philosophy* 76 (May 1979): 275.

PRINCIPLISM AND THE ETHICAL APPRAISAL 413

Given the proposal outlined above, it is not clear to us why Clouser and Gert's best case interpretation of the value of principles could not be restated in a more positive light. "At best", they suggest, "principles operate primarily as checklists naming issues worth remembering when considering a biomedical moral issue".[40] We recognize that they are holding out for a more deductivist theory that gives clearer action guides, and is thus more determinate.[41] This is similar but not identical to what we mean by a heuristic; similar in that principles might operate as important reminders of the several moral aspects of a bioethical issue. A heuristic might function in this way as well, to stimulate thinking. However, a heuristic is more than simply a prompt; it is an internalized strategy that can be imposed on a set of facts to facilitate ordered decision making. This activity seems to approximate the goals of research ethics review described above. Given that research protocols are complicated documents, and that ethical considerations will similarly be multi-faceted, depending (for example) on the type of research proposed, the type of patients who will be participating, and the degree of risk imposed, REBs could benefit from adopting strategies that help to ensure that these multiple factors are regularly considered.

E. WHAT GETS SPECIFIED? INCORPORATING SENSITIVITY TO CONTEXT

We initially suggested that the ethical principles provide a reasonable grounding for the ethical assessment of clinical trials but that they lack both sufficient content and a method of application. We proposed that the action of specifying both general and specific norms in clinical research can be accomplished using the principles as heuristics in a dialectical process. We were then left in the position, however, of having to presume that the content of this activity simply emerges from the participants themselves. This is unsatisfying because it fails to provide an account for the source of the particular description of the norms.

We believe that a reasonable next step is to acknowledge that principlism need not constitute a static set of requirements but might be further improved by emphasizing its role in a dialectical relationship with specific contextual considerations that arise in the actual process of research ethics review. We propose that this latter strategy would be a reasonable next step if emphasis was given to the

---

[40] Clouser and Gert, *op. cit.* p. 220.
[41] We are grateful to David DeGrazia for discussing this interpretation with us.

414   ERIC M. MESLIN ET AL

importance of a concept we call *sensitivity to context* in research ethics review.

Since our goal was not to defend principlism as much as explain how it might be sufficient as a basis for research ethics review, it will now be evident that principlism may be found to be somewhat lacking in its appreciation of the contextual features of cases. It is not entirely lacking, however. For example, in the third edition of *Principles of Biomedical Ethics* Beauchamp and Childress suggested that "Which principle overrides in a case of conflict will depend on the particular context, which always has unique features" (p. 61). This position is further reflected in their defense of the relevance of principles arising from, and in turn reinforcing, certain fundamental social and political values:

> Moral principles are not disembodied rules, cut off from their cultural setting. Most, if not all of our moral beliefs have arisen from shared experiences and through social agreements or arrangements. Morality is by its very nature, not an individual-centred phenomenon (p. 61).

In the fourth edition, they indicate the direction they believe principles will take us, and how much supplementary work is left for context:

> The more accurate estimate is that principles point us in the right direction, but we then typically encounter a host of other considerations that must be accommodated, such as institutional practices, limited resources, judgments about acceptable risk, religious beliefs, and personal projects and aspirations (p. 108).

By context, we mean the facts, situations, relationships and circumstances that arise for given individuals at given points in time.[42] Sensitivity to context may be a neglected aspect of REB review. Without sensitivity to context, the ethical appraisal of clinical trials will be devoid of any meaningful consideration about the individual persons, specifically the patients and health care professionals who are participating in research. Without sensitivity to context, ethical appraisal will lack consideration of the particular interests of families and friends of current and future patients, and about the effect on society from the development of scientific knowledge. Without sensitivity to context, the ethical realities of clinical research will be nothing more than descriptions of standards

---

[42] For an important discussion of the place of context in deliberations in bioethics, see Barry Hoffmaster, "Can ethnography save the life of medical ethics?" *Social Science and Medicine*, 1992, vol. 35: 1421–31.

PRINCIPLISM AND THE ETHICAL APPRAISAL 415

that must be satisfied without consideration of who will be satisfying them.

Context does not belong to any particular moral theory or perspective, although two different approaches to context have been suggested in bioethics. The first arises from recent developments in feminist moral theory and the ethic of care (which overlap but are not identical); the second from the contemporary defense of casuistry. Sherwin has suggested that while scholars in feminist ethics and bioethics may differ regarding the use of context, "both perceive a need to focus on the contextual details of actual situations that morally concerned persons find problematic".[43] While the meaning of context also differs for different feminist philosophers, some common themes can be described:

- a general acknowledgement that appeals to deductivist models of moral analysis are insufficient to solve moral problems;
- the pedagogical need to refer to case study to highlight the important details of moral problems;
- agreement that matters of character and responsibility are morally significant;
- a recognition of the necessity to take explicit account of the details of specific relationships of those involved.

In their edited volume, Kittay and Meyers have identified a range of perspectives on how principles and feminist moral theory might interact. Some authors explicitly reject principlism as a source for ethical deliberation, maintaining instead that "a distinctive feature of a care morality is a contextual and narrative method rather than a deductive application of general principlism".[44] Others maintain that ethical principles may have a place in moral decision making, but that they differ with respect to the source, content and implementation of them.[45] We find ourselves persuaded by this latter approach. For example, Helen Holmes has argued that feminist values amplify principlism for appraisal of the ethics of clinical trials:

> I define an action (in this case clinical research) as "ethical" if it is just, is beneficent, and respects autonomy. Drawing upon the insights of feminist ethics, I amplify this definition by proposing that clinical research is ethical if it respects all humans — even if female, poor or of color — fully allows them to make informed

---

[43] Susan Sherwin *No Longer Patient: Feminist Ethics and Health Care*. Philadelphia: Temple University Press, 1992, p. 76.

[44] Kittay, Eva F. and Meyers, Diana T. eds. *Women and Moral Theory*. New York: Rowman and Littlefield, 1987, p. 11.

[45] See for example, Virginia Held, "Feminism and moral theory", in Kittay and Meyers, pp. 111–128.

416   ERIC M. MESLIN ET AL

choices, and at the same time cares for them, recognizes their place in relationships that are vital parts of their lives, and is situation- and context-sensitive.[46]

The relevance of feminist perspectives in health research is made abundantly clear by Jevne and Oberle who suggest that the traditional scientific paradigm rejects, as confounding, those variables relating to an individual's social, psychological or cultural experience.[47] Moreover, a significant proportion of research — specifically clinical trials — has systematically excluded women. This underrepresentation has been the focus of recent discussions.[48]

The role of context is found in the clinical ethics literature[49] and in recent discussions of casuistry.[50] The object of moral deliberation is the *case*, the collection of facts, values, and personalities that comprise the situation about which judgment is to be applied. The classical casuistic method was that of rhetoric. The new casuistry involves three elements: reliance on paradigm cases, reference to broad consensus, and acceptance of problem certitude.[51]

The circumstances and facts under which research involving human subjects is conducted is an example of the contextual features described above. Research ethics review might benefit from the casuistic approach: the protocol could easily be regarded as a "case" to be evaluated; there are numerous paradigm cases against which to compare a study;[52] most REBs adopt the consensus approach to protocol review, preferring it to the more regimented procedure of voting;[53] and many who are involved in research ethics review recognize that even paradigmatic examples of scientifically sound research may be ethically questionable. Thus, the case-based reasoning of casuistry lends itself directly to REB deliberations,

[46] Helen Holmes, "Can clinical research be both 'ethical' and 'scientific'?" *Hypatia*, 1989; 4: 157.

[47] Ronna Jevne and Kathleen Oberle, "Enriching health care and health care research", *Humane Medicine* 9(3), 1993.

[48] Sue V. Rosser, "Revisioning clinical research: gender and the ethics of experimental design", *Hypatia* 1989; 4: 107–124.

[49] Albert R. Jonsen, Mark Siegler, and William Winslade. *Clinical Ethics* 3rd. ed., New York: McGraw-Hill, 1992.

[50] Albert Jonsen, "Casuistry and clinical ethics", *Theoretical Medicine* 1986; 7: 69; Albert R. Jonsen, and Stephen Toulmin. *The Abuse of Casuistry*. Berkeley, CA: University of California Press, 1988.

[51] Jonsen, *op. cit.*

[52] Typically, the cases discussed in the literature are of unethical research. See for example, Beecher, op. cit.; Alastair V. Campbell, "A report from New Zealand: an 'unfortunate experiment'". *Bioethics*, pp. 59–66, 1989 (1). Jay Katz, *Experimentation with Human Beings*. New York: Russell Sage, 1972.

[53] Miller, *op. cit.*

PRINCIPLISM AND THE ETHICAL APPRAISAL   417

since the process of review is as important as its substance. It is in this respect that we see harmonization between the activity of specification described above and the role of context: *the contextual features of a case provide the content for the activity of specification.*

The methods by which contextual details of a protocol are obtained may be varied. We have proposed elsewhere that it may be useful to consider the role of patient preferences in clinical trials.[54] Others have suggested that increased consultation with potential subjects in advance of protocol development would provide important additional information.[55] In fact, it can be argued that sensitivity to context, or considerations of the ethically relevant details of a given protocol, *is* the practical process of research ethics review. In such an environment, REBs approach each new protocol against a backdrop of facts and values pertinent to the participants in a clinical trial (including investigators and subjects).

This process is not simply an application of principles to cases, nor is it simply an appeal to principles to justify certain contextual features. Rather, it is a dialectical process, one not defined by a particular direction of logical flow, but by a continuous testing of contextual features against certain practical standards or criteria-paradigm cases or the insights of other REB members, for example — all within the purview of the principles. In this way, for example, a randomized trial involving an emergency surgical procedure for incompetent patients which, at first glance, appears to be disrespect-ful of the potential subject's autonomy and therefore unacceptable, may, upon further consideration of other specific features of the protocol, be deemed to be acceptable — with certain conditions — precisely because the research design offers the best hope of discovering useful data, in keeping with a more broadly construed principle of beneficence. In such a case, both the moral framework and the actual process of review must be flexible enough to accommodate reasonable solutions. We think the proposed model provides this flexibility without sacrificing moral substance.

F. CONCLUSION

The widespread acceptance of fundamental ethical principles as the source for ethical evaluation has created a tension. On the one hand

[54] James E. Till, Heather J. Sutherland, Eric M. Meslin, "Is there a role for preference assessments in research on quality of life in oncology?" *Quality of Life Research*, 1993; 1: 31–40.
[55] Carol Levine, Nancy Dubler, Robert J. Levine, "Building a new consensus: ethical principles and policies for clinical research on HIV/AIDS", *IRB: A Review of Human Subjects Research* 1991; 13: 1–17.

418   ERIC M. MESLIN ET AL

the ethical principles derived from utilitarian and deontological theory collectively provide a comprehensive but not particularly exhaustive background for evaluating clinical trials. These principles provide a useful template against which to compare human research as conceived and conducted for the past two decades. On the other hand, while the contribution of the National Commission's work cannot be overstated, little subsequent progress was made in providing a justification for using the principles as sources of ethical appraisal. Given both the changing face of research (e.g., large multicentre trials, new designs, epidemiologic investigations), and the increasing sophistication of the philosophic assessment of the ethical principles themselves, the foundation for the ethical appraisal of research involving human subjects may be in jeopardy.

We have suggested that principles should function as heuristics that can be specified in the context of clinical trials, acting not as formal rules for decision making, but rather as cognitive prompts for thinking about the types of considerations that research involving human subjects ought to accommodate. We further proposed that by supplementing the principles with a concept we called sensitivity to context, REBs would have access to a more useful and philosophically satisfying account of their responsibilities in research ethics review.

Acknowledgement

This research is supported by a grant from the Social Sciences and Humanities Research Council of Canada (#806-91-0002). The Centre for Bioethics is supported by a Health-Systems Linked Research Unit Grant from the Ontario Ministry of Health and by the Bertha Rosenstadt and William C. Harris Estates. We would like to acknowledge the helpful comments of David DeGrazia on an earlier version of this paper, and to the two anonymous reviewers for *Bioethics*. We wish also to acknowledge the careful typing of several drafts of this manuscript by Margot Smith.

Centre for Bioethics, University of Toronto,
Department of Philosophy, University of Toronto
Sunnybrook Health Science Centre, New York, Ontario,
Ontario Cancer Institute/Princess Margaret Hospital, Toronto, Ontario

[4]

The Nuremberg Code in Light of Previous Principles and Practices in Human Experimentation

David J. Rothman

In the fifty years since the issuance of the Nuremberg Code, the ethics of human experimentation has assumed such centrality in social thought and public policy that it requires an act of imagination to recall just how novel this event was. Nuremberg represented the first attempt to set forth and enforce an explicit set of principles, literally a code, in the conduct of human experimentation. Whatever weaknesses commentators would later identify, and whatever refinements marked the content of successor codes, Nuremberg was the pioneer effort to implement standards that clinical investigators were required to observe.

Its originality as a code notwithstanding, Nuremberg was certainly not the earliest effort to analyze the ethics of human experimentation. Already in the thirteenth century, the English philosopher Roger Bacon had explained that progress in medicine would never come as quickly as in the natural sciences because scientists could "multiply their experiments till they get rid of deficiency and errors". The physician, on the other hand, was unable to do this "because of the nobility of the material in which he works".[1] Over the years, many individuals proposed appropriate standards for investigators to follow and decried particular abuses in practice. But until Nuremberg, there was practically no professional or public governance of human experimentation.

Thus, to appreciate the degree to which Nuremberg built on the past precedents and the degree to which it represented a novel departure, it is necessary to examine the state of clinical research and ethics in the pre-1947 period. First, in terms of principles, what obligations did the investigator owe the subject? What information was to be shared? What degree of consent, if any, was necessary? Second, in terms of practice, were the principles respected by investigators? Did they live up to the standards? Finally, to the extent that practice diverged from principle, what efforts were made at enforcing standards? Were penalties levied on errant researchers, either by legally constituted bodies or professional organizations?

All of these questions are of obvious relevance to the history of medicine. But no less important, particularly as we observe its fiftieth anniversary, they are essential to framing the contribution of the Nuremberg Code
itself. At the trial of the Nazi doctors, defense attorneys claimed that before
World War Two the ethics of human experimentation were undeveloped,
both in the United States and Germany. Principles of voluntariness and of
consent, they argued, were poorly understood and usually ignored. American physicians, no less than German ones, paid no heed to consent and frequently carried out experiments on ignorant and unwilling subjects. These
points certainly establish Nuremberg's novelty, but at the price of finding a
fatal flaw in the prosecution of the Nazi doctors. Nuremberg becomes an
exercise in ex post facto punishment, setting new standards and then imposing them on the defendants. To be sure, the conviction and punishment
of the offenders could easily be justified by ruling that their acts were so
horrendous that they constituted a crime against humanity. They had committed war crimes, including the murder of innocent civilians; indeed, the
Nuremberg court offered this very judgment: "the record clearly shows the
commission of war crimes and crimes against humanity". But instead of
stopping there it continued on to address the issue of "Permissible Medical
Experiments". Ultimately, it condemned the Nazi doctors for unethical
research; they were guilty as physicians, not as civilians, of "violating
moral, ethical and legal concepts", not in a more straightforward sense, of
murder. Precisely why the court eschewed war crimes and addressed human experimentation as such has never been satisfactorily explained. But
whatever the reason, the court's posture brought unprecedented attention to
the ethics of human experimentation.

Ethical Principles in Human Experimentation before Nuremberg

The modern history of the ethics of human experimentation begins with
Claude Bernard's 1865 book, *An Introduction to the Study of Experimental
Medicine*. No one more cogently than Bernard delineated the potential
contribution that clinical research could make to medicine. So vital was it
that Bernard regarded human experimentation as the third pillar of medical
knowledge. As he traced it, physicians first based their treatments upon
findings made through their senses, that is, what they saw and heard
through direct and intimate encounters with the patient. They felt the pulse,
noted the color of the face, examined the urine, and listened to the chest,
initially by putting their ear to it, later by using a stethoscope. Physicians,
Bernard continued, learned to do more than rely upon their senses. They
also "observed", by which he meant that they grouped facts together and
formulated hypotheses; they made predictions about treatment outcomes
and then studied whether they proved right. In this way, observation was
essential to determining which interventions were effective. From Bernard's perspective, however, this exercise was essentially passive. The

physician stood back and collected data, wisely and shrewdly, but from a distance.

It was the third form of knowledge that Bernard celebrated, what might be called "active observation". To clarify its meaning and implications, Bernard invoked the French naturalist, Georges Cuvier: "the observer listens to nature; the experimenter questions [nature] and forces her to unveil herself". In his own terms:

> Experimenters must be able to touch the body on which they act, whether by destroying it or by altering it, so as to learn the part which it plays in the phenomena of nature...It is on this very possibility of acting, or not acting, on a body that the distinction will exclusively rest between sciences called sciences of observation and sciences called experimental.

The very language with which Bernard describes experimentation establishes its potency, not only in terms of its ability to create knowledge but to generate ethical problems as well. Bernard's experimenter "touches" parts of the body, not gently, but to destroy it or alter it so as to learn more about its biological function. In this way, the investigator forces nature to "unveil herself", and in the process, he himself becomes an aggressor, indeed, something of a sexual molester as he strips nature of her secrets.

Had Bernard stopped his analysis of clinical research there, the development of human experimentation in the nineteenth century would appear as an exercise in the ruthless accumulation of knowledge, one that was deaf to the decencies of humanity or principles of ethics. But Bernard went on, and after exploring the epistemology and methods of clinical research, he declared in passages now famous:

> Experiments, then, may be performed on man, but within what limits? It is our duty and our right to perform an experiment on man whenever it can save his life, cure him or gain him some benefit. The principle of medical and surgical morality, therefore, consists in never performing on man an experiment which might be harmful to him to any extent, even though the result might be highly advantageous to science, i.e., to the health of others.

Bernard provides a frank and full recognition of the power of human experimentation to do good and to do harm. And with this double-edged potential in mind, he insists that research must always be in the best interests of the subject. If an experiment has the potential to cure, it may be carried out. But if it has no therapeutic potential and may injure the subject, it must not be conducted, regardless of how important the findings might be for others.

Obviously, Bernard's maxims are not fully in accord with contemporary principles, particularly given the scant attention he paid to the idea and meaning of consent. But others among his contemporaries not only echoed his insightful judgments but on occasion went beyond them, incorporating principles of consent into their own frameworks.

This was certainly true of the great American clinician, William Osler. Properly credited with bringing scientific methods into medical education and clinical practice, Osler, as would be expected, was fully appreciative of the vital role of human experimentation. In 1907, he addressed "The Evolution of the Idea of Experiment in Medicine", sounding very much like Claude Bernard, and when it came to consent, superseding him.[2]

Like Bernard, Osler emphasized both the enormous capacity of clinical medicine to generate new knowledge and its highly invasive characteristics. In his formulation, "Man can interrogate as well as observe nature", and through this process, lighten many of "the burdens of humanity." Even more consistently than Bernard, Osler believed that experimentation was part and parcel of the conduct of clinical practice: "Every dose of medicine given is an experiment as it is impossible in every instance to predict what the result may be". Even so he, too, insisted on setting limits on human experimentation. First, experiments on man must never be carried out before they had been tried on animals. Second, and here departed from Bernard, Osler not only ruled out non-therapeutic research but required investigators to obtain the consent of the subject:

> For man absolute safety and full consent are the conditions which make such tests allowable. We have no right to use patients entrusted to our care for the purpose of experimentation unless direct benefit to the individual is likely to follow. Once this limit is transgressed, the sacred cord which binds physician and patient snaps instantly.

In effect, Osler enunciated the principles of consent well in advance of this proposition in the Nuremberg Code.

The viewpoints expressed by Bernard and Osler were shared widely. In 1886, a less prominent Boston physician, Charles Francis Withington, published an essay entitled, *The Relation of Hospitals to Medical Education*. The position he advocated were regarded as so important that his contribution won the prestigious Boylston Prize from Harvard University. Withington posed the ethical question in terms of the "possible conflict between the interests of medical science and those of the individual patient, and the latter's indefeasible rights". He was not at all confident that investigators satisfactorily resolved the conflict, and in truth, he himself had some trouble drawing boundaries between the needs of science and the "rights" (his term) of patients. But in the end, he came down staunchly on the side of rights, to the point of suggesting a remedy of a patient "Bill of Rights" which would not be adopted for another 90 years:

> In the older countries of Europe especially, where the life and happiness of the so-called lower classes are perhaps held more cheaply than with us, enthusiastic devotees of science are very apt to encroach upon the rights of the individual patient in a manner which cannot be justified. In this country, we

are less likely to fall into this error than those living under monarchical institutions, but even with us it may be well to draw up, as it were, a Bill of Rights which shall secure patients against any injustice from the votaries of science.

Withington insisted that patients had "a right to immunity from experiments merely *as such*, and outside the therapeutic application. This right is one that is especially liable to violation by enthusiastic investigators". Researchers who wished to try a new drug had to rely upon volunteers. In his view, "They had no right to make any man the unwilling victim of such an experiment".[3] He then concluded with a sentence that encapsulated the core principals of medical ethics: "The occupants of hospital wards are something more than merely so much clinical material during their lives and so much pathological material after their death".[4]

Although other texts reiterating these same principles could be easily marshalled, these three make apparent that the ethical dimensions of clinical research were recognized by physicians who advanced the development of modern medicine. Such a conclusion ought not to be surprising, for the bedrock principle on which they rested their analyses was as old as medical ethics itself: do not harm, neither to the patient nor to the subject. Experimentation was bound by the ethics of the doctor-patient relationship, which, as we shall see, was a useful starting point, although not an altogether adequate model upon which to base the regulation of human experimentation.

All these writings drew a sharp distinction between therapeutic and non-therapeutic research, and were far more concerned with the latter than the former. They had little difficulty in condemning non-therapeutic research, especially when it placed the subject-patient at risk. But what was almost completely absent from their analysis was a discussion of the ethical principles that should govern experiments with a therapeutic potential. What was the physician obliged to tell the patient about an experiment that might benefit him? Was consent required? Who was to make the calculus of risk of harm versus benefit of cure? By ignoring this set of issues and focusing so exclusively on non-therapeutic research, these commentators make the intent and motive of the physician-researcher the critical determinant. Were he seeking new knowledge and not attempting to benefit the patient, then he was obliged to share information with the subject and obtain consent. But were his intentions to cure or to treat, then apparently he did not have to divulge the facts or obtain the patient's acquiescence to the procedure. Thus, the position adopted (which would remain intact for many decades) was consistent with the tradition in medical ethics of trusting to the integrity of the physician, not requiring formal collegial oversight or consultation or the patient's agreement. So long as the researcher's self-styled purpose was to benefit the patient, he enjoyed an ample discretion unfettered by colleagues or patients. In brief, the mindset of the physician, not the autonomy of the subject, drove the ethical analysis.

The Practice of Human Experimentation before Nuremberg

The uniformity that marked the discussions of the ethical principles in research disappears when one examines the actual practices of investigators, and the reactions to them by the medical profession and the public. Here one finds countless examples of research conduct that blatantly violates the prevailing ethical norms. In a similar vein, one finds some observers outraged by the transgressions and others far more complaisant. The one generalization that can be offered is that no matter how grievous the ethical misconduct in research, professional disciplinary action or some collective expression of censure or disapproval almost never occurred. With a handful of exceptions, investigators who freely disobeyed all the norms set forth by a Bernard or an Osler paid no price for it.

The historical record, particularly as explored by Susan A. Lederer, makes abundantly clear that many investigators demonstrated scant regard for the rights or well-being of subjects. They conducted non-therapeutic research on unknowing or incompetent persons, putting them at risk and causing direct and serious harms. In 1904, a southern physician, Claude Smith, purposefully infected blacks with hookworm to study the transmission of the disease and did not give them the slightest hint as to what he was actually doing. "The patient", Smith stated in his published report, "seemed to have an idea that it was some medicine preparatory to the operation, as nothing was said to him about it".[5] In 1883, George Fitch, resident physician at an Hawaiian leper colony, purposely infected some unknowing 18 leprosy patients with syphilis to prove the similarities between the two diseases.[6] Another of his colleagues infected relatives of leprosy patients who themselves were free of the disease with the leprosy organism to study transmission. "A splendid field for experimental work was at hand", he candidly wrote, "and stretching all questions of professional ethics, I did not hesitate to avail myself of the opportunities afforded me for testing the inoculability of leprosy".[7]

Some research protocols inflicted such egregious harm on subjects as to earn the condemnation of other investigators. The research by the Italian bacteriologist Guiseppe Sanarelli was a case in point. To prove that he had isolated the bacillus that caused yellow fever, he infected five Montevideo hospital patients with it and claimed (mistakenly) that he had produced the disease in them. William Osler led the attack on the ethics of his research: "[T]o deliberately inject a poison of known high degree of virulency into a human being, unless you obtain that man's sanction, is not ridiculous, it is criminal".[8] In a later and fuller elaboration of this point, Osler explained:

> The limitations of deliberate experimentation upon human beings should be clearly defined. Voluntarily, if with full knowledge, a fellow-creature may submit to certain tests, just as a physician may experiment upon himself. Drugs, the value of which has been carefully tested in animals and are found harmless may be tried on patients, since in this way alone may progress be made, but deliberate experiments such as Sanarelli carried on with cultures of

known and tested virulence, and which were followed by nearly fatal illnesses, are simply criminal.[9]

In much these same terms, Osler, and many other colleagues as well, condemned the cancer research that had been conducted by two German surgeons, both of whom took malignant cells from the diseased breast of a patient and injected them into the other, healthy, breast, to study the transmissibility of cancer cells. *The Journal of the American Medical Association* reported the incidents, applauding the subsequent refusal of a French medical academy to discuss the findings because they were obtained in so unethical a fashion. It hoped that "the storm of indignation which has been aroused, shall deter others who might have in view, in their zeal for science, [conducted] similar unjustifiable experiments".[10]

The roster of non-therapeutic research on uninformed subjects could be extended almost indefinitely. In 1911, Hideyo Noguchi injected several hundred residents of a New York orphan asylum with an experimental substance, Luetin, to learn whether it might serve to indicate the presence of syphilis. Other researchers used orphans to test the efficacy of tuberculin as a vaccine against tuberculosis as well as to trace the development of such dietary deficiencies as scurvy. So too, researchers subjected black infants at an Atlanta, Georgia hospital to lumbar punctures without the permission of their parents. One investigator even went so far as to infect an infant with the herpes virus for experimental purposes. As with orphans, prisoners were used as subjects in non-therapeutic and harmful protocols, including one protocol that imposed a diet designed to cause pellagra, and another that injected ameba in order to study the course of dysentery. Finally, investigators in the 1920s used prisoners in San Quentin, California to study the effects of implants of testicles taken from executed prisoners and rams.[11]

The Disparities between Ethics and Practice

The research protocols that so flagrantly violated the existing ethical precepts in human experimentation were not carried out covertly or kept hidden from view. To the contrary, the findings were published in the major and widely read medical journals. Nevertheless, the conduct did not incite professional criticism, let alone discipline, except in a handful of cases. To be sure, Osler and several colleagues forcefully condemned some of the protocols described here, including the yellow fever and breast cancer examples. But these were individual reactions and the occasional efforts made to move beyond that to a more official condemnation or censure failed.

Why this professional passivity before these violations of ethics? First, such bodies as the American Medical Association had little authority or organizational standing. Well into the opening decades of the twentieth century, when the profession had managed to impose some standards on medical education and medical licensing, it still did not yet enjoy sufficient status or cohesion to act in concert in the arena of human experimentation. Second, and closely related to its lower status, the profession was unwilling to draw greater attention to ethical misdeeds for fear of arming its critics, particularly the outspoken members of anti-vivisection societies. To concede that some investigators acted irresponsibly was to give ammunition to those who thought that all investigators acted irresponsibly, and thereby subvert the entire research enterprise. Commenting on a recent discussion in the German parliament on research which purposefully infected prostitutes with syphilis, the *Journal of the American Medical Association* joined in the condemnation of the research but, apprehensive about lay reactions, added: "If laymen would divert their attention to charlatans...the world would be benefited, while these attacks on the regular profession tend to impair the confidence of the public in trained physicians and thus they fall easy prey to unscrupulous quacks".[12] The contention was by no means ill-founded. There was a popular and widespread suspicion about what went on in medical laboratories. Even so, the professional response to the violations was exceptionally timid.

Third, the absence of collective action may reflect the fact that the human subjects put at risk and harmed were almost always marginal to the society. They were poor Southern blacks, or prison inmates, or residents of orphan asylums, themselves vulnerable in all so many ways to abuse but outside the net of public concern. To mount a campaign on their behalf would have been extraordinary, and a reluctance to do so - particularly if it might lower the prestige of medical research - is not altogether surprising. The researchers, in the end, were abusing *other* peoples's bodies.

Human Experimentation in the United States, 1940-1945

The record that we have explored here provides the context for understanding the conduct of human experimentation in the United States during World War Two. The challenges that military needs posed for American medicine were pressing, including how to protect soldiers against malaria, particularly when the Japanese controlled the supply of quinine; how to protect them against influenza, especially in the wake of the 1919 pandemic; and how to protect them against dysentery. Investigators diligently attempted to develop vaccines or antidotes and to these ends, human experimentation was vital. There were few useful animal models available and to compound the difficulties, malaria was not naturally occurring in the United States, dysentery was rare, and influenza unpredictable. For obvious reasons, the diseases could not be researched where they were found, that is, under battlefield conditions. This meant that researchers had to create the very conditions that they had to study. Put more directly, they had to infect subjects with the disease organisms and test their preparations against them for efficacy.

How did the investigators recruit subjects for their research and were they respectful of the norms of consent and do no harm? In the over-whelming majority of cases, the answer is no. The subjects were typically made up of institutionalized mentally disabled persons (suffering from mental illness or mental retardation), institutionalized orphans, and prison-ers. None of them were truly capable of giving consent, certainly not the mentally incompetent or the orphaned children, and (although this point has been debated) not convicts deprived of liberty, living in conditions of severe deprivation, and under total state control. Thus, the researchers violated long-standing ethical norms by carrying out non-therapeutic ex-periments that were dangerous and lacked subject's consent.

In specific terms, researchers conducted their studies on dysentery in state institutions for the retarded. Indeed, government research grants fa-vored investigators who had "access to various state institutions where fa-cilities for study of dysentery are unexcelled", precisely because hygienic conditions were so primitive. Researchers also carried out their investiga-tions in orphan asylums; the boys at the Ohio Soldiers and Sailors Orphan-age, were injected with "killed suspensions for various types of shigella group of bacteria", to see whether the compounds would protect against dysentery. Unfortunately, the preparations proved highly toxic, causing fe-vers on the average of 104 degrees Fahrenheit and leaving the boys ex-hausted.

The influenza research used subjects residing in state facilities for the retarded, in correctional centers for juvenile offenders, and in state hospi-tals for the chronic mentally ill. The protocols divided the residents in two - one group received the trial vaccine, the other a placebo, and then both were challenged with influenza virus. The vaccines proved to be of varying efficacy, but all the control group and for many of the active agent group contracted high fevers and suffered aches, pains, and debilitation.

The bulk of the malaria research went on in state mental hospitals and prisons. In one series of experiments, psychotic, backward patients were infected with malaria through blood transfusions and then given experi-mental anti-malarial therapies. A psychiatrist was a member of the team, but his function was not to determine the subjects' competency to give consent but to explain their symptoms to the investigative team.[13]

Thus, the marked disparity between the principles of research ethics and the reality of laboratory practices prior to the issuance of the Nuremberg Code confirms the import of promulgating a formal code. In its absence, individuals cogently and persuasively defined the rules of conduct that should govern human experimentation, but their precepts lacked formal standing or authority. What was so crucial, then, about the Nuremberg Code was not so much its content as its form. Its authors correctly insisted that the guidelines expressed well known and established values. Its uniqueness lies in the fact that these principles were formally endorsed by a court and presented as a code.

Thus, to understand the history of human experimentation immediately after Nuremberg, it must be remembered that this codification of principles owed little to organized medical bodies. The prosecutors called physicians as witnesses and used them as consultants, but the document stood as the work of judges and its stipulations were realized through a court, not through professional medical bodies. In essence, the initial regulatory effort in human experimentation was external to medicine - which helps to account for both its weaknesses and strengths in the post-World War Two period. This circumstance enables us to understand, on the one hand, why Nuremberg exerted so little impact on the practice of human experimentation. In the United States, for example, the Code seemed aimed at Nazis and madmen, not at bone fide physicians and researchers. But on the other hand, the Code helped to bridge the gap between medicine and other disciplines, initiating a concern for medical ethics among legal scholars, religious ethicists, and philosophers. Finally, the Code set an example that eventually influenced the policies of medical organizations. Nuremberg was the critical precedent for the formal and collective pronouncements of such bodies as the American Medical Association and the World Medical Association. What began outside the domain of medicine came, in time, to be integrated into medicine.

Notes

1   Quoted to Bull, J.P. (1959), 'The Historical Development of Clinical Therapeutic Trials', *Journal of Chronic Diseases*, 10, p. 222.
2   *Transactions Cong. Am. Phys. Surg.*(1907), 7, 1, pp. 7-8.
3   Withington was also alert to the possibilities of non-therapeutic experiments on terminally ill patients. An investigator, he insisted, "has no right to take advantage of the patient's extremity to *recommend* a procedure which can have no other advantage than to enhance the operator's reputation for boldness".
4   Withington, Charles Francis. (1886), *The Relation of Hospitals to Medical Education*, Boston, Cupples, Uphman, p. 15.
5   Smith, Claude A. (1904), 'Uncinariasis in the South with Special Reference to Mode of Infection', *JAMA*, 43, p. 596.
6   Lederer, Susan E. (1995), *Subjected to Science: Human Experimentation in America before the Second World War*, New York, Oxford University Press, pp. 17, 16.
7   Mouritz, A. A. St. M. (1951), 'Human Inoculation Experiments in Hawaii including Notes of Arning and Fitch', condensed, arranged and annotated by W. Wade, *International Journal of Leprosy*, 19, p. 205.
8   Sternberg, George M. (1898), 'The Bacillus Icteroides (Sanarelli) and Bacillus X (Sternberg)', *Transactions of the Association of American Physicians*, 13, p. 71 (discussion of paper by Osler).
9   Quoted by Lederer. (1995), *Subjected to Science*, p. 63.
10 'Grafting Cancer in the Human Subject'. (1891), *JAMA*, 17, p. 234.
11 Lederer, Susan E. (1995), *Subjected to Science*, pp. 110-111.
12 'Experiments on Human Beings' (1900), *JAMA*, 34, p. 1359.
13 For further details of the American wartime research see, David J. Rothman. (1991), *Strangers at the Bedside*, New York, Basic Books, chapter two.

[5]

NUREMBERG'S LEGACY: SOME ETHICAL REFLECTIONS

*JAMES F. CHILDRESS**

The Nuremberg Code: Its Context and Content

The Nuremberg Code was promulgated by four American judges at the Doctors' Trial at Nuremberg, in the case of the *United States of America v. Karl Brandt et al.* in 1946 to 1947. Twenty-three defendants, all but three of them medical doctors, were tried for truly horrendous "crimes alleged to have been committed in the name of medical or scientific research" (both war crimes and crimes against humanity), including the horrific high altitude, freezing, malaria, and mustard gas experiments, among others, which resulted in countless severe injuries and deaths [1]. Fifteen were found guilty; seven received the death sentence. The court's judgment included the "Nuremberg Code," consisting of 10 "basic principles" to govern permissible medical experiments.

This code, which received substantial input from two American physicians—Leo Alexander and Andrew Ivy—was an attempt to close the gap created by the relative absence of formal statements of ethics in human experimentation by a more or less authoritative body. Several times in this essay I will use the metaphor of gaps to indicate how various efforts to formulate ethical principles, rules, and procedures seek to fill or close or cover holes in the protections of research subjects' rights and welfare. This metaphor certainly fits the promulgation of the Nuremberg Code. The judges probably adopted this Nuremberg Code, as Leonard Glantz suggests, because of "their shock in finding that there were essentially no written standards for human experimentation that had been adopted by an authoritative institution" [2]. Hence the 10 rules, a modern-day decalogue for human experimentation, so that no one could plead ignorance of ethical obligations.

The 10 Nuremberg principles were not created ex nihilo. There were few earlier codes, but, ironically, two German regulations earlier in this century (a 1900 Prussian directive and a 1932 Reich Circular) offered

*University of Virginia, Cocke Hall, Room 101, Charlottesville, VA 22903.
Email: childress@virginia.edu.

strong statements of ethical obligations and rights in research (see [3, pp. 127–32]). Unfortunately, codes do not guarantee ethical conduct. And several physicians had already articulated ethical standards to guide human experimentation [3, pp. 121–26]. There is debate, however, about whether they represented only "occasional voices" (Jay Katz) or actually constituted "a powerful tradition in ethical thought" (David Rothman) [4, 5]. At any rate, the two physicians who served as expert medical witnesses for the prosecution drew on earlier formulations including, somewhat inappropriately, the Hippocratic tradition, which doesn't really address the issues raised by research with human subjects [3, pp. 132–37].

WHY THE NUREMBERG CODE?

Glantz is probably right about the judges' shock at not finding a written, authoritative code and about their felt need to close that gap. They clearly did not need the Nuremberg Code in order to state principles by which they could condemn the doctors' actions: they had sufficient grounds to do so in existing laws, even German laws, that prohibited murder, mayhem, and maiming, which the physicians (and others) had not extended to Jews and to others they viewed as less than human (and then subjected to actions that were even prohibited by a 1933 German law for protecting animals) [3, p. 132]. The guilty verdicts were, in short, overdetermined, and they did not presuppose a code for human experimentation—the verdicts were adequately justified by other rules against war crimes and crimes against humanity.

The court and others, such as Telford Taylor, the chief counsel for the prosecution, viewed the Nuremberg Code as a summary of common medical morality, at least as affirmed even if not always practiced. It expressed putatively universal standards with "many antecedents" [6, p. 150]. The Code's prefatory statement notes that human experimentation can "yield results for the good of society that are unprocurable by other methods or means of study." "*All* agree, however," the prefatory statement continues, "that certain basic principles must be observed in order to satisfy moral, ethical and legal concepts" [7, p. 102]. The 10 principles then followed.

CONTENT OF THE NUREMBERG CODE

1. "The voluntary consent of the human subject is absolutely essential." The statement then specifies the meaning of this first principle to include the requirement that the "person involved should have the legal capacity to give consent; should be so situated as to be able to exercise free power of choice, without the intervention of any element of force, fraud, deceit, duress, overreaching, or other ulterior form of constraint or coercion; and should have sufficient knowledge and com-

prehension of the elements of the subject matter involved as to enable him to make an understanding and enlightened decision." This last requirement is itself further specified, along with the insistence that the one who initiates, directs or engages in the experiment has the "personal duty and responsibility" to ascertain the quality of the subject's consent.

2. "The experiment should be such as to yield fruitful results for the good of society, unprocurable by other methods or means of study, and not random and unnecessary in nature."

3. "The experiment should be so designed and based on the result of animal experimentation and a knowledge of the natural history of the disease or other problem under study that the anticipated results will justify the performance of the experience."

4. The fourth principle requires the avoidance of "all unnecessary physical and mental suffering and injury."

5. The fifth principle rules out experiments in which there is "an a priori reason to believe that death or disabling injury will occur." It recognizes a possible exception in experiments in which "experimental physicians also serve as subjects."

6. This principle requires proportionality between the risks and probable benefits of the research: "The degree of risk to be taken should never exceed that determined by the humanitarian importance of the problem to be solved by the experiment."

7. "Proper preparation should be made and adequate facilities provided to protect the experimental subject against even remote possibilities of injury, disability, or death."

8. This principle limits research to "scientifically qualified persons" who should be required to exercise the "highest degree of skill and care" throughout.

9. "During the course of the experiment the human subject should be at liberty to bring the experiment to an end if he has reached the physical or mental state where continuation of the experiment seems to him to be impossible."

10. This last principle indicates that the "scientist in charge must be prepared to terminate the experiment at any stage" if there is probable cause to believe that its continuation "is likely to result in injury, disability, or death to the experimental subject."

Two of these 10 principles (numbers 1 and 9) deal with the potential or actual subject's right to consent or refuse—voluntarily and with adequate information—to participate in research, and to withdraw from it, while the remaining eight deal with the subject's welfare in the context of the protocol, its design, its necessity, and its balance of risks and benefits and with ways to protect that welfare.

RECEPTION IN THE UNITED STATES

For many years the Nuremberg Code played virtually no role in ethical discussions, public policies, and legal decisions in the United States. It was effectively circumscribed and even marginalized in various ways. As formulated in the context of a criminal trial, it could be considered a code for barbarians, the Nazis, who were guilty of brutal excesses, not a code for civilized researchers. Another line of dismissal considered codes with sanctions unnecessary and insufficient because research subjects are truly protected only by virtuous professionals [8]. And yet adopting the Nuremberg Code's principles would have challenged several practices in the United States, including the use of prisoners in certain experiments. Ruth Faden and colleagues conclude: "the Code, at the time it was promulgated, had little effect on mainstream medical researchers engaged in human subjects research" [9].

In short, both bad and good reasons led to the Code's relative neglect. An indefensible reason was the failure by many physicians and investigators to view voluntary, informed consent as very important, especially in therapeutic research, in part because medical paternalism still reigned in therapeutic contexts. A more defensible (but still inadequate) reason is that the Code itself is imperfect and incomplete. While designed to close a gap—to articulate a formal, authoritative code of common medical morality in experimentation—it also left some gaps and filled others with rigid and unyielding principles. A few examples will illustrate the Code's deficiencies.

First, the Court conceded that it was mainly concerned with "those requirements which are purely legal in nature—or which at least are so clearly related to matters legal that they assist us in determining criminal culpability and punishment" [10]. Such a focus necessarily omits or at least downplays concerns that are more ethical in nature and have little to do with criminal culpability and punishment.

Second, the Nuremberg Code considered only non-therapeutic research, and it ruled out all research involving incompetent subjects because of its absolute rule of subject consent—only the subject could consent to his or her participation in research. (Incidentally, Dr. Alexander's memorandum for the court included proxy consent for incompetent subjects, but this was omitted by the judges [3, pp. 135-36]. The Code's omissions are certainly understandable in light of the terrible non-therapeutic experiments the court had to address, but these gaps almost certainly contributed to the Code's "marginalization in modern medicine" [11, p. 308].

The Declaration of Helsinki

"Most discussions begin with Nuremberg," George Annas and Michael Grodin observe, but "almost none end there, and there has been a consistent and insistent movement away from the directness of the Code toward more flexible forms of judging the conduct of human experimentation" [11, p. 307], I want to test their judgment with respect to the Declaration of Helsinki adopted by the World Medical Association in 1964.

FEATURES OF THE DECLARATION OF HELSINKI

Most interpreters of medical research ethics concur that the Declaration of Helsinki was "greatly influenced by the Nuremberg Code," despite its significant departures from the earlier code [6, p. 158]. The Declaration has been revised and updated several times since its adoption in 1964 (1975, 1983, and 1989). Perhaps one major reason is that Helsinki I (as the first is now called) failed to include informed consent as one of its "basic principles," even though it did incorporate informed consent into its requirements for both non-therapeutic and therapeutic research. And, in contrast to the Nuremberg Code, it stressed (in 3c) that "consent should as a rule be obtained in writing."[1]

The Declaration of Helsinki represents at least two major developments in ethics in research involving human subjects. First, it offers a less stringent requirement of the research subject's own voluntary, informed consent: it allows some incompetent subjects to be enrolled in some research protocols on the basis of a legal guardian's consent or permission. Second, the Declaration distinguishes therapeutic research (what it calls "clinical research combined with professional care") from "non-therapeutic clinical research." And it clearly extended its basic principles along with the requirement of voluntary, informed consent to therapeutic research.

Helsinki II in 1975 further strengthened informed consent by making it a basic principle. It also mandated independent ethical review committees, and insisted that reports of experimentation violating its ethical principles not be accepted for publication. Hence, it recommended procedures for protecting human subjects, not simply substantive standards.

ORDER OF PRINCIPLES

Debate continues about whether these codes, singly or together, adequately covered, or filled, important gaps in the protection of human research subjects. Jay Katz vigorously defends the Nuremberg Code over the Declaration of Helsinki, even in its later versions. For him Helsinki is partially responsible for "the unfulfilled legacy of the Nuremberg Judges" because it stresses the advancement of science rather than voluntary, informed consent (the Nuremberg Code's first principle) [4, p. 1665].

---

1. For different versions of the Declaration of Helsinki, see Appendix 3 in [7].

Katz also criticizes the later, revised versions of the Declaration that do include voluntary, informed consent among the "Basic Principles." His criticism continues because these revised codes list consent ninth rather than first—that is, consent follows principles concerning research protocols, qualified researchers, and balancing risks and potential benefits.

Katz's complaint forces us to consider the moral rhetoric of codes and declarations. In doing so, we need to distinguish three possible ways to arrange principles: order of presentation; order of practical consideration; and rank order. The *order of presentation* within a code—i.e., which principles are listed first, second, etc.—must be distinguished from the *order of practical consideration*—i.e., which factors the code indicates should be considered first, second, etc., in practice. And both must be distinguished from the *rank order*—i.e., the respective weights of different principles. What is critically important is how much weight or strength codes assign to their principles, even to principles listed later. It is possible, for instance, to list a principle—such as voluntary, informed consent—ninth rather than first but also to make it indispensable and even absolute.

A code's order of presentation may reflect the order of practical consideration, which is important when investigators propose or review boards examine particular protocols. For instance, I believe we should in practice consider, and ethically evaluate, the research protocol's design, the research's risks, its probable benefits and their balance, as well as the fair selection of research subjects, before we consider and ethically evaluate the protocol's form and process of voluntary, informed consent. Why? If the research protocol is ethically unsatisfactory on these other grounds, we don't even need to inquire into proposed subject consent. And potential subjects should not be asked to participate in research that fails to satisfy these principles; indeed, it would be unethical to do so. But even if a protocol is ethically satisfactory on all the other grounds, it shouldn't go forward without voluntary, informed consent. In short, it shouldn't matter if a code lists the requirement of voluntary, informed consent in some position other than first place, as long as consent has an essential role in the consideration and evaluation of a protocol.

In contrast to what Katz and others sometimes seem to suggest, voluntary, informed consent is not "a sufficient safeguard" for human subjects [4, p. 1666]. Even if it is the most important safeguard, it is only one such safeguard, and its function has less to do with protecting subjects from harm and more to do with respecting their autonomy. Other safeguards are also very important and even necessary—only when taken together do they provide sufficient protection for research subjects' rights and welfare. The egregious violation of the principle of consent/refusal in the Nazi experiments provided a reason for the judges who formulated the Nuremberg Code to place subject consent first and to make it absolute.

PROFESSIONAL FOUNDATIONS AND PUBLIC PARTICIPATION

Some commentators also note the different professional foundations of the two codes: the Nuremberg Code was written by lawyers, by judges, in the context of a criminal trial; while the Declaration of Helsinki was written by physicians for physicians [12]. These differences should not be overstated, however, because physicians provided important materials for the judges in the Nuremberg Doctors' Trial and because the judges insisted that the 10 principles reflected medical ethics. Nevertheless, the court, as I previously noted, concentrated on legal requirements and the determination of criminal culpability and punishment. Furthermore, many physicians found the Nuremberg Code problematic because of its rigid set of "legalistic demands," in contrast to the Declaration of Helsinki's "set of guides." Whereas the Nuremberg Code represented a "legalistic document," the Declaration of Helsinki represented an "ethical" one that was "more broadly useful" [13].

Neither Nuremberg nor Helsinki adequately reflects what, in my judgment, has become increasingly important: the role of the public. Of course, researchers and others often assume a public role, but it is also important to recognize the role of the public in deliberation about principles of research ethics and in the function of review boards, such as the Declaration of Helsinki included. The public should have such a role in part because research subjects are drawn from the public. In the United States public participation has been increasingly emphasized in the continuing development and application of federal regulations and guidelines for investigators and IRBs. I will now turn to selected developments in the United States, with particular attention to issues currently before the National Bioethics Advisory Commission (NBAC).

Selected Developments in the United States[2]

Human subjects research in the United States has not always followed either the Nuremberg Code or the Declaration of Helsinki. Revelations in the late 1960s and early 1970s about several unethical experiments, including the notorious U.S. Public Health Service's "Tuskegee Study of Syphilis in the Negro Male," led to the formation of the National Commission for the Protection of Human Subjects of Biomedical and Behavioral Research (hereafter the National Commission), which made several substantive and procedural recommendations for protecting research subjects. Procedurally, the National Commission relied on institutional review boards (IRBs), which had already emerged as important mechanisms to protect human subjects; substantively, it formulated several principles and guidelines, many

---

2. Some ideas and paragraphs in this third section are drawn from [14].

of which became formal regulations in the Department of Health, Education, and Welfare (later the Department of Health and Human Services) and were later incorporated into what became the "Common Rule." (Below I will discuss the National Commission's principles of beneficence, respect for persons, and justice, as expressed in its Belmont Report.) With these developments, along with the work of the President's Commission for the Study of Ethical Problems in Medicine and in Biomedical and Behavioral Research and other structures and mechanisms, research with human subjects seemed both ethically settled and secure.

Indeed, in the 1980s, discussants commonly observed that the major controversies in research concerned the use of animals rather than the use of humans. However, in a fine prophetic statement in 1989, Alexander M. Capron observed: "today the subject [of research involving human subjects] is often naively viewed as one of settled ethical principles, detailed statutory and regulatory requirements, and multifaceted procedures. History suggests that such claims must be viewed skeptically: the principles may be less conclusive and the guidelines less protective than they appear" [15].

The Advisory Committee on Human Radiation Experiments (ACHRE), chaired by Ruth Faden of the Johns Hopkins University School of Public Health, was established by President Clinton in response to stories that put a human face on information that had circulated for years. For instance, a series of reports in the *Albuquerque Tribune* disclosed the names of Americans who had been injected with plutonium, the manmade material that was a key ingredient of the atom bomb. The ACHRE itself examined the records of several thousand experiments funded and conducted by different branches of the federal government, mostly in secret, as part of the Cold War. These experiments included feeding cereal with minute amounts of radioactive material to the science club at the Fernald School for the Retarded, total body irradiation of cancer patients, and testicular irradiation of inmates in Oregon and Washington prisons; many of the experiments clearly violated the Nuremberg Code and the Declaration of Helsinki. Following its review, the ACHRE recommended how the federal government should respond to its past actions and also indicated how it could learn from the legacy of these cold war experiments [16].

THE NBAC

The National Bioethics Advisory Commission (NBAC) was one result of the ACHRE's report. It was designed not only to respond to some specific issues the ACHRE had raised but also, more generally, to provide a national public forum for dialogue on ethical issues in research involving human subjects. Established by Presidential Executive Order in 1995 (though it did not meet until October 1996), the NBAC is required to "provide advice and make recommendations to the National Science and

Technology Council [in the White House], other appropriate entities and the public, on bioethical issues arising from research on human biology and behavior, including the clinical applications, of that research" [17]. According to its charge, NBAC must give first priority to two main areas: (1) protection of the rights and welfare of human research subjects; and (2) issues in the management and use of genetic information, including but not limited to human gene patenting.

Extensive and substantial governmental regulations and guidelines already exist for research involving human subjects, in contrast to genetics, along with relatively settled professional standards. Here the task is to examine what appears in law, regulations, guidelines, and practices to determine where there are important gaps. Hence, in research involving human subjects, the NBAC has to identify and plug gaps, often by modifying or adding to what already exists. The NBAC's progress has been slower than desired, in part because of two scientific breakthroughs that led to presidential requests for specific reports. The first was the 1997 announcement of Dolly's birth several months earlier; following this announcement, President Clinton requested a report on and recommendations about cloning within 90 days [18]. The second was the report by scientists in late 1998 that they had isolated pluripotent stem cells from fetal tissue after deliberate abortions and from embryos left over after in vitro fertilization; President Clinton again requested a report and recommendations, the preparation of which consumed much of a year [19]. As a member of the NBAC, will briefly consider some possible gaps in human subject protections, some of which the NBAC hopes to plug.

The Protection of Research Subjects with Mental Disorders. One gap, many agree, appears in the protection of vulnerable or special populations. Guidelines already exist for some vulnerable populations: prisoners, children, and pregnant women. From the very first meeting of the NBAC's subcommittee on human subject research, concerns were registered about another possibly vulnerable population in need of additional protections: those with decisional or cognitive impairments.

The National Commission had proposed guidelines for those institutionalized as mentally infirm, but those guidelines were never adopted for various reasons, including additional and, to many, burdensome mechanisms, such as the use of consent auditors and possibly a subject advocate, which the DHEW had added in proposing regulations. Although the lack of specific regulations and guidelines may not have caused major harms and wrongs to research subjects, the NBAC believed that it needed to address the uncertainties and confusion surrounding research with subjects with mental disorders that may affect decision-making capacity. Its substantive and procedural recommendations departed from the Nuremberg Code's absolute insistence on the research subject's own voluntary, informed consent, at least for research with low levels of risk and for research that offers a possibility of direct therapeutic benefit. Nevertheless, the NBAC recommended stringent and controversial requirements for research that involves persons who lack the capacity to decide for themselves about participation, that offers no prospect of direct medical benefit to research subjects, and that involves more than minimal risk for those subjects [20, 21].

Shifting Paradigms of Research. Another gap has emerged in the protection of human subjects because of a shift in paradigms of research and, consequently, in perceptions of injustice in research. The earlier paradigm, prominent from Nuremberg on, focused on the risks and burdens of research and on the need to protect potential and actual research subjects from harm, abuse, exploitation, and the like. Ethical guidelines for this paradigm emphasize voluntary, informed consent—that's where the Nuremberg Code begins.

Our basic approach in the United States, according to Carol Levine, "was born in scandal and reared in protectionism" [22]. The dominant model in protectionist policies is non-therapeutic research, i.e., research that doesn't offer the possiblity of therapeutic benefit to the subject. In the paradigm shift, however, attention turns from non-therapeutic to therapeutic research (e.g., clinical trials of promising new therapeutic agents), from protection to access, and from risks and burdens to possible benefits. This shift resulted particularly (but not only) from the epidemic of HIV infection and AIDS, as, for example, activists pressured the FDA to expand access to new treatments.

This inclusionist paradigm is important—it continues the shift from Nuremberg to Helsinki and beyond. However, we should not totally abandon the protectionist paradigm. The hard ethical task is to combine what is valuable in both in order to protect subjects' rights and welfare in light of a principle of justice that now rejects exclusion as well as exploitation. Other gaps, beyond the overly protectionist construal of justice, may also appear in the Belmont principles and their traditions of interpretation.

The Belmont Principles. The NBAC is not supposed to review and approve or disapprove particular research projects but rather to examine the "broad, overarching principles to govern the ethical conduct of research" [17]. One big question is whether major gaps exist in our heritage of ethical principles for research.

Three broad principles, articulated by the National Commission in the 1970s, particularly in its *Belmont Report*, still govern research involving human subjects [23]. Various guidelines and regulations specify these principles, and, where those guidelines and regulations are incomplete or unclear, IRBs further interpret the principles to determine whether to approve or reject particular research protocols. Those principles are:

1. *Respect for persons.* This principle requires that researchers respect the autonomous choices of those who are autonomous, and protect those

with diminished autonomy. Rules of consent/refusal specify this principle.

2. *Beneficence.* This principle requires benefiting and not harming, but since both parts often cannot be fully realized simultaneously research ends up with balance of benefits (to subjects and others) and harms (to subject). The rules that specify this principle require not harming and maximizing possible benefits and minimizing possible harms.

3. *Justice.* This principle entails fairness in distributing burdens and benefits, especially in protecting from exploitation those who might be selected because of "easy availability . . . compromised position, or . . . manipulability, rather than for reasons directly related to the problem being studied." (I have already noted how an inclusionist model also focuses on justice in terms of access to research.)

Versions, or at least aspects, of these principles also appeared earlier in the Nuremberg Code and the Declaration of Helsinki, usually stated as more specific rules, such as informed consent.[3] However, the NBAC can't simply repeat these principles and rules in a fundamentalist way. Instead, it—and other groups and individuals—must continue to probe them, to see whether they need to be modified or supplemented.

At the NBAC's first meeting, Ezekiel Emanuel, then a commissioner, contended that these three principles and related guidelines do not adequately address *community*. Attending to community could mean, among other possibilities, that we should add community as a fourth principle, or that we should interpret all these principles in a communitarian rather than a merely individualistic manner. This second approach would involve reexamining the Belmont principles and other guidelines through the lens of community. A good case can be made that the NBAC should rethink these principles to make sure that community is sufficiently included. Following are a few illustrations of what this might entail.

Beneficence already includes attention to the society's welfare, within the benefit to be balanced against the risks to subjects. However, attention to community might also require, as has become more widespread in practice, attention to potential harms to particular communities such as Indian or Jewish communities, rather than only harms to individuals. An example is the possible harm to a group identified with particular genes that are considered deleterious, such as cancer genes.

---

3. The distinction between principles and other normative formulations, such as rules, often hinges on their level of generality, with principles often being view as more general than rules and other more specific formulations (and terms such as guidelines referring to both of them). Hence, in current discourse, the requirement to obtain voluntary, informed consent from potential research subjects might be considered a rule, while respect for personal autonomy might be considered a principle. Nevertheless, the Nuremberg Code's specific formulations are considered principles. Hence, in this paper, I have not operated with a precise distinction between principles and rules. See, for instance, [24].

Reinterpreted through the lens of community, the principle of respect for persons would consider persons not merely as isolated individuals, who consent or refuse to consent to participate in research, but also as members of communities. However, we need to be cautious in such a move because it is not possible or justifiable to determine an individual's wishes and choices by reading them off communal traditions, beliefs, and values, or merely to subordinate the individual's autonomy to the community's will. And there is vigorous debate about how we should interpret the principle of respect for persons in cultures that are less individualistic than our own; this debate recently erupted in controversies about international research [25, 26].[4]

Finally, justice concerns more than fairly selecting research subjects and fairly distributing the benefits and burdens of research participation. It may include the participation by various communities in the design and evaluation of research. It could also include compensation for research-related injuries, as an expression of the community's solidarity with those who suffer injuries in research after assuming a position of risk on behalf of the community. From this standpoint, it is not enough to disclose on the consent form whether there will be any compensation for research-related injuries that are non-negligently caused; instead, compensation should be provided. In meeting with representatives of bioethics commissions around the world, the NBAC learned that most other countries, with a commitment to universal access to health care, do not view compensation for research-related injuries as a problem—such injuries would be routinely covered, at least for medical expenses. (The NBAC has not to this point endorsed a proposal by some commissioners to address compensation for research-related injuries, in part because some other commissioners thought that this was a solution in search of a problem.)

In short, it is important to revisit the Belmont principles in light of concerns about community, as well as other concerns, but the NBAC needs to do so in a way that does not neglect or distort what was important in earlier, more individualistic interpretations. It is not clear yet what might emerge if the NBAC takes this route. Even though the NBAC sponsored a conference, with other groups, in April 1999—the 20th anniversary of the *Belmont Report*'s publication in the *Federal Register*—to revisit the Belmont principles, some commissioners would like to see the NBAC issue a new, succinct report on basic principles.

Institutional Structures and Mechanisms. Obviously principles, rules, and guidelines are not self-implementing—they require various structures, mechanisms, and agents for their implementation. And the NBAC is looking into the adequacy of some of these. Its one specific mandated task in the area of research involving human subjects is to examine the adequacy

---

4. I will not deal here with the important issues raised by international and crosscultural research, particularly issues of universalism and pluralism. For a very helpful discussion, see [27, 28].

of the policies and procedures for protecting human subjects in each executive branch department and agency conducting, supporting, or regulating research involving human subjects.

The NBAC has also affirmed the ideal of protecting all research subjects, including those in privately funded and conducted research, through the twin mechanisms of institutional review and informed consent, but it hasn't defended a particular way to extend protections to such subjects. And serious questions have emerged about whether IRBs, which currently constitute the frontline protection for research subjects, can and do perform this task adequately.

Over the last 20 years in the United States, research involving human subjects has greatly expanded, and the number of protocols has increased dramatically. In addition, many are now multi-site protocols, which involve several teams of investigators and large numbers of research subjects. Regulations have also increased; institutional support is often minimal; individual members feel overworked and underappreciated; conflicts of interest are not uncommon; and so forth. As a result, fears abound that IRBs may not be able adequately to protect research subjects. In light of such concerns, the NBAC is preparing a report on the U.S. system for protecting the rights and welfare of research, but it is too early to anticipate the report's precise recommendations about ways to strength or supplement IRBs.

Some commentators suggest that efforts to protect human research subjects through the IRB system may fail because substantive and procedural guidelines are too complete and thus too burdensome, rather than because of gaps in those guidelines. As a result, many believe that investigators and IRBs spend too much time, energy, and resources on what is not so important and too little on what is really important, such as risky research. Hence some propose that if the NBAC tries to bridge some gaps in substantive and procedural guidelines, it should also try to eliminate or reduce what is less important or indicate that it should receive less attention or lower priority.

Conclusions

Because of various gaps and other deficiencies, the Nuremberg Code does not provide a timeless and sufficient ethical guide to research involving human subjects—hence, Nuremberg "fundamentalists" are mistaken (as fundamentalists often are). The Code's real legacy, at a higher level of generality, is its vision of a fundamental and absolute commitment to the rights and welfare of research subjects, whatever the prospect of scientific advancement.

Appropriating and extending this legacy requires that we continue to reflect sensitively, imaginatively, and rigorously on ethical standards for research with human subjects, just as Helsinki did, just as the National Commission did, just as CIOMS did, and just as other bodies have done and continue to do. This ethical reflection takes place in a continuing societal conversation about the foundations, meaning, weights, and implications of various ethical principles, rules, and procedures in research, in light of various changes in research and its context. This conversation must be broad based and open; it must include the public as well as professionals; and it must involve various segments of the public, including those who view themselves as socially marginal. It also must continue into the future as we seek ways to protect subjects' rights and interests and to generate valuable scientific knowledge. Only by doing so can we continue Nuremberg's remarkable legacy.

REFERENCES

1. Taylor, T. Opening statement of the prosecution. In *The Nazi Doctors and the Nuremberg Code: Human Rights in Human Experimentation*, edited by G. J. Annas and M. A. Grodin. New York: Oxford Univ. Press, 1992. 70.
2. Glantz, L. H. The influence of the Nuremberg Code on U.S. statutes and regulations. In *The Nazi Doctors and the Nuremberg Code: Human Rights in Human Experimentation*, edited by G. J. Annas and M. A. Grodin. New York: Oxford Univ. Press, 1992. 197.
3. Grodin, M. Historical origins of the Nuremberg Code. In *The Nazi Doctors and the Nuremberg Code: Human Rights in Human Experimentation*, edited by G. J. Annas and M. A. Grodin. New York: Oxford Univ. Press, 1992.
4. Katz, J. The Nuremberg Code and the Nuremberg Trial: A reappraisal. *JAMA* 20:1662–66, 1996.
5. Rothman, D. J. Letter to editor *JAMA* 277(9):709, 1997; Katz, J. In reply. *JAMA* 277(9):709–10, 1997.
6. Perley, S., et al. The Nuremberg Code: An international overview. In *The Nazi Doctors and the Nuremberg Code: Human Rights in Human Experimentation*, edited by G. J. Annas and M. A. Grodin. New York: Oxford Univ. Press, 1992.
7. See prefatory statement to Nuremberg Code. In *The Nazi Doctors and the Nuremberg Code: Human Rights in Human Experimentation*, edited by G. J. Annas and M. A. Grodin. New York: Oxford Univ. Press, 1992.
8. Beecher, H. Ethics and clinical research. *New Engl. J. Med.* 274:1354–60, 1966.
9. Faden, R., S. E. Lederer, and J. D. Moreno. U.S. Medical Researchers, the Nuremberg Doctors Trial, and the Nuremberg Code. *JAMA* 276(20):1667, 1996.
10. See the tribunal's judgment in *The Nazi Doctors and the Nuremberg Code: Human Rights in Human Experimentation*, edited by G. J. Annas and M. A. Grodin. New York: Oxford Univ. Press, 1992. 103.
11. Annas, G. J., and M. A. Grodin. Where do we go from here? In *The Nazi Doctors and the Nuremberg Code: Human Rights in Human Experimentation*, edited by G. J. Annas and M. A. Grodin. New York: Oxford Univ. Press, 1992.
12. Annas, G. J. The Nuremberg Code in U.S. courts: Ethics versus expediency. In *The Nazi Doctors and the Nuremberg Code: Human Rights in Human Experimentation*, edited by G. J. Annas and M. A. Grodin. New York: Oxford Univ. Press, 1992. 205.
13. Beecher, H., as quoted by Refshaauge, W. The place for international standards in conducting research for humans. *Bull. WHO* 55(supp.):133–35, 1977; which in turn is quoted in [12].

14. Childress, J. F. The National Bioethics Advisory Commission: Current challenges and future directions. *J. Health Care Law Policy* (forthcoming).

15. Capron, A.M. Human experimentation. In *Medical Ethics*, edited by R. M. Veatch. Boston: Jones and Bartlett, 1989. 128.

16. Advisory Committee on Human Radiation Experiments. *Final Report*. Washington, DC: U.S. GPO, 1995. Ch. 18.

17. National Bioethics Advisory Commission. Charter. 26 July 1996.

18. NBAC. *Cloning Human Beings: Report and Recommendations of the National Bioethics Advisory Commission.* Rockville, MD: 1997.

19. NBAC. *Ethical Issues in Human Stem Cell Research. Vol. 1: Report and Recommendations of the National Bioethics Advisory Commission.* Rockville, MD: 1999.

20. NBAC. *Research Involving Persons with Mental Disorders that May Affect Decisionmaking Capacity.* Rockville, MD: 1998.

21. Childress, J. F. An introduction to NBAC's Report on Research Involving Persons with Mental Disorders that May Affect Decisionmaking Capacity. *Accountability in Research* 7:101–15, 1999.

22. Levine, C. Changing views of justice after Belmont: AIDS and the inclusion of "vulnerable" subjects. In *The Ethics of Research Involving Human Subjects: Facing the 21st Century.* edited by H.Y. Vanderpool. Frederick, MD: University Publishing Group, 1996. 106.

23. National Commission for the Protection of Human Subjects of Biomedical and Behavioral Research. *The Belmont Report: Ethical Guidelines for the Protection of Human Subjects.* DHEW publication no. (OS) 78-0012. Washington, DC: U.S. GPO, 1978.

24. Beauchamp, T. L., and J. F. Childress. *Principles of Biomedical Ethics*, 4th ed. New York: Oxford Univ. Press, 1994.

25. Council for International Organizations of Medical Sciences (CIOMS), in Collaboration with the World Health Organization (WHO). *International Ethical Guidelines for Biomedical Research Involving Human Subjects.* 1993.

26. Vanderpool, H. Y., ed. *The Ethics of Research Involving Human Subjects: Facing the 21st Century.* Frederick, MD: University Publishing Group, 1996. 501–10.

27. Levine, R. J. International codes and guidelines for research ethics: A critical appraisal. in *The Ethics of Research Involving Human Subjects: Facing the 21st Century,* edited by H. Y. Vanderpool. Frederick, MD: University Publishing Group, 1996. 235–59.

28. Macklin, R. Universality of the Nuremberg Code. *The Nazi Doctors and the Nuremberg Code: Human Rights in Human Experimentation,* edited by G. J. Annas and M. A. Grodin. New York: Oxford Univ. Press, 1992. Ch. 13.

[6]

Allen Buchanan

The Controversy over
Retrospective Moral Judgment

ABSTRACT. The mandate of the U.S. Advisory Committee on Human Radiation Experiments required that the Committee take a position on the validity of *retrospective moral judgments*. However, throughout its period of operation, the Committee remained divided on the question of whether sound judgments of individual culpability and wrongdoing should be included in its *Final Report*. This essay examines the arguments that various committee members marshalled to support their opposing views on retrospective moral judgment and explains the significance of the controversy.

T HE MANDATE OF THE ADVISORY COMMITTEE on Human Radiation Experiments was to determine the appropriate criteria for ethical evaluation and then to evaluate ethically the radiation experiments conducted by or under the auspices of the U.S. Government between 1944 and 1974. From the beginning of the Committee's work, there were voices both within and outside of it that expressed serious reservations about the central task of ethical evaluation. They challenged the validity of *retrospective moral judgments,* if not generally, then at least in the case of judgments of *individual* wrongdoing and culpability.

A significant proportion of the Committee's reflections on the ethics of the experiments—as distinct from its purely historical research into the facts—was occupied with recurrent discussions about the problem of retrospective moral judgment. The most active participants in those discussions polarized into two factions: those who believed that the Committee's *Final Report* (ACHRE 1995) could and should make judgments of individual wrongdoing and judgments that ascribed culpability to identified individuals and those who had strong, but sometimes not clearly articulated, objections to doing so.

In the first weeks of the Committee's deliberations it became evident that this controversy was not likely to be resolved without a systematic analysis of the scope and limits of retrospective moral judgment. Accordingly, a background paper was commissioned on the topic and its results were presented to the Committee.[1]

The ethical framework that the Committee adopted is based on the view that there is no special problem of retrospective moral judgment. Instead, the framework takes the position that, at most, differences in the cultural context in which past events occurred, not the mere passage of time, can *in some instances* affect the ethical judgments we make about the past. The framework provides an account of what sorts of differences in cultural context can influence the validity of various distinct types of retrospective moral judgments. The main elements of the framework are (1) a classification of types of retrospective moral judgment and (2) a specification of the conditions that can limit the ability to make sound retrospective moral judgments of the various sorts.

The types of retrospective moral judgments identified include: (a) judgments about the moral qualities of institutions and policies, (b) judgments concerning the moral qualities of actions, (c) judgments that particular agents acted wrongly (not just that wrongs occurred), (d) judgments about the culpability, and degree of culpability, of agents, both institutional or collective, and individual, and (e) judgments about the character of individual agents.

The framework then identifies three types of ethical criteria that in principle are relevant to the evaluation of the experiments: (1) general ethical principles that are so basic to morality that we assume they were applicable in the past as well as today, (2) obligation-generating principles that were adopted by government agencies at the time the experiments were being conducted and were clearly intended to govern the way in which the experiments were conducted, and (3) central principles of professional ethics (including the ethics of the medical profession and the ethics of administration). The fundamental conclusion of Chapter 4 is that each of these three types of criteria can serve as standards for making valid retrospective moral judgments of *all* types, including judgments of individual wrongdoing and culpability.

As noted earlier, Chapter 4 also identifies factors that can mitigate or in some cases entirely undercut the various types of retrospective moral judgments. The crucial point is whether these factors are present in a

BUCHANAN • RETROSPECTIVE MORAL JUDGMENT

particular case. For example, we may simply lack sufficient evidence of what actually transpired in a particular case to be able to apply one of the ethical standards, or the culture in which the agent operated may have generated what the Committee calls moral ignorance, which prevented agents from seeing what they ought to have done. Or, even if such cultural moral ignorance is not so deep and persuasive as to exculpate an individual entirely, it may reduce the degree or magnitude of his or her blame. Perhaps just as importantly, the framework acknowledges that we may have a basis for making one kind of judgment, but not another—e.g., we may have sufficient evidence to judge that a particular person acted wrongly, and even that he was blameworthy for having done so, but have no basis for concluding that he was a person of generally bad moral character.

Thus, while there are specific circumstances in which some retrospective moral judgments would be invalid, there is no *general* prohibition against retrospective moral judgments, including judgments that attribute wrongdoing to particular individuals and that assign moral blame to those individuals for the wrongs they did. In other words, the ethical framework the Committee developed was committed to the view that it is possible not only to say that wrongs occurred, but that individuals acted wrongly, and that at least in some cases they were morally blameworthy for the wrongs they committed.

Yet in spite of the fact that the Committee "signed off" on this ethical framework, controversy persisted. Some committee members still remained unwilling to make judgments of individual wrongdoing or of individual culpability, even though they were willing to say that institutions were defective and that wrongs were committed. It is worth emphasizing that the committee members who were unwilling to make judgments of individual wrongdoing and culpability did not develop a position paper to support their view and did not circulate any attempt to refute the arguments of the background paper that led to the formulation of the ethical framework. For this reason, the following account of the controversy is inevitably highly reconstructive.

Although the controversy continued to surface from time to time during public meetings of the Committee, the nature of the disagreement seemed to shift. Perhaps because they found the arguments of the evolving ethical framework difficult to answer, the committee members who had all along expressed a reluctance to blame individuals for the wrongs committed in the course of the experiments, took a different tack. At first, at least some of them suggested that even if it were possible to make well-grounded judgments of individual culpability about past agents, there was no *need* to do so. Instead, the Committee should focus on the future—on making well-crafted recommendations designed to reduce the chance of future occurrences of wrongdoing.

At this point, some individuals on the other side of the controversy replied that there were three reasons not to focus on the future to the exclusion of making judgments of individual culpability in the past. First, they argued, more effective deterrence is likely to be achieved if individuals are put on notice that they will be held accountable *as* individuals—i.e., that they will not be able to hide behind the organizational or institutional veil, as they could if judgments of culpability and wrongdoing were limited to collectivities such as government agencies or the medical profession. Second, it was suggested that part of what is required for doing justice to those whose rights were violated in the course of the experiments is to identify as blameworthy the individuals who violated those rights. To fail to fix blame on particular individuals, where sound factual evidence and appropriate ethical standards enabled the Committee to do so, would be to fail to show proper respect for those whose rights were violated. Third, by failing to make decisions of individual wrongdoing the Committee would undercut the strongest case for compensating the victims of the experiments—one based on justice, on the premise that the rights of the subjects were violated. (This conclusion rests on the rationale that if A has a right, then there is a correlative obligation on others and that A's right is violated—and compensation for this violation is owed—only if others fail to fulfill their obligations, i.e., if they act wrongly).

Once these arguments were voiced, the character of the controversy seemed to shift again, or, to put the matter more neutrally, it became clear that a different concern was motivating at least some of those who were unwilling to make judgments of individual wrongdoing and culpability. The issue of *standards of evidence* came to the fore. According to some committee members, even if there was in principle no bar to making retrospective moral judgments of individual wrongdoing and culpability, in the case of the radiation experiments there was insufficient factual evidence to do so. The disagreement then became one over *how strong* the evidence of wrongdoing or culpability must be before a well-grounded judgment could be made.

BUCHANAN • RETROSPECTIVE MORAL JUDGMENT

This dispute was never resolved. However, those who had been advocating that the *Final Report* include some judgments of individual wrongdoing and culpability offered one last argument in favor of doing so. They emphasized the ethical framework's distinction between judgments of wrongdoing and culpability, on the one hand, and judgments about the *character* of agents, on the other. They noted that one can state that a person acted wrongly and even that he or she was blameworthy for doing so, without implying any global condemnation of the person as having a flawed character. The suggestion was that a proper humility in the face of the undeniable complexity of human motivation, and a due recognition of the fact that even good people can act badly in some circumstances, is better expressed by distinguishing between judgments of culpability or wrongdoing and judgments about character, than by setting excessively high standards of evidence for judgments of the former sorts. Their opponents apparently rejected this conclusion. Perhaps, even when the distinction between judgments of character and those concerning wrongdoing and culpability is duly acknowledged, they believed very strongly that the Committee lacked sufficient evidence to say that particular individuals acted wrongly or that they were morally blameworthy. It should be emphasized that the controversy over standards of evidence was not a dispute about the legitimacy of *retrospective* moral judgment as such. There is every indication that the disagreement over standards of evidence would have persisted even if the actions in question had been contemporary rather historical.

In the following article, Tom L. Beauchamp argues that the *Final Report* failed to make some judgments of individual wrongdoing and culpability that it should have made. The preceding reconstruction of the Committee's disagreements over the scope and limits of retrospective judgment not only provides an explanation of the discrepancy that Beauchamp portrays; it also shows why, if Beauchamp is correct, the mistake he reveals is an important one. For if in fact the *Final Report* should have made but did not make judgments of individual wrongdoing and culpability, then it is defective on two distinct accounts. As those who advocated the inclusion of such judgments argued, if it failed to hold individuals responsible who should have been judged responsible, the *Report* did not do all it could have done to prevent further occurrences of the unethical behavior it exposes; it also did not achieve full justice toward those whose rights were violated.

[249]

NOTE

1. This author, who served as a staff consultant to the Committee, and Ruth Macklin, who was a member of the Committee, each wrote drafts of background papers. Material from Macklin's draft was incorporated into later drafts of a longer background paper for which this author was principally responsible and which benefitted from important contributions from Ruth Faden, Jeffrey Kahn, Ruth Macklin, and Jonathan Moreno.

REFERENCES

ACHRE. Advisory Committee on Human Radiation Experiments. 1995. *Final Report*. Washington, DC: U.S. Government Printing Office.

[7]

Tom L. Beauchamp

Looking Back and Judging Our Predecessors

ABSTRACT. The Advisory Committee on Human Radiation Experiments has correctly argued that persons and institutions can sometimes be held responsible for actions taken more than a half-century ago, when practices and policies on the use of research subjects were strikingly different. In reaching its conclusions, the Committee did not altogether adhere to the language and commitments of its own ethical framework. In its *Final Report,* the Committee emphasizes judgments of *wrongdoing,* to the relative neglect of *culpability;* it discusses mitigating conditions that are exculpatory, but does not provide a thoroughgoing assessment of either culpability or exculpation. However, the Committee's shortcomings are mild in comparison to the deficiencies in the "Report of the UCSF Ad Hoc Fact Finding Committee on World War II Human Radiation Experiments" of the University of California at San Francisco. The latter report reaches no significant judgments of either wrongdoing or culpability. The findings that should have been reached by both committees are discussed.

IT IS WIDELY BELIEVED, AS THE CHAIRMAN of the Chemical Manufacturers Association recently opined, that "You cannot judge people or a company based on today's standards or knowledge for actions taken 40 to 60 years ago" (Ex-owner 1994). The claim is that people cannot be judged or held responsible for forms of waste disposal, research practices, types of marketing, and the like that were common and rarely challenged a half-century ago. The Advisory Committee on Human Radiation Experiments has shown that this thesis cannot be sustained, at least not without heavy qualification.

The Committee's framework of distinctions and principles is found in Chapter 4 of its *Final Report,* entitled "Ethics Standards in Retrospect" (ACHRE 1995). I accept the major components of the framework presented by the Committee, but I will argue that the Committee does not altogether adhere to the language and commitments of that framework in later chapters of the *Final Report*. My concern is with how the Committee's framework was used and how it could and should have been used to make retrospective judgments about *wrongdoing* and *culpability*. Because of space constraints, I will limit my comments to the plutonium cases (see ACHRE 1995, Chapter 5), largely the University of California at San Francisco (UCSF) case. However, these conclusions are generalizable to the entire report, especially to the "Findings" located in Chapter 17.

Although there are imperfections in the Committee's use of its own framework in reaching judgments of culpability, these shortcomings are significantly offset by its persuasive and well-documented judgments of wrongdoing. Furthermore, even this committee's weaknesses look like strengths in comparison to the deficiencies in the "Report of the UCSF Ad Hoc Fact Finding Committee on World War II Human Radiation Experiments" of the University of California at San Francisco (UCSF 1995). The latter report, I will argue, effectively has no framework and reaches no significant judgments of either wrongdoing or culpability, although it should have done so.

STANDARDS FOR RETROSPECTIVE JUDGMENT

In its *Final Report,* the Advisory Committee presents a well-developed set of distinctions, principles, explanations, and arguments pertinent to retrospective moral judgments. The Committee delineates "An Ethical Framework" (ACHRE 1995 [GPO, pp. 197-212; Oxford, pp. 114-24]), which I will call "the framework." Its core, for my purposes, is (1) a distinction between *wrongdoing* and *culpability;* (2) the identification of three kinds of ethical standards relevant to the evaluation of the human radiation experiments (basic principles, government policies, and rules of professional ethics); and (3) an account of culpability and exculpation, including mitigating conditions that are exculpatory. I will briefly review what the *Final Report* says about these three parts of the framework.

The Wrongness of Actions and the Culpability of Agents

The distinction between the wrongness of actions and the culpability of agents derives from the need to distinguish whether one is evaluating the moral quality—in particular, the wrongness—of actions, practices, policies, and institutions or evaluating the blameworthiness (culpability) of agents. The Committee correctly concluded that past actions regarding the conduct of human radiation research can be judged instances of wrongdoing without at the same time judging the agents who performed them to be culpable. From the fact that an action was wrong or that someone was wronged by the action, it does not follow that the agent(s) who performed the actions can be fairly blamed, censured, or punished. This distinction is of the highest significance and is rightly given a prominent position in the Committee's Ethical Framework (ACHRE 1995 [GPO, pp. 208-12; Oxford, pp. 121-24]).

Universal Moral Principles and Contemporaneous Policies and Rules

Second, the Advisory Committee identified six basic ethical principles as relevant to its work: "One ought not to treat people as mere means to the ends of others;" "One ought not to deceive others;" "One ought not to inflict harm or risk of harm;" "One ought to promote welfare and prevent harm;" "One ought to treat people fairly and with equal respect;" and "One ought to respect the self-determination of others" (ACHRE 1995 [GPO, p. 198; Oxford, p. 114]). These principles state general obligations. The Committee held that they are widely accepted and that the validity of the principles is not time-bound. A hundred years or a thousand years ago would not alter their moral force (ACHRE 1995 [GPO, p. 199; Oxford, p. 115]). By contrast, policies of government agencies and rules of professional ethics do not have this ahistorical quality, but instead are specific as to time and place (ACHRE 1995 [GPO, pp. 214-21; Oxford, pp. 125-30]).

Culpability and Exculpation

Third, building on the wrongdoing-culpability distinction, the Advisory Committee added an account of culpability and exculpatory conditions (ACHRE 1995 [GPO, pp. 208ff; Oxford, pp. 121ff]). The Committee found that several factors limit our ability to make judgments about the blameworthiness of agents. These include lack of evidence; the presence of conflicting obligations; factual ignorance; culturally induced moral ignorance, in which "cultural factors . . . prevent individuals from discerning what they are morally required to do" (ACHRE 1995 [GPO, p. 209; Oxford, p. 121]); an evolution in the delineation of moral principles; and indeterminacy in an organization's division of labor and designation of responsibility.

[253]

KENNEDY INSTITUTE OF ETHICS JOURNAL • SEPTEMBER 1996

Although these conditions are exculpatory—i.e., they *mitigate* or *tend to absolve* of alleged fault or blame—satisfaction of the conditions does not always exculpate and only two of the conditions affect judgments of wrongdoing (ACHRE 1995 [GPO, p. 204; Oxford, p. 118]). The conditions are satisfied by degrees, and exculpation can involve balancing several different considerations (ACHRE 1995 [GPO, p. 210; Oxford, p. 122]). Presumably at the heart of the Committee's work is an examination of whether these exculpatory conditions were present in particular cases in order to determine whether the persons involved are exculpated —that is, are free or relatively free of blame for what they did.

The Committee understood "its first task" to be that of evaluating the rightness or wrongness of actions, practices, and policies. However, it also emphasized the importance of discovering whether judgments ascribing blame to individuals or groups can and should be made. It noted that "unless judgments of culpability are made *about particular individuals,* one important means of deterring future wrongs will be precluded" (ACHRE 1995 [GPO, p. 212; Oxford, p. 123], emphasis added).

THE UCSF CASE

One case considered by the Advisory Committee, and the only one I will consider in detail, originates at UCSF and eventuates in the Ad Hoc Committee report previously mentioned. I will use this case as an example of the Advisory Committee's application of its framework to assess a case and as a means of evaluating the UCSF Ad Hoc Committee's judgments.[1]

Plutonium Injections from 1945 to 1947

The salient facts in this case are as follows. From April 1945 to July 1947, 17 patients were injected with plutonium at three university hospitals—UCSF, the University of Chicago, and the University of Rochester—and 1 at Oak Ridge Hospital in Tennessee. Three of the 18 (known as CAL-1, 2, and 3) were injected at UCSF. Eventually allegations surfaced that the injections of plutonium were toxic to the patients and that they never consented to involvement as subjects of the research.

These patient-subjects were part of a secret research protocol initiated by the Manhattan Engineer District, a government program responsible for the production of atomic weapons. The purpose of this scientific research was to determine the excretion rate of plutonium in humans so that the government could establish safety levels and standards for work-

BEAUCHAMP • JUDGING OUR PREDECESSORS

ers who handled this radioactive element. Although performed largely in secret, some of this work was known publicly as early as 1951. It was discussed in the 1970s and 1980s, but did not generate a substantial controversy until 1993, as a result of the work of a persistent investigative reporter in Albuquerque, N.M.

The 1995 Report of the UCSF Ad Hoc Committee

On January 7, 1994, UCSF Chancellor Joseph Martin appointed an Ad Hoc Committee to investigate these allegations by studying the history of UCSF involvement. After a year of investigating documents and debating the issues, this committee filed its report in February 1995. The Ad Hoc Committee confirmed UCSF involvement and confirmed that at least one of the three initial patients had been included in the secret government protocol. The UCSF report notes that the "injections of plutonium were not expected to be, nor were they, therapeutic or of medical benefit to the patients" (UCSF 1995, p. 27).[2]

The Ad Hoc Committee found that written consent was rare, disclosure narrow, and the permission of patients not typically obtained even for nontherapeutic research during this period. They found that it is not known and that we "cannot know" exactly what these research subjects were told or what they understood (UCSF 1995, pp. 26, 34). They also found that the word "plutonium" was classified at the time; it is therefore certain that it was not used in any explanations that might have been made to patient-subjects. The committee noted that in a recorded oral history in 1979, Kenneth Scott, one of the three original UCSF investigators, said that he never told the first subject what had been injected in him. Scott went on to say that the experiments were "incautious" and "morally wrong" (UCSF 1995, pp. 26-27).[3]

Nonetheless, the Ad Hoc Committee wrote, "At the time of the plutonium experiments, [today's issues about proof of consent] were not discussed. The Committee is hesitant to apply current-day standards to another historical period," although "overall, the Committee believes that practices of consent of the era were inadequate by today's standards, and even by standards existing at the time . . . . [T]he Committee believes that researchers should have discussed risks with potential subjects" (UCSF 1995, pp. 32, 34).

The Ad Hoc Committee concluded that this experimentation offered no benefit to subjects but also caused no harm because patients did not

Human Experimentation and Research

develop any medical complications. It also found that the experiments themselves were "consistent with accepted medical research practices at the time" (UCSF 1995, p. 33). The Ad Hoc Committee concluded that the subjects were *wronged* and the experimentation was "unethical" *if* the patients did not understand or agree to the interventions; in this event, they were wronged because their integrity and dignity were violated. However, the Ad Hoc Committee found that since it could not establish what the patients understood, no basis existed for saying that they actually were wronged (UCSF 1995, pp. 28-34).

In an appendix to the Ad Hoc Committee's report, a lawyer and committee member, Elizabeth Zitrin, concluded that even if the experiments were consistent with accepted medical practices at the time, "it does not make them ethical. And they were not consistent with the highest standards of the time articulated by the government, the profession, or the public." The Chairman of the Ad Hoc Committee, Roy Filly, responded that this comment by the lawyer held investigators to an unrealistically high research standard.[4] I will consider this issue momentarily, but first one further development in this case merits attention.

One day after the Ad Hoc Committee filed its report in February 1995, it received a recently declassified memorandum about this research that had been written on December 30, 1946. The memo was written by the Chief of the Operations Branch, Research Division, at the Oak Ridge Atomic Facility. His subject was the preparations being made "for injection in humans by doctors [Robert] Stone [one of the three original UCSF investigators] and [Earl] Miller." The memo reports that:

> These doctors state that the injections would probably be made *without the knowledge of the patient* and that the physicians assumed full responsibility. Such injections were not divergent from the normal experimental method in the hospital and the patient signed no release. (Chapman 1946, p. 1)

This memorandum and other known facts in the UCSF case indicate, despite an excessively restrained Ad Hoc Committee report (see below), that these patients were seriously wronged, even if they were not physically or mentally harmed (ACHRE 1995 [GPO, pp. 249-52, 256-58, 264-69; Oxford, pp. 149-52, 154-55, 160-63]). The UCSF committee was unwilling to reach conclusions about wrongdoing, preferring, like the chairman of the Chemical Manufacturers Association, the position that it is too demanding to judge people or institutions for actions taken a half-century ago. Nowhere did the Ad Hoc Committee consider culpability, but its conservative conclusions strongly hint at exculpation (largely because of the limited evidence available to the committee).

I believe that no analysis of this case or the other plutonium cases can be adequate if it evades examination of questions of both wrongdoing and culpability. The Advisory Committee's framework makes exactly this demand. But how does the Advisory Committee fare in making the judgments its framework calls for, and does it fare better than the Ad Hoc Committee?

THE ADVISORY COMMITTEE'S FRAMEWORK

A section entitled "Applying the Ethical Framework" in the Advisory Committee's *Final Report* evaluates "human radiation experiments conducted between 1944 and 1974" (ACHRE 1995 [GPO, pp. 212-21; Oxford, pp. 124-30]). I will first outline what, in my judgment, the Committee could be expected to have decided in light of its framework and, second, ways in which the Committee deviated from what could be expected.

The Committee's framework and discussion of its application indicate that the Committee undertook three assignments:

(1) to locate moral wrongdoing that violates either basic moral principles or guidelines in the government policies and professional ethics of the period;

(2) to place the violations in the context of mitigating or exculpatory conditions (as appropriate); and

(3) to decide which persons and institutions are culpable and which exculpated (as well as which lie on a continuum between the two).

Through a resourceful and historically innovative examination of the actual policies of government agencies and rules of professional ethics of the period, the Committee unhesitatingly addressed the first assignment:

> [T]hese experiments were unethical . . . . [T]wo basic moral principles were violated—that one ought not to use people as a mere means to the ends of others and that one ought not to deceive others . . . . The egregiousness of the disrespectful way in which the subjects of the injection experiments and their families were treated is heightened by the fact that the subjects were hospitalized patients . . . . [leaving] them vulnerable to exploitation. (ACHRE 1995 [GPO, pp. 267-68; Oxford, p. 162])

This evaluation of wrongdoing contrasts with the vacillation and indecisiveness in the UCSF Ad Hoc Committee report. Although, with the exception of the memo, both committees had basically the same documentary evidence before them, the ways in which that evidence was used for retrospective judgments is striking. This contrast makes for an excellent bioethics case study of different approaches to the evidence for retrospective moral judgment.

The Advisory Committee tackled the second assignment with the same decisiveness and conscientious use of historical documents. In the UCSF case and other radiation cases, it noted that judgments of excusability, culpability, and the like depend, at least to some extent, on whether proper moral standards for research involving human subjects were acknowledged in government agency policies and in the culture of medicine. If relevant standards and duties were entirely undeveloped at the time, this lamentable circumstance becomes exculpatory for persons accused of wrongdoing. Such circumstances would be very different from a situation in which there existed well developed and officially endorsed policies for human subjects research.

The Committee determined, however, that exculpation does not come easily, because policies that included vital elements that would today be considered central to the ethics of research involving human subjects existed even in the mid-1940s. For example, the Committee concluded from the evidence before it that "it was common to obtain the voluntary consent of healthy subjects who were to participate in biomedical experiments that offered no prospect of medical benefit to them" and that ill subjects were not a relevantly different class of subjects (ACHRE 1995 [GPO, p. 217; Oxford, p. 127]). The Committee also found that "even fifty years ago, [the six basic] principles were pervasive features of moral life in the United States" that every medical investigator could be expected to observe (ACHRE 1995 [GPO, p. 204; Oxford, p. 118]).

In light of these discoveries and conclusions, the Committee often reacted to proposed exculpatory conditions with the same strength and decisiveness with which it reacted to violations of principles. An example is found in its conclusion that the mitigating condition of culturally induced moral ignorance does not apply to many government officials, because they simply failed to implement or communicate requirements that were already established as their responsibility: "The very fact that these requirements were articulated by the agencies in which they worked is evidence that officials could not have been morally ignorant of them" (ACHRE 1995 [GPO, p. 215; Oxford, p. 126]).

Throughout its assessments under assignment (2), the Committee relied on the above-mentioned cluster of factors, including factual ignorance and culturally induced moral ignorance, that limit the ability to make judgments of agent culpability. These criteria and the conclusions drawn from them contrast markedly with the work of the UCSF Ad Hoc Committee, which attempted to place a maximal distance between the policies of the 1940s and those of the 1990s, rather than to locate their similarities. The Ad Hoc Committee was willing to find mitigating conditions that either exculpate or suggest exculpation at almost every point in the trail of evidence, whereas the Advisory Committee placed the evidence in a broader and more revealing context.

The mood and strategy shift, however, in the Advisory Committee's handling of the third assignment; there is a sharp deviation from what I have outlined as the expected path. Instead of assessing culpability and exculpation for individuals and institutions, the Committee focused almost entirely on the wrongness of actions. Despite its statement, previously quoted, that "judgments of culpability [should be] made *about particular individuals,*" no such judgment is reached in the *Final Report*—not about the plutonium cases or any other cases—apparently because the Committee found the trail of warranting evidence to run out at just this point.

This outcome is surprising in light of the Committee's assessment that many of the individuals involved in these cases had an obligation to the norms governing conduct and yet often failed to take them seriously. For example, the Committee found that various physicians could and should have seen that using sick patients as they did in the plutonium cases was

> morally worse than using healthy people, for in so doing one was violating not only the basic ethical principle not to use people as a mere means but also the basic ethical principle to treat people fairly and with equal respect. (ACHRE 1995 [GPO, p. 219; Oxford, pp. 128-29])

Following these indictments of the *actions* of physicians—and government officials, in corresponding passages—the reader is poised for the next step: a treatment of mitigating conditions that are exculpatory, followed by an assessment of culpability or exculpation. Surprisingly, this analysis never develops—or at least does not develop for the evaluation

KENNEDY INSTITUTE OF ETHICS JOURNAL • SEPTEMBER 1996

of specific individuals. Only in the final sentence of Chapter 5 does the Committee hint at the issue, using a new language of "accountability." It determined that responsible officials at government agencies and medical professionals responsible for the plutonium injections were *"accountable* for the moral wrongs that were done" (ACHRE 1995 [GPO, p. 269; Oxford, p. 163], emphasis added).

Clearly these professionals were accountable (responsible and answerable), but were they culpable (blameworthy and censurable)? One could argue that the term "accountable" is functioning in the above quotation to blame, but the terms do not have the same meaning, and the subtlety of the point will escape even close readers. The Committee makes no connection in its *Final Report* between being accountable and being culpable; nor does it present an argument to indicate that in reaching the above judgment of accountability the Committee is blaming the individual physicians responsible for the injections or any of the other parties mentioned.

Some of this lost ground is recovered in the Committee's "Finding 11" in Chapter 17, where the Committee finally restores the language of blame and returns to its earlier style of reaching decisive conclusions:

> The Advisory Committee finds that government officials and investigators are blameworthy for not having had policies and practices in place to protect the rights and interests of human subjects who were used in research from which the subjects could not possibly derive medical benefits (nontherapeutic research in the strict sense). By contrast, to the extent that there was reason to believe that research might provide a direct medical benefit to subjects, government officials and biomedical professionals are less blameworthy for not having had such protections and practices.
>
> We also find that, to the extent that research was thought to pose significant risk, government officials and investigators are more blameworthy for not having had such protections and practices in place. (ACHRE 1995 [GPO, pp. 787-88; Oxford, pp. 503-4])

This passage is particularly important for understanding what the Committee believed it could and could not conclude in light of the massive body of evidence before it. The Committee apparently thought that it could blame only individuals and groups of individuals in institutions such as government agencies and the medical establishment. While this blaming is amorphous and anonymous, the Committee managed to reach an extremely important general assessment:

BEAUCHAMP • JUDGING OUR PREDECESSORS

[G]overnment officials and biomedical professionals should have recognized that when research offers *no prospect* of medical benefit, whether subjects are healthy or sick, research should not proceed without the person's consent. It should have been recognized that despite the significant decision-making authority ceded to the physician within the doctor-patient relationship, this authority did not extend to procedures conducted solely to advance science without a prospect of offsetting benefit to the person. (ACHRE 1995 [GPO, p. 788; Oxford, p. 504])

These forms of blame are improvements over the weaker conclusions in Chapter 5 about the plutonium cases. They also, once again, contrast noticeably with the inconclusiveness in the UCSF Ad Hoc Committee report, which assesses no form of blame, general or particular. Nonetheless, nowhere in the Advisory Committee's *Final Report* is a named agent (other than the federal government and the medical profession) ever found culpable. This is true not only in the Advisory Committee's discussion of the plutonium cases, but throughout the Committee's report. Such an outcome is not what one would have expected after the Committee's indictments of the intentional actions of wrongdoing mentioned throughout its *Final Report,* and it raises questions of what might have been decided within the Committee's framework had the Committee not held out for exceptionally high standards of historical and testimonial evidence before assessing individual blame (as discussed in the Conclusion below).

WHAT FINDINGS SHOULD HAVE BEEN REACHED ABOUT THE VIOLATIONS OF STANDARDS?

I will now consider what judgments the Committee should have reached, given its framework and objectives. In some cases, it did reach these judgments; in others it did not. Again the UCSF case will serve as the principal example.

In asking whether the UCSF investigators violated moral standards, we could be asking one or both of two questions, as the Advisory Committee notes. A first question is whether these investigators violated well-articulated *rules of professional ethics* or *government policies.* A second question is whether any *universal rights* or *principles* were violated. The Advisory Committee offers convincing answers to both questions. However, its answer to the second needs assessment before proceeding to the more important questions of mitigating conditions.

KENNEDY INSTITUTE OF ETHICS JOURNAL • SEPTEMBER 1996

Were Universal Standards Violated?

The Committee specifically notes that the first *two* of its principles were violated, namely, that persons may not be used as mere means to the ends of others and that persons may not be deceived by others; elsewhere in the *Report* it adds a violation of its fifth principle, namely, "one ought to treat people fairly and with equal respect" (ACHRE 1995 [GPO, pp. 219, 267; Oxford, pp. 128-29, 162]). The claim that three principles were violated is clearly justified, but the mention of only three principles is puzzling. The evidence assembled in the UCSF case, and in other cases before the Committee, is sufficient to conclude that *all six* of the principles identified by the Committee were violated.

The third principle is, "one ought not to inflict harm or risk of harm." Given what was known and not known about plutonium at the time, it is reasonable to infer that the physicians involved placed their patients at risk of harm, though perhaps a risk at an uncertain level. Whether this principle was violated was a matter of debate during the Advisory Committee's deliberations, but the available evidence seems to warrant a conclusion that violations of the principle did occur. It is not credible that a physician could inject a patient with plutonium without any awareness that doing so involved risk for the patient. The fourth principle is, "one ought to promote welfare and prevent harm." In the context of the plutonium experiments, it does not appear that a serious attempt was made to prevent harm from occurring. There was an attempt to refine the methods used so as to reduce the likelihood and magnitude of harm, but no more. Finally, the sixth principle is, "one ought to respect the self-determination of others." This principle was violated beyond a reasonable doubt, because the investigators routinely ignored the right to consent to bodily invasions following adequate disclosures.

I believe that it would not require much ingenuity to show that the Advisory Committee *implicitly* recognized that all six of its principles were violated in the plutonium cases. However, the Committee's failure to reach the explicit conclusion that all six principles were violated is not insignificant. The Committee identified its set of principles in order to provide a comprehensive account of what could be reasonably expected of persons. It aimed for a complete assessment of past practices in order to reduce the risk of errors and abuses in future human experimentation. The Committee insisted that, in light of these goals, a "complete and accurate diagnosis requires not only stating what wrongs were done, but also explaining who was responsible for the wrongs occurring" (ACHRE 1995 [GPO, p. 212; Oxford, p. 123]).

Underassessment of the number of principles violated is an unfortunate outcome. Perhaps it is but a minor error in the Advisory Committee's report, but I note that the same type of error afflicts the report of the UCSF Ad Hoc Committee.[5] If the Advisory Committee hoped to affect the thinking of future committee members on committees like the one at UCSF, it would have been instructive to show that and how all six principles had been violated.

WHAT FINDINGS SHOULD HAVE BEEN REACHED ABOUT EXCULPATORY CONDITIONS?

Is the ineffectual professional ethics during the period in question a condition that mitigates blame (an exculpatory condition)? Yes. Does this condition erase the wrongs done to research subjects? No. Judgments of wrongdoing are not affected by exculpatory conditions. Does the ineffectual professional ethics exculpate the agents involved? No. A weak professional ethics merely mitigates (tempers, lessens the severity of) blame; it does not clear of blame or exculpate. I will address exculpation in a moment. The immediate question is about exculpatory conditions and how they are related to the void in professional standards: What conditions are exculpatory? Why are they exculpatory? To what degree do they exculpate?

As previously noted, the Committee identified a set of exculpatory or mitigating conditions: lack of evidence; the presence of conflicting obligations, including obligations to protect national security; factual ignorance; culturally induced moral ignorance; an evolution in the delineation of moral principles; and indeterminacy in an organization's division of labor and designation of responsibility. To these conditions we might add that blame could be mitigated by culturally induced misunderstandings, by a person's good character, and by what in law is called "excusable neglect" (caused by an unavoidable hindrance or accident).

Only three of these conditions need assessment here because of the role they play in the plutonium cases: (1) factual ignorance, (2) culturally induced moral ignorance, and (3) obligations to protect national security.

Factual Ignorance

The Advisory Committee never argues that a significant measure of nonculpable factual ignorance was operative in the UCSF case. The

Committee is commendably clear that claims of nonculpable factual ignorance can too easily function as an excuse for wrongful actions (and, by inference, for failures to make retrospective moral judgments):

> [J]ust because an agent's ignorance of morally relevant information leads him or her to commit a morally wrong act, it does not follow that the person is not blameworthy for that act. The agent is blameworthy if a reasonably prudent person in that agent's position should have been aware that some information was required prior to action, and the information could have been obtained without undue effort or cost on his or her part. (ACHRE 1995 [GPO, p. 208; Oxford, p. 121])

Culturally Induced Moral Ignorance

A claim of culturally induced moral ignorance also lacks credible backing in the UCSF case. Even if we grant that there were no strong cultural incentives to abstain from the research and little instruction in medical ethics, it is not too much to expect these physicians to have been aware that their actions required a justification other than the experiment's utility for others. Never in the history of civil medicine has it been permissible to exploit patients by using them to the ends of science in nontherapeutic research that carries risk of harm. It is worth remembering that in the plutonium cases, the problem is not merely that no *informed* consent was obtained. No consent at all was obtained.

Culturally induced beliefs, such as the belief that consent is not morally required in a hospital setting, are most likely to constitute a valid excuse for wrong actions when alternative views are unavailable or are not taken seriously in the context. But alternative views were available and were considered matters of the utmost significance in sources available to the relevant parties. It was known or easily knowable at the time: (1) that a debate had occurred during the mid-1940s about experimentation in Nazi Germany; (2) that the AMA Judicial Council had sided in 1946 with what would soon be the Nuremberg view that voluntary consent to participation in research is essential; (3) that the Hippocratic tradition required physicians to put the care of patients first, not to deviate radically from accepted therapies, and not to risk harm to patients through nontherapeutic interventions; and (4) that there was a long tradition of post-Hippocratic writings in medical ethics that included Thomas Percival, Claude Bernard, and Walter Reed, each of whom recognized nontherapeutic experimentation as valid only if subjects had consented.

Thus, requirements such as voluntary consent to experimentation and protection against harmful interventions had long been present in the medical community and even were present in some government policies traceable to the early 1940s (see Lederer and Moreno 1996).

In light of this history, the UCSF physicians could not plausibly appeal to nonculpable moral blindness, because they and the officials at their institutions, as well as responsible higher officials in medicine, could have been expected to remedy contextual moral ignorance. There was ample opportunity for remediation of inadequate moral beliefs and therefore culpability for the continuance of those beliefs. The excuse of *nonculpable ignorance,* then, is not credible.

Conflicting Obligations—The National Security Exception

The matter of mitigating conditions is, however, more complicated than nonculpable ignorance, because it might be argued that there was reason to believe that the research constituted a justifiable *exception* to ordinary physician obligations and government policies requiring compliance with established standards. In the UCSF case and others considered by the Advisory Committee, obligations to protect national security might be viewed as conflicting with and overriding obligations to protect human subjects. The so-called "national security exception" suggests that in order to survive as a nation and preserve a culture of freedom we can justifiably forfeit some measure of individual rights and interests—a classical utilitarian justification that promotes the public interest by asking for some sacrifice on the part of individual citizens. The Cold War struggle in the late 1940s could magnify the importance of this proposed exception; perhaps it could even serve as the sole justification for the research done with human subjects.

The Advisory Committee considers this argument in Chapter 4 and rightly blunts its force. The Committee maintains that appeals to national security would have unjustifiably caused investigators to lose sight of firm requirements of voluntary consent. Those requirements could have been satisfied by asking subjects for their permission after telling them that they would be injected with a radioactive substance that might be dangerous and would not be beneficial, but would help protect the health of persons involved in the war effort.

The culpability of agents in the plutonium cases might be mitigated by their conscientious and understandable interpretation of the need to protect workers in projects of great national significance, leading them to authorize or to perform the research. Government officials and possibly the physicians with whom they contracted could perhaps be found blameless because of the massive confusion surrounding the Cold War commitments and their general lack of familiarity with research medicine, but the Advisory Committee rightly rejected the plausibility of this claim, especially for government employees.

In some respects this defense is even less plausible for physicians. The special nature of the patient-physician relationship places a more stringent obligation on physicians to attend to the welfare of the patient, not merely their patients, but any patient with whom they are professionally involved. In clinical circumstances, patients defer to their physicians' judgment, and it seems transparent that these physicians capitalized on this deference and failed to adequately protect the welfare of their patients (a violation of the Advisory Committee's fourth principle).

The Advisory Committee also discredited the thesis that national security was ever formally invoked to justify these research efforts.

> [I]n none of the memorandums or transcripts of various agencies did we encounter a *formal* national security exception to conditions under which human subjects may be used. In none of these materials does any official, military or civilian, argue for the position that individual rights may be justifiably overridden owing to the needs of the nation in the Cold War. (ACHRE 1995 [GPO, p. 206; Oxford, p. 120])

In short, the evidence does not indicate that the agents themselves viewed their actions in this light, and even if they did, there were alternatives to the forms of exploitation of patients that occurred in the plutonium cases.

Culpability or Exculpation?

The final problem is whether judgments of exculpation or judgments of culpability follow from the foregoing analysis. Were the mitigating conditions sufficient to exculpate the agents? To this question, I believe the answer is, emphatically, "No." Weak training in professional ethics, embryonic federal policies, and parallel forms of ignorance, together with other mitigating conditions, temper the reach of possible judgments of blame, but they are not sufficient conditions of exculpation. Indeed, these conditions are only weakly exculpatory. Violation of the six basic universal principles is, by itself, sufficient for a judgment of culpability.

BEAUCHAMP • JUDGING OUR PREDECESSORS

Any intentional act of taking patients who were seriously ill and placing them at risk without their knowledge or consent in nontherapeutic research indicates culpability. The evidence suggests both that the physician-investigators knowingly exploited these patients and that sufficient opportunities existed for physicians to obtain relevant information in order to determine whether their actions were warranted. Even if responsibilities were not clearly assigned to individuals in institutions, and even if the effort involved numerous persons, sufficient guidelines and historical precedents still existed to make judgments of culpability. That federal officials and physicians associated with the plutonium cases were culpable seems to follow from the Advisory Committee's thesis that if the means to overcome cultural biases or relevant forms of ignorance are available to an agent, and the agent fails to take advantage of these means, the agent is culpable.

In reaching such conclusions, the Advisory Committee was right to insist that we can and should assess persons other than the UCSF investigators, including persons in positions of authority or responsibility for initiating the research and for overseeing it—government authorities as well as those with oversight responsibilities in medical and research institutions. Those responsible for setting, implementing, and overseeing standards for the conduct of research are at least as culpable as those who conducted the research.

CONCLUSION

All things considered, the performance of the physicians and government officials involved in the plutonium cases seems inexcusable. At the same time, the fairest conclusion in these cases may be that the various exculpatory conditions I have considered excuse the agents involved *to some degree*. The moral culpability of agents admits of degrees, and there are many degrees on the scale, depending upon what is known, what is believed, what is intended, and what is widely recognized and disseminated. For example, there are degrees of culpable moral ignorance in these cases, and it would be difficult to pinpoint the degree of culpable ignorance for any particular agent.

Perhaps it is enough, however, to be able to conclude that whatever the degrees of culpability, culpability there must be. A milder conclusion holds that it is enough in these cases to judge persons or institutions to be deficient in conduct, which itself carries a loss of status and reputation, without attaching the stigma of blame or inflicting punishments

KENNEDY INSTITUTE OF ETHICS JOURNAL • SEPTEMBER 1996

such as formal censure, invalidation of a license, or fines. Which among these possible conclusions did the Advisory Committee reach, and was it correct to take the course it did?

The Committee's even-handed Findings 10 and 11 (ACHRE 1995 [GPO, pp. 785-89; Oxford, pp. 502-4]) provide a clue. Here the Committee determines that physicians and government officials were "morally responsible in cases in which they did not take effective measures to implement" available government and professional standards. The most favorable interpretation of these findings, in light of the rest of the *Final Report,* is that the Committee is *blaming* government officials and associated physicians for moral failures. Despite its relatively polite language of "accountability" and "responsibility," the Committee's view strongly suggests that government officials and physicians in positions of leadership were culpable for their serious moral failures.

At the same time, in the attempt to be even-handed and not to stretch beyond the evidence—a key consideration in the Committee's deliberations and findings (Buchanan 1996)—the Committee reached conclusions that do not extend all the way to the culpability of individual physicians and government officials. In eschewing questions of individual culpability, the Advisory Committee risks reproach for indecisiveness, not unlike the criticisms I have offered of the UCSF Ad Hoc Committee. However, in assessing the fairness of such criticism of both the Advisory Committee and the UCSF committee, it should be remembered that these committees had a responsibility not to overstep the evidence, a task that becomes increasingly difficult in assessing the culpability of particular individuals.

It would also be rash to judge the Advisory Committee harshly for not investigating each government official and physician who might be blamed for wrongdoing. The Committee existed for little more than a year and did not have the means for a broadscale investigation of individuals. Nonetheless, I believe that sufficient evidence exists (and was available to the Committee) for judgments of culpability in the case of a number of individuals involved in the human radiation experiments. In the UCSF case alone, investigator Kenneth Scott himself strongly suggested physician culpability during the above-mentioned interview. The evidence in this case also indicates that principal investigator Robert Stone was guilty of the kind of negligence, errors of judgment, and moral failures that are sufficient for culpability.

If we cannot judge particular persons blameworthy in a case as clear as that of the UCSF plutonium injections, it is hard to see how to stop

BEAUCHAMP • JUDGING OUR PREDECESSORS

short of either exculpation or paralysis of judgment in a great many cases of serious past moral wrongs. This problem of line-drawing cannot be dismissed, as the Advisory Committee recognized, on grounds that it is too difficult for human judgment. We should be cautious but not incapacitated in the work of retrospective moral judgment. Cautiousness in making claims to have sufficient evidence of culpability is a virtue, but suspending judgment in the face of sufficient evidence is simply a failure to make the proper judgment.

The matter is complicated, of course, by questions of the proper criteria of sufficient evidence. More than one standard of evidence can be defended, and significant epistemological problems surround the defense of one standard over another. All evidence gathering assumes a theory of what counts as evidence, and two or more theories may support competing standards, making assertions of sufficiency inherently contestable. While this problem is of indisputable relevance to assessments of culpability, it does not provide an adequate reason to doubt the availability of a reasonable standard for making such assessments. In the present case, I do not believe that the standard would vary significantly from those used by the Advisory Committee for assessing wrongdoing.

The bigger problem is the amount of time it would have required to assemble the evidence properly in each particular case, given the lapse of 50 years and the many gaps of information as to what did and did not happen at the time. Time was not available for all cases to be handled appropriately, nor could all the desired evidence have been acquired (Buchanan 1996). Since it generally is less time-consuming to assemble evidence of sufficient quality to assess culpable nonperformance within the professions than to assemble comparable evidence for culpable wrongdoing on the part of each individual, it is easy to understand why the Advisory Committee reached the conclusions it did. But with more careful collection and sifting of the evidence in individual cases, the quality of the evidence may turn out to be as good as the evidence of general institutional culpability in medicine and government.

A judgmental person is a fool, but fear of rendering a foolish judgment sometimes induces an unwarranted reserve. Such restraint appears to have unjustifiably inhibited decision making by the UCSF Ad Hoc Committee. The Advisory Committee cannot be similarly evaluated, because it was decisive beyond what might reasonably have been anticipated in light of its broad and diverse mission. However, it seems likely that the Advisory Committee's revealing findings are no more than a starting point for judgments of individual culpability that we can expect and should encourage in the ongoing work on the subject of the human radiation experiments.

NOTES

1. In presenting the facts in the UCSF case, some parts of my discussion derive from the Advisory Committee's Final Report, but most derive from the Ad Hoc Committee's Report. All the facts were well known to the Advisory Committee, which discusses the UCSF case in Chapter 5.
2. The amount of plutonium injected was approximately 0.1 percent of the LD50 in rats and 0.35 percent of the LD50 in dogs.
3. The oral history was conducted by medical historian Sally Hughes.
4. See Elizabeth A. Zitrin and Roy A. Filly. UCSF, "Report of the UCSF Ad Hoc Fact Finding Committee," Letters, Appendices. Filly's response is reported by Keay Davidson (1995).
5. For an excellent example of this error, see the personal statement by UCSF committee member Mack Roach III (UCSF 1995, Appendices).

REFERENCES

ACHRE. Advisory Committee on Human Radiation Experiments. 1995. *Final Report.* Washington, DC: U.S. Government Printing Office. Subsequently published as: *The Human Radiation Experiments.* New York: Oxford University Press, 1996. [Pagination for both volumes is provided in the text cites.]

Buchanan, Allen. 1996. The Controversy over Retrospective Moral Judgment. *Kennedy Institute of Ethics Journal* 6: 245–50.

Chapman, T. S. 1946. Memorandum: To Area Engineer, Berkeley Area (30 December). ACHRE No. DOE-112194-D-3.

Davidson, Keay. 1995. Questions Linger on 1940s UCSF Plutonium Shots. *The San Francisco Examiner* (23 February): A6.

Ex-owner of Toxic Site Wins Ruling on Damages. 1994. *New York Times* (18 March): 5B.

Lederer, Susan E., and Moreno, Jonathan D. 1996. Revising the History of Cold War Research Ethics. *Kennedy Institute of Ethics Journal* 6: 223-37.

UCSF. University of California at San Francisco. 1995. *Report of the UCSF Ad Hoc Fact Finding Committee on World War II Human Radiation Experiments.* (February, unpublished but released to the public.)

[8]

T wenty years ago Peter Buxtun, a public health official working for the United States Public Health Service, complained to a reporter for the Associated Press that he was deeply concerned about the morality of an ongoing study being sponsored by the Public Health Service—a study compiling information about the course and effects of syphilis in human beings based upon medical examinations of poor black men in Macon County, Alabama. The men, or more accurately, those still living, had been coming in for annual examinations for forty years. They were not receiving standard therapy for syphilis. In late July of 1972 the *Washington Star* and the *New York Times* ran front-page stories based on Buxtun's concerns about what has been called the longest running "nontherapeutic experiment" on human beings in medical history and "the most notorious

Arthur L. Caplan is director, Center for Biomedical Ethics, University of Minnesota, Minneapolis, Minn.

Arthur L. Caplan, "When Evil Intrudes," *Hastings Center Report* 22, no. 6 (1992): 29-32.

When Evil Intrudes

by Arthur L. Caplan

case of prolonged and knowing violation of subject's rights"—the Tuskegee study.[1]

Buxtun went public with his ethical concerns after years of complaining to officials from the Centers for Disease Control and the Public Health Service with no apparent effect. His decision to blow the whistle led to a series of sensational congressional hearings chaired by Senator Edward Kennedy in February and March of 1973. Legislators and federal officials expressed outrage over the immorality of a study in which poor, illiterate men had been deceived and given placebo treatment rather than standard therapy so that more could be learned about syphilis. Americans

found it hard to believe that the Public Health Service had intentionally and systematically duped men with a disease as serious as syphilis—contagious, disabling, and life-threatening—for more than forty years.

The level of outrage about the Tuskegee study was enormous. One CDC official labeled the experiment akin to "genocide."[2] As a result of public anger over the immorality of the study, Congress created an ad hoc blue ribbon panel to review both the Tuskegee study and the adequacy of existing protections for subjects in all federally sponsored research. Even though the panel did not receive all the information about the study that the government had available,[3] they were still concerned enough about what had taken place to recommend the creation of a national board with the resources to reexamine all aspects of human experimentation in the United States. Congress, in 1974, created the National Commission for the Protection of Human Subjects of Biomedical and Behavioral Research which, in its seventeen reports and numerous appendix volumes, laid the foundation for the ethical requirements that govern the conduct of re-

Hastings Center Report, November-December 1992

"SYPHILIS VICTIMS GOT NO THERAPY"

The experiment, called the Tuskegee Study, began in 1932 with about 600 black men, mostly poor and uneducated, from Tuskegee, Ala., an area that had the highest syphilis rate in the nation at the time.

. . .

As incentives to enter the program, the men were promised free transportation to and from hospitals; free hot lunches; free medicine for any disease other than syphilis and free burial after autopsies were performed.

. . .

Of the decision not to give penicillin to the untreated syphilitics once it became widely available, Dr. Miller [chief of the venereal disease branch of the Centers for Disease Control in 1972] said, "I doubt that it was a one-man decision. These things rarely are. Whoever was director of the VD section at that time, in 1946 or 1947, would be the most logical candidate if you had to pin it down".

New York Times
26 July 1972

search on human subjects in the United States to this day.

Syphilis continues to challenge America's and the world's medical, public health, and moral resources. While there are a variety of antibiotics available to treat the disease, it has proven to be a stubborn and resilient foe. The Centers for Disease Control has found steady and alarming increases in the incidence of primary and secondary syphilis over the past decade. It is still a major public health problem in the United States today, especially among young black males.

The rise in the incidence of the disease has ensured that writings about the diagnosis, management, and treatment of syphilis are prominently featured in the professional literature of public health and biomedicine as well as in standard textbooks about venereal and infectious diseases. Ongoing concern about syphilis has led physicians and public health officials to draw upon as much information as they can about the course of the disease. One of the bitter if generally unacknowledged ironies of the Tuskegee study is that, while it now occupies a special place of shame in the annals of human experimentation, its findings are still widely cited by the contemporary biomedical community.

In looking at instances of scientific misconduct and moral malfeasance with respect to research it is quite common to find the position advanced that good science is incompatible with bad ethics. When one wrestles with the horror of the medical abuse of vulnerable human beings it is somewhat comforting to believe that those who engage in such abuse could not produce anything of real value to medicine. Yet the continuing invocation of the findings of the Tuskegee study by those who diagnose, study, or treat syphilis shows that it is sometimes impossible to avoid a confrontation with the question of the ethics of relying on knowledge obtained in the course of immoral research.

The "bad ethics, therefore bad science" argument actually has two distinct components. One part of the argument holds that researchers engaged in obvious immoral conduct with their subjects could not generate useful or valid scientific findings. The second part holds that when the ethical conduct of research is egregiously immoral then any findings obtained ought not to be admitted into the body of scientific knowledge. While it may often be true that it is difficult to trust findings obtained using subjects who were abused or harmed (as was the case in Nazi concentration camp studies),[4] this part of the argument is not always true. Even a cursory glance through the literature of health care reveals that the Tuskegee study was and remains a key source of information about the diagnosis, signs, symptoms, and course of syphilis. No effort has been made to impugn its findings, and the biomedical community has relied upon them for decades.

James Jones, in his landmark book on the Tuskegee study, *Bad Blood*, notes that no researcher involved in the study ever published a single, comprehensive summary of its findings. The absence of such a review paper may have fostered the impression that no substantive findings of any real significance were obtained. But Jones also notes in the appendix to his book that Public Health Service scientists, physicians, and nurses associated with the study published a total of thirteen articles between 1936 and 1973 based solely upon its findings. These papers appeared in a wide variety of peer-reviewed journals, including *Public Health Reports*, *Milbank Fund Memorial Quarterly*, *Journal of Chronic Diseases*, and *Archives of Internal Medicine*.

It is a relatively simple matter to establish the importance assigned to the findings of the Tuskegee study by the contemporary biomedical community. The computerization on large data bases of the majority of the world's professional biomedical journals allows searches to be conducted to see which, if any, recent journal articles cite any of the thirteen papers presenting the findings of the Tuskegee study. An initial database search for the period January 1985 to February 1991 produced twenty such citations from a wide spectrum of journals, including American, British, and German publications. The twenty citations make reference to seven of the original thirteen papers.

A visit to any large medical library will also quickly reveal the importance assigned to the findings of the Tuskegee study in recent years. An informal random selection of twenty medical textbooks on sexually transmitted diseases, infectious disease, human sexuality, and public health published after 1984 turned up four books that made explicit reference to the study and cited at least one of the same thirteen articles. Three textbooks were published in the United States, one in England.

The range of journals in which contemporary articles on syphilis, venereal disease, and dementia directly cite the papers reporting the findings of the Tuskegee study is quite large. Direct citations of the Tuskegee study papers appear in articles in the

30

Hastings Center Report, November-December 1992

Journal of Family Practice (1986), *The Lancet* (1986), *British Heart Journal* (1987), *New England Journal of Medicine* (1987), *Journal of the American Geriatrics Society* (1989), *The American Journal of Medicine* (1989), *American Journal of Public Health* (1989), and *Medical Clinics of North America* (1990), among others.

Nearly all the references in both the periodical literature and the medical textbooks use the Tuskegee study to describe the natural history of the disease. A recent review article on cardiovascular syphilis is typical of the way in which the Tuskegee study and its findings are cited:

In 1932, the United States Public Health Service initiated the Tuskegee Study to delineate further the natural history of untreated syphilis. A total of 412 men with untreated syphilis and 204 uninfected matched controls were followed prospectively. Vonderlehr (15), reviewing the autopsy material from the first years of the study, noted that only one-fourth of the untreated patients were without evidence of any form of tertiary syphilis after 15 years of infection. Moreover, cardiovascular involvement was the most frequently detected abnormality. Peters (16) analyzed the autopsy data from the first 20 years of the study. He found that 50% of patients who had been infected for 10 years had demonstrable cardiovascular involvement. Of the 40% of syphilitic patients who died during this period, the primary causes of death were cardiovascular or central nervous system syphilis (16). Of the 41% of survivors at 30 years of follow-up, 12% had clinical evidence of late, predominantly cardiovascular syphilis (17). Most of these patients had evidence of cardiovascular syphilis at the 15-year analysis (17). These data . . . indicate that . . . complications are usually evident 10 to 20 years after primary infection, and cardiovascular syphilis is the predominant cause of demise in those patients who die as a direct result of syphilis.[5]

The reference numbers 15, 16, and 17 in the excerpt are to three of the thirteen papers reporting the findings of the Tuskegee study.

Yet another representative example from the contemporary periodical literature of health care invoking the findings of the Tuskegee study appears in a review of neurosyphilis and dementia:

Neurosyphilis is rare as a manifestation of syphilis. Tertiary and late latent syphilis have been decreasing in incidence since the 1950s. There have been two studies of untreated syphilis: in the Oslo study neurosyphilis eventually developed in 7% of the patients, and in the Tuskegee study, syphilitic involvement of the cardiovascular system or the central nervous system was the primary cause of death in 30% of the infected patients, with cardiovascular involvement being much more common than neurosyphilis.[6]

Textbook references are quite similar to those that appear in the periodical literature. In giving an overview of the natural course of untreated syphilis one recent text states:

A prospective study involving 431 black men with seropositive latent syphilis of 3 or more years' duration was undertaken in 1932 (the Tuskegee study, 1932-1962) (16). This study showed that hypertension in syphilitic black men 25-50 years of age was 17 percent more common than in nonsyphilitics. Cardiovascular complications including hypertension were more common than neurologic complications were, and both were increased over control populations. Anatomic evidence of aortitis was found to be 25-35 percent more common in autopsied syphilitics, while evidence of central nervous system syphilis was found in 4 percent of the patients.[7]

Reference number 16 is to one of the thirteen papers in which the Tuskegee findings were presented.

These examples clearly illustrate the continuing importance assigned to the Tuskegee study by those concerned with understanding and treating syphilis. The case for the study's importance could be further bolstered by tracking down secondary and tertiary references to its findings. There can be no disputing the fact that contemporary medicine has accepted the findings as valid and continues to rely on them as a key source of knowledge about the natural history of the disease.

The acceptance of the Tuskegee study findings as valid refutes the argument that bad ethics is always incompatible with valid science, but the question still remains as to whether the data of the Tuskegee study should continue to be utilized. It may make sense in some situations to argue that data obtained by immoral means should not be used purely on ethical grounds. But even if it were wrong to cite data acquired by immoral means there is simply no way to purge the knowledge gained in the Tuskegee study from biomedicine. Too much of what is known about the natural history of syphilis is based upon the study, and that knowledge has become so deeply embedded that it could not be removed.

Still, the view that the study was immoral and therefore worthless has flourished. This is a cause for concern, because the belief that not much of value came from the Tuskegee study allows both medicine and bioethics to avoid examining such troubling questions as how immoral research could be conducted by reputable scientists under the sponsorship of the American government for forty years, how such research could be allowed to continue long after the promulgation of the Nuremberg and Helsinki Codes, and what the moral duties and responsibilities are of those in biomedicine who continue to cite the study's findings today.

While one of the textbooks that discusses the Tuskegee study does make reference to the ethical shadow hanging over the findings,[8] none of the others and none of the articles in the peer-reviewed periodical literature that directly cite the papers based on the study do so. Should the results of the Tuskegee study continue to be invoked in review articles and texts without some accompanying discussion of the manner in which the findings were obtained and the ethical impact that the study had on the subsequent responsibilities of re-

Hastings Center Report, November-December 1992

searchers? Given that the study played a crucial role in causing Americans to rethink the ethics of human experimentation, it would seem morally incumbent upon those who discuss its findings in the context of textbooks and review articles to allot some space for a discussion of the ethical problems associated with it.

There are obvious limits to the extent to which anyone writing a scientific paper or book can review the circumstances and conditions under which scientific knowledge was obtained. The history of medicine is replete with examples of research, certainly considered immoral by contemporary standards, that generate findings still widely accepted and cited. Not every article in a scientific journal can be used as a vehicle for educating the reader about the morality of human experimentation.

But there are obvious forums in biomedicine, such as textbooks and review articles, where it makes sense for authors to include some discussion of the ethical circumstances surrounding morally dubious or blatantly immoral research. The obvious immorality of research methods should not blind us to the importance of noting and discussing them. If no place is made for discussions of the morality of studies such as Tuskegee, the research community may become complacent about the importance of its responsibilities toward human subjects at the same time as the public comes to believe that good science cannot emerge from immoral research.

References

1. Stephen B. Thomas and Sandra C. Quinn, "The Tuskegee Syphilis Study, 1932 to 1972: Implications for HIV Education and AIDS Risk Education Programs in the Black Community," *American Journal of Public Health* 81, no. 11 (1991): 1498-1505, at 1501; Ruth Faden and Tom Beauchamp, *A History and Theory of Informed Consent* (New York: Oxford, 1986), p. 165.

2. James H. Jones, *Bad Blood: The Tuskegee Syphilis Experiment* (New York: Free Press, 1981), p. 207.

3. Jay Katz, personal communication, 1991.

4. See Arthur Caplan, ed., *When Medicine Went Mad* (New York: Humana, 1992).

5. J. D. Jackson and J. D. Radolf, "Cardiovascular Syphilis," *The American Journal of Medicine* 87 (October 1989): 428-29.

6. J. A. Rhymes, C. Woodson, R. Sparage-Sachs, and C. K. Cassel, "Nonmedical Complications of Diagnostic Workup for Dementia: University of Chicago Grand Rounds," *Journal of the American Geriatrics Society* 37, no. 12 (1989): 1157-64, at 1160.

7. G. L. Mandell, R. G. Douglas, Jr., and J. E. Bennett, eds., *Principles and Practice of Infectious Diseases*, 3rd ed. (New York: Churchill Livingstone, 1990), p. 1797.

8. K. K. Holmes, P. Mardh, P. F. Sparling, and P. J. Wiesner, *Sexually Transmitted Diseases*, 2nd ed. (New York: McGraw-Hill, 1990).

T wenty years ago, when the *Washington Star* told the public that the United States Public Health Service had, since 1932, maintained a study of untreated syphilis in the Negro male that was *still* going on, my reaction was, How could people have done this? I later worked on the participants' lawsuit, and I learned of the study's many complexities. In the end, though, the best explanation of "how" it could have happened is the obvious one: the researchers did not see the participants as part of "their" community or, indeed, as people whose lives could or would be much affected by what the researchers did.

Looking back on those events after two decades, there are a number of observations I'd like to make.

Tuskegee under the Law

First, I should like to describe some aspects of the legal landscape of the

Harold Edgar is Julius Silver Professor of Law, Science and Technology at The Columbia University Law School, New York, N.Y.

Harold Edgar, "Outside the Community," *Hastings Center Report* 22, no. 6 (1992): 32-35.

[9]

Sissela Bok

Shading the Truth in Seeking Informed Consent for Research Purposes*

> Much of our lives is taken up by truth-seeking, imagining, questioning. We relate to facts through truth and truthfulness, and come to recognize and discover that there are different modes and levels of insight and understanding.
>
> Iris Murdoch, *Metaphysics as a Guide to Morals*

ABSTRACT. I want to argue for two propositions. First, I suggest that what some researchers may take to be a simple trade-off between minor violations of the truth for the sake of access to far greater truths represents a profound miscalculation with far-reaching and cumulative reverberations. Second, I submit that today's research environment, as demanding, competitive, and sometimes bewildering as it is, offers genuine scope for what Murdoch calls truth-seeking, for imagining and questioning, and for relating to facts through both truth and truthfulness; but that, in so doing, it presents hard choices with respect to methods, and, in turn, to personal integrity—not only in particular research projects but also with respect to that fragile research environment in its own right.

IN EXPLORING THE problems of shading the truth in research, I want to draw on Iris Murdoch's view, expressed in the passage above, of human beings as engaged in "truth-seeking, imagining, questioning," and as relating to facts "through truth and truthfulness" (Murdoch 1992, p. 26). It may appear paradoxical that investigators should shade the truth in order to gain greater insight into the truth: that they should invent elaborate scenarios for hiding or distorting the truth in their dealings with human subjects in order to shine a more powerful light on truths that might otherwise remain concealed. But there is no paradox in

---

*This article is based on the 1994 André Hellegers Lecture at the Kennedy Institute of Ethics. An earlier version of this lecture was presented at a June 1994 Symposium on "Issues in the Conduct of Research: What Is Happening to American Science?" at the Harvard Program in the Practice of Scientific Investigation.

KENNEDY INSTITUTE OF ETHICS JOURNAL • MARCH 1995

so doing, least of all if we see their effort at truth-seeking rather as an attempt to relate to facts, in Murdoch's terms, through truth but at the expense of truthfulness.

I want to argue for two propositions. First, I suggest that what some researchers may take to be a simple trade-off between minor violations of the truth for the sake of access to far greater truths represents a profound miscalculation with far-reaching and cumulative reverberations. Second, I submit that today's research environment, as demanding, competitive, and sometimes bewildering as it is, offers genuine scope for what Murdoch calls truth-seeking, for imagining and questioning, and for relating to facts through both truth and truthfulness; but that, in so doing, it presents hard choices with respect to methods, and, in turn, to personal integrity—not only in particular research projects but also with respect to that fragile research environment in its own right.

Scientists have long insisted on the need for scrupulous honesty in the reporting of research *results*. The entire scientific undertaking rests on the degree to which investigators communicate their results accurately to one another and to the public at large. Otherwise, the testing of new results will be obstructed and efforts to build on them for further research will be undermined. But the call for scrupulous honesty with human subjects has been far less insistent. It is no accident that the requirement for adequate informed consent of subjects has made such a tardy appearance in the armamentarium of research ethics, when compared with the long-standing stress on veracity and accuracy in the communication of research results. Furthermore, stricter regulation of how informed consent is actually sought in practice has come about only after repeated revelations of abuses of the rights of human subjects.

It is only right, in view of such abuses, that the informed consent requirement, when it was finally taken seriously, should have been stressed primarily for the sake of the subjects themselves. But there is no reason to think only of averting potential risks to them; indeed, doing so has relegated to the penumbra—to the shade—questions about the risks that the practice of bypassing fully informed consent might carry both for investigators and for the research environment in which they operate.

Leaving such questions out of account can be especially tempting to investigators who believe that fully informed subjects would either refuse to take part in an investigation or would respond in misleading ways. Say you are seeking important information regarding the effects on children of parental alcoholism or abuse and need to supplement it with probing interviews with parents and children. Will you provide adequate information about the aims and methods of your study to the participants? And if you do, how trustworthy do you imagine their responses will be?

But isn't that the role of IRB's? Isn't it up to them to flag research proposals that conceal the true aims of studies from subjects? IRB's do indeed flag many such proposals, but not all (Mishkin 1994). We all know the horror stories, some very recent, of subjects misled about research in which they would have had every reason to refuse to participate. My concern here, however, is with the far more numerous proposals for shading the truth that seem so innocuous that they slide through IRB's with little or no debate.

I shall consider such proposals in biomedical research and in psychology separately, since the acceptance of deceptive research in psychology is so much more out in the open. To use an analogy from the period of the Iran-Contra scandal: the hesitant, roundabout, often secretive proposals for misleading subjects in *biomedical research* call to mind the approach of John Poindexter, National Security Adviser under President Ronald Reagan, whereas the flamboyant acknowledgment of outright lying along with more subtly deceptive schemes in *social psychology* are more like the brazen statements by Oliver North, staff member in the National Security Council at the time. Poindexter indicated, in explaining his actions, that "Our objective here all along was to withhold information;" Colonel North minced no words in declaring that "We had to choose between lives and lies" (Truth... 1987). And just as both Poindexter and North took for granted that the overriding rationale legitimizing deceit was the advancement of national security, so researchers defending duplicitous research may invoke as their rationale the advancement of knowledge, or even of truth itself.

BIOMEDICAL RESEARCH

In January 1992, I was asked to write an editorial in the *Journal of the American Medical Association,* on the occasion of the publication in that journal of a study raising questions about shading the truth for research purposes (Bok 1992b).[1] The study's stated objective was "To determine the prevalence of recent cocaine use and the reliability of patient self-reported cocaine use" (McNagny and Parker 1992, p. 1106). The participants were "male patients, aged 18 to 39 years, presenting to the triage desk for immediate care" in an inner-city walk-in clinic in

[3]

KENNEDY INSTITUTE OF ETHICS JOURNAL • MARCH 1995

Atlanta, Georgia (p. 1106). These men, over 90 percent of whom were black, were asked to participate in a study about asymptomatic carriage of sexually transmitted diseases and were told that their urine would be tested for STDs. Unbeknownst to them, their urine would also be tested for illicit drugs. All information linking their names to drug testing results would be removed. A local human studies committee had approved both studies. The information about drug use obtained in the second study was then compared to answers the subjects gave on a questionnaire. The authors concluded that the results of the study "…underscore the magnitude of cocaine abuse among black, inner-city men. Patient self-report of illicit drug usage is highly inaccurate. Accuracy of self-report may be increased by asking less specific questions" (McNagny and Parker 1992, p. 1106).

The methodology of this study has to intrigue anyone concerned with questions of truth, truthfulness, and deceit in research. It involved these factors at three levels: it aimed, first, to reveal the truth about the subjects' cocaine use and, second, to test the degree of truthfulness or deceit in their responses. Third, in order to achieve these two aims, subjects were to be deceived about both. There were to be no outright lies, but the truth would be shaded in one of the dictionary senses of "to shade": "To conceal from view, to hide partially, as by a shadow; to veil, obscure; to disguise" *(Oxford English Dictionary)*.

As the authors stated in their article: "Patients were not told that their urine would be analyzed for cocaine metabolites; however, patients were never told that their urine would *not* be tested for drugs" (McNagny and Parker 1992, p. 1106). In other words, the investigators were not planning to lie outright, in the sense of making a statement they knew to be false with the intent of misleading their subjects. But in concealing the aim of their study, they would be attempting to deceive unwary subjects about this aim as fully as if they had lied.

Ordinarily, research protocols that bypass informed consent in such ways would be dismissed out of hand by human studies committees. Imagine if investigators in one of the radiation experiments that has recently come to light (McCally, Cassel, and Kimball 1994) explained that: Patients were not told that their testicles would be exposed to radiation to determine the effects, if any, of such radiation; however, patients were never told that their testicles would *not* be thus exposed to radiation.

What, then, could have been the justification for bypassing informed consent in the Atlanta study? No one can know for sure without being

[4]

BOK • SHADING THE TRUTH

privy to the IRB deliberations about the study. But one or more of four claims may have been advanced. The first is that there could be no serious problem with the informed consent procedure employed, since the participants had been asked to consent both to give a urine specimen and to submit to being interviewed about illicit drug use. True, they had not been told that there was to be a study connecting the two elements, much less about the study's aims; but why would that be necessary so long as they had consented to the different elements of the study?

This interpretation of informed consent is inadequate, however; for so long as subjects do not know the aims of the second study, they cannot weigh its risks to themselves. This is precisely why the canons of research ethics, such as the Nuremberg Code or the Declaration of Helsinki, traditionally insist that the *aims* of a study must be explained to prospective subjects along with the methods to be employed and the anticipated benefits and potential risks.

A second argument is equally specious: that by coming to the clinic the subjects had somehow consented in advance to studies about which they would agree to ignore the aims. By no stretch of the imagination can such consent be presumed. Unlike placebo trials, properly conducted, in which subjects do give their fully informed consent to the very fact that they will be kept ignorant of certain aspects of the study, no such prior consent had been asked of the men in the Atlanta study.

A third argument for viewing the Atlanta research proposal as acceptable despite its bypassing of genuine informed consent holds that the participants did not need to be able to weigh risks to themselves since the study carried no such risks. To be sure, it concerned sensitive information regarding illicit drug use that the subjects might well have taken to present risks had they been asked for genuine consent; but the investigators aimed to eliminate those risks by removing the identity number linking study subjects and consent forms prior to the urine drug testing (McNagny and Parker 1992, p. 1107).

This argument fails on several grounds, however. Efforts to preserve confidentiality and remove links between participants and study data are far from foolproof; the point about the informed consent requirement is precisely that subjects ought to have the right to weigh risks for themselves *even* if they turn out to be wrong from an objective point of view. When it comes to highly sensitive information, participants, once informed of a study's aims, ought to have the right to refuse to participate for whatever reasons they choose to take seriously. Their freedom

[5]

KENNEDY INSTITUTE OF ETHICS JOURNAL • MARCH 1995

to do so serves not only to protect their autonomy but also to guard against errors and possible abuses that can creep into the research process and the review process, when it is left up to investigators and human studies committees to decide when to bypass informed consent.[2] Once investigators begin to take for granted that they can ignore the requirement for informed consent regarding sensitive information on risk-benefit grounds, the traditional protections for human subjects will themselves be threatened.[3]

To be sure, there are types of medical research where informed consent is unnecessary or impossible to obtain or beside the point, as in many statistical and other studies of past medical records or body fluids routinely gathered and part of existing databases. There will also always be difficult borderline cases between adequate and inadequate consent procedures. But by no stretch of the imagination can one argue that misleading people intentionally about the aims of a prospective study concerning sensitive information renders them adequately informed.

In this particular study, moreover, it would not have been far-fetched for participants to have looked quite differently at the risks. They may have had reason to be leery of assurances about confidentiality and anonymity, above all where violations of the law, such as cocaine consumption, were involved. They may have felt targeted, as inner-city black men, and concerned that the publication of the test results might contribute to their being labeled as a group in a discrediting manner. Furthermore, to the extent that they learned, after the fact, of deceptive studies such as the one to which they had unwittingly been subjected, they would have greater reason than before to be skeptical of the hospital in question—where, after all, they had come for medical help, not to take part in any studies—and possibly of health professionals more generally. Such doubts could add to their reluctance to seek medical help in the future and to speak candidly enough with health professionals to receive the best possible advice.

A traditional response to such objections, familiar from debates in anthropology and the social sciences, is to say there is no need to consider the risks that certain categories of participants will learn about the results of invasive studies in which they have unwittingly participated. Too many investigators and members of IRB's take for granted that participants, to the extent that they are poor, ill, uneducated, and culturally isolated, are unlikely to have access to scholarly journals or books. But, as Margaret Mead (1961) and others[4] have pointed out, discredit-

[6]

ing information published about members of any group or society, however distant, has an astounding way of traveling back to them.

The final argument for proceeding with the study even in the face of
such objections admits that preference should ideally be given to nondeceptive studies of "patient reliability" on sensitive issues, such as cocaine
use; but holds that the deceptive bypassing of informed consent is nevertheless called for, given the importance of the information sought,
when nondeceptive methods cannot achieve the desired results. In such
a case, would not the possible contribution of such a study to the scientific knowledge outweigh whatever minor or remote risks investigators
envisage for participants?

The implicit basis for this argument is, once again, the initial cost-benefit weighing made by investigators. In the concern for truth-seeking, the
overriding of traditional requirements of truthfulness toward subjects
may seem a small price to pay. Again, however, such an argument overlooks the requirement that prospective participants, not only investigators and members of IRB's, be included among those who make the cost-
benefit evaluations, especially in studies involving sensitive information.
Given that this weighing of risks and benefits must also be allowed to
prospective participants, the question of whether to deal honestly with
persons asked to be in a study cannot legitimately be *part* of the investigators' weighing of benefits and risks.

In addition, it is important for everyone who plans or reviews studies
to examine with the greatest care both the claim regarding potential contributions to knowledge and the claim that no alternative, nondeceptive
study designs can achieve the same results. Doing so requires, in its own
right, truth-seeking and imagining, especially when ethical questions are
raised about a particular study. What is the genuine need for, and value
of, the information sought in proposals for each new study? And by
what means does one best cast about for imaginative, nondeceptive
approaches to study designs?

The latter question was at the center of the debate when I presented
my conclusions regarding the Atlanta proposal to a broadly interdisci-
plinary group of biostatisticians and other experts on study design (Bok
1992a). A number of nondeceptive research designs were discussed:
among them were variations of "randomized response" designs, which
allow investigators to probe sensitive questions without violating the
requirement for informed consent (see, e.g., Greenberg, Abernathy, and
Horwitz 1986); comparisons of different surveys of illicit drug usage

[7]

without urine testing, similar to the surveys often done of students and cheating; and a design in which people could be inducted into two entirely separate studies—one of questionnaire responses, the other of urine samples—and then told that there would be no connection, no matching, just a study of the proportions of correlations, to see whether there would be any discrepancies.

I conducted a miniature informal study with this group of experts. I asked them to reply, anonymously and untraceably, to the question of whether they would have passed the Atlanta study had they been members of the appropriate human studies committee. The results show that it is far from an open-and-shut case: eight would have voted to go ahead with the study; nineteen would have said no; and five would have abstained (Bok 1992a).

The arguments that qualify the informed consent requirement on the basis of cost-benefit analyses and estimates of risks to subjects by investigators and the absence of alternative study designs will not be found in the Nuremberg Code, the Declaration of Helsinki, or any codes of medical or scientific ethics. The authors of these documents likely would have been surprised, therefore, to find precisely these qualifications in a 1993 document published by the Office for Protection from Research Risks (OPRR). Concerning deceptive research, the OPRR guidelines indicate that

> [s]ometimes, particularly in behavioral research, investigators plan to withhold information about the real purpose of the research or even to give the subjects false information about some aspect of the research. This means that the subject's consent may not be fully informed. (OPRR 1993, p. 3–18—3–19)

In such cases, according to the OPRR, IRB's must consider risks to subjects. To receive a waiver of consent requirements, a study must present no more than minimal risk; the waiver must not adversely affect the rights and welfare of subjects; the waiver must be essential to the ability to carry out research; and "debriefing," or explaining the matters concealed from subjects to them afterwards, must "take place where possible" (OPRR 1993, p. 3–19).

PSYCHOLOGICAL RESEARCH

Can it be an accident that these same qualifications on requirements for informed consent, which are absent from traditional codes of medical research ethics, are nearly identical to qualifications long taken for

BOK • SHADING THE TRUTH

granted in psychological research? They are unequivocally set forth as guidelines for psychological research in the American Psychological Association's (APA) "Ethical Principles of Psychologists and Code of Conduct" (APA 1992). This document looks benignly at certain forms of deception, so long as they are directed only at research subjects. Even as the "Ethical Principles" insist that psychologists "not make *public* statements that are false, deceptive, misleading or fraudulent" [emphasis added] about their training or their publications, for example, it goes on to explain when deception is permitted in their *research* (APA 1992, 3.03, 6.15).

> (a) Psychologists do not conduct a study involving deception unless they have determined that the use of deceptive techniques is justified by the study's prospective scientific, educational, or applied value and that equally effective alternative procedures that do not use deception are not feasible.

> (b) Psychologists never deceive research participants about significant aspects that would affect their willingness to participate, such as physical risks, discomfort, or unpleasant emotional experiences. (APA 1992, 6.15 a, b)

According to the Code, any deception must be explained to participants as early as possible, preferably at the conclusion of their participation. But if "scientific or humane values justify delaying or withholding this information, psychologists take reasonable measures to reduce the risks of harm" (APA 1992, 6.18 b).

It stands to reason that prospective subjects would prefer to have the opportunity to judge for themselves the possibility of harm they run in psychological research—as, for instance, in Stanley Milgram's 1963 obedience study, which has since been replicated with variations on countless campuses across the world. Furthermore, it is unlikely that individuals who have been subjected to research they find intrusive, degrading, or otherwise objectionable would be sanguine about the assurances regarding psychologists' ability to "take reasonable measures to reduce the risks of harm." Given the range of severity of the impact on subjects of the knowledge they may acquire about themselves or others, the greater vulnerability of some subjects, the minimal amount of time usually devoted to debriefing, and the peculiar explanatory structures with which many investigators operate, the bland notion of "reduc[ing] the risks of harm" appears naive at best.

The APA guidelines, moreover, do not concern rare exceptions to standard provisions regarding informed consent. On the contrary, surveys of the social psychology literature indicate that the proportion of

KENNEDY INSTITUTE OF ETHICS JOURNAL • MARCH 1995

studies resorting to deceptive experimentation has increased from 36.8 percent in 1963, when Stanley Milgram published his original obedience studies, to 47 percent in 1983 (Fisher and Fyrberg 1994, p. 417). The vigorous debate that has ensued about the effects of deceptive studies on subjects has not impeded the growth in popularity of deception techniques. Indeed, the imagination that has gone into designing deceptive research scenarios has resulted in a proliferation of studies that go far beyond any simple form of shading the truth. Even if shading were defined, in this context, not merely as concealment, veiling, and disguise, but also in terms of penmanship, as penciling in shadows and light, many such scenarios involve the most vivid coloration.

While the risks to *subjects* from such scenarios, and the subjects' right to determine whether to take part in them, are treated cavalierly in the APA's code, two further sorts of risk are omitted from it altogether: possible damage to trust from deceptive practices, and possible risks run by the researchers engaging in such practices.

In contrast to the APA code, the Canadian Psychological Association's (CPA) "Canadian Code of Ethics for Psychologists" addresses the first of these types of risk. It adds an important caution to its paragraphs about deceptive research, namely, that psychologists, before proceeding with such research, ought to seek an independent review of the risks of a particular project to public or individual trust (CPA 1991, III.29). It is a caution that, if taken seriously in the United States, would surely argue for a vast retrenchment in the number of deceptive studies.[5]

Trust in most United States institutions has diminished, sometimes abruptly, since the 1960's. Science and social science are no exceptions. It would matter more than ever, therefore, for future authors of the APA "Ethical Principles" to weigh, as have their Canadian colleagues, the long-range cumulative effects of deceptive research practices on trust; and thus the effects of the conduct of individual researchers as well as of the standards set by the profession as a whole in its code of conduct. In so doing, psychologists in the United States might consult the writings of social theorists such as Kenneth Arrow (1974), Partha Dasgupta (1988), and Anthony Giddens (1994), who have studied the institutional costs of practices destructive of trust (see also, Bok 1989b, Ch. 2; 1990a). These authors have argued that trust is a public good, much like water and air, that can increase the efficiency of any system but also can atrophy or be depleted.

I share this view of trust as a social good (Bok 1990b, 1989b, forth-

BOK • SHADING THE TRUTH

coming 1995). Every human relationship, whether in families, on city blocks, in communities, or in professional contexts, thrives only as long as a minimum of trust can be maintained. When trust is damaged, through dishonesty, betrayal, or incompetence, these relationships suffer. It is far harder to regain trust, once lost, than to squander it in the first place.

Anthony Giddens has pointed, in *Beyond Left and Right* (1994, p. 4), to a shift with respect to trust in present-day societies. Time was when office-holders, scientists, professors, and others in positions of authority could count on a measure of initial respect and trust consonant with their positions. This is no longer the case, in part because that trust has been too often violated in the past, and in part because the institutions themselves generate less respect. Public officials, for example, can no longer count on automatic respect or trust merely as a result of their social position or authority. Rather, they have to earn what Giddens (1994, p. 4) calls "active trust:"

> Active trust is trust which has to be won, rather than coming from the tenure of preestablished social positions or gender roles. Active trust presumes autonomy rather than standing counter to it, and is a powerful source of social solidarity, since compliance is freely given rather than enforced by traditional constraints.

The same is true in biomedicine and in the social sciences: distrust may be unwarranted in the case of particular individuals, but is fed by reports of the abuses engaged in by others. Trust in a profession or an institution is lost through a combination of widely publicized misconduct by a few and innumerable infractions by a great many—all seemingly insignificant individually, but with a mounting cumulative effect.

Distrust of health professionals as well as of social scientists is already high. The difficulties in gathering census data and other types of information indicate how many in the public are suspicious of the motives of those who design and execute such studies. College students, who supply the majority of the subjects for social science research, have developed their own defensive strategies to confound investigators targeting them for deceptive research: if asked, many will recount their own imaginative counter-scenarios for tripping up research projects they find invasive or manipulative. They have learned to give as good as they get—something that generates, among those who devise deceptive research designs, still more ingenious efforts to catch students unaware.

Thus, for professionals, as for public servants, it is more important than ever to win back the active trust that they no longer can count on

[II]

KENNEDY INSTITUTE OF ETHICS JOURNAL • MARCH 1995

receiving automatically. Moreover, winning this active trust requires them to conduct themselves in a way that leaves no doubt about their acceptance of ordinary standards of honesty and fair treatment. From this point of view, there should be no difference between the honesty expected of researchers toward their colleagues and the public at large, on the one hand, and toward the subjects of their research, on the other; nor between the integrity expected of them with respect to their research *results* and their research *procedures*.

DECEPTION AND CHOICE

Anyone can make mistakes when it comes to lying and shading the truth, and be influenced by all manner of forces and temptations. But it is altogether different to *choose* to be someone who deals with people through deceit; and it is especially troubling when this choice seems to be imposed on individuals by their professions.

On this subject, Immanuel Kant and John Stuart Mill, whose moral views are often contrasted, agree. They both stress the deleterious effects of choosing deception and the importance of veracity, or truthfulness. In *Utilitarianism*, Mill speaks of the "cultivation in ourselves of a sensitive feeling on the subject of veracity" as a "sacred rule," since that feeling is

> one of the most useful, and the enfeeblement of that feeling one of the most hurtful, things to which our conduct can be instrumental; and [...] any, even unintentional, deviation from truth does that much toward weakening the trust-worthiness of human assertion, which is not only the principal of all present social well-being but the insufficiency of which does more than any one thing that can be named to keep back civilization, virtue, everything on which human happiness on the largest scale depends.... (Mill [1861] 1961, p. 349)

Mill contends that anyone who helps to diminish the reliance people can have in one another's word, "acts the part of one of their worst enemies." Advocates of deceptive research may not agree with Mill's judgment; but the fact is that they rarely even take into account the risk of damaging the climate of trust in which they have to operate. The same is true of the risks such research poses for *themselves* as moral agents, especially when they not only undertake practices of deceit, but also plan them and even teach such procedures to others.

The psychologist and bioethicist Thomas Murray has written about his experience, as a graduate student in social psychology, with the

BOK • SHADING THE TRUTH

socialization process connected to deceptive research and about the possible costs to the researchers themselves:

> In trying to make our laboratory so much like the world, do we sometimes succeed in making the world like the laboratory? When we learn to stage events and manage impressions, are we led to do the same with our other relationships? Do we eventually come to see people as so easily duped outside the laboratory as within it? (Murray 1980, p. 14)

What about "learning to lie with a completely straight face *and* a clear conscience" (Murray 1980, p. 14)? What psychic price, Murray asks, does the individual social psychologist pay? And what happens to the perceptions of graduate students, whose objections are wafted aside and whose path of professional advancement may appear to call for accommodation rather than critique of existing practices?

Immanuel Kant ([1798] 1978) could have been speaking to these graduate students, among others, on the choices open to them, in his last book, *Anthropology from a Pragmatic Point of View*. It represents his summing up of a course he had taught for many years on "anthropology" in the sense of what it means and should mean to be a human being. He considers, in Part II, the various meanings of "character," and the question of how to live with "the gift of morality"—the extraordinary possibility of *making* moral choices that no other living beings possess.

Character, Kant insists, is not carved in stone or imprinted upon us, like the characters of the alphabet from which the concept of moral character is derived; it is not traced into our personalities from our earliest years; it cannot be transmitted to us even by the finest schools, and often, in fact, does not develop at all. But when it does develop, it involves a choice: a chosen moral stance, free to all to make at all times: "A certain solemn resolution," as Kant put it, to be a principled person out of respect not only for other people but also for oneself (Kant [1798] 1978, p. 206).

In the absence of making the choice to lead a principled life, it is worthless, in his view, merely to wish somehow to become a better person. And just weighing arguments for and against particular actions, or making subjective cost-benefit calculations, is equally unlikely to provide trustworthy guidance. Individuals who do are like loose cannons, acting according to poorly understood requirements of the moment.

In this regard, Kant saw a complex interaction between dishonesty toward others and incomplete or twisted honesty toward oneself. The lie

KENNEDY INSTITUTE OF ETHICS JOURNAL • MARCH 1995

to others relies on and calls forth poor estimates about one's own responsibility, motives, and *treatment* of others as well as of oneself. In turn, such poor estimates diminish one's caution regarding further lies and ways of shading the truth.

As a result, the highest maxim, or subjective rule of life, for someone who wants to lead a principled life and to be someone of character, turns out to be, for Kant ([1798] 1978, p. 207), "uninhibited truthfulness toward oneself as well as in the behavior toward everyone else." This, Kant maintains, is the minimum requirement for treating people with the respect due them and oneself; and also the fullest expression of human dignity—trying to live up to that dignity in one's own life and respecting it enough in others not to knowingly mislead them or manipulate them.

Though Mill would have pointed to certain rare exceptions to what he called "the sacred rule" of veracity, he might well have concurred with Kant's linking internal and external truthfulness in this way. Likewise, Kant would have agreed with Mill about the cumulative deleterious effects on the climate of trust of individual departures from such a rule.

Two important challenges confront this view of two-way truthfulness, toward others and oneself. One concerns the notion of truth in its own right. Since it is never possible to know the full truth, why should it matter if we lie occasionally to serve some important purpose, such as the advancement of knowledge?

This argument blurs the concepts of truth and truthfulness, however; and I take it that Iris Murdoch, in stating that we are truth-seeking beings who relate to facts through both truth and truthfulness, had a distinction between the two very much in mind. The distinction is that between the epistemological domain of truth and falsity, and the moral domain of intended truthfulness or deception. We surely can never exhaust the domain of truth; but we can know far more clearly whether we intend to deal truthfully with others or to mislead them.[6]

The second challenge to Kant concerns his insistence on *uninhibited* truthfulness with oneself as well as with others. Surely it is impossible to avoid all self-deception, even if we can do much more to avoid deceiving others. Bombarded as we are with sensory impressions, we filter and shield ourselves from the outset, and do indeed "shade" ourselves from fuller knowledge of much that we might otherwise learn. We can deal with only a fraction of the information that comes our way, and manage even to distort a good deal of that.

BOK • SHADING THE TRUTH

In light of all that we now know about memory distortion and the brain mechanisms whereby we filter information, Kant might have amended his view somewhat. He might have spoken, not simply of uninhibited truthfulness toward oneself, but of *striving* for it rather than intentionally inhibiting it still further. I believe that he would have continued to insist that doing so is the only way to know whether we care about ourselves as moral agents, as persons of genuine responsibility and character.

Sometimes it is necessary to shield ourselves against intolerable or unwieldy knowledge. But the cumulative burden of unexamined shielding and distortion is great. It is true that we could not survive if bombarded ceaselessly by information of a useless, threatening, or unduly burdensome nature. But we struggle with such thick layers of bias and rationalization, compartmentalization and denial, that our choices suffer immeasurably unless we do our best to counteract their effects.[7] As Iris Murdoch wrote in an earlier book, *The Sovereignty of Good* (1985, p. 59): "The chief enemy of excellence in morality (and also in art) is personal fantasy: the tissue of self-aggrandizing and consoling wishes and dreams which prevents one from seeing what is there outside one."

We are misinformed often enough, blunder often enough, shield ourselves enough, and live in deep enough self-imposed shade. We must not add to those forms of distortion by intentionally choosing to engage in deception or self-deception. This is as true in biomedical and social science research as in all other fields. Kant's view of the link between truthfulness with oneself and with others and Murdoch's cautioning against personal fantasy are of crucial relevance for evaluating policies of shading the truth in seeking what must remain *informed* consent.

NOTES

1. The study in question was: Sally E. McNagny and Ruth M. Parker (1992), "High Prevalence of Recent Cocaine Use and the Unreliability of Patient Self-report in an Inner-city Walk-in Clinic." Additional discussion of this study appears in Beauchamp and Childress (1994, pp. 154–55).
2. I draw, in this paragraph and the following ones, on my editorial "Informed Consent in Tests of Patient Reliability" (Bok 1992b).
3. For a discussion of weighing risks in research, see Bok (1978).
4. See discussion and other references in Bok (1989a).
5. It speaks in more modulated and less self-congratulatorily bombastic terms

KENNEDY INSTITUTE OF ETHICS JOURNAL • MARCH 1995

than the APA document. It does not simply declare, in the indicative, that psychologists abide by moral principles or respect the rights of clients and subjects, for example, but holds that they *should* do so, or that they would do certain things if they seek to observe a certain principle.

6. I have discussed this distinction in "Is the Whole Truth Attainable?", in *Lying: Moral Choice in Public and Private Life* (Bok 1990b, Ch. 1).

7. Sentence quoted from Bok (1982, p. 71).

REFERENCES

APA. American Psychological Association. 1992. Ethical Principles of Psychologists and Code of Conduct. *American Psychologist* 47: 1597–1611.

Arrow, Kenneth. 1974. *The Limits of Organization.* New York: Norton.

Beauchamp, Tom L., and Childress, James F. 1994. *Principles of Medical Ethics.* 4th ed. New York: Oxford University Press.

Bok, Sissela. 1978. Freedom and Risk. *Daedalus* 107 (Spring): 117–27.

———. 1982. *Secrets: On the Ethics of Concealment and Revelation.* New York: Pantheon Books.

———. 1989a. Intrusive Social Science Research. In *Secrets: On the Ethics of Concealment and Revelation,* 2d ed., pp. 230–48. New York: Vintage.

———. 1989b. *A Strategy for Peace: Human Values and the Threat of War.* New York: Pantheon Books.

———. 1990a. Can Lawyers Be Trusted? *University of Pennsylvania Law Review* 138: 913–33.

———. 1990b. *Lying: Moral Choice in Public and Private Life,* 2d ed. New York: Vintage.

———. 1992a. Informed Consent and Prospective Studies of Patient Reliability. Address to the Stanford Biostatistics Seminar, 27 February, unpublished manuscript.

———. 1992b. Informed Consent in Tests of Patient Reliability. Journal of the American Medical Association 267: 1118–19.

———. Forthcoming 1995. *Cultural Diversity and Shared Moral Values.* Columbia: University of Missouri Press.

CPA. Canadian Psychological Association. 1991. Canadian Code of Ethics for Psychologists, Revised. Old Chelsea, Québec: CPA.

Dasgupta, Partha. 1988. Trust as a Commodity. In *Trust: Making and Breaking Cooperative Relations,* ed. Diego Gambetta, pp. 49–71. New York: Blackwell.

BOK • SHADING THE TRUTH

Fisher, Celia, and Fyrberg, Denise. 1994. Participant Partners: College Students Weigh the Costs and Benefits of Deceptive Research. *American Psychologist* 49: 417–27.

Giddens, Anthony. 1994. *Beyond Left and Right.* New York: Blackwell.

Greenberg, B. C.; Abernathy, J. R.; and Horwitz, D. C. 1986. Randomized Response. In *Encyclopedia of Statistical Sciences,* IV, ed. S. Kotz and N. L. Johnson, pp. 540–46. New York: John Wiley & Sons, Inc.

Kant, Immanuel. [1798] 1978. *Anthropology from a Pragmatic Point of View,* trans. Victor Lyle Dowdell. London: Feffer and Simons, Inc.

McCally, Michael; Cassel, Christine; and Kimball, Daryl G. 1994. U.S. Government-Sponsored Research on Humans 1945–1975. *Medicine and Global Survival* 1 (March): 4–17.

McNagny, Sally E., and Parker, Ruth M. Parker. 1992. High Prevalence of Recent Cocaine Use and the Unreliability of Patient Self-report in an Inner-city Walk-in Clinic. *Journal of the American Medical Association* 267: 1106–8.

Mead, Margaret. 1961. The Human Study of Human Beings. *Science* 133: 163.

Mill, John Stuart. [1861] 1961. *Utilitarianism.* In *The Philosophy of J. S. Mill,* ed. Marshall Cohen. New York: The Modern Library.

Mishkin, Barbara. 1994. It's IRB's All Over Again. *Professional Ethics Report* (Spring): 4–6.

Murdoch, Iris. 1985. *The Sovereignty of Good.* London: Ark Paperbacks.

———. 1992. *Metaphysics as a Guide to Morals.* New York: Allen Lane/ Penguin Press.

Murray, Thomas H. 1980. Learning to Deceive. *Hastings Center Report* 10 (2): 11–14.

OPRR. National Institutes of Health, Office of Intramural Research, Office for the Protection from Research Risks. 1993. *Protecting Human Research Subjects: Institutional Review Board Guidebook.* Washington: U.S. Government Printing Office.

Truth, Public Service and Accountability. 1987. *Time* (3 August): 14.

[10]

Trust

The Fragile Foundation of Contemporary Biomedical Research

by Nancy E. Kass, Jeremy Sugarman, Ruth Faden, and Monica Schoch-Spana

It is widely assumed that informing prospective subjects about the risks and possible benefits of research not only protects their rights as autonomous decisionmakers, but also empowers them to protect their own interests. Yet interviews with patient-subjects conducted under the auspices of the Advisory Committee on Human Radiation Experiments suggest this is not always the case. Patient-subjects often trust their physician to guide them through decisions on research participation. Clinicians, investigators, and IRBs must assure that such trust is not misplaced.

I n addition to its investigation of research conducted in the past, the Advisory Committee on Human Radiation Experiments also examined the current status of research with human subjects to ensure that research today and in the future be conducted in accord with the highest ethical standards. To that end, the Advisory Committee conducted three projects that examined *contemporary* human subjects research. Among these was the Subject Interview Study, a project that enrolled almost 1,900 outpatients nationwide to determine their experiences with and attitudes about research.[1] Approximately one hundred of the patients who enrolled in this study and reported having personal experience in medical research were interviewed a second time and in greater depth to gain further insight into their reasons for participating and their understanding of the research enterprise. This paper describes the findings from these interviews and their implications for conducting ethically sound research with human subjects.

These in-depth interviews were conducted at fourteen institutions across the country, including academic research institutions, Veterans' Affairs hospitals, community hospitals, and federal government hospitals. Patients were recruited from the waiting rooms of medical oncology, radiation oncology, and cardiology outpatient clinics at each of the participating institutions. During interviews, which averaged forty-five minutes, patients were asked to describe the research project in which they were enrolled, how they had learned about it, how they had decided to partici-

pate, consent procedures, how they felt about the experience, and how they felt about research more broadly. Interviewers encouraged respondents to speak freely about each topic and also to raise additional topics that were of relevance to their experience in medical research.[2]

Of the 103 patients who were interviewed, there were almost equal numbers of women and men. Patients tended to be Caucasian (74%), to be high school but not college graduates (52%), and to have private health insurance (65%). Participants also were significantly more likely to be in research evaluating a therapy (65%), than in survey research or studies evaluating a diagnostic test. In this report, we will focus predominantly on the experiences of patients enrolled in therapeutic research.

Why Patients Become Subjects

Many factors influenced patients' decisions to participate in research. And as one might expect, those in therapeutic research cited different reasons for participating than did those in other types of research. Among the more prominent motivations for subjects enrolled in therapeutic research was a sense that the experimental intervention was better than any existing alternative, and indeed offered some hope of personal benefit.[3] Patients made comments such as, "If there's something new on the market that might be better than the traditional program they've been using, why not try it?" (Subject 333208-7), or "I was more interested in something more advanced and potentially better" (443247-2).

The theme of hope was often wedded to despair. For many patients, research came after they had tried other standard or experimental interventions and either had exhausted those treatments' effectiveness or had experienced little benefit at all. Often, they viewed the investigational "treatment" as a last hope for improvement or amelioration of their conditions. As one respondent said, "Well, what was driving me to say 'yes' was the hope that this drug would work . . . When you reach that stage . . . and somebody offered that something

Nancy E. Kass, Jeremy Sugarman, Ruth Faden, and Monica Schoch-Spana, "Trust: The Fragile Foundation of Contemporary Biomedical Research," *Hastings Center Report* 26, no. 5 (1996): 25-29.

Hastings Center Report. September-October 1996

that could probably save you, you sort of make a grab of it, and that's what I did" (332250-0). Less typical were the comments of one respondent who said, thoughtfully, "You don't know what that cancer's gonna do. God, I don't . . . think anybody can

Such reflexive decisionmaking regarding research is indicative of the immense trust that patients placed in their physicians; participating in research was simply the right thing to do if their doctor recommended it. "There's not a lot that you can con-

and "I do not feel like the drug would be on the market if it were going to harm me, and if it would help in any way . . . I'm very willing to participate in this and perhaps other studies" (443241-5). Perhaps the most blatant expression of this trust was the patient who said, "I don't believe they would offer me anything that isn't beneficial to me, in my condition" (221106-8). Much more unusual was a patient who believed he should be more in charge of his own treatment decisions: "I sort of take my own treatment in my head and tell them that I'm his client. It's not the other way around" (552143-0).

These stories suggest that the current emphasis in research ethics on analyses of benefits and risks and on subjects' autonomous decisionmaking is insufficient.

---

guarantee you any benefits" (552126-5). Clearly, many patient-subjects hope for personal benefit when they enroll in research, hope that this intervention might offer them longer life, less pain, or fewer symptoms.

Yet many participants who had tried other interventions without success felt more that there simply were no alternatives left. They characterized the decision to participate as a matter of little choice: "My doctor told me if I do not take the drug, in a couple of months I [will] die. So, I had no choice. Who wants to die? Nobody" (333215-2). Similarly, one patient said, "Well, he [the oncologist] said he'd already been through everything he knew what to do. He would try to keep me as comfortable as he could. That's when he told me about this new treatment. I told him we would try it" (443250-6). One respondent said, "They didn't pressure me, but I felt pressure because there isn't anything else" (334110-4).

Physicians' recommendations were also powerful factors influencing patients' decisions to become research subjects. The comments of two respondents are typical: "My personal reasons [for enrolling] were because I was advised to do it" (335227-5); and, "He asked me if I wanted to go on it, and I said 'If it's what you think I should do, yes, because you know more about it than I do.' . . . [H]e said, 'I think it would be a good idea to try it'" (552264-4).

trol when you're sick, so you have to rely on your doctors . . . if he suggests that you should go into a research project, I think you should really take his advice or her advice . . . because if you take the time to get yourself a good doctor and they're involved in research, they would never steer you wrong" (552244-6). Perhaps the most extreme comment along these lines was from a respondent who described her doctor's role in her decision to participate, "Oh, I love that man. He has kept me alive and I obey him and I do what he tells me to do" (114217-3).

Patients also placed a good deal of trust in the hospitals in which they were receiving care. Their belief was that if you come to the right place, you get whatever is the best available treatment. You can *trust* that if they're conducting this research at that hospital, it must be state-of-the-art. "I think I've got the best treatment down there at [named hospital]. I don't think I could get any better" (333208-7). Similarly, "If it's not through [named hospital], I wouldn't touch it" (442304-2).

Finally, respondents expressed trust in the research enterprise as a whole. There seemed to be a widespread belief that checks and balances were in place, and oversight ensured that no harms could be done. For instance, one respondent said, "They know what they're doing. They wouldn't have you do this if they didn't know what they were doing" (332324-3);

Comments about the consent process underscored the importance of trust in the experiences of these patients. Many participants expressed that their decision to participate had been made before they had been given the consent form to sign. They knew they wanted to participate, they trusted that it was right, and the details described in the form were not particularly relevant. "[T]o me, they are the doctors, and once I had gotten those doctors and I trusted them . . . it was pretty much up to them. I wanted to know what I was going to be going through as far as what to expect . . . but a lot of the little nitty-gritty detail, I did not even want to know" (114250-4). Even those who tried to understand what they were being given to read about the study expressed a similar feeling: "I read some of the literature and it didn't mean a hill of beans to me because I didn't know anything about medical science but, like I say, if it's to help me, I'll go in" (332324-3). Patients assumed that they need not pay attention to what was written in a consent form, or suggested that although the form was not particularly readable, it did not matter because they knew they wanted to participate in research regardless.

This belief seems to hinder the adequate fulfillment of the informed consent process, however. The comment by one patient-subject that when offered the possibility of being in a medical research project, "you make a grab for it" is quite revealing. The stories these patient-subjects told about why they decided to participate in research suggest that the current

Hastings Center Report, September-October 1996

emphasis in research ethics on analyses of benefits and risks and on subjects' autonomous decisionmaking is insufficient. The paradigm must be enriched with a sensitivity to the profound trust participants place in researchers and the research enterprise.

The Significance of Trust

The concept of trust has been addressed in the literature in reference to the physician-patient relationship both generally,[4] and in the specific context of research.[5] Edmund Pellegrino suggests that trust is essential to all human relationships and functions to reduce complexity.[6] On Pellegrino's view, a climate of mistrust— that might ensue if violations of trust are experienced—cannot sustain itself. He notes, "We must trust that our vulnerability will not be exploited for power, profit, prestige, or pleasure" (p. 73). He also claims that patients only should entrust to doctors that piece of their "good" that is medical:

> Medical good is only one of the components of the complex notion of patient good . . . patients should not entrust to the physician the responsibility for determining the totality of their good, [and] physicians must not assume they are entrusted with such a broad mandate. (pp. 80-82)

This is particularly relevant in the research context since there are many nonmedical consequences of being in research. Changes in quality of life, interference with work or home life, and demands on a patient's time all can contribute to what constitutes the patient's overall "good."

Annette Baier asserts that when trust exists, harm as well as good can result: "Not all the things that thrive when there is trust between people . . . are things that should be encouraged to thrive . . . There are immoral as well as moral trust relationships."[7] To the extent that patients' vulnerabilities are taken advantage of in research—even as a result of well-intentioned inaccuracies in descriptions of the research or exaggeration of the likelihood of benefit—the boundary into an "immoral" trust relationship has been crossed.

Investigators face extraordinary challenges in maintaining their integrity. If desperate patients come in search of help, and an investigational intervention is available that is targeted for their condition, it is very difficult to present information about the risk and value of that intervention without in some way stimulating patients' hope. Yet there is a morally critical fine line between allowing or even encouraging a patient's hope because of the beneficial value hope itself can provide and misleading the patient to a point where hope is raised inappropriately and harms are created.

Respecting this line necessitates understanding the difficulties in distinguishing medical research from treatment. For many of the patients interviewed in this project, medical research and medical treatment were closely connected. On the one hand, respondents seemed to be quite capable of distinguishing which interventions were associated with the research, separate from their regular clinical care. Similarly, they were clear in pointing out what the unique goals of a research intervention are, asserting, for example, that "[Research is] the only way advancement is made in the medical field . . . [I]t's gotta be done at some point in time on human beings" (551334-6). Such statements suggest that respondents recognize that the goal of research is to help society broadly, while the goal of medical care is to advance the best interests of the individual patient.

Through further discussion, however, it was evident that most respondents, while able to articulate the broad goals of research, viewed their own participation as simply another treatment option. One respondent, when asked to describe her research experience, replied, "I think of it as a means of treating what I have" (335227-5). Another's comments suggested a similar belief, "[participating in research] was through necessity . . . The thought never entered my mind that I would withdraw from this program" (553215-5).

Such results ought not to be surprising perhaps, given the documented tendency of some physicians to inflate the potential benefits of research interventions. In one study, virtually all physicians thought their

patients would benefit from investigational treatments, and 43 percent said they had "no doubts at all about benefits of treatment" despite a statement in the consent form that benefit could not be assured.[8] In another study, physicians consistently overestimated the likelihood of benefit from clinical trials.[9]

Nevertheless, altruism clearly also played a role in respondents' decisions to participate. Although for some altruism seemed to be their primary motivator, for most others it was just a component of their overall decision. For example, some respondents conveyed that while they were hoping for personal benefit, it could not be guaranteed, and that at least good would come to someone else as a result of their having participated. As one remarked, "I was hoping, if not for me, at least something for the next people coming along" (223212-2). Another respondent who had a hereditary condition was quite deliberate in wanting to join an effort that might help others in the future:

> because if it's hereditary and it sure seems [to be] in my situation . . . I'm concerned about my daughter. I'm concerned about her kids, and [it] goes on and on and on . . . [W]ithin my generation I've had three cousins die of the same thing (221240-5).

Another respondent indicated that her own approach to research had changed as her illness had progressed:

> [I]t will never cure me . . . I'll be dead in the next couple of years . . . but if they can find something that can save someone else [I'll be happy] . . . I don't have the expectations that . . . I did . . . seven or eight years ago . . . I'm realistic. It might help. It might not. But, you know, they're going to find out something that's going . . . to help somebody else and you have to think of it that way (335213-5).

Still others viewed participation as almost a civic responsibility. "I feel like [participating in research] is a moral obligation as a citizen. You put back into your community" (443218-3).

Hastings Center Report, September-October 1996

Not surprisingly then, patients conceptualize research participation in quite complex ways. On the one hand, patients described themselves as sincerely motivated to help others, while, on the other, they suggested that they would not have participated benefits. That is, research should not be presented simply as a new intervention with possibilities for beneficial effects, but as an intervention with little evidence suggesting whether effects will be beneficial or harmful. In the end, physicians, even with paternalistic stance of IRBs not only is warranted, but is expected.

IRBs should also take measures to assure that investigators do not overrepresent the benefits of research and that all consequences of the research that relate to the patient's "good" be explained. For example, when reviewing consent forms for Phase I research, IRBs should strike out comments suggesting the likelihood of personal benefit to participants. Such actions send a clear message to investigators, and those potential participants who choose to read these forms, about the investigative nature of such trials. Similarly, IRBs should assure that potential subjects are provided with information about the duration of the trial, any associated discomforts, and information concerning how the trial could affect their ability to function in daily life.

> Clinicians should be mindful of the tremendous influence they have over their patients, given that the mere suggestion of enrollment in research by a patient's personal physician was interpreted by many patients to be an endorsement.

It is essential to recognize that the trust which patient-subjects place in their physicians and the research enterprise is likely to be quite fragile. As Sissela Bok has written, "It is far harder to regain trust, once lost, than to squander it in the first place."[10] Examples from the past highlight that abuses of human subjects have a lasting and devastating effect not only on individuals' trust of biomedical research, but also on entire communities.[11]

Human subjects research allows scientific and medical progress to move forward, which is in the best interests of all of us. To be entrusted with the authority to conduct human subjects research is a privilege. Yet only through vigilance and humility will we as investigators be able to live up to the trust that is placed in us; and only if that trust is deserved can the research enterprise survive.

on that basis alone. Most patients were aware of the broader stated purpose of research and could discuss research as an endeavor that advances science and helps future patients; yet patients also expressed that they would not have joined if they had not believed that some personal benefit might result as well.

Implications for the Conduct of Research

These findings have significant implications for individual clinicians, investigators, and those who evaluate and regulate clinical research. Clinicians should be mindful of the tremendous influence they have over their patients, given that the mere suggestion of enrollment in research by a patient's personal physician was interpreted by many patients to be an endorsement. This is not to suggest that, absent certainty (which obviously is an impossibility), physicians should not offer patients options, including research participation; but physicians should be sensitive to the extraordinary power of their remarks. If research is one in a series of options for a patient, and research offers a possibility of benefit, but a minuscule one given existing evidence, then that intervention should be described in a manner that is consonant with a realistic portrayal of these risks and the best of intentions, do their patients a disservice if they are inaccurate in their portrayal of what it means to be a subject of research.

Investigators, on the other hand, should make it clear that their primary loyalty is to future patients. While investigators also unequivocally have an obligation to minimize harm to subjects and to respect their wishes, patients who enroll as research subjects must understand this shift in loyalties that is inherent to the role of investigators, in contrast to that of patients' personal physicians.

So too those who oversee research should be humbled by the trust patient-subjects have in the research enterprise and should continue to do their best to live up to that trust. The findings of the Subject Interview Study are a cogent reminder for institutional review boards (IRBs) to take seriously their responsibility to review research on subjects' behalf, and not to allow research to be approved with the assumption that patient autonomy and informed consent will provide sufficient protection. Patients assume that research into which they enter is safe, trusting that the research enterprise protects them from harm. They often do not read consent forms carefully because they assume that someone else has scrutinized the risks and benefits on their behalf. These findings suggest that a

Acknowledgments

Drs. Kass and Sugarman and Ms. Schoch-Spana worked on the staff of the Advisory Committee on Human Radiation Experiments, and Dr. Faden was chair of the committee. The views presented are those of the authors and do not represent the views of the Advisory Committee. The findings, recommendations, and analysis of the Advisory Committee are detailed in *The Final Report of the Advisory Committee on Human Radiation Experiments,* available from the Government Printing Office.

Hastings Center Report, September-October 1996

References

1. This study is described in detail in Chapter 16 of the *Final Report of the Advisory Committee on Human Radiation Experiments* (Washington, D.C.: U.S. Government Printing Office, 1995), pp. 724-57.

2. Interviews were audiotaped, transcribed, and analyzed using qualitative techniques and text analysis computer software. Copies of all transcripts and TALLY analysis segments are available through the records collection of the Advisory Committee on Human Radiation Experiments maintained at the National Archives and Records Center, Washington, D.C. Quotations from interviews presented in this article are identified by subject number in the text.

3. Similar findings have been reported from other studies, for example, Barrie R. Cassileth et al., "Attitudes Toward Clinical Trials Among Patients and the Public," *JAMA* 248, no. 8 (1982): 968-70; Sjoerd Rodenhuis et al., "Patient Motivation and Informed Consent in a Phase I Study of an Anticancer Agent," *European Journal of Cancer and Clinical Oncology* 20, no. 4 (1984): pp. 457-62; Christopher Daugherty et al., "Perceptions of Cancer Patients and Their Physicians Involved in Phase I Trials," *Journal of Clinical Oncology* 13, no. 5 (1995): 1062-72.

4. See, for example, Richard M. Zaner, "Phenomenon of Trust and the Patient-Physician Relationship," in *Ethics, Trust, and the Professions: Philosophical and Cultural Aspects*, ed. Edmund D. Pellegrino, Robert M. Veatch, and John P. Langan (Washington D.C.: Georgetown University Press, 1991), pp. 45-63; Joseph P. Lyons, "The Doctor in the Current Milieu," *Perspectives in Biology and Medicine* 37, no. 3 (1994): 442-59; Annette Baier, "Trust and Antitrust," *Ethics* 96 (January 1986): 231-60.

5. Sissela Bok, "Shading the Truth in Seeking Informed Consent for Research Purposes," *Kennedy Institute of Ethics Journal* 5, no. 1 (1995): 1-17.

6. Edmund D. Pellegrino, "Trust and Distrust in Professional Ethics," in *Ethics, Trust, and the Professions*, pp. 69-85.

7. Baier, "Trust and Antitrust," pp. 231-32.

8. Doris Penman et al., "Informed Consent for Investigational Chemotherapy: Patients' and Physicians' Perceptions," *Journal of Clinical Oncology* 2, no. 7 (1984): 849-55.

9. Sudha Rajagopal, Phyllis J. Goodman, and Ian F. Tannock, "Adjuvant Chemotherapy for Breast Cancer: Discordance Between Physicians' Perception of Benefit and the Results of Clinical Trials," *Journal of Clinical Oncology* 12, no. 6 (1994): 1296-1304.

10. Bok, "Shading the Truth," p. 11.

11. James H. Jones, "The Tuskegee Legacy: AIDS and the Black Community," *Hastings Center Report* 22, no. 6 (1992): 38-40.

❖

[11]

QUESTING FOR GRAILS: DUPLICITY, BETRAYAL AND SELF-DECEPTION IN POSTMODERN MEDICAL RESEARCH

George J. Annas, JD, MPH*

Contemporary physicians and scientists often describe their experiments as part of a search for the "Holy Grail." Sometimes this quest is expressed more specifically, as when the Human Genome Project is described as a search for the "Holy Grail of biology."[1] This rhetoric suggests that experimental work is holy, God's work, and that the results will prove miraculous and good for everyone. But this type of blind devotion produces uncritical action that can ultimately destroy values essential to human dignity.

As Tennyson tells us in his poem, "The Holy Grail," "an excessively zealous pursuit after spiritual truth can be as destructive to social order as an indulgence in the materialistic qualities of life."[2] In Tennyson's poem, for example, a monk tells the questing Sir Percivale that forsaking his life at court for the hardship of the search for the Holy Grail was a choice he made at a time Percivale thought he could have both, a "double life," but that his dream of a better life was also a plague:

> but O the pity
> To find thine own first love once more—to hold,
> Hold her a wealthy bride within thine arms,
> Or all but hold, and then—cast her aside,

---

* Edward R. Utley Professor and Chair, Health Law Department, Boston University Schools of Medicine, Law, and Public Health. A.B., Harvard College, 1967, J.D., Harvard Law School, 1970, M.P.H., Harvard School of Public Health, 1972. An early version of this Article was presented at "Humans in Experiments" Conference, Hamburger Institut für Sozialforschung, Hamburg, Germany, June 28-30, 1995.

1. *See, e.g., Those Who Forget Their History: Lessons for the Human Genome Quest*, in GENE MAPPING: USING LAW AND ETHICS AS GUIDES 46, 47-48 (George J. Annas & Sherman Elias, eds., 1992) (discussing this use of language by Judith P. Swazey).

2. TENNYSON'S POETRY 354 n.7 (Robert W. Hill, Jr., ed., 1971).

> Forgoing all her sweetness, like a weed!
> For we that want the warmth of a double life,
> We that are plagued with dreams of something sweet
> Beyond all sweetness in a life so rich,—[3]

Contemporary medical researchers often lead "double lives" in pursuit of their research goals, exhibiting the same determination and desperation as the questing knights of the Holy Grail. Like the knights of old, a medical researcher's quest of the good, whether that be progress in general or a cure for AIDS or cancer specifically, can lead to the destruction of human values we hold central to a civilized life, such as dignity and liberty.[4]

Doubling and duplicity in both language and action have become the hallmark of experimentation on humans in the United States and most of the developed world. We have come to this pass, like King Arthur's knights, with good intentions and worthy goals. Neither our intentions nor our goals, however, can justify the duplicitous use of language in human experimentation nor the betrayal of the Hippocratic ethic of "do no harm" in the physician (researcher)/patient (subject) relationship.

This Article explores the evolution of the rationales physicians, from the Nazi doctors to contemporary experimenters, have used to justify experiments on their patient/subjects. The goal of this exploration is to articulate the destruction concealed by duplicitous language, including role ambiguity and overt deception. In conclusion, some remedial actions will be proposed. Although the scale and justification for research on humans is different when sponsored by the government or by private industry, language distortions and role ambiguities have infected both. This will be demonstrated by examining past government-sponsored, war-justified ex-

---

3. *Id.* at 368.

4. The most articulate, and most often quoted, statement of this principle is by Hans Jonas and it deserves quotation here. Jonas understood that some of his suggested protections for human subjects might lead to slower medical progress, but nonetheless accepted this as a reasonable price to pay for the maintenance of important human values:

> Let us not forget that progress is an optional goal, not an unconditional commitment, and that its tempo in particular, compulsive as it may become, has nothing sacred about it. Let us also remember that a slower progress in the conquest of disease would not threaten society, grievous as it is to those who have to deplore that their particular disease be not yet conquered, but that society would indeed be threatened by the erosion of those moral values whose loss, possibly caused by too ruthless a pursuit of scientific progress, would make its most dazzling triumphs not worth having.

Hans Jonas, *Philosophical Reflections on Human Experimentation*, 98 DAEDALUS 219, 245 (1969).

periments (as exemplified by the radiation experiments), and current drug company-sponsored, profit-justified experiments (as exemplified by cancer and AIDS experiments).

I. A POSTMODERN CRITIQUE

Most scholars date postmodernism from Hiroshima and the Holocaust, one an instantaneous annihilation and the other a systematic one. Together, they represent the death of our civilization's dream of moral and scientific progress that had characterized the modern age. The postmodern world is much more ambiguous and uncertain. Postmodern criticism seeks to subvert our culture and our beliefs. Nonetheless, by seeing culture and beliefs as subjects worthy of study and critique, it simultaneously legitimizes them. "It is . . . this doubleness that prevents any possible critical urge to ignore or trivialize historical-political questions."[5] The "double discourse" of the postmodern world is both illustrated and illuminated in our post-World War II discourse on human experimentation; a discourse that simultaneously condemns the Nazi experiments as barbaric, while demanding access to contemporary experiments as a human right. Use of a double discourse in this context obscures what should be illuminated and marginalizes what should be privileged. Exposing the pervasiveness of the double discourse at least gives us the option of confronting the ambiguities in our motivation and our actions and (re)forming, or at least (re)framing, current rules governing research on humans.

The concepts of doubling and "doublethink" live in contemporary human experimentation. For example, psychiatrist and author Robert Jay Lifton, has suggested that the way in which the Nazi physicians at Auschwitz could continue to see themselves as healers while killing concentration camp inmates was through a process of "doubling." He describes it as "the division of the self into two functioning wholes, so that a part-self acts as an entire self."[6] Lifton's psychiatric assessment of the

---

5. LINDA HUTCHEON, THE POLITICS OF POSTMODERNISM 15 (1989).

6. ROBERT JAY LIFTON, THE NAZI DOCTORS: MEDICAL KILLING AND THE PSYCHOLOGY OF GENOCIDE 418 (1986). Lifton also discusses the "healing-killing paradox" in which Nazi physicians kill for the sake of the health of the state, the "German biotic community." He goes on to explain:

Since the healing-killing paradox epitomized the overall function of the Nazi regime, there was some truth in the Nazi image of Auschwitz as the moral equivalent of war. War is the only accepted institution . . . in which there is a parallel healing-killing paradox. One has to kill the enemy in order to preserve—to "heal"—one's people, one's military unit, oneself.

Nazi doctors need not be accepted. Nonetheless, there is a long history of the double in literature, including, for example, *Frankenstein* (between the creator and his creature) and *Dr. Jekyll and Mr. Hyde.* As Dr. Jekyll puts it:

> Though so profound a double-dealer, I was in no sense a hypo-crite; both sides of me were in dead earnest; . . . . With every day, and from both sides of my intelligence, the moral and the intellectual, I thus drew steadily nearer to that truth, by whose partial discovery I have been doomed to such a dreadful ship-wreck: that man is not truly one, but truly two.[7]

Doubling, of course, produces double standards; even "double think-ing." This latter concept is well described in George Orwell's *1984*, where power, "'the capacity to inflict unlimited pain and suffering on another human being[,]'"[8] is an end in itself. Orwell was writing primarily about totalitarian dictatorships, such as the Soviet Union under Stalin and Ger-many under Hitler. In Orwell's view, the key to a successful totalitarian system is abolishing truth as objective reality. When successful, "anyone who is a minority of one must be convinced that he is insane."[9] The dom-inant mode of thinking in this type of a society is denoted "doublethink," which means "'the power of holding two contradictory beliefs in one's mind simultaneously, and accepting both of them.'"[10]

The party's slogans in *1984* illustrate the concept of doublethink: "War is Peace, Freedom is Slavery, and Ignorance is Strength."[11] We tend to recognize these pairings as nonsensical, and think we could never be vic-tims of such blatant propagandistic sloganeering. But even a cursory his-tory of modern human experimentation demonstrates the pervasiveness of three doublespeak concepts: experimentation is treatment, researchers are physicians, and subjects are patients. Indeed, we have encapsulated all three into a "newspeak" word, "thereapeauticresearch" (although we retain a space between the c and the r).

This doublespeak allows us to use double standards as they suit our purposes. It permits us to treat truth as negotiable and then allows us to act irrationally. We act in the best interest of patients. The experiment is justified as therapy or potential therapy. But if the experiment produces

---

Id. at 431.
    7. ROBERT L. STEVENSON, DR. JEKYLL AND MR. HYDE 79 (1981).
    8. GEORGE ORWELL, 1984 at 263 (*Afterward* by Erich Fromm).
    9. *Id.* at 264.
   10. *Id.*
   11. *Id.* at 7.

harm, it was after all, only an experiment and thus nonetheless a "success" because we learned something from it that could benefit others. It should be of only slight comfort that the term therapeutic research was not invented by a totalitarian government, but rather by physicians who were responding to a legal condemnation of experiments performed under the authority of a totalitarian government—the Nuremberg Code (the "Code").

II. THE NUREMBERG CODE AND THE DECLARATION OF HELSINKI

The Nuremberg Code was formulated by United States judges at the end of the 1946-47 trial of twenty-three Nazi physician-experimenters. The Nazi experiments involved murder and torture; systematic and barbarous acts with death often the planned endpoint. The subjects of these experiments were concentration camp prisoners, mostly Jews, Gypsies, and Slavs. The Nuremberg Code was articulated in response to horrendous nontherapeutic, nonconsensual concentration camp research. Nonetheless, the judges meant the application of the Code to be universal. As we near its fiftieth anniversary, the Nuremberg Code remains the most authoritative legal and ethical document governing international research standards and one of the premier human rights documents in world history.[12]

The judges based the Nuremberg Code on natural law theory. They derived it, with the help of expert witnesses from universal moral, ethical, and legal concepts. The Code protects individual subjects first by protecting their rights. Voluntary, informed, competent, and understanding consent is required by the first principle of the Code, and principle 9 gives the subject the right to withdraw from the experiment. The consent of the subject is necessary under the Nuremberg Code, but consent alone is *not sufficient*. The other eight principles of the Code are related to the welfare of subjects and must be satisfied *before* consent is even sought from the subject. The subject cannot waive these provisions. The requirements of these eight welfare provisions include a valid research design to procure information important for the good of society that cannot be obtained in other ways; the avoidance of unnecessary physical and mental suffering and injury; the absence of an *a priori* reason to believe that death or disabling injury will occur; risks that never exceed benefits;

---

12. THE NAZI DOCTORS AND THE NUREMBERG CODE: HUMAN RIGHTS IN HUMAN EXPERIMENTATION (George J. Annas & Michael Grodin, eds., 1992) [hereinafter THE NAZI DOCTORS AND THE NUREMBERG CODE].

and the presence of a qualified researcher who is prepared to terminate the experiment if it "is likely to result in the injury, disability, or death" of the subject.[13]

---

13. The Nuremberg Code:
    1. The voluntary consent of the human subject is absolutely essential.

This means that the person involved should have legal capacity to give consent; should be so situated as to be able to exercise free power of choice, without the intervention of any element of force, fraud, deceit, duress, overreaching, or other ulterior form of constraint or coercion; and should have sufficient knowledge and comprehension of the elements of the subject matter involved as to enable him to make an understanding and enlightened decision. This latter element requires that before the acceptance of an affirmative decision by the experimental subject there should be made known to him the nature, duration, and purpose of the experiment; the method and means by which it is to be conducted; all inconveniences and hazards reasonably to be expected; and the effects upon his health or person which may possibly come from his participation in the experiment.

The duty and responsibility for ascertaining the quality of the consent rests upon each individual who initiates, directs or engages in the experiment. It is a personal duty and responsibility which may not be delegated to another with impunity.

    2. The experiment should be such as to yield fruitful results for the good of society, unprocurable by other methods or means of study, and not random and unnecessary in nature.

    3. The experiment should be so designed and based on the results of animal experimentation and a knowledge of the natural history of the disease or other problem under study that the anticipated results will justify the performance of the experiment.

    4. The experiment should be so conducted as to avoid all unnecessary physical and mental suffering and injury.

    5. No experiment should be conducted where there is an *a priori* reason to believe that death or disabling injury will occur; except, perhaps, in those experiments where the experimental physicians also serve as subjects.

    6. The degree of risk to be taken should never exceed that determined by the humanitarian importance of the problem to be solved by the experiment.

    7. Proper preparations should be made and adequate facilities provided to protect the experimental subject against even remote possibilities of injury, disability, or death.

    8. The experiment should be conducted only by scientifically qualified persons. The highest degree of skill and care should be required through all stages of the experiment of those who conduct or engage in the experiment.

    9. During the course of the experiment the human subject should be at liberty to bring the experiment to an end if he has reached the physical or mental state where continuation of the experiment seems to him to be impossible.

    10. During the course of the experiment the scientist in charge must be prepared to terminate the experiment at any stage, if he has probable cause to believe, in the exercise of the good faith, superior skill, and careful judgment required of him, that a continuation of the experiment is likely to result in injury, disability, or death to the experimental subject.

Physician-researchers viewed the Nuremberg Code as constraining and inapplicable to their practices because (1) it was promulgated as a human rights document by judges at a criminal trial and (2) the judges made no attempt to deal with clinical research on children, healthy volunteers, patients, or mentally-impaired people. The Code, after all, applied only to Nazis. Moreover, the Code has no explicit rules for many modern research agendas. The answer to the first concern is that the Code is universal; the response to the second lies in an interpretation of the Code, rather than in its abandonment. A reasonable analogy is the way we interpret the United States Constitution to apply to changes in technology.

The World Medical Association, nonetheless, has consistently tried to displace the Code with The Declaration of Helsinki, a more permissive alternative document, first promulgated in 1964 and amended three times since. The Declaration of Helsinki is subtitled "recommendations guiding doctors in clinical research" and is just that, recommendations by physicians to physicians. The Declaration's goal is to replace the human rights-based agenda of the Nuremberg Code with a more lenient medical ethics model that permits paternalism.

U.S. researcher Henry Beecher probably best expressed medicine's delight with the Declaration of Helsinki's ascendancy when he said in 1970, "'The Nuremberg Code presents a rigid act of legalistic demands. . . . The Declaration of Helsinki, on the other hand, presents a set of guides. It is an ethical as opposed to a legalistic document, and is thus a more broadly useful instrument than the one formulated at Nuremberg.'"[14]

The core of the Declaration of Helsinki is a doubling, dividing research into therapeutic ("Medical Research Combined with Professional Care") and nontherapeutic, thus blurring the line between treatment and research. The physician (researcher?) need not obtain the subject's (patient's?) informed consent to "medical research combined with professional care" if the physician submits the reasons for not obtaining consent to the independent review committee.[15] The current trend seems to seek to go even further, abolishing the distinction between research and therapy, researcher and physician, and subject and patient altogether.

The Nuremberg Code, *reprinted in* THE NAZI DOCTORS AND THE NUREMBERG CODE, *supra* note 12, at 2.

14. Sir William Refshauge, *The Place for International Standards in Conducting Research for Humans*, 55 BULL. WORLD HEALTH ORG. 133-35 (Supp. 1977) (quoting H.K. BEECHER, RESEARCH AND THE INDIVIDUAL: HUMAN STUDIES 279 (1970)). The full text of all four versions of the Declaration of Helsinki appear in THE NAZI DOCTORS AND NUREMBERG CODE, *supra* note 12.

15. THE NAZI DOCTORS AND THE NUREMBERG CODE, *supra* note 12, at 342.

In this new regime, research becomes treatment, the researcher becomes the healer, and the subject becomes a patient. The way language is used to obscure the truth and justify the unjustifiable can be illustrated by some cold war radiation experiments performed in the United States in the 1940s, 1950s, and 1960s, and contemporary experiments on terminally ill cancer and AIDS patients.

III. THE COLD WAR RADIATION EXPERIMENTS

In 1986, Representative Edward J. Markey (D. Mass.) released a report from the House Subcommittee on Energy Conservation and Power entitled "American Nuclear Guinea Pigs: Three Decades of Radiation Experiments on U.S. Citizens."[16] The report detailed 31 experiments conducted on more than 700 Americans by the federal government from the 1940s to the 1970s, most designed to test the effect on the human body of exposure to radiation. The experiments included injection of plutonium or uranium into terminally ill patients; irradiation of the testicles of prisoners to study the impact of radiation on fertility; exposure of nursing home residents to radium or thorium, either injected or ingested, to measure the passage of these radioactive substances through the body; and feeding of radioactive fallout to human subjects to see how the human body would excrete it. Although the 1986 report was carefully documented and cited specific published reports on the studies, it went virtually unrecognized and unheralded[17] primarily because the administration of President Ronald Reagan dismissed it as overblown.

Under the administration of President Bill Clinton, the reaction to similar disclosures, involving thousands of Americans, was dramatically different. In October 1993, reporter Eileen Welsome of the *Albuquerque Tribune* wrote a series of articles about five individuals who, without their knowledge or consent, had been injected with plutonium from 1945-47 as part of an Atomic Energy Commission ("AEC") study of the impact of plutonium on human beings.[18] The information was sought to help determine how to treat workers and scientists exposed to plutonium at weap-

---

16. STAFF OF HOUSE SUBCOMM. ON ENERGY CONSERVATION AND POWER OF THE COMM. ON ENERGY & COMMERCE, 99TH CONG., 2D SESS., AMERICAN NUCLEAR GUINEA PIGS: THREE DECADES OF RADIATION EXPERIMENTS ON U.S. CITIZENS (Comm. Print 1986).

17. A similar response greeted a later report of the STAFF OF SENATE COMM. ON VETERANS' AFFAIRS, 103D CONG., 2D SESS., IS MILITARY RESEARCH HAZARDOUS TO VETERANS' HEALTH? LESSONS SPANNING HALF A CENTURY (Comm. Print 1994).

18. Eileen Welsome, *The Plutonium Experiment*, ALBUQUERQUE TRIB., 1993 (A special reprint of a three-day series of articles originally published Nov. 15-17, 1993).

ons development and production plants. In one case, plutonium was injected into the leg of a thirty-six-year-old man who was thought to have bone cancer. The leg was then amputated for study. As a result of the amputation, the man could no longer work and was dependent upon his wife to support him. He died forty-five years later in 1991. Another subject was misdiagnosed as having stomach cancer and was injected with plutonium in 1945. He lived to age seventy-nine, dying in 1966. The subjects were not told the purpose of the experiments, either at the time or when follow-up studies were conducted later.

When these stories became public, Hazel O'Leary, Secretary of the U.S. Department of Energy ("DOE"),[19] said she was "appalled and shocked" by the plutonium experiments.[20] She took steps to begin an investigation of other radiation experiments conducted by the AEC and suggested that a way should be found to compensate the victims. This reaction was shared by President Clinton, who established an interagency task force to conduct a similar review of all federal agencies that might have been involved in radiation experiments during the cold war. The President also formed an Advisory Committee to the Task Force, which issued its final report in October 1995.[21]

The Advisory Committee's 900 page report detailed a number of specific experiments and made recommendations regarding radiation experiments in particular, and research on human beings in general. Two specific experiments—one dealt with superficially by the Advisory Committee, the other in detail—illustrate the pervasive problems in the government-sponsored radiation experiments. The first was funded by the AEC and conducted at Boston's Massachusetts General Hospital in the mid-1950s. The experiment was designed to find the dose of uranium that could be tolerated by humans. The primary published report involved five terminally ill patients with brain tumors who were injected with uranium (U^{235}).[22] Four of the five were semicomatose or in a coma at the

---

19. The Department of Energy is the successor to the Atomic Energy Commission.

20. Welsome, *supra* note 18, at 47.

21. ADVISORY COMMITTEE ON HUMAN RADIATION EXPERIMENTS, FINAL REPORT (1995) [hereinafter FINAL REPORT]. The President not only accepted the Report in a White House ceremony on October 3, 1995, he also signed an Executive Order creating a National Bioethics Advisory Commission to advise the government on matters on research with human beings as well as other "bioethical issues." Executive Order, No. 12,975, 60 Fed. Reg. 52,093 (1995).

22. A.J. Luessenhop et al., *The Toxicity in Man of Hexavalent Uranium Following Intravenous Administration*, 79 AM. J. ROENTGENOLOGY 83-100 (1958). There were 11 subjects altogether. *See* FINAL REPORT, *supra* note 21, at 262-69.

time; most died within two months, but one lived for seventeen months. There is no evidence of consent by anyone, although permission to perform an autopsy was refused by the family of the only woman in the study. The published report of the experiment (which indicated that the subjects had been exposed to a range of ten percent to thirty percent of a lethal dose of uranium) concluded, "Of the common laboratory animals, man appears to correspond most closely to the rat in regard to intravenous tolerance to uranium."[23] Human subjects were used in the experiment because they were captive and available. No consent was sought or obtained, apparently because the researchers believed that terminally ill individuals could not be harmed. No disrespect to the subjects is intended by noting that they were treated no better than laboratory rats would have been. This was apparently not unusual in the 1950s. As one eminent physician, Louis Lasagna, told the Advisory Committee's investigators in an oral history interview, "Mostly, I'm ashamed to say, it was as if[,] and I'm putting this very crudely purposely[,] as if you'd ordered a bunch of rats from a laboratory and you had experimental subjects available to you."[24]

The Advisory Committee concluded that even if one of the purposes of the study had been to see if large doses of uranium localized in brain tumors, one of the patients had no such tumor.[25] "Even for the patient-subjects with brain cancer, there was no expectation on the part of investigators that the experiment would benefit the subjects themselves."[26] The Committee concluded that although these patients were dying, and thus presumably were "not likely to live long enough to be harmed[,] it d[id] not justify failing to respect them as people."[27] Even though the Committee found no evidence that informed consent was obtained from the subjects (it clearly could not be from those who were comatose), the Committee nonetheless stopped short of condemning the experiment, saying simply, "Unless these patients [subjects?], or the families of comatose or incompetent patients, understood that the injections were not for their benefit and still agreed to the injections, this experiment . . . was unethical."[28]

---

23. Luessenhop, *supra* note 22, at 100.

24. *See* Karen MacPherson, *Radiation Tests in Past Decades Broke Ethics Rules*, SACRAMENTO BEE, Jan. 23, 1995, at A5 (quoting Dr. Louis Lasagna, reporting to the White House Advisory Committee on Human Radiation Experiments).

25. FINAL REPORT, *supra* note 21, at 263.

26. *Id.*

27. *Id* at 269.

28. *Id.*

But much more could—and should—have been said: Treating people like rats is unethical, even if relatives think it is acceptable. There are limits to what even dying patients can consent to if one takes the eight welfare principles of the Nuremberg Code seriously.[29]

The next experiment, the Cincinnati Whole Body Radiation Experiment, was conducted a decade later. By then, simply asserting that the patient was dying was no longer seen as sufficient justification for using them for your own purposes. The Cincinnati Experiment, which involved eighty-eight subjects from 1960 to 1971, is described in a 1973 medical report by the investigators.[30] The study was financed by the U.S. Defense Project Support Agency "to determine whether amino acids or other biochemicals in the urine could 'serve as an indicator of the biological response of humans to irradiation.'"[31] Like the Massachusetts General Hospital study, this experiment was designed to test a hypothesis for the U.S. military on subjects selected primarily because they were available and thought to be terminally ill with cancer.

In the medical literature, the researchers attempted to transform this military research study into a civilian treatment series: "[t]he purpose of these investigations [was] to improve the treatment and general clinical management and if possible the length of survival of patients with advanced cancer."[32] It was alleged that, "[a]ll patients gave informed consent."[33] The patients were "eligible for this form of treatment if they ha[d] advanced cancer for which [a] cure could not be anticipated."[34] Later in the article, the experimental protocol itself is transformed into "the therapeutic regime."[35] Whether therapy or experimentation, however, serious problems were apparent even in this self-serving rendition:

---

29. The justification for treating human beings like rats was the same as one of the major justifications used by the Nazi doctors at Nuremberg: it was wartime (albeit a cold war) and "extreme circumstances demand extreme action." In addition, these subjects were "already condemned to death" and thus were not harmed by the experiments. Michael A. Grodin, *Historical Origins of the Nuremberg Code*, in THE NAZI DOCTORS AND THE NUREMBERG CODE, *supra*, note 12, at 132.

30. FINAL REPORT, *supra* note 21, at 385-406; Eugene L. Saenger et al., *Whole Body and Partial Body Radiotherapy of Advanced Cancer*, 117 AM. J. ROENTGENOLOGY RADIUM THERAPY & NUCLEAR MED. 670, 670-85 (1973). The principal investigator, Eugene L. Saenger of the University of Cincinnati, wrote his first (and last) description of the study in the medical literature (yearly reports had been provided to the U.S. Defense Atomic Support Agency).

31. FINAL REPORT, *supra* note 21, at 386 (citation omitted).

32. Saenger, *supra* note 30, at 670.

33. *Id.* at 671.

34. *Id.*

35. *Id.* at 672.

eight subjects (almost ten percent) could have died directly from the radiation exposure; none were told of the risk of death nor of the common and devastating side effects of nausea and vomiting (fifty-six percent experienced it); and most patients were poor, black, and at least twelve percent had IQs under seventy.[36]

The principal investigator, noted radiologist Eugene Saenger, continues to defend this experiment as therapy. He has said that total body irradiation ("TBI treatments") "were given as a 'palliative cancer therapy' for people for whom there was no better alternative."[37] This assertion is simply not credible.[38] The Committee seems to have had considerable difficulty in deciding (1) whether these patients were subjects, (2) whether this intervention was innovative treatment (or experimental), and (3) whether the physicians were trying to help their patients. These are, of course, the ambiguities in research that are attenuated by duplicitous language. Nonetheless, the Committee ultimately concluded:

> The impact of the research protocol on the care of the patient-subjects cannot be construed as beneficial to the patients; in addition, there is evidence of the subordination of the ends of medicine to the ends of research. The decisions to withhold information about possible acute side effects of TBI as well as to forgo pretreatment with antiemetics were irrefutably linked to advancing the research interests of the DOD. To the extent that this deviated from standard care, and caused unnecessary suffering and discomfort, it was morally unconscionable.[39]

The Committee went on to raise, but not answer, a question at the core of our inquiry: "Whether the ends of research (understood as discovering

---

36. *Id.* at 680; *In re* Cincinnati Radiation Litig., 874 F. Supp. 796, 803 (S.D. Ohio 1995).

37. Final Report, *supra* note 21, at 387.

38. Nor should it, given the other types of studies that were conducted on these subjects. *See, e.g.,* Louis A. Gottschalk et al., *Total and Half Body Irradiation: Effect on Cognitive and Emotional Processes,* 31 Archives Gen. Psychiatry 574, 574-80 (1969) (discussing the effect of whole body radiation on their cognitive ability in a study done for the Defense Atomic Support Agency); Fred G. Medinger & Lloyd F. Craver, *Total Body Irradiation with Review of Cases,* 48 Am. J. Roentgenology & Radium Therapy 651, 651-71 (1942) (discussing a study, which Saenger himself cites in his 1973 article, indicating that whole body radiation is useless for cancers that involve localized tumors).

> Except for transient relief of pain in a few cases, the results in these generalized carcinoma cases were discouraging. The reason for this is quickly apparent. Carcinomas are much more radio resistant than the lymphomatoid tumors, and by total body irradiation the dose cannot be nearly large enough to alter these tumors appreciably [without killing the patient].

Id. at 668.

39. Final Report, *supra* note 21, at 405.

new knowledge) and the ends of medicine (understood as serving the interests of the patient) necessarily conflict and how the conflict should be resolved when it occurs are still today open and vexing issues."[40]

Before the Committee's *Final Report* was issued, a federal judge, relying on the Nuremberg Code, permitted a lawsuit by the families of these subjects against the researchers to proceed, stating:

> The allegations in this case indicate that the government of the United States, aided by officials of the City of Cincinnati, treated at least eighty-seven (87) of its citizens as though they were laboratory animals. If the Constitution has not clearly established a right under which these Plaintiffs may attempt to prove their case, then a gaping hole in that document has been exposed. The *subject of experimentation* who has not volunteered is merely an object.[41]

Because the Committee recommended compensation for only a handful of injured subjects, the ultimate decision about monetary compensation for injury will be made in the courts.

IV. CANCER AND AIDS

Writer Susan Sontag has noted that cancer and AIDS have become linked as perhaps the two most feared ways to die in the developed world. In her words, "AIDS, like cancer, leads to a hard death. . . . The most terrifying illnesses are those perceived not just as lethal but as dehumanizing, literally so."[42] Philosopher Michel Foucault was not speaking

---

40. *Id.*

41. *In re* Cincinnati Radiation Litig., 874 F. Supp. 796, 822 (S.D. Ohio 1995) (emphasis added). It is heartening that the judge relied heavily on the Nuremberg Code as a basic human rights document in reaching her decision and was not swayed by the doublethink in the 1973 article. *Id.* at 820. This case, however, is most noteworthy for its uniqueness. Usually, experimentation is successfully disguised as therapy. For example, immediately prior to the Gulf War, the U.S. Department of Defense sought and received permission from the Food and Drug Administration not to obtain informed consent from soldiers who were to be given drugs and vaccines under an "investigational new drug" protocol. The justification for this exemption was that consent was "not feasible" although no objective evidence was presented to support this assertion. Instead, it was simply alleged that these investigational agents were really "preventative or therapeutic treatment[s] that might save" lives. Request for Exemption from Informed Consent Requirements for Operation Desert Shield, Department of Defense, 55 Fed. Reg. 52,813-17 (1990). *See generally* George J. Annas, *Changing the Consent Rules for Desert Storm*, 326 NEW ENG. J. MED. 770, 770-73 (1992) (discussing the rule and the legal challenges to it and recommending that it be withdrawn by the FDA).

42. SUSAN SONTAG, ILLNESS AS METAPHOR AND AIDS AND ITS METAPHORS 126 (1990).

of the medicalization of death by cancer and AIDS, nonetheless his chronicle of the shift of power over life and death to government, is equally applicable. "Now it is over life, throughout its unfolding, that power establishes its domination; death is power's limit, the moment that escapes it . . . ."[43] In human experimentation on the terminally ill, we have Foucault's vision of public power played out in private; researchers take charge of the bodies of the dying in an attempt to take charge of the patient's lives and prevent their own personal deaths and death itself. One of the Nazi doctors' chief defenses at Nuremberg was that experimentation was necessary to support the war effort.[44] Now combating disease has itself become a "war" as we speak of a "war on cancer" and a "war on AIDS." And in that war, patients, especially terminally ill patients, are conscripted as soldiers. As former editor of the *New England Journal of Medicine* Franz Ingelfinger stated: "[T]he thumb screws of coercion are most relentlessly applied . . . [to] the most used and useful of all experimental subjects, the patient with disease."[45] But as Sontag reminds us, war metaphors are dangerous in disease because they encourage authoritarianism, overmobilization, and stigmatization. In her words:

> No, it is not desirable for medicine, any more than for war, to be "total." Neither is the crisis created by AIDS a "total" anything. We are not being invaded. The body is not a battlefield. The ill are neither unavoidable casualties nor the enemy. We— medicine, society—are not authorized to fight back by any means whatever.[46]

The self-deception inherent in seeing experimentation as treatment, especially in terminally ill cancer patients, is well-illustrated by contemporary Phase I drug studies with anticancer agents. Are they research or therapy? Food and Drug Administration ("FDA") regulations state that Phase I studies are intended to have no therapeutic content, but are to determine "toxicity, metabolism, absorption, elimination, and other pharmacological action, preferred route of administration, and safe dosage range."[47] Nonetheless, National Cancer Institute ("NCI") researchers

---

43. 1 MICHEL FOUCAULT, THE HISTORY OF SEXUALITY 138 (Robert Hurley trans., 1990)

44. Grodin, *supra* note 29, at 132.

45. Franz J. Ingelfinger, *Informed (but Uneducated) Consent*, 287 NEW ENG. J. MED. 465, 466 (1972).

46. SONTAG, *supra* note 42, at 182-83.

47. PRESIDENT'S COMMISSION FOR THE STUDY OF ETHICAL PROBLEMS IN MEDICINE

have insisted on calling them "potentially therapeutic."[48]

The self-deception problem is that in a terminally ill person, virtually any intervention, even a placebo, can be described as "potentially therapeutic." Once this misleading label is applied, the nonbeneficial Phase I study is *de facto* eliminated and transformed into therapy, now labeled "experimental therapy." Any distinction between experimentation and therapy is lost. This "phase I-doublespeak" has invaded even pediatric research, even though no cures or remissions for longer than a year have been documented in Phase I studies, and even though remissions occur less than six percent of the time and most last less than two months.[49] Thus, the conclusion that "[a]dministration of chemotherapy in Phase I pediatric oncology trials should be considered a *therapeutic research* intervention because there is some likelihood of modest benefits accruing to *participating subjects*"[50] is untenable. Parents consenting on behalf of their dying children seem to be doing so because they are provided with false hope and unrealistic expectations. Moreover, ninety-four percent of investigators concede that patients (adults) enroll in Phase I studies "mostly for the possible medical benefit."[51]

Self-deception permits both researchers and subjects to "double" themselves: it permits researchers to see themselves as physicians and subjects to see themselves (and their children) as patients. When physician and researcher are merged into one person, it is unlikely that patients can ever draw the distinction between these two conflicting roles because most patients simply do not believe that their physician would knowingly harm them or would knowingly use them as a means for their

---

AND BIOMEDICAL AND BEHAVIORAL RESEARCH, PROTECTING HUMAN SUBJECTS 65 (1981).

48. *Id.* (quoting letter from Edward N. Brandt, Jr., Assistant Sec. for Health, Dept. of Health & Environment (Nov. 20, 1981, at 3-4)).

49. Wayne L. Furman et al., *Mortality in Pediatric Phase I Clinical Trials*, 81 J. NAT'L CANCER INST. 1193, 1193 (1989). This review of 31 phase I clinical trials in children involving 577 "patients," found "34 objective responses (11 complete and 23 partial) to . . . 27 Phase I agents, yielding an overall response rate of 5.9%. . . . The duration of the 11 complete responses ranged from 12 to 300 days, with a median of 60 days." *Id.* at 1193.

50. Terrence F. Ackerman, *The Ethics of Phase I Pediatric Oncology Trials*, IRB, Jan.-Feb. 1995, at 1, 5 (emphasis added).

51. Eric Kodish et al., *Ethical Issues in Phase I Oncology Research: A Comparison of Investigators and Institutional Review Board Chairpersons*, 10 J. CLINICAL ONCOLOGY 1810, 1812 (1992); Mortimer B. Lipsett, *On the Nature and Ethics of Phase I Clinical Trials of Cancer Chemotherapies*, 248 JAMA 941, 941-42 (1982). For a discussion of the limits of parental authority to consent on behalf of their children, see Catherine L. Annas, *Irreversible Error: The Power and Prejudice of Female Genital Mutilation*, 12 J. CONTEMP. HEALTH L. & POL'Y 325 (1996).

own end. Because of the almost blind trust patients have in their physicians, the Helsinki Declaration's theoretical division between therapeutic and nontherapeutic research is meaningless. This is, of course, clearest for terminally ill patients who have "exhausted" all therapeutic options.

AIDS has always been perceived as the disease in which there literally is *no* distinction between treatment and experimentation. This is because, even though we are moving toward making AIDS a chronic condition, there is still no cure for AIDS. The disease primarily strikes the young, leading to a death that is premature. Existing treatments that can prolong life are far from satisfactory. ACT-UP's (AIDS Coalition to Unleash Power) political slogan, "A Drug Trial is Health Care Too," for example, serves to duplicitously conflate experimentation with therapy. It also encourages people with AIDS to seek out experimentation as treatment and physician-researchers to view AIDS patients as potential subjects who have "nothing to lose." Under this rationale, all types of experiments are performed under the guise of treatment. At the extreme are the experiments of Henry Heimlich in China, who used malaria infection to stimulate the immune system of AIDS patients. Anthony Fauci, director of the National Institute of Allergy and Infectious Disease and one of the nation's top authorities on AIDS, characterizes Heimlich's experiment as "'quite dangerous and scientifically unsound.'"[52] Heimlich, on the other hand, says it is "'safe for patients,'" and he gets their consent.[53]

The most potentially far-reaching work in human experimentation is in the area of genetics. French Anderson, one of the leaders in the field, has argued that even the initial genetic experiments on humans should really be regarded as therapy:

> There exists a fundamental difference between the responses of clinicians [physicians] and basic scientists [researchers] to the question: Are we ready to carry out a human gene therapy clinical protocol? . . .
>
> The basic scientist objectively analyzes the preclinical data and finds it wanting. . . .
>
> Clinicians look at the situation from a different perspective. Every day they are expected to provide their patients with the

52. Tim Bonfield, *Heimlich Uses Malaria in Research on AIDS*, CINCINNATI ENQUIRER, Nov. 7, 1994, *available in* LEXIS, News Library, Gannett News Service File.

53. *Id.* This "treatment" was also used in an episode of Chicago Hope. *See* George J. Annas, *Sex, Violence and Bioethics: Watching ER and Chicago Hope*, HASTINGS CENTER REP., Sept.-Oct. 1995, at 40, 42.

best treatments for disease. When they deal with incurable diseases, they must watch their patients die. . . . The urge to do something, anything, if it might help is very strong. . . .

. . . A clinician's reaction to a *new therapy protocol* tends to be: If it is relatively safe, and it might work better, then let's try it. Historically, much of medical innovation has resulted from trial and error experimentation

. . . What's the rush? The rush is the daily necessity to help sick people. Their (our) illnesses will not wait for a more convenient time. We need help *when* we are sick.[54]

Anderson concludes his argument, "It will take many years of clinical studies before gene therapy can be a widely used treatment procedure. The sooner we begin, the sooner patients will be helped."[55] The distinction between experimentation and treatment is lost in this discussion, with the ethics of the inapplicable doctor-patient treatment model dominating the scientist-subject model. Likewise, the use of a baboon heart in the Baby Fae transplant was considered lifesaving therapy by the surgeon even though it was the first operation of its kind in the world.[56] It should be obvious that the fact that the patient is dying does not transform experimental interventions into standard treatment modalities and does not eliminate the necessity for informed consent. It is the nature of the intervention and the data that support its use, not the medical status of the patient or the intent of the physician-researcher, that determine the nature of the intervention. Likewise, consent can be asked for only after a justifiable research protocol has been developed. Just as consent is no

---

54. French Anderson, *What's the Rush?*, 1 HUMAN GENE THERAPY 109, 110 (1990) (emphasis added); *see also New Zealand's Leap into Gene Therapy*, 271 SCIENCE 1489 (1996) (describing a first of its kind genetic experiment as "therapy"); Larry Thompson, *Should Dying Patients Receive Untested Genetic Methods?*, 259 SCIENCE 452 (1993).

55. *Id.* That genetic therapy (experimentation) has been oversold was recognized by an NIH review panel set up by Director Harold Varmus to study the current state of the technology. In their December 1995 report, the panel concluded that "gene therapists and their sponsors are 'overselling' the technology, promoting the idea that 'gene therapy is further developed and more successful than it actually is.'" Eliot Marshall, *Less Hype, More Biology Needed for Gene Therapy*, 270 SCIENCE 1752 (1995). In fact, the panel concluded that "'[c]linical efficacy has not been definitively demonstrated at this time in any gene therapy protocol . . . despite anectdotal claims of successful therapy' . . . ." *Id.*; *see also* Meredith Wadam, *Hyping Results 'Could Damage' Gene Therapy*, 378 NATURE 655 (1995) (discussing view by a panel at the National Institute of Health that U.S. biomedical researchers have been "overselling" the result of somatic gene therapy trials).

56. George J. Annas, *Baby Fae: The Anything Goes School of Human Experimentation*, HASTINGS CENTER REP., Feb. 1985, at 15.

justification for the torture, it is no justification for improper research.
As I have put it previously:

> We must stop treating terminally ill cancer and AIDS patients as
> subhuman by [irrationally] offering them questionable experi-
> ments in the guise of treatment. We cannot justify this behavior
> on the basis of either their demand for it or our belief that the
> ultimate good of mankind will be served by it. Researchers who
> believe their subjects cannot be hurt by experimental interven-
> tions *should be disqualified* from doing research on human sub-
> jects on the basis that they cannot appropriately protect their
> subjects' welfare with such a view. Likewise, subjects who be-
> lieve they have "nothing to lose" and are desperate because of
> their terminal illness should also be disqualified as potential re-
> search subjects because they are unable to provide voluntary,
> competent, informed or understanding consent to the experi-
> mental intervention with such a view. It should be emphasized
> that these are proposed *research* rules that would not necessarily
> apply to treatment in a doctor-patient relationship untainted by
> conflicts of interests.[57]

V. WHY LANGUAGE MATTERS

Language can clarify, but it can also obscure. The project of at least
some leading medical researchers since Nuremberg seems to have been
to use language to obscure; to blur or eliminate the distinctions between
research and therapy, scientist and physician, and subject and patient.
This doublethink is the essence of "therapeutic research," a concept that
has been used to disguise the true nature of experimental protocols and
to obscure the ideology of science (which follows a protocol to test a hypothesis) with the ideology of medicine (which uses treatments in the best
interests of individual patients).[58] The motivation for disguising the distinction between interventions executed to test a hypothesis to gain
generalizable knowledge and those performed for the benefit of the individual, seems to be to lower the standards for obtaining informed consent. To the extent that physicians have been permitted to withhold
certain risk information from patients under the "therapeutic privilege,"

---

57. George J. Annas, *The Changing Landscape of Human Experimentation: Nuremberg, Helsinki and Beyond*, 2 HEALTH MATRIX 119, 135 (1992).

58. *See* Alexander Capron, *Informed Consent in Catastrophic Disease Research*, 123 U.
PENN L. REV. 340, 350 (1974); Jay Katz, *Human Experimentation and Human Rights*, 38
ST. LOUIS U. L.J. 7, 12 (1993); Nancy King, *Experimental Treatment: Oxymoron or Aspira-
tion?*, HASTINGS CENTER REP., July-Aug. 1995, at 6.

this view has received at least some legal sanction. Modern informed consent doctrine, however, is meant to safeguard the patient's interest in both decision-making autonomy (liberty) and dignity. Thus, it is no longer appropriate to have separate disclosure requirements for therapy and research. Whatever differences currently exist in practice should be abolished because the rationale for information disclosure is identical in both cases.

There should be only one standard of informed consent, applying to both research and therapy, and it should be as set forth in article one of the Nuremberg Code: voluntary, competent, informed, and *understanding*. Courts have seemed to place the emphasis in the treatment arena on disclosure alone (*i.e.*, the "informed" part of informed consent) rather than on the understanding of the information by the patient. Nonetheless, because the test of competence is the ability to understand and appreciate the information needed to give informed consent,[59] it is fair to conclude that the requirement of understanding the material information has always been an implicit part of the informed consent doctrine.

Consent requirements should also include all of the elements spelled out in the leading informed consent cases, such as *Cobbs v. Grant*[60] and their progeny,[61] and the federal rules for research on human subjects. Of course special rules can (and should) apply to those individuals who cannot consent for themselves, and these rules of substituted consent should be uniform (although there may be times when substitute consent is *not* permitted at all in the case of research because of its lack of benefit to the subject).[62] In this way, researchers should not be tempted to see their work as treatment so that they can avoid the requirements of informed consent—which in any event should be universal.

Informed consent is necessary in both contexts to protect the rights of the individual, but it is not sufficient. Consent, for example, has been transformed from a shield to protect subjects to a sword to be used against them in contemporary research. The consent (or demand) of the

---

59. George J. Annas & Joan Densberger, *Competence to Refuse Medical Treatment: Autonomy vs. Paternalism*, 15 TOLEDO L. REV. 561, 578 (1984).

60. 502 P.2d 1 (Cal. 1972).

61. For a discussion of these cases, see George J. Annas & Frances H. Miller, *The Empire of Death: How Culture and Economics Affect Informed Consent in the U.S., the U.K., and Japan*, 20 AM. J.L. & MED. 357 (1994) and Heather Goodare & Richard Smith, *The Rights of Patients in Research*, 310 BRITISH MED. J. 1277 (1995).

62. *See, e.g.*, CHILDREN AS RESEARCH SUBJECTS: SCIENCE, ETHICS AND LAW (Michael Grodin & Leonard Glantz eds., 1994); *infra* note 95 and accompanying text (providing recommended rules for terminally ill research subjects).

research subject is now often seen as sufficient justification in itself to perform the experiment on a human being.[63] But the consent of the research subject does not transform an experimental protocol into a therapeutic intervention. Consent speaks to liberty and dignity, not to reasonableness or risks and benefits. Choice, however, has been so reified in our society that we seldom ask "choice for what purpose?" Thus, Americans clamor for a "right to choose" virtually every consumer item and have already transformed medicine into a consumer commodity. Is it any wonder that Americans not only want to "choose" experimental, first-of-their-kind interventions, or that many have gone even farther and insist on choosing death itself with the assistance of a physician?[64] Consent does not justify killing a person anymore than it justifies an otherwise unjustifiable experiment. In the scientific research context, more safeguards are needed to protect the welfare of individual subjects. The "more" is, at minimum, the eight subject welfare precepts (updated as necessary) of the Nuremberg Code that the doublethink language seeks to obscure.

VI. MARKET IDEOLOGY

Two ideologies have been explored: (1) the ideology of science, which puts the requirements of the research protocol designed to objectively test a hypothesis as the highest priority and (2) the ideology of medicine, which puts the best interests of the patient as the highest priority. Medicine, however, is currently faced with a new dominate ideology—the ideology of the marketplace, which puts profit-making (sometimes denoted by its method, cost-containment) as its highest priority. For example, it has never been a secret that the pharmaceutical industry has been the most consistently profitable industry since World War II.[65] Now, however, as competition in this industry has heated up, and as the new

---

63. This seems to be especially true in AIDS research. *See, e.g.,* George J. Annas, *Faith (Healing) Hope and Charity at the FDA: The Politics of AIDS Drug Trials*, 34 VILL. L. REV. 771 (1989) (providing examples of FDA actions in the AIDS area that were politically motivated).

64. *See, e.g.,* Quill v. New York 1996 U.S. App. LEXIS 6215 (2d Cir. April 2, 1996) (no distinction between refusing life-sustaining treatment and committing suicide); Compassion in Dying v. Washington, 1996 U.S. App. LEXIS 3944 (9th Cir. March 6, 1996); George J. Annas, *Death by Prescription; The Oregon Initiative,* 331 NEW ENG. J. MED. 1240 (1994) (on the provisions of Oregon's ballot measure); Margaret Sommerville, *The Song of Death: The Lyrics of Euthanasia,* 9 J. CONTEMP. HEALTH L. & POL'Y 1 (1993) (on the use of language in the euthanasia debate).

65. Brian O'Reilly, *Drugmakers under Attack,* FORTUNE, July 29, 1991, at 48.

biotechnology industry is emerging with great promises of future profits, the role of a successful clinical experiment has become central to the profitability of an entire industry. In this domain, both scientific truth and the best interests of patient-subjects can often find themselves sacrificed in the name of the bottom line. As one observer of the new biotechnology noted of the current state of medical science in the United States, "To do science you need money, but to raise money competitively you need to project illusions that are the antithesis of science."[66] Selling illusions to investors has replaced selling illusions to patients.[67]

A contemporary example combining cancer research and U.S. atomic research effectively illustrates the continuing pervasiveness of double-think and its dangers to human subjects in an atmosphere governed not by war metaphors, but by market metaphors.[68] The Brookhaven National Laboratory is currently pursuing an experimental protocol to redo, in a more sophisticated manner, a radiation experiment conducted between 1951 and 1960. The experiment tests the use of a boron compound delivered to the brain in a stream of neutrons (generated by a nuclear reactor). The hope of this experiment is that the boron will become radioactive and deliver its radiation selectively to a brain tumor. This approach, termed "boron neutron capture therapy," proved either useless or fatal in the 1950s.[69]

The first subject, Joann Magnus, had a terminal brain tumor (a glioblastoma) and was admitted to the new experimental protocol before it was ready (in September 1994) because she had strong political connections.

---

66. BARRY WERTH, THE BILLION DOLLAR MOLECULE 355 (1994).

67. Of course, illusions may be protected by both parties in the human experimentation context. As Christopher Hitchens notes in his iconoclastic biography of Mother Teresa, he is more interested in understanding the public's reaction to her alleged sainthood than Mother Teresa's own views of herself. In his words,

> What follows here is an argument not with a deceiver but with the deceived. If Mother Teresa is the adored object of many credulous and uncritical observers, then the blame is not hers, or hers alone. In the gradual manufacture of an illusion, the conjurer is only the instrument of the audience. He may even announce himself as a trickster and a clever prestidigitator and yet gull the crowd. *Populus vult decipi — ergo decipiatur.*

CHRISTOPHER HITCHENS, THE MISSIONARY POSITION 15 (1995).

68. *See, e.g.,* George J. Annas, *Reframing the Debate on Health Care Reform by Replacing Our Metaphors*, 332 NEW ENG. J. MED. 744 (1995).

69. *See, e.g.,* L.E. Farr et al., *Neutron Capture Therapy of Gliomas Using Boron, in* TRANSACTIONS OF THE AMERICAN NEUROLOGICAL ASSOCIATION 110-13 (1954); W.H. Sweet et al., *Boron-Slow Neutron Capture Therapy of Gliomas*, 1 ACTA RADIOLOGICA 114 (1963); Scott Allen, *Radiation Experiments Coming Back to Haunt Researches*, BOSTON GLOBE, May 29, 1995, at 27, 28.

As Ms. Magnus herself said, "'I had nothing to lose.'"[70] Her physician said, "'I do what I think is best for each individual patient,'. . . . Without this treatment, 'she'd be dead.'"[71] Reporter Andrew Lawler's description of this first of its kind experiment in *Science* exemplifies the victory of doublethink. In his words, what happened involved "an improved version of a therapy," an "updated treatment," and simply, "the therapy."[72] Although only two subjects (of a planned protocol of twenty-eight) have undergone this experiment, Brookhaven National Laboratory is described as "bracing for a flood of requests from dying patients," having to devise "a lottery to choose from among those who meet stringent initial requirements for treatments . . . ."[73] "The procedure" is viewed as "a tremendous cash cow" for the laboratory.[74]

In our postmodern world, it seems to have struck no one as strange that DOE Secretary Hazel O'Leary, the very person who demanded (and received) a serious and sustained investigation into cold war radiation experiments, was also the person who sponsored the first subject for this U.S. Government experiment.[75] In this case, Secretary O'Leary adopted the rationale of treatment of a terminally ill patient when she said, "There's a passion in the hearts of people who know they are terminal with a disease for which there seems to be no cure."[76] However, this particular experiment is about research, not treatment, and about giving the nuclear reactors made irrelevant by the end of the cold war a new lease on life (not "patients") by engaging them in, what O'Leary terms, "'the positive side of nuclear technology.'"[77] Just how positive this procedure is remains to be seen. At least one critic, Princeton physicist and former head of the DOE's Office of Energy Research, William Happer, has noted that demand for experimentation with this procedure has existed for years and has been led by the "reactor mafia" who hope "to find some

---

70. Faye Flam, *Atomic Medicine's Second Chance: Brain Cancer Case Revives Boron Radiation Therapy Method Using Nuclear Reactor*, WASH. POST, Dec. 13, 1994, (Health Magazine), at 9.

71. *Id.* A parallel example involves the use of genetic experiments for glioblastoma. *See* Larry Thompson, *Should Dying Patients Receive Untested Genetic Methods?*, 259 SCIENCE 452, 452 (1993).

72. Andrew Lawler, *Brookhaven Prepares for Boron Trials*, 267 SCIENCE 956, 956 (1995).

73. *Id.*

74. *Id.*

75. *Id.*

76. James Warren, *Positive Side of Nuclear Science: Energy Officials Find Themselves Playing in Life and Death Dramas*, CHI. TRIB., Apr. 23, 1995, §5, at 2.

77. *Id.*

way to keep the reactors going."[78] What is obscured in this language is the experiment itself and that the "requirements" are those of science, not of medicine. This experiment is often viewed as a last resort therapy, demonstrating the continuing ambiguity of postmodern experimentation on the terminally ill.[79]

Although the Advisory Committee decided not to explore contemporary radiation experiments like the one at Brookhaven, the Committee did do the most comprehensive study to date on current research consent practices in the United States. Specifically, the Advisory Committee reviewed a random sample of eighty-four research protocols, consent forms, and IRB deliberations involving ionizing radiation funded from 1990 through 1993, and compared them with a sample of forty-one nonionizing radiation studies from the same period.[80] In a separate study, 1,900 patients at medical institutions across the country were interviewed.[81] Advisory Committee member Professor Jay Katz of Yale conducted an independent review of ninety-three of these proposals.[82] No significant differences were found between radiation and nonradiation protocols or consent forms.[83] Of the 125 studies, 78 were rated as involving greater than minimal risk.[84] Of these, the Committee concluded that about one-half raised serious or moderate ethical concerns, mostly affecting such things as the ability to understand the experiment, knowledge that participation is voluntary, and the ability to understand the potential risks involved. Professor Katz's separate study of the ninety-three proposals identified forty-one that posed greater than minimal risk. Of these, Katz identified thirty (or seventy-five percent) that raised serious ethical concerns, ten borderline, and twenty more serious.[85] In the Committee's words:

Katz found that the most striking element of the troublesome

---

78. Earl Lane, *A Treatment Before its Time*, NEWSDAY, Sept. 4, 1994, at A7, A67.

79. Nor should it surprise us that even before her death, when Ms. Magnus suffered her first set back, the medical director at Brookhaven announced: "'None of us view this as a failure in any sense.'" Arguing that what was going on was research, not treatment, he continued by noting that "the initial goals of the research are to show that treatment is safe and has no unintended side effects. 'Hopefully we get some information as to the effectiveness' as well." Earl Lane, *Pioneer Patient Hospitalized, Setback for Woman in Neutron therapy*, NEWSDAY, May 3, 1995, *available in* LEXIS, News Library, Newsday File.

80. FINAL REPORT, *supra* note 21, at 695-97.

81. *Id.* at 724-25.

82. *Id.* at 711.

83. *Id.* at 701.

84. *Id.* at 700.

85. *Id.* at 712.

consent forms was the lack of a forthright and repeated acknowledgment that patient-subjects were *invited* to participate
in human experimentation. All too quickly the language shifted
to *treatment* and *therapy* when the latter was not the purpose
and was only, at best, a by-product of the research.[86]

Katz described his own reaction to his study and the report in a "statement" in the body of the Advisory Committee's Final Report. On examining the informed consent process, Katz stated:

> I had expected to discover problems, but I was stunned by their
> extent. . . . The obfuscation of treatment and research, illus-
> trated most strikingly in Phase I studies, but by no means lim-
> ited to them; the lack of disclosure in randomized clinical trials
> about the different consequences to patient-subjects' well being
> if assigned to one research arm or the other; the administration
> of highly toxic agents, in the "scientific" belief that only the
> knowledge gained from "total therapy" will *eventually* lead to
> cures, but without disclosure of the impact of such radical inter-
> ventions on quality of life or longevity.[87]

Katz concluded that although we all officially acknowledge that informed
consent is central to the protection of subjects, we have "failed . . . to take
responsibility for making these requirements meaningful ones."[88]

The message from this study is that the IRB and informed consent
mechanisms adopted to displace the Nuremberg Code's "rigid" requirements have failed. In almost half of all cases, this failure can be documented by a review of records alone—a review of actual consent
discussions with the subjects would likely have been even more devastating. In its patient interview and survey, for example, the Advisory Committee found direct evidence of language choices are used to deceive
potential research subjects. The patients were asked to compare the
terms "clinical trial," "clinical investigation," "medical study," and "medical experiment" with "medical research."[89] It will probably surprise no
one that the term medical experiment "evoked the most striking and negative associations" and was the only term ranked worse than medical research.[90] "Clinical investigation" and "clinical trial" were somewhat
better than "medical research," but the term "medical study" got the

---

86. *Id.* at 713.
87. *Id.* at 853.
88. *Id.* at 854.
89. *Id.* at 734 (emphasis omitted).
90. *Id.*

most favorable ratings of all.[91] Such studies were viewed as "less risky, as less likely to involve unproven treatments, and as offering a greater chance at medical benefit."[92] The study also indicated that many patients identify and conflate research with treatment.[93] In short, for many potential research subjects, deception or self-deception is inherent in our current research endeavors.

VII. SOME SUGGESTIONS

It is no wonder that Americans demand experimentation as treatment and insist that their insurance companies and health care plans pay for experimental interventions. There is, of course, a continuum from (scientific) experiment to (therapeutic) treatment,[94] but few interventions are in the gray zone and an objective distinction can almost always be made between an experimental intervention and a treatment. An experiment, for example, does not become therapy simply because no conventional (validated or invalidated) intervention exists any more than subjects become patients simply because they are given a terminal diagnosis. I have proposed elsewhere that we adopt special regulations to protect the rights and welfare of terminally ill patients from exploitative experimentation.[95]

---

91. *Id.*

92. *Id.*

93. *Id.* at 747-50.

94. *See, e.g.*, RENEE FOX & JUDITH SWAZEY, THE COURAGE TO FAIL (1974).

95. Proposed Regulations Governing Research on Terminally Ill Patients:

1. For the purpose of these regulations a "terminally ill patient" is one whose death is reasonably expected to occur within six months even if currently accepted and available medical treatment is used.

2. In addition to all other legal and ethical requirements for the approval of a research protocol by national and local scientific and ethical review boards (including IRBs), research in which terminally ill patients participate as research subjects shall be approved only if the review board specifically finds that:

(a) The research, if it carries any risk, has the intent and reasonable probability (based on scientific data) of improving the health or well-being of the subject, or of significantly increasing the subject's length of life without significantly decreasing its quality;

(b) There is no *a priori* reason to believe that the research intervention will significantly decrease the subject's quality of life because of suffering, pain, or indignity attributable to the research; and

(c) Written informed consent will be required of all research participants over the age of 16 in research involving any risk, and such consent may be solicited only by a physician acting as a patient rights advocate who is appointed by the review committee, is independent of the researcher, and whose duty it is to fully and objectively inform the potential subject of all reasonably foreseeable risks and benefits inherent in the research protocol. The patient rights advocate will also be empowered to monitor the actual research itself.

I continue to believe that this is necessary. Like the Nuremberg Code's consent requirement, however, it is not sufficient.

To confront not only our mortality, but also our morality, we must use language to clarify rather than obscure what we do to one another. Minimally, we must correctly identify and describe roles and responsibilities in human experimentation. In our postmodern world, it may not be realistic to think we can always distinguish research from therapy, physicians from scientists, or subjects from patients. Nonetheless, it is morally imperative to use language to clarify differences because ignoring these differences undermines the integrity of scientific research, the integrity of the medical profession, and the rights and welfare of patients and subjects.

This conclusion seems unremarkable and is not likely to be controversial. Putting it into practice, however, will require changes in the way we conduct contemporary experiments on humans that will likely cause controversy. Nonetheless, if we take the dignity, rights, and welfare of the subjects of human experimentation seriously in the clinical medicine arena, we should take at least the following minimal steps:

1. Research must always be identified as research, and its purpose (to gain generalizable knowledge) always spelled out and differentiated from medical treatment designed only to benefit the patient.

2. Patients should always continue to be patients, even if they also volunteer to serve as research subjects. It is unlikely that it will ever be possible—in our death-denying and death-defying world—for patients not to indulge in self-deception by imagining that research is really treatment and that they are patients, not research subjects. We cannot separate the subject into two persons. *But we can assure that the subject-patient always has a physician whose only obligation is to look out for the best interests of the patient.* Thus, we can (and should) prohibit physicians from performing more than minimal risk research on their patients, and as a corollary, only permit physician-researchers to recruit the patients of other physicians for their research protocols. In this way, at least the "doubling" of physician and researcher can be physically (and perhaps psychologically) eliminated.[96]

---

3. The vote and basis for each of the findings in subpart (2) shall be set forth in writing by the review board and be available to all potential subjects and the public.

4. All research protocols (including the financial arrangements between the sponsor and the researcher) involving terminally ill subject shall be available to the public, and the meetings of the scientific and ethical review boards on these protocols shall be open to the public. Annas, *supra* note 57, at 138.

96. This suggestion has been made many times in the past. The primary objections to it

3. There should be strict disqualification rules for both subjects and researchers to engage in the research enterprise. At the extremes, for example, subjects who believe they have "nothing to lose" should be disqualified from participation because they are unable to give understanding (and perhaps voluntary) consent. Researchers who feel subjects have "nothing to lose" by participating should also be disqualified from doing research on them because they are not able to protect the dignity and welfare of their prospective research subjects with this attitude.[97]

4. The term "therapeutic research" and all of its progeny, such as "experimental treatment" and "invalidated treatment," should be abolished from research protocols and informed consent processes and forms. Research is research, designed to test a hypothesis and performed based on the rules of the protocol; treatment is something else, designed to benefit a patient, and subject to change whenever change is seen in the patient's best interest. Confusing research with treatment confuses both the researcher and subject and permits self-interested self-deception by both of them. The doubling and doublethink phenomena are difficult enough to control even when language itself is not used to disguise ambiguity.[98]

5. To help expose the new market ideology of experimentation, the researcher should be required to disclose any and all financial incentives involved in the research to both the IRB and to the potential subjects. This information should be presented to the subject in a separate written disclosure form so that the subject knows what financial incentives (*i.e.,* conflicts of interest) may be affecting the scientific judgment or medical judgment of the researcher.[99]

---

have not been philosophical but practical. In major cancer centers, for example, virtually every patient has been referred for "new" or experimental protocols because conventional therapy has failed. Their primary care physician may be from another city or state. Who is to be their physician (with only their best interests in mind)? Simply appointing someone at the cancer research hospital may not be sufficient because it can be assumed that this person will share the general research/science ideology of the institution itself. But the logistics can be mastered if the goal is taken to be one of high priority—and in this setting, there can be no higher priority than protection of the patient's welfare. One approach, for example, is to use retired or semi-retired physicians as patient advocates whose only job is to look out for the patient's welfare. *See* FINAL REPORT, *supra* note 21, at 140-41.

97. It is not just the use of the magic words "nothing to lose" that would trigger the disqualification (since both researchers and subjects would quickly learn not to use them), but an objective evaluation of the experiment and the researchers and/or subject's evaluation of it. The example of inducing malaria to treat AIDS necessarily requires both a researcher who thinks the patient has nothing to lose and a patient-subject who agrees with this assessment. *See supra* note 52.

98. *See* King, *supra* note 58.

99. *Cf.* Moore v. Regents of the Univ. of Cal., 793 P.2d 479, (Cal. 1990). This case is

6. Institutional Review Boards should be radically overhauled. We now have more than fifteen years experience with them, and they continue to support both doublethink and the double nature of the researcher physician. In this regard, they have primarily engaged in legitimizing ambiguity and deception and have betrayed the research subjects they are charged to protect. The explanation may be found in both the federal regulations that govern IRBs and the membership of these bodies. Reform on at least three levels is required. We need to (1) form a national human research agency to set the rules for research on humans, monitor their enforcement, and punish those who fail to follow them;[100] (2) rewrite current research rules to reflect the problems of doubling outlined in this Article; and (3) restructure IRBs so that their role is to protect the subjects of research (not the researcher) and to hold researchers accountable to a national body (the proposed National Human Research Agency), not their own institution. At a minimum, this will require democratizing the IRBs by requiring a majority of members be community members and by opening all meetings to the public.

Changing our ways in our postmodern world will not be easy. Our quest for the Holy Grail of medicine (immortality?), as honorable as it is in theory, can become destructive in practice. As Bertolt Brecht has Galileo say in the version of his play he rewrote following Hiroshima:

> I take it that the intent of science is to ease human existence. . . . Should you, then, in time, discover all there is to be discovered, your progress must become a progress away from the bulk of humanity. The gulf might even grow so wide that the sound of your cheering at some new achievement would be echoed by a universal howl of horror.[101]

---

discussed in GEORGE J. ANNAS, STANDARD OF CARE: THE LAW OF AMERICAN BIOETHICS 167-80 (1993); *see also* Harold Edgar & David J. Rothman, *The Institutional Review Board and Beyond: Future Challenges to the Ethics of Human Experimentation*, 73 MILBANK Q. 489, 501 (1995) (recommending the preclusion of research on patients of a product in which the researcher has a commercial stake).

100. *See, e.g.*, FINAL REPORT, *supra* note 21, at 855-56; FINAL REPORT OF THE TUSKEGEE SYPHILLIS STUDY AD HOC ADVISORY PANEL, U.S. DEPT. OF HEALTH EDUCATION AND WELFARE 23-24 (1973) (recommending a national review panel).

101. BERTOLT BRECHT, GALILEO 18 (Charles Laughton, trans. & Eric Bentley ed., 1992).

[12]

Roles and Fictions in Clinical and Research Ethics

*David N. Weisstub**

This paper was originally presented as The Honorourable Mr. Justice O'Byrne/Alberta Heritage Foundation for Medical Research Lecture on Law, Medicine and Ethics, at the University of Alberta and the University of Calgary in March 1996.

Introduction

Although the bioethics movement is a burgeoning system of diplomates, medical doctors in search of more reflective career activities, lawyers who are prepared to commit themselves to a more socially responsible and integrated professional life, philosophers who are zealous about wanting to apply abstractions to real-life situations, and theologians who, with or without faith, want to remain in a position of prudential authority for life and death decision-making, it should be borne in mind that bioethics, as a phenomenon, is a newly created attempt at a discipline of concepts and professional activities. The commentary following will reveal certain cautions about the development of this field. The issues with which these professionals are engaged are not only relevant but pressing in the context of our advanced industrialized economies.

In the earliest period of writing and reflection associated with bioethics, which gathered force in the late 1950s, thoughtful generalists alongside theologians and philosophers, began to pose serious questions about the limits of technical medicine, given the humanistic burdens inherited from the monstrous period of dehumanization during the Second World War that showed the capacity of medicine in general, and the research enterprise in particular, for gross violations against humanity. These pioneer efforts were not unconnected to attacks against medical elitism, and became associated in the 1960s with a pervasive negativism in the popular culture about "hard" medicine and the self-serving patterns of professional conduct connected to corporativism in the health system.

David N. Weisstub is Philippe Pinel Professor of Legal Psychiatry and Biomedical Ethics, Faculté de médecine, Université de Montréal, Montréal, Quebec.

In the second generation of bioethics formation, more generalized philosophical efforts were sustained, contributing to the foundation of special centres of reflection such as Hastings and Kennedy. Since that time in the early 70s, the movement has come a far way. Our point here is to query whether this rapid expansion of power and territory is altogether clear in its production of philosophical mantras and power elites. Our purpose here is not to debunk the seriousness of the overall endeavour, given, as we have already observed, the great importance of its target area of inquiry; nor do we wish to question the integrity of the proponents of an association of intellectuals and practitioners who are bent on cooperating as multi-disciplinarians in some resolution of moral dilemmas presented in medical practice and research. Rather, it is to ask whether the achievements of the movement lead us in any particular way to an improved notion of how to make meaningful ethical decisions, how to fashion laws with an appropriate medico-ethical content and direction, and how to train the advocates of bioethics who are so fulsomely present in our hospitals and committees.

Bioethics entered by the late 1970s into the precincts of medical research, and represented the major influence on studies undertaken by the US government to work out the general principles of that discipline. In 1967, the National Institutes of Health produced the system of surveillance for institutional review boards, and by the mid-1970s a full-scale presentation was made available to the public of how to begin to think as experts about the rights and wrongs of medical ethics in research.

The picture we have been confronted with since the late 1980s, and the full maturation of our *fin de siècle*, is vastly different from the eager and expansive contributions of earlier decades. Although bioethics experts can now be found everywhere, and are present as the key experts to advise research ethics committees, we must take time to reflect on the criteria and the role models guiding these experts. Our notions of the common good, responsibility, attitudes towards vulnerable persons, perceptions about communications styles, transformations of moral sensibilities on end-of-life matters, restructuring of familial models, and an overall tendency towards more egalitarian exchanges of information between professional elites and consumers, have all to be factored into our recalculation of benefits and risks in both therapy and the research enterprise.

The world of research ethics cannot be dissociated from its foundations in the broader bioethics movement. And it is through the importation of core bioethics principles that research ethics has been predominantly fashioned as a way of perceiving moral thresholds and decisions about priorities. Our manner of thinking, informed by the Kantian and utilitarian polarities afforded by philosophy,[1] has led us to assume that failure to achieve expressed value formulations leads directly to moral turpitude and/or pragmatic failure. This results from the position of our philosophical differences in rigid and uncompromising frameworks. For example, Kantians would have us conclude that violations of human dignity are the necessary outcome of utilitarian calculi; and for the utilitarians, Kantian commitments to the autonomous will are seen to miscalculate the rationales that are part of our state of compromised rationality. In reality, our ethical thinking proceeds along the lines of our attempt to defer, in balance, to treat persons as ends and not as means, and to measure the good, both in theory and practice, when we take into account outcomes of an array of health interventions.[2] As we bear down more carefully on these familiar polarities and realize accommodations are inevitable, we come to agree with Macklin and Sherwin in situations where linkages are made to social contexts:

> In any case, it follows from either theory that we have a prima facie obligation to treat other persons honestly, to seek their consent in matters affecting them, and to be sensitive to their interests.[3]

We should conclude that representative theories of pure form are appreciably present for our consideration, but that in applying our actual decision-making models, for example in dealing with difficult cases of ethically permissible experimentation, our analyses and conclusions are foreshadowed by aspects and conflations of the value schemes that are associated with conscionable behaviour in liberal democracies. The challenge for us is to avoid exaggerated views, which albeit given in good intentions, can lead in the name of Kantianism to excessive paternalism or the outright redefinition and denigration of humans deemed to be incomplete. It is not inconceivable that Kantians may will as a universal law that persons with genetic defects or specific racial characteristics should be either denied access to certain health services, or policed, in order to facilitate the social buttressing of our so-called rights by pushing substandard levels of rationability beyond the pale of citizenship. In cases of extreme utilitarianism, the rationalized sacrifices of individual persons for the greater good are part of presentations of theory.

When we are forced to live and decide about cases in the domain of applied ethics, we must challenge ourselves to conjoin empathy with fundamental values,

---

[1] L.W. Sumner, "Utilitarian Goals and Kantian Constraints" in B.A. Brody, ed., *Moral Theory and Moral Judgments in Medical Ethics* (Boston: Reidel, 1988) 15.

[2] E.H. Loewy, "Kant, Health Care and Justification" (1995) 16:2 Theoretical Medicine 215; D.C. Thomasma, "Assessing Bioethics Today" (1993) 2:4 Cambridge Quart. Healthcare Ethics 519; S.H. Furness, "Medical Ethics, Kant and Mortality" in R. Gillon, ed., *Principles of Health Care Ethics* (New York: Wiley, 1994) 159-171.

[3] R. Macklin & S. Sherwin, "Experimenting on Human Subjects: Philosophical Perspectives" (1975) 25 Case Western Law Review 434 at 457-458.

for without such, the social integration of persons without full capacity will not be guaranteed. Rather than emanating from any existing philosophical system, with preferred value schemes attached, our ethical humanism is better located within the experience of empathy. In fact, when we are in the midst of actual ethical decision-making, it is rare even in our professional and cultured social environment to see value systems presented, defined, and logically justified apart from general statements of commitment to tolerance and respect for certain key values such as autonomy and personhood. Having committed in principle to such values, we must advance our protections through affording thorough and far-reaching guidance-rules upon which we can base a legal framework for regulation.

In my final report, as Chairman of the *Enquiry on Research Ethics* for the Government of Ontario, I asserted the following:

> Neither the established principles which dominate bioethics discussions on research, such as beneficence, respect for persons, and justice, nor legal remedies such as informed consent, have been found to be of any substantial practical use in resolving the conflicts of interests that present themselves in the field of research ethics. In ideal terms, these principles and legal remedies, to which we wish to subscribe as a matter of moral commitment and preferred values, do not translate easily into effective remedies. The most generalized moral principles have little predictive value. In the field of the protection of vulnerable populations, beneficence, which motivates us to interventionist policies, does not sit well with the complementary principle of respect for persons which should instantiate policies to enhance autonomy and self-determination, even at the expense of the best interests of subjects. The world of moral principles comes into contact with the universe of legal principles insofar as the law has developed certain instruments, or doctrines, to protect the autonomous life of subjects. Insofar as the application of legal principles has resulted in such autonomous actions causing harm to individuals and their extended social bodies such as the family, the conflict of principles of law has become the subject of scrutiny and disquiet in parallel with the conflicts experienced at the more abstract levels of discussion by philosophers, theologians, and ethicists. With regard to legal remedies it may be seen that the doctrine of informed consent has not been followed with any credibility and its cost in the quality of human relations or economy has not been empirically documented in any significant way to date. In fact, legal remedies have been highly selective and irregular, are after the fact,

and have in any event not proven to protect the special populations to which such doctrines were initially directed.[4]

It is against this background perception that we pursue our further inquiry here. What we will attempt to show is that the dilemmas we are facing in making priority decisions about the elderly and other high-cost groups of citizens, including specific groups of vulnerable persons, have led us quite naturally to make, arguably in good faith, a set of both moral and legal fictions in order that our social needs have respectable "justificatory" ethics. We are not suggesting here that such fictions are mere rationalizations. On the contrary, much of what happens in the life of our moral and legal fictions falls into the domain of what we can term "white lies" and "soft fictions". These are meant to balance our need to fulfill different goals, some of which are in implicit or explicit conflict with one another. The resolution of these conflicts can be directly linked to how we view the doctor/patient or researcher/subject relationship, and to our perspectives about the extent to which we can hold citizens morally liable to act on behalf of others, or for that matter, expect a society to accept the burden of incapacitated citizens. Insofar as philosophers and legal doctrine have afforded us some of the tools that assist us in our public discussion, we must remain both grateful and accommodating. However, unquestioning reliance on such expertise or on legal regimes can not only be misleading, but also a contributing factor to the kind of dependency where moral failures can be most pronounced. Disfavouring a real public debate on controversial matters related to medical ethics, for example in research, is a sacrifice that no civilized democracy should allow. We turn then to consider the role models that are part of the active world of bioethics, as we have constituted it, and thereafter to the field of research ethics as the applied terrain upon which bioethics has already left indelible marks and patterns.

Part I

In ethics consultations, committees, and informal exchanges which occur among professionals and their patients, there is a high degree of incertitude about two matters: firstly, whether there is integrity to the body of knowledge called "bioethics"; and secondly, whether from this existing material there emerges a clear directive about the best method of training people to benefit a potential group of clients to make, or have made for them, the most "beneficial" ethical decisions. Often, the jump is made quickly into the second category, where a polemicism has a tendency to replace scientific inquiry. Given where people are situated, often out of self-interest in this professional arena, there is the

---

[4]   Ontario, Enquiry on Research Ethics, *Final Report: Enquiry on Research Ethics* (Toronto: Queen's Printer, 1995) (Chair: D.N. Weisstub) at 2.

assumption that choosing the wrong model, either in professional role-playing or in a concept of education, will lead to adverse ethics.

Without entering into a full inquiry into the integrity of the body of knowledge underlying this movement, we might have a more modest beginning to an improvement of our understanding by turning to the distinctive roles that emerge in the ordinary course of discussion found among clinicians. The three dominant models could be described as: the ethicist as tranquillizer; the ethicist as advocate; and the ethicist as a conscience surrogate. In all these modalities, there are a set of assumptions and implications for what is perceived to be correct professional-ethical behaviour. Choosing one course of action is not necessarily mutually exclusive of correlative roles, but certainly in many circumstances, the roles stand in opposition and lead to different ways of conducting relationships between professionals and their clients, and to profoundly different views about how to educate a generation of informed professionals and a specific group of experts.

At the root of these modalities is the presumption that we have in mind an ideal type or product. If, in the case of searching for an integrated paradigm of expertise, we think inevitably of specialized knowledge or experience, we must probe in the case of each of our modalities the link between taking on a role and a certain species of professionalism, either by way of background or according to the building-block model of achieving a justified hybrid. Put simply, questions must be posed about whether the "ethicist" is the goal or the problem; whether clinical experience is the necessary pre-requisite or condition for acting responsibly when ethical conflicts are presented; whether clinical ethicists are best placed or found in the context of committees, multidisciplinary consultation groups, or one-to-one hands-on consultations with families or patients in an informal structure within a hospital or clinical environment; and finally, whether they find their best ultimate role in an educational process meant to improve the dialogic between health professionals and their subjects.

One thing is certain. The need for clinical ethicists is pronounced in hospitals and in the health environment at large, due either to the extended life span realized in most industrialized societies (influenced by the utilization of new technologies), or as a necessary input to stem the tide of social inquietude attributed to the evaporation of a consensus morality previously found in more cohesive social orders, either driven by collective appreciation of either religious or political values. The pressures towards reliance upon clinical ethicists have arguably been recent and never stronger than now. It is unclear, however, whether our preoccupation about having a need for clinical ethicists will be long term (so that their evolution will be concretized and better defined), or whether clinical ethicists, after a generational trend has been exposed, will be rendered obsolete and regarded as ethical transition objects in a period of major social upheaval. Arguably, clinical ethicists may eventually be viewed in a similar way to the advocacy group which dominated the thinking of minorities and consumers, until it was replaced by more autonomous, independent and politically assertive self-advocates who rejected the notion of dependency on experts.

One of the dynamics which lies behind all the options of role-playing is the presence or absence of the ethicist in terms of the direct contact either visual or emotional, which occurs between professional and subject. This raises in part the question of whom the ethicist serves. Is the role of the ethicist to facilitate the value-formation of a group of professionals who, in the forum of a committee structure, decide ethical outcomes among themselves? How important is the act of communicating and assisting in the clarification of communication, and for a value which is subject-oriented? Many professionals may even fear opening up imponderables relating to pain, life-threatening decisions, the management of one's loved ones, and personal affairs with a subject or a family group in distress. Ethicists may often be poorly trained in the emotional dimension of the process of communicating values. On the other hand, mental health professionals, or physicians for that matter, may be modest in their understanding of the kinds of values which are at stake and should be articulated in order to arrive at meaningful decisions. People faced with moral dilemmas want to be assisted with the gathering of relevant knowledge, enhanced in their capacity for self-reflection, placed in a position to articulate shared values, and prepared to assess the impact of these values (and the decisions flowing from them) on those parties who are relevant to their own constituted sense of personal or social well-being. It seems as if one of the greatest threats to all of us is our sense of inadequacy in, on the one hand, being able to reflect on intra-psychic conflicts that are part and parcel of our sense of physical or spiritual health, and on the other, once we are equipped with such self-reflection, being able to move out again into the world, with a sense of freedom and lack of shame, to share thoughts, and eventually decisions, with others who have been, are, or will be, part of a reconstituted universe which has a life beyond any mortal unit.

In the face of the pressures and requirements placed on the shoulders of ethicists who live the daily life of decisions, there is a need to explore how roles represent a set of reference points around which professional practices occur and are justified.

The Ethicist as Tranquillizer

It may well be that the overwhelming purpose and function of clinical ethicists is to calm an environment which is already inflated emotionally due to the need to make a decision where every alternative is connected to, or will result

Human Experimentation and Research

in, serious pain (physical or emotional) for a person, family or group. The call for an ethicist is catalyzed by the absence of a pastoral or professional authority figure, who could present a moral resolution to the issue at hand. In some instances, there will be a great sense of satisfaction to see the appearance of an expert, perhaps in the actual physical guise of a doctor, robed in white, and under the command of a beeper unit, indicating the dependency of patients on the professional's immediate availability to respond to a call of urgency. The content or ethical rationalization in such a picture is surely secondary to the pronounced emotional need of the dependent party. Depending upon the communication orientation of the clients, professionals often learn to fulfill this mandate with considerable social skill. In some cultural contexts, certainty is the measure of professionalism, whereas in others, an affected modesty and the soft approach of merely facilitating an exchange through the role of arbitrator or mediator represents an appropriate comfort zone to the consumers. In any event, the ethicist is there to create the conditions for a scaling down of conflict, and to facilitate leading the parties to resolution.[5]

Some professionals see their roles as clinicians thusly: as participation in a mask, or worse, a fraudulent undertaking. A want or need does not, in and of itself, produce integrity for professionals who have serious intellectual doubt about both their mandate, and the body of knowledge upon which advice or guidance is based. From the intellectual point of view, some ethicists who do applied work still persist in the view that without a set of principles, which are the mainstay of any operational activity, there will always be the gnawing disbelief in being able to establish moral connectors between thought and practice. The black box problem in clinical ethics in its embryonic stage may not be dissimilar to the conditions of medicine at an earlier time. Medicine in the pre-industrial era, although limited in science, still had a calming-placebo effect, even where the fear level of the party in need was not at issue. But whereas medicine has always demonstrated some basis in science for offering effective remedies where something had to be proved causatively, ethicists, who are pressed upon to make associations between knowledge and practice, are arguably on weaker ground. This is not to say that we need to achieve a positivistic ethics which is measurable or provable, in order to be able to function in a useful and credible manner as ethicists, nor do we wish to suggest as an expressed difficulty here that we are prepared to declare moral bankruptcy because, as a society, we should admit that we suffer from the extremities of moral relativism. Such radical conclusions are neither what we should necessarily admit, or accept, as a given. Rather, in our

---

[5]   See also J.J. Glover, D.T. Ozar & D.C. Thomasma, "Teaching Ethics on Rounds: the Ethicist as Teacher, Consultant and Decision-Maker" (1986) 7:1 *Theoretical Med.* 13-32; D.C. Thomasma, "The Role of the Clinical Medical Ethicist: the Problem of Applied Ethics and Medicine" in M. Braide *et al.*, eds., *The Applied Turn in Contemporary Philosophy* (Bowling Green: Bowling Green State University Press, 1983) 137-157.

search for general principles, we may clarify the limitations of the state of our science and what it leads to thereafter practically. Otherwise, we can only turn in circles on some form of professional intuition, which is dangerously close to an appeal to authority or paternalism.[6] Such elitism is out of synchrony with the increasing level of popular education about health matters, and with the heightened awareness about life-and-death matters in medicine which are widely discussed in our popular culture. Therefore, we should conclude that regardless of how much the population, even when educated and aware, wants to be tranquillized by a new elite corps of professionals, such professionals and their critics are well-advised to exercise caution, simply because the process has become self-aggrandizing, self-justifying and based upon emotional need.

The Ethicist as Advocate

There is an ongoing ambiguity about which set of skills best serves the enhancement of empowerment, the mainstay of the deontological movement that views the ideal subject as a fully rational and autonomous party who should always strive to maximize principled decision-making. With such a model in mind, the challenge to the ethicist is to bend to the legal will or model of the rational citizen, an orientation which also affects our view of how to treat incapacitated or dependent individuals. Thus, some ethicists find themselves functioning as "in-hospital" lawyers, and armed with an effective legal apparatus, prepare themselves to act as intermediaries or ombudspersons between or among complainants in the health system. With exposure, it is rare that legally trained persons can avoid a natural inclination towards collusion where there is an identification, if not over-identification,[7] with a caring or paternalistic ethic that is in conflict with the traditional role of a legal professional. It is not unusual to see ethicists with a legal background functioning through and for a mind set normally associated with the medical model, where intervention is directed to protect the patient from self-destructive decision-making. Ironically, the legally trained professional, who originally identified with a rational deontological substructure, is transformed into a paternalistically-oriented intermediary within a system that is health-based and directed, and for which the advocate has had no significant, or even relevant, preparation. Interestingly, however, as we have observed in the case of ethicist as tranquillizer, the need of patients to be secure

---

[6]   B.A. Brody, "Autonomy and Paternalism—Some Value Problems; a Utilitarian Perspective; a Deontological Perspective" in B.A. Brody, ed., *Ethics and Its Applications* (New York: HBJ, 1983) 159.

[7]   D. Barnard, "Reflections of a Reluctant Clinical Ethicist: Ethics Consultation and the Collapse of Critical Distance" (1992) 13:1 Theoretical Med. 15.

in a foreign and threatening environment may be equally strong *vis-à-vis* the lawyer as a symbolization of certitude and rectitude.

Legalities have everywhere intruded into the pristine domain of both "ethics" and "professional practice". There is such a vast jurisprudence of health law, with elaborate judicial reflections on social values pertaining to health, that it is impossible for anyone presuming to function as an applied ethicist to forget, even for a moment, the momentous impact that legal decisions have on our ethical thinking about health matters and on the way in which we conduct our professional practices. These legal decisions are part of a larger picture of codification and legislation as well as an extensive literature where lawyers and legal philosophers associate their thinking with the major trends extant in philosophy and political theory. To think of law as isolated in the health area from ethics and politics is to associate either law or practical philosophy with abstractions, or other social eras inapplicable to our current time and place.

The advocacy movement, apart from matters of theory, is a mirror of political attitudes which burgeoned in the 1960s and led to dramatic reinvestigations into our belief in professional elites. The association therefore of a newly created elite group of ethicists with the advocacy movement represents an odd alliance of bedfellows. For at once we may see that the advocacy movement, which was meant to subvert elitism, evolved in its various guises into a specific group of experts, many of them para-professionals, who then led their legally oriented expertise in the direction of taking on tasks which emerged from the health system from a different set of premises, that were often contradictory to the ones behind the advocacy movement. Now we are faced with advocates and ethicists who share two sets of problems: firstly, how to define their roles professionally; and secondly, how to orient themselves to their knowledge-base in such a way that a sense of professional integrity is preserved from an intellectual point of view in the definition and purposiveness of the ongoing roles encountered.

The dialectical play between advocacy, ethics clarification and health system paternalism presents a dramatic challenge to all participants who wish to locate a professional role. As team-playing is so strongly part of the consultation process in which health advocates participate, any restrictive view of a legalistic role ceases to make practical sense. However, once the legally-oriented advocate begins to apply the craft of informing parties about the law, putting steps into motion to assess mental capacity or dealing with claims on the system of rights and benefits, advocates cannot separate their tasks from their responsibility of social judgement, accountability to health providers, and responsive behaviour towards family members and public institutions. Finding one's way back to a professional role, or learning how to justify morally a hybrid of activities, can become conflictual, challenging and deeply confusing. Bluntly stated, it is often difficult for advocates who have found their way into the universe of clinical ethics to know whether it is in the undoing of their professional training or in the efficacy of a mature application of their background, that good is brought to patients who depend on their counsel.

The Ethicist as a Conscience-Surrogate

Even stronger than the need for tranquillity or advocacy, is the desire on the part of persons to find a reference towards moral superiority. It is not true that we are able to operate in a moral vacuum. On the contrary, there is great moral anxiety in the modern world where acts of violence and disrespect are present and threaten our social order. Coupled with the prolongation of life and the vulnerability of an aging population is the celebration, in popular culture, of physical health and youthfulness. With fiscal crises and the privatization trend in health care services, something near a panic-level of concern can be seen; there is a social recognition that in the process of prioritizing health entitlements, we will need to find a ground for ethics that will be collectively tolerated even as it remains respectful to traditionally stated deontological systems which underline the need to respect persons as ends in themselves. Such universal principles are being tested and attacked insofar as clinical ethics comes into contact with scarcity of resources. As tensions rise in this sector, the requirement for the ethicist to take on the role of conscience-surrogate accelerates.

In this way, the ethicist is the replacement for and embodiment of the traditional role of the Church. In search of conscience, hospitals and medical institutions, no less than governments, seek experts to set the limits of individual sacrifice required by a novel communitarian ethic. Clinical ethics in this light is pulled between crass pragmatism and the impulse to preserve a humanistically-centred liberalism. As we realize that liberalism as a political philosophy is on the wane, and that in advanced industrialized societies we have a stark mainstream commitment to *laissez-faire* social arrangements and the privatization of publicly-centred institutions, clinical ethicists find themselves at the heart of social transformation. They are often consulted as a new species of experts of last resort. Although burdensome in the extreme to be the moral conscience of a confused society, it also can be not only enticing, but heady. Therefore, it should be the mandate of clinical ethicists to guard against moral narcissism. Time and time again, even the most distinguished professionals in medicine will join patients in moral desperation to locate an expert who will relieve either or both of the parties from exercising moral judgement when there is a limited understanding of the values involved, and even less, of the values implicated in the outcome of the decision to be arrived at. To be the moral conscience in such situations is not as difficult as might appear at first glance, because there is little investment in requesting details from the parties involved in justifying acts of conscience. Rather, the commitment is to give relief from the guilt engendered by even a self-reflected move which is not grounded in consensus. Reliance on ethicists often springs from the depths of human-moral misery and inadequacy. Taking over ethically is no different than mental health professionals being overly directive in circumstances where their patients are truly fragmented and dependent. It is necessary, then, for clinical ethicists to define their relationship with those who receive their delivery of moral goods, and to make sure that such pronouncements are virtuous and empowering of patient autonomy, rather than manipulative and dependency-creating.

Clinical ethicists should be trained in moral modesty. The creation of the clinical ethics movement can be directly attached to the reality that contemporary society has nowhere else to turn. Where physical health transcends spirituality, and hedonism has been the dominant ideal of our social fabric for a number of generations, clinical ethicists will not easily be able to convince the public that ethicists embody desirable codes of principles and behaviour practices. Clinical ethicists are part of the conditioning of society at large. How then, in such a universe, can clinical ethicists assist patients and health professionals to enter into a dialogue of mutuality and concern? The creation of the conditions among medical trainees and other professionals that will allow them to approach patients so that there can be an honest exchange of risks and benefits, of a moral as well as of a medical nature, is what conscience should dictate. The role of clinical ethicists should be, through training and facilitating a process of dialogue between health professionals and patients, to raise the level of consciousness in our health-related decision-making to the point where conscience is heightened among all parties. The ethicist should not remain disembodied or disengaged. Clinical ethics, if it is to have meaning, should be the living process of locating conscience through dialogue, namely through caring communication. In this way humanism or liberalism can be re-enlightened, even in economies of scarcity, and where political and social values have been found wanting.

Part II

We turn now to consider the role and function of clinical ethics in the. specific domain of research, where we can observe the testing out and crystallization of a mature formation of a generalized movement of ethics training and concept building. After a number of decades during which philosophers and clinicians attempted to formulate a core of organizing concepts, the research industry became the recipient of a framework according to which, presumably, "applied ethics" could be named with a requisite level of respectability. Why research in medicine became the focal point of the ethics movement is an interesting social question in itself, arising as it did in the environment of industrialized and highly developed medical centres: the Germany of the 1930s and the America of the 1950s. In either milieu, we are driven to consider how abuses were destined to have occurred in a scandalous manner against the interests of vulnerable persons, and where, in any event, the lapse of moral fortitude within the medical fraternity should be regarded as nothing less than legendary.

The analysis here will have three focal points: firstly, research and multi-ethics, a consideration of issues raised by our preferred model of group decision-making; secondly, a reflection on informed consent as an organizing concept and its attendant myths and misunderstandings; and finally, a commentary on how fictions have penetrated our approaches to vulnerable populations in the area of research ethics.

Research and Multi-Ethics

The idea of committee decision-making sits well with our democratic notion that a paternalistic "one man show" is marked with the arrogance of a bygone era. However, the "doctor knows best" concept, which permeated ethical decision-making until only a few decades ago has been bypassed by a dependency, of a similar nature, on technical expertise. This has been done with the override that, in matters which cast up moral differences, society should guarantee a fair dialogue, ruled by principles of administrative justice that obligate researchers to professional standards of disclosure and care.

In putting together a committee whose mandate is not only to occupy itself with whether the research under review has achieved a minimal level of scientific integrity, but is also to see that "ethics are fulfilled", we are warranted in questioning how the team effort contributes to the process of acquiring and disseminating a consensus of informed morality based upon some appreciation of expertise. In the discourse of research ethics committees, there is an almost startling repetition of certain catch phrases: beneficence, respect for persons and justice. Normally, members of such committees are not particularly well informed about the philosophical content surrounding these principles, and it is not clear whether referring to them advances in any significant way the goal of attaining shared moral precepts for making hard decisions. In fact, the reverse may be true, that these terms have become slogans behind which experts provide justifications and the tie-ins between principles and actions are not even questioned by committee members. We should not underestimate the investment that committee members have in avoiding responsibility for ethical dilemmas which are confusing and guilt-producing.

272   Health Law Journal Vol.4, 1996

Committee members acting on research matters all bring some mode of professional training to their work, and carry the normal citizen's package of ethical impulses, as these arise from familial, environmental, cultural, professional, and socio-political inputs. Given that we are not a homogeneous society with respect to the format of these influences, it is not surprising that our impulse on these committees is to avoid opening up Pandora's box, lest we be prompted to enter debates which would expose disturbing matters for exchange. Such matters would include questioning the extent to which the committee in question is already weighted in the direction of a particular outcome, whether the research industry or a selected interest within the research endeavour is overly represented in the group, the style of decision-making dominant in the committee (for example, whether it is adversarial or mediational), and the key expert's orientation in theology or philosophy, which could make a serious difference in influencing the social attitudes of the other participants and the eventual outcome of the committee decision. If the prism of these questions is expanded to allow for identification of how the ethics formation of each of the committee members really presents itself, we would achieve a rare dialogue about "ethics controversies and priorities".

In many institutions we can still find committees ruled by the researchers themselves, where the ethics could be best described as those of self-interest. In others, there is excessive reliance on the oracular presence of an ethicist. In some instances, we can still find provocative examples of members of extended research teams who sit in judgment on their own research. We should disallow such extreme cases, given the clear lack of ethical integrity. But in the great majority of cases, persons of goodwill are meant to grapple as a team in search of a viable morality consensus. Reasonable persons should not come to unreasonable disagreements, except in a minority of circumstances in which true moral quandaries are present. The question is how to prepare committees to locate the right brand of ethics in passing judgment when they are confronted with such inevitable divisions of emotion and opinion.

The multi-ethical dimension of committees is both good and bad. In a positive light, we presumably have a better representation of the spread of public opinion in the divergence of personalities appointed for the task. This is only a presumption, however, because we certainly are not surprised to find an in-house quality in many of the existing committees. In most cases, we will not find any members from the group of research subjects. Nor will we have any significant feedback from subjects about how they have been handled by research ethics committees, even though we might assume, given the ubiquitous reliance on the mantras of autonomy and respect for persons, that the researcher/subject relationship would have been a first priority. From this point of view, the ethical ideal of the multi-ethics committee structure seems to have been a failed reality.

Quite apart from the lack of consistency in both the analysis of ethical principles, and how these principles can be and are applied in practice, there is the endemic problem of achieving uniformity among research committees in hard cases. The issue is whether we should aspire to such consistency given the difficult nature of the problems. From the points of view of planning and research, consumer expectations about entitlements, and obtaining access to research where there may be a correlative therapeutic benefit (short or long term), consistency becomes a meaningful requirement. Also, a lack of consistency allows some research ethics committees to be considered lax with respect to ethical standards which affect certain institutional practices, so we can expect research funds to flow in an overly determined fashion to certain institutions, provinces or countries.

In order to realize a desirable level of consistency, guidelines should be formatted by overseeing bodies, and regulated by regional political authorities. We are not prepared to submit that rigid national standards should be put into place, because a new set of issues arise once research ethics decision-making is taken over by any aloof and overly regimented body that might fail to take into account justified local differences. Nevertheless, given the uncertainty of leaving research committees to their own devices, the lack of clarity in how we connect theory and practice in research ethics, and to the variances of decision-making styles among professional elites, we should avoid *ad hoc* reliance on the committee structure. Perhaps the greatest value of the best-constituted committees is that they afford a period of reflection for interested and affected parties to meet face to face, in order to make ethics a result of a collective exchange rather than collective interest. The strength of the committee is not, and should not be, in the unanimity of ethics, but in the potential for a meaningful and truthful division of expressed opinion that first attracts controversy, and thereafter human-centred compromise in the hard cases, which are the only truly relevant ones for reflection.

Informed Consent as an Organizing Concept: Myths and Misunderstandings

The "core issue" directing how research ethics committees make decisions can be tied directly to primary input from the bioethics tradition of the 1960s, namely the doctrine of informed consent. Through this instrument, the core values of the bioethics movement were deemed realized, so much so that informed consent should rightfully be regarded as the high watermark of the great period of bioethics expansionism in the 1970s and 80s. Despite the fact that informed consent represents a major improvement over the preceding era of overt medical paternalism, we should be cautious in over celebrating its achievement, both in

274   Health Law Journal Vol.4, 1996

relationship to its originally stated goals, and with regard to the most important group that it was aimed to protect, namely vulnerable persons. To some extent, we might say that informed consent is, at least partially, a myth produced by the bioethics movement: one which has regrettably distracted research ethics committees from confronting moral realities.

As an example of practical and legal ethics, consent mushroomed as an all-pervasive line of defense against the prospects of paternalistic abuse. In a brief period of twenty years, from courtroom to ethics committees, it became a basic assumption that both legal and moral problems were acceptably resolved if the conditions of legal consent were realized. To accomplish this, an elaborate system of legal decisions established outright bans on certain forms of medical practice, while drafting the permissible rationales for modifying the need for informed consent through the defining of mental capacity, best-interests, guardian and substitution rules, maturation levels for children, and more recently, criteria for providing advance consents. All this work was surely not in vain, much of it motivated by a real desire on the part of courts and legal commentators to ensure that, to the best of our institutional abilities, we would enshrine the consent doctrine as a protection against past evils.

Without wishing to return to a pre-consent universe, we might nevertheless expose the mythic characteristic of the doctrine, insofar as it should be seen to be useful but limited, not unlike abstract philosophical systems that in their application seemingly fail to deliver requisite protections. Over-reliance on the law of consent in fact carries with it the risk that we may willfully blind ourselves to the real exchanges of power and benefits between researchers and subjects. To begin with, consent is a model based on a contractual relationship, which in its pristine form is rare both in medical practice and research.

Recently, Shuck observed:

> A priori, there are strong reasons to suspect that informed consent, at least the law in books, is often honored in the breach and almost impossible to enforce as a practical matter. Most of the existing empirical studies on informed consent support this intuition. These studies reveal three related impediments to implementation of informed consent doctrine: (1) most physician-patient discussions appear to be rather perfunctory and reinforce physician control; (2) the treatment context discourages patients form exploiting the information that physicians do provide; and (3) the nature of the tort system makes it difficult for patients to establish an effective legal claim.[8]

---

[8]   P.H. Schuck, "Rethinking Informed Consent" (1994) 103 Yale L. J. 899 at 932-33.

The practical limitations of the informed consent doctrine have now been fully documented by empirical research that has assessed the link to subject understanding.[9] By and large, we have established the fact that subjects are often unaware that they are even participating in experimentation, despite the physician's adherence to well-worked legal requirements.[10] This limitation persists even where institutional review boards have taken their supervisory role seriously.[11]

Apart from the issue that our procedures rather systematically disfigure the cognitive capacity needed to make informed consent meaningful, we are also prey to the fact that, more often than not, the subordinates of researchers manage the informed consent process. This does not mean to say that subordinates are inferior communicators to researchers; the contrary may sometimes be true, and indeed revealing. As an ideal, however, we should commit ourselves to the prospects of moral relationships occurring between researchers and subjects in as personal a manner as possible, in order to avoid the depersonalization of the research enterprise.

Model informed consent presumes that a rational decision-maker is mobilized after being exposed to the relevant information that will allow risks and benefits to be assessed in the light of a specific set of personal values. This idealization can have the impact of misdescribing not only reality, but also the requirements of effective decision-making in the system.[12] After having made critical decisions about 'trustability', research subjects are frequently called upon to commit to a process at large, and often are not given details at various stages,

---

[9]   There has been considerable criticism of these studies because of their conceptual and methodological deficiencies. While this may tend to limit their practical usefulness in terms of constructing an adequate practical model of informed consent, the studies nonetheless point to serious problems with the way in which informed consent currently operates. A comprehensive critique of the informed consent research may be found in A. Mazel & L.H. Roth; "Toward an Informed Discussion of Informed Consent: A Review and Critique of the Empirical Studies" (1983) 25 Arizona L. Rev. 265. See also P.S. Appelbaum, L.H. Roth & C. Lidz, "The Therapeutic Misconception: Informed Consent in Psychiatric Research" (1982) 5 Int. J. L. & Psych. 319; P.S. Appelbaum & L.H. Roth, "The Structure of Informed Consent in Psychiatric Research" (1983) 1:4 Behavioral Sci. and the Law 9; and P.R. Benson, L.H. Roth & W.J. Winslade, "Informed Consent in Psychiatric Research: Preliminary Findings from an Ongoing Investigation" (1985) 20 Society, Sci. & Med. 133.

[10]   P.R. Benson & L.H. Roth, "Trends in the Social Control of Medical and Psychiatric Research" in D.N. Weisstub, ed., *Law and Mental Health: International Perspectives*, Vol. 4 (New York: Pergamon Press, 1988) 1 at 24.

[11]   B.H. Gray, *Human Subjects in Medical Experimentation* (New York: Wiley-Interscience, 1975). A comprehensive survey of the consent research can be found in Benson & Roth, *ibid.* at 24-31.

[12]   C.H. Fellner & J.R. Marshall, "Kidney Donors - The Myth of Informed Consent" (1970) 9 Am. J. Psych. 79.

276   Health Law Journal Vol.4, 1996

as would be required, in order to be part of an ongoing commitment to a particular course of action.[13]

It is often difficult to establish how subjects use information to make actual participation decisions, given that the overwhelming variable is a matter of predisposition and the primacy of emotional factors rather than a logical or rational process. Even when rationality is available for our assessment and deconstruction, further reflection reveals a high level of distortion owing to psycho-pathological factors.[14] The aforementioned difficulties amalgamate to make informed consent in many diverse contexts meaningless, abstracted, or misguided.

> All of these factors, it can be argued, interfere sufficiently with the rational deliberation that is at the core of at least some autonomy-related conceptions of informed consent that the purpose of the doctrine is vitiated. Informed consent then comes to be considered a "myth" [according to Fellner and Marshall's 1970 study], which can only act as an impediment to the delivery of health care without producing any benefits of its own.[15]

If we squarely face the power imbalance between researchers and subjects, it is farfetched to consider informed consent as anything more than an open-ended legal mechanism for checking and controlling unsuspected or untrammeled power.[16] This redressing of power imbalances should be both the aim and outcome of the informed consent doctrine, rather than the provision of a detailed contract of disclosure, which is the normal ideal supported by the diversified legal doctrines that have come under its broad penumbra. If we see our ideal as the creation of power equilibria and regard it as a matter of process rather than one of conclusion, we will accept that protections can only be realized through a commitment to the idea that parties should be involved in an ongoing exchange. This inevitably will raise questions of competing interests for different groups found within the system.

---

[13]   R.R. Faden & T.L. Beauchamp, "Decision-making and Informed Consent: A Study of the Impact of Disclosed Information" (1980) 7 Social Indicators Research 314; Fellner & Marshall, *ibid.*

[14]   W.C. Thompson, "Psychological Issues in Informed Consent" in President's Commission for the Study of Ethical Problems in Medicine and Biomedical and Behavioral Research, *Making Health Care Decisions: The Ethical and Legal Implications of Informed Consent in the Patient-Practitioner Relationship*, vol. III (Washington, D.C.: U. S. Government Printing Office, 1982) 83.

[15]   P. Appelbaum, "Informed Consent" in D. N. Weisstub, ed., *supra* note 10 at 78. The author cites C.H. Fellner & J.R. Marshall, *supra* note 14.

[16]   R.A. Burt, *Taking Care of Strangers: The Rule of Law in Doctor-Patient Relations* (New York: The Free Press, 1979). See also J. Katz, *The Silent World of Doctor and Patient* (New York: The Free Press, 1984).

The largest problem which looms above and beyond informed consent doctrinalism is the fact that health services systems, now under severe constraints and revamping, leave increasingly less time to health care providers to develop meaningful dialogues with the consumers of health treatments or research protocols. We are forced to question whether the doctrine is an actual disincentive to the effective use of resources that can objectively be linked to positive outcomes for the recipients.[17] The problem is seen therefore as structural, showing an "informed consent gap ... [which] reflects the constraints imposed by human psychology, the physician-patient relationship, the tort law system, and an increasingly cost-conscious health care delivery system - and that these constraints are largely intractable."[18]

Certain arguments have been represented by Veatch to show that the law of informed consent in the treatment area is shamefully inadequate to cope with anything more than a trivial exchange of facts in relation to risk. As Veatch rightfully indicates, there is much beyond the shadow of facts in consent decision-making. Of greater importance are the host of values that make up a person's constellation of beliefs, attendant upon factors such as family life, religious upbringing and belief systems, and attitudes about fundamental values that pertain to the fabric of one's social and political environment. Until physicians understand their own inadequacy to articulate disclosure that is relevant for a meaningful response, in the largest sense of the word, informed choice will either be an empty abstraction or a hollow configuration. In fact, Veatch suggests that informed consent is based upon liberalism, namely the respect for acute autonomy, and is a myth in a vacuum without the support structure of liberal values. Veatch argues that over time a more mature idea of decision-making about medical matters will emerge, as patients choose institutions and medical practitioners based on a rooted understanding of how the latter may act as partners, sharing a value-scheme that reaches to the heart of critical, human conflicts and their resolution.[19]

---

[17]   See Schuck, *supra* note 9.
[18]   *Ibid.* at 905.
[19] R.M. Veatch, "Abandoning Informed Consent" (1995) 25:5 Hastings Center Report 5.

An unsympathetic accounting of such a partnership or covenantal bond[20] would note that the inherent imbalance in power would place the stronger party in a paternalistic role over the subject. Such an accounting would fail to appreciate the significant attribute of the fiduciary and evolutionary nature of the covenantal concept. It is the obligation of the stronger party to make every effort at all points in the relationship to maximize the autonomous reach of the assertive power of the subject; failure to do so is a violation of the covenant. The subject is also required to push back the paternalistic arm to the maximum extent possible, while showing a realistic appreciation of the other person's mandate. Rather than seeing the relationship as one between parent and child, the covenantal archetype is closer to that of a parent preparing and dealing with the emancipatory movements of an adolescent approaching adulthood, whose space increases until free choice is respected and acknowledged. In this way, the second party of the covenant can be held morally responsible for the enactment of meaningful choice.

It is interesting to explore the parameters of Veatch's observations about the limitations of informed consent, as we know it within the reality of the research context, because his analysis is even more compelling when surrogate decision-making is considered. When one turns to research, often dealing with incapacitated or profoundly vulnerable parties, one has to ask how realistic it is to speak about choices and pairing of value systems between researchers and subjects. As an ideal type or model, Veatch's point of view is compelling. Certain classical defenders nonetheless continue to advocate the viability and relevance of informed consent. But even those are forced to admit that short of thoroughly integrating the doctrine into a meaningful process of exchange that is reflected in the ethos of medicine, the law of informed consent is destined to remain nothing more than a fairy tale.[21] As a safeguard against the tyranny of elitist decision-makers, the doctrine of informed consent, based on a complete disclosure of facts relating to risk, should be regarded as a protective device in the area of research.

---

[20]   The idea of covenant is not a stranger to either the medical profession or to the Western legal or moral tradition. The medical profession itself has grown up with the idea of covenant as part of the Hippocratic Oath *vis-à-vis* the physicians' obligations and indebtedness owed to his teacher and his progeny for the service of the knowledge given. See W.F. May, "Code and Covenant or Philanthropy and Contract?"in S.J. Reiser, A.J. Dyck & W.J. Curran, *eds., Ethics in Medicine: Historical Perspectives and Contemporary Concerns* (Cambridge, Mass.: The MIT Press, 1977) 65. See also L.R. Tancredi & D.N. Weisstub "Malpractice in American Psychiatry: Toward a Restructuring of Psychiatrist-Patient Relationship" in D.N. Weisstub, *ed., Law and Mental Health: International Perspectives, Volume 2* (Oxford: Pergamon Press, 1986) 83 at 90-94.

[21]   See J. Katz, "Informed Consent - Must it Remain a Fairy Tale?" (1994) 10 J. Contemporary Health L. & Policy 69 at 90-91. However, he argues that we should allocate the requisite resources, and generate the necessary commitment for the doctrine to fulfill its mandate effectively.

In actuality, for many parties who are part of research protocols, to speak of an articulated value system is a luxury which is not supported by fact.

In research, safeguards are critical, and the rationalizations made on behalf of others, however much motivated by the ideal of values in concert, are a luxury we are ill-advised to entertain before our society achieves a threshold of listing, exchanging, and clarifying the nature of the risks that subjects may endure. Of course, values come into play in research and are at times even more important than in normal cases of therapy. But realism about the history of violations of rights and abuses with regard to subjects should lead us to extreme caution in experimenting with the concept of individual, professional, and societal values working in a synchronized relationship. Rather, we should continue to emphasize the foreseeable, the need for protecting the individual through laying out the level of risk measured against the perceived benefit to be obtained from a positive research outcome in as forthright a manner as possible. Taking such a risk should then be the choice of the subject whose body is being offered for the good of others. Where there are surrogate decision-makers involved, the burden should be great to minimize risk where the vulnerability of the subject is at issue. There is greater latitude for an exchange of philosophical values where treatment brings an immediate benefit to the patient.

Vulnerability and Fictions

Many of us are comfortable in indulging the fiction that the most significant human characteristic is rationality. A commitment to rationality as the first value of humanness leads us quickly either to prejudicial reactions that favour certain individuals who are blessed with natural intellectual superiority, or to respect more highly those individuals whose social conditioning has equipped them with more effective tools for acquiring and applying rational discourses. We can avoid these inherited or accultured differences by inviting citizens to think of an equal playing field where differentiations are not part of our permissible calculations.[22] Within more elaborate statements of metaphysical or philosophical systems, we are invited again to fictionalize the entitlements and participation of citizens in perfected systems or evolutionary moralities of a wide variety, such as those of Plato, Aristotle, Hegel and St. Thomas. In the elaboration of these internally consistent and closed systems, we are brought into the higher range of fantasy by being in contact with divine knowledge or absolute truth. Regrettably, none of these philosophical visions have clearly equipped or been linked to societies in world history so as to afford consistently protections for the more vulnerable

---

[22]   For the original statement of such a proposed veil of ignorance, see J. Rawls, *A Theory of Justice* (Cambridge, Mass.: Belknap Press of Harvard University Press, 1971) at 136-142.

populations. Caring ethics have stemmed more from acts of charity and benevolence than from systemic philosophical reflection.

The inability of formalistic philosophy to discernibly impact on our capacity for socially protective acts remains a warning for our future practices affecting vulnerable populations. Without the provision of specific procedural steps that guarantee a societal duty against sacrificing individuals for higher ethical or utilitarian goals, we remain at risk. In their defense, Kantians would surely submit that committing our treatment of humans to an ends analysis rather than a calculation of consequences would be a sufficient condition for protection. But Kantian formalism, as we have observed, in and of itself, and perhaps due to its excessive formalism, cannot contain our assertive tendencies to redefine persons who are not to our liking and for whom we have no respect. Such persons are then placed under the regime of a universalizable judgement, to their detriment. The only real protection that we have in civilized societies is to request citizens be placed in imaginative experiments where they force themselves to stand in other person's shoes. But that itself cannot be professed as anything more than an experiment, because it does not necessarily counteract the dissociative tendencies that persons have who believe that, in the event of inferiority, they would resist defending the rights of or even punishing their own family members that suffer from certain defects.

Because the benefits of research are so obviously attractive to societies, particularly where special populations are viewed as a drain on limited resources, we find in such instances that our social sensibilities are strained to the limit. It is facile to say that because of these propensities we should simply locate the strongest members of our communities to be subjected to experimentation involving high risk. We commit ourselves to this view because there is an obvious fear that once we turn down the road of using vulnerable populations in research, our logic can rapidly lead us to human denigration and tragedy. The capacity of biological engineering is exponentially increasing, and affords us the possibility and even vision of producing a servant class whose organs and subjective behaviours could be harnessed for the interests of a new social order.

How then do we begin to rationalize in a morally credible way the inclusion of handicapped persons, whose own rationality is clearly at issue, in research endeavours? Here, we indulge a specific fiction which suggests the following: if it is morally elevating for persons of normal intelligence to participate in research beneficial to others, we should elevate persons of limited capacity by taking them into this world of beneficial exchanges. By such a rationale, and indeed fiction, we can decide to ask handicapped persons to give their organs to siblings in need, thereby making whole as moral beings persons who have been given lesser evaluations with respect to their worth for other purposes in the social system.

In a recent report of the UK Medical Research Council the following statement was made:

> [I]t is not in the public interest for persons suffering from mental incapacity to be excluded from socially responsible behaviour purely through lack of consent competence. Where the risk attending participation in non-therapeutic research into mental disorder is minimal and a reasonable person with that disorder but able to consent is likely to accept that risk, when told that such research might lead to advances in treatment, it would be strange if a person unable to consent because of that disorder should be imputed with a wholly different attitude to the welfare of the class of persons of which he is a member.[23]

How should we properly define the moral transaction or trade-off that is occurring here? Are we saying that if a society agrees to care for its vulnerable populations, then at the very least, we should be able to enlist such recipients in assisting our community to benefit individuals suffering from the same class of illnesses, or if it is our will, the society at large? We say this with some moral comfort, because we are ready to assume the view that where minimal risks are at issue, reasonable citizens would participate, without hesitation, in the majority of cases. We see this as part of a minimal cooperativist ethic that is part of what it means to be constituted as a morally functioning individual within a larger society. In this way we choose to reject individuals for their moral irresponsibility and lack of sociability when they refuse to assist in our progressive stand against disease and suffering. When we enlist handicapped or vulnerable persons in the research endeavour, we choose a model of citizenship rather than capacity as our normative term of reference. Our paternalistic intervention for their elevation where no serious risk is entailed, in the final analysis should not fail to meet the criteria offered by classical utilitarian or ethically normative models. If we see participation as a fiction of morally justified enhancement in conduct associated with higher ethical activity, namely sacrifice, a net gain is experienced on two grounds of calculation: our regard for human worth *qua* moral actor, and the material benefit accruing to society at large. In many cases, the benefactor/actor is treated better by the social system as a result of these minor sacrifices, given the reality of the scarcity of resources.

Once we step on the pathway of fictionalizing the moral enhancements of vulnerable populations, we are told to heed the slippery slope arguments made by lawyers: the steps of our logic can quickly take us to dark and dangerous corridors. Whenever crisis looms, such as in war conditions, we do not hesitate

---

[23]   Working Party on Research on the Mentally Incapacitated, *The Ethical Conduct of Research on the Mentally Incapacitated* (London: Medical Research Council, 1991) at 20.

to bring persons forward to defend neighborhoods, cities, or indeed, even the larger and more abstract construct of country and state. In times of peace and more careful planning, are we allowed to participate in a siege mentality in which the denial of participation is tantamount to saying that we will not ask all members, regardless of capacity, to be enlisted in the production and defense of a healthier and therefore better society. In smaller and tighter units of social fabric, such as the family, or limited populations such as villages or tribes, it would be odd to contemplate that vulnerable persons would not be listed as truly valued family members in an action of defense. Unlike the larger units in our reference system, which are a part of technologically oriented living, we do not search in such small units for moral arguments to dissuade us from making handicapped members real citizens. In fact, we might see the abandonment of vulnerable persons in such moments of impending defeat or attack as disrespectful to their inclusiveness in a tightly woven social fabric. Our challenge is to locate the true reasons for why we fear the inclusion of the vulnerable in circumstances where persons of normal capacity would be enlisted without hesitation or reservation.

In modern democracies, our distrust of state and public institutions has left us with great disquiet about enlisting persons for any form of socially desirable benefits without the application of strict standards of capacity and appreciation. It is only in the family, in our contemporary liberal environments, that we are prepared to give limited leeway for decision-making that warrants the inclusion of vulnerable members. Even there, distrust is so great that most of our Western legal systems are prepared to place strict limits on familial sacrifices, lest miscarriages of respect are rationalized by stronger or more superior family members. The issue, therefore, becomes who the guardians should be: loved ones such as the family; depersonalized and institutionalized administrative review structures that reflect a diversity of professions and populations within our society; or the judiciary, our most respected organ of social decision-making, which is trained to debrief and assess as generalists not only information inputs, but the submissions of adversarial parties. If we conclude that there has to be room for each of the aforementioned groups to participate in different aspects of the research enterprise, we should recognize that two requirements are necessary on an ongoing basis: the availability of procedural mechanisms for scrutinizing the protocols and policies of researchers, and society's participation in an ongoing dialogue with the major actors in research, in particular, the subjects themselves. Without such ingredients being put into place, and carefully proceduralized, any notion that we are giving an elevated moral standard or status to vulnerable persons by including them in research goes beyond fiction and myth-making to abuse itself. Equally, to abandon vulnerable persons as irrelevant or incapable of participation in research with minimal risk, should be regarded as morally irresponsible behaviour on the part of enlightened societies.

Part II
Protecting Human Subjects

[13]

HUMAN EXPERIMENTATION AND HUMAN RIGHTS*

JAY KATZ**

I. INTRODUCTION

$\mathbf{A}$ dilemma confronts physician-investigators in the conduct of research with patient-subjects. As physicians they are dedicated to caring for their patients, healing their pain, reducing their suffering. As investigators they are dedicated to caring for their research, advancing knowledge for the benefit of science and future patients. These two commitments conflict whenever an individual physician-investigator comes face to face with an individual patient-subject. Indeed, in this encounter between two persons, four personae confront one another: the physician, the investigator, the patient in need of immediate

* A revised and extended version of a paper presented at St. Louis University School of Law on March 19, 1993, and as the Ipolitas Benedict Bronushas Lecture at the University of Maryland School of Medicine on April 2, 1993.

I want to express my thanks to George J. Annas, Robert A. Burt, Jesse A. Goldner, Robert J. Levine, Lainie F. Ross, Elizabeth van Dusen, Katherine Weinstein and Alan J. Weisbard for their helpful comments on earlier drafts of this article. My current research assistant, Steven D. Lavine, assisted me in preparing this article for publication and his thoughtful observations shaped its final version. I am particularly indebted to my former research assistant, Peter D. Mostow, with whom over the past two years I discussed everything contained in this article. His contributions influenced my thinking and I cannot thank him enough. Finally, I want to express my gratitude to my wife Marilyn A. Katz. From the first draft to its final version I discussed with her everything contained in this article, and her critical wisdom, though not specifically acknowledged, is reflected throughout.

** Elizabeth K. Dollard Professor Emeritus of Law, Medicine and Psychiatry, and Harvey L. Karp Professorial Lecturer in Law and Psychoanalysis, Yale Law School.

help, and the subject who may himself be helped or who may help future patients.

This dilemma is new to the practice of medicine, which in the past only served patients' individual therapeutic needs. Only during the last fifty years, subsequent to World War II, did medical research increase in magnitude unprecedented in the millennia of medical history.[1] Indeed, in today's world medical practice often encompasses both research and therapeutic aspects. The research component of any medical intervention, however, may not serve the individual therapeutic interests of patients. Instead, their well-being is subordinated to the dictates of a research protocol designed to advance knowledge for the sake of future patients.

In the aftermath of World War II the world was also confronted, as it had never been before, with the terrible human costs which human experimentation could entail. The revelation of the medical experiments conducted by Nazi physicians during the war,[2] and, twenty-five years later the discovery of the Tuskegee Syphilis Study conducted by Public Health Service physicians in the United States[3] before, during, and after the Nazi concentration camp experiments had taken place, led to the realization that even medical progress can exact an intolerable price. Both revelations, and others as well, had a decisive impact on the promulgation of codes and regulations for the protection

---

1. *See* DAVID J. ROTHMAN, STRANGERS AT THE BEDSIDE, 53-54 (1991).
Congress gave the [National Institutes of Health] (NIH) . . . the budgetary resources to expand on the work of the [Committee on Medical Research]. In 1945 the appropriation to NIH was approximately $700,000. By 1955 the figure had climbed to $36 million; by 1965, $436 million; and by 1970, $1.5 billion, a sum that allowed it to award some 11,000 grants, about one-third requiring experiments on humans.
Id.

2. *See* TRIALS OF WAR CRIMINALS BEFORE THE NUREMBERG MILITARY TRIBUNAL, Volumes I & II, The Medical Case, U.S. Government Printing Office (1948) [hereinafter TRIALS OF WAR CRIMINALS]; THE NAZI DOCTORS AND THE NUREMBERG CODE, (George J. Annas & Michael A. Grodine eds. 1992).

3. From 1932 until 1972, physicians of the U.S. Public Health Service conducted an experiment, the so-called Tuskegee Syphilis Study, in Macon County, Alabama, involving 399 black persons afflicted with syphilis. The subjects had not been informed that they were participating in an experiment to study the natural history of untreated syphilis. Instead, they thought that they were under the medical care of the U.S. Public Health Service. The study was terminated in 1972 at the recommendation of the Tuskegee Syphilis Study Ad Hoc Advisory Panel. For detailed accounts, see U.S. DEPARTMENT OF HEALTH, EDUCATION, AND WELFARE, PUBLIC HEALTH SERVICE, FINAL REPORT OF THE TUSKEGEE SYPHILIS STUDY AD HOC ADVISORY PANEL (1973) [hereinafter TUSKEGEE SYPHILIS STUDY]; JAMES H. JONES, BAD BLOOD (1981); and Alan Brandt who discovered evidence unavailable to the Panel which documented the deceptions practiced by the U.S. Public Health Service physicians throughout the course of the study. Alan M. Brandt, *Racism and Research: The Tuskegee Syphilis Study*, 8 HASTINGS CENTER REPORT 21-29 (Dec. 1978).

of subjects of research. The requirements of consent[4] and informed consent,[5] based on principles of autonomy and self-determination,[6] became central prescriptions for the protection of subjects of research.

What transpired at Auschwitz and Tuskegee would not have led to regulations of the human experimentation process had these events been viewed as isolated occurrences, ascribable to causes utterly distinct from ordinary contemporary research practices. The regulations were a response to an appreciation that important lessons could be learned from these events of relevance to contemporary research. They were also a response to the realization, questioned by some,[7] that reliance on the ethical conscience, inculcated in physician-investigators during their medical education, provided insufficient protection to the human rights of subjects of medical research.

In this article I shall argue that these newly promulgated requirements and other safeguards—for example, Institutional Review Boards (IRBs) charged with the obligation to review and approve research proposals[8]—still do not satisfactorily protect the rights of patient-subjects to inviolability of personhood and body. In exploring this problem my ultimate intent is to stimulate discussion on the need to provide greater protection to patient-subjects' rights to self-determination and bodily integrity whenever they are used as means for the ends of human progress. I shall argue that respect for individual autonomy and for self-determination, which informed consent is intended to safeguard, will remain hollow aspirations until the nature and quality of the conversations between physician-investigators and patient-subjects about participation in research are radically transformed.[9] Inviting such participation for the sake of science, society, and future patients is an awesome request which, in a democratic society committed to respect for human rights, requires the most punctilious attention to disclosure and consent.

Before proceeding, I should make it clear that I do not intend to discuss research with vulnerable groups, such as children or the mentally impaired,

---

4. *See infra* notes 50-51 and accompanying text.

5. *See infra* notes 52-54 and accompanying text.

6. For a discussion of the principle of autonomy, see *infra* note 66.

7. *See* Henry K. Beecher, *Ethics and Clinical Research*, 274 NEW ENG. J. MED. 1354 (1966).

The ethical approach to experimentation in man has several components, two are more important than the others, the first being informed consent. . . . Secondly there is *the more reliable safeguard* provided by the presence of an intelligent, informed, conscientious compassionate responsible investigator.

Id. at 1360 (emphasis added).

8. *See infra* notes 92-93 and accompanying text.

9. For a detailed discussion of the kind of conversations I envision in therapeutic settings, see JAY KATZ, THE SILENT WORLD OF DOCTOR AND PATIENT (1984) [hereinafter THE SILENT WORLD], particularly Chapter 6, *Respecting Autonomy: The Obligation for Conversation, id.* at 130-164.

who do not have the capacity to give their consent. *My focus is on the many patient-subjects who have the capacity to consent.* Nor shall I say a great deal about investigators' ethical obligations to consider carefully whether the research project is important enough, and based on solid methodological grounds, to warrant asking human beings to join them in their endeavors. Clearly, consent is a necessary, but not sufficient, justification for using human beings as subjects for research; they deserve only to be used for experimental purposes when an important research question is in need of careful elucidation. Finally, I also shall not address the problem of physical harm which patient-subjects may suffer whenever they are parties to research. While some of the subjects are inevitably harmed, I grant the point frequently made, that as a group they may be harmed physically less, or at least not more, than are patients with similar diseases in therapeutic settings.[10] I exclude consideration of physical harm, however, for another important reason. I want to distract attention from the prevalent and extensive debate on the permissible limits of physical harm to subjects[11] and, instead, draw attention to the neglected and scant debate on the justifications for encroachments on subjects' rights to decisional authority in the conduct of research.[12]

---

10. P.V. Cardon et al., *Injuries to Research Subjects*, 295 NEW ENG. J. MED. 650-54 (1976). *See also* ROBERT J. LEVINE, ETHICS AND REGULATION OF CLINICAL RESEARCH 39-40 (2d ed. 1986) [hereinafter ETHICS AND REGULATION].

11. Wikler identified as the central moral problem in human experimentation "the possibility of subjects being injured or hurt." He went on to say that "[t]he other issues involved [such as informed consent] are far from negligible; but I believe that if [physical injury] were not a factor, human experimentation would not be the moral issue of the same order as it is now." Daniel Wikler, *The Central Ethical Problem in Human Experimentation and Three Solutions*, 26 CLIN. RES. 380 (1978). If Wikler is correct, then this article seeks to raise the consciousness of the medical community and the public about the great harm done by the disrespect accorded to the dignitary rights of subjects of research.

12. Two recently reported experiments which received considerable press attention are examples in point.

(1) Hepatitis B Study: During a drug trial conducted at the National Institutes of Health, five out of fifteen participants died some time after the administration of an experimental drug, Fialuridine (FIAU), that had shown promise in the treatment of Hepatitis B. Lawrence L. Altman, *Fatal Drug Trial Raises Questions about 'Informed Consent'*, N.Y. TIMES, Oct. 5, 1993, at B7 [hereinafter *Fatal Drug Trial*]. The principal investigator correctly averred that "the public must understand that 'drugs can do harm just as much as they do good,'" for despite the best intentions and care, injuries will accompany experimental investigations as they do therapeutic interventions. *Id.* at col. 4. Questions, however, were also raised about the adequacy of the informed consent process. For example, "Dr. [Judith] Swazey [co-director of a major study of review boards and consent forms for the National Institutes of Health] said that the term 'new medication' was misleading. [The principal investigator] should have used the term 'experimental anti-viral compound' on the form and underlined it." *Id.* at cols. 4-5. My reading of the Clinical Research Protocol and the Informed Consent Form suggests that it adequately disclosed the risks of the study. *See* Jay H. Hoofnagle, Six-Month Course of FIAU for Chronic Hepatitis B (Feb. 10, 1993) (on file with author) [hereinafter Research Protocol]. At the same time, and in agreement with

More importantly, I shall argue throughout this article that the protection of the rights of research subjects to self-determination cannot be safeguarded until a number of underlying problems affecting the informed consent process in decisive ways have been resolved. The underlying problems are these: (1) The obfuscation of the distinction between therapy and research and the

---

Swazey but generalizing on her observation, the informed consent form did not make crystal clear that this was purely an experimental study. To be sure, if the promise of therapeutic benefit materializes the subjects will benefit, but for now they must appreciate that, similar to other experimental interventions, their participation could expose them to grave unknown risks. In this instance, such a forthright acknowledgement was particularly important since in the prior pilot study "[p]otential side effects of FIAU were seen in two patients but in both cases FIAU did not clearly appear to play a major role." *Id.* at 5. The death of one of the patients in the pilot project was ascribed to other causes and, from the vantage point of hindsight, was probably an incorrect assessment. The death of five participants, of course, deserved investigation and from my reading of the protocol would have established that the investigators took great care to avoid such a possibility. The question, however, remains whether the patient-subject knew that they had agreed to join the experimenters on a voyage into the unknown that could shatter their limbs or lives. That fact should also have been highlighted, as it was not, in the informed consent form. The unfortunate and perhaps unavoidable death of five subjects thus can easily divert attention from a crucial issue: the importance of paying the most punctilious attention to disclosure and consent.

(2) The IL-2 Study: In another experiment, prominent cancer researchers confessed to injecting a drug, IL-2, into "the brain tumors of dying patients to see if it would help them." Philip J. Hilts, *Researchers Admit Study With Drugs Had No O.K.*, N.Y. TIMES, Oct. 28, 1993, at B5 col. 1. The drug had not been approved for such use by the FDA and the investigators had not submitted their protocol to the hospital's Institutional Review Board (IRB). The newspaper account does not mention whether the patient-subjects were informed about their participation in an experiment and the circumstances surrounding it. What particularly caught my attention in reading the story was that "the United States Attorney's office in Manhattan investigated the case [and decided] not to prosecute . . . at least in part because no apparent harm was done to the patients, who were near death from brain tumors." *Id.* Again the focus is on physical harm and not on the harm inflicted by disrespecting the decisional authority of the patients involved. If the investigators had discussed with their patients the investigational nature of the study and the patients, aware of their desperate condition, had agreed, then, beyond infractions of federal regulations, a major question that remains is when, if ever, can unapproved drugs be used with subjects' consent? The same question has arisen in research with unapproved drugs for AIDS patients. In my view, both they and terminally ill patients can be apprised of the status of such drugs and such patients who are so aware of their desperate, well nigh hopeless, situation, may then be quite willing to opt for participation. As long as they are protected from physician-investigators' spurious promises and other deceptive exploitations of their necessitous circumstances, there may be nothing wrong with honoring their consent. Indeed, respect for autonomy may dictate it. Since it will give them a measure of hope—and what else is left to them at this most agonizing time in their lives—why deprive them of such solace? The danger of unscrupulous invitations, of course, remains but careful review of both the reasonableness of the scientific proposal *and* the forthrightness of the informed consent process can do much to ensure that the patient-subjects know to what they are consenting.

accompanying confusion of patients and subjects;[13] (2) the impact of the ideology of medical professionalism on the conduct of human experimentation;[14] (3) the unclarity about the different tasks of medicine and research;[15] and (4) the impact on the informed consent process on the mindset of physician-investigators and the principles that govern the invitation to participation in research.[16] Finally, I shall suggest that the resolution of any inevitably persisting tensions between the inviolability of person and the acquisition of knowledge cannot be left to the discretion of physician-investigators or local IRBs. If any encroachments on citizen-patient-subjects' rights to self-determination prove to be necessary, it should require a thoroughly considered and explicit congressional mandate which now does not exist. It should also require the establishment of a national body with the authority to formulate rules for, as well as to administer and review, the human experimentation process.[17] A recent research project conducted with schizophrenic patients will illustrate these contentions.[18]

II. THE RESEARCH-THERAPY DISTINCTION

Physician-investigators have long maintained that clinical research and therapy, more often than not, are indistinguishable; that the drugs or therapies they subject to scientific study frequently are, or could be, proffered to patients in therapeutic settings; and that the only difference between their scientific endeavors and clinical practice resides in the objective evaluation of efficacy and risk-benefits to which they submit their interventions. Thus, since vast uncertainties and ignorance about effectiveness and risk-benefits are ubiquitous in the practice of medicine, every medical intervention, therapeutic or investigative in intent, constitutes an experiment.[19] Moreover, investigators

---

13. *See infra* notes 19-34 and accompanying text.
14. *See infra* notes 35-55 and accompanying text.
15. *See infra* notes 56-63 and accompanying text.
16. *See infra* notes 64-90 and accompanying text.
17. *See infra* notes 91-101 and accompanying text.
18. *See infra* notes 102-136.
19. For example, Thomas Chalmers stated: "It is extremely hard to distinguish between clinical research and the practice of good medicine. Because episodes of illness and individual people are so variable, every physician is carrying out a small research project when he diagnoses and treats a patient." *Quoted in* ETHICS AND REGULATION, *supra* note 10, at 3. While Levine is correct that in recent years new definitions of what constitutes research have been formulated, the obfuscation of subject and patient described in this section continue to obliterate the research/therapy distinction, at least in investigators' interactions with research subjects. *Id.* at 3-10. More generally, Royall documented the convictions of many investigators who continue to defend the ethics of clinical trials on the basis of the unsatisfactory state of clinical practice:

[I]f therapy A were known to be better than B, then there would be no need for a [clinical trial]. And if it is not known, then the physician who believes that A is better has no sound basis for recommending A; his belief represents only a personal opinion, an

are apt to argue that in clinical practice patients are exposed to unnecessary, scientifically unproven, ineffective, and at times dangerous therapies about which patients learn little because their physicians believe in the therapies and their unwarranted beliefs are shared by many of their professional peers. In this view, clinical research differs from practice only in its endeavors not to perpetuate these uncertainties, but to resolve them once and for all for the benefit of future patients and perhaps even for the patient-subjects involved in clinical trials. Indeed, investigators maintain that clinical research is an enterprise more moral than clinical practice because ultimately it will safeguard patients and future patients from the slings and arrows of useless, if not dangerous, therapies. Therefore, it is grossly unfair not to extend the considerable discretion which doctors enjoy in making decisions on behalf of patients in therapeutic settings to investigators, and instead subject them to onerous review procedures regarding informed consent.

These contentions speak to the latitude physicians are given generally in making decisions on behalf of patients, despite the requirement for informed consent. For even in clinical practice the doctrine of informed consent continues to be an empty ritual not only because it does not require physicians to disclose the uncertainties inherent in their interventions, about which investigators are so correctly concerned, but also because the doctrine remains so inattentive to its underlying *idea* that patients and physicians must make decisions jointly, with ultimate decision-making authority residing in the patient and *not* in the physician.[20] Yet, all these problems notwithstanding, the doctrine of informed consent, as currently articulated, imposes similar disclosure and consent obligations for therapy and research,[21] with the only

---

unscientific hunch, and is not a proper basis for responsible professional judgment.
Richard M. Royall, *Ethics and Statistics in Randomized Clinical Trials*, 6 STAT. SCI. 51, 55 (1991). He then quotes Freund who shares these views:

> [M]uch of what the surgeon assumes he knows is not based on solid scientific data, but rather on training, experience, and reinforcement. The choice of treatment is neither more nor less likely to be correct if made arbitrarily than if assigned randomly in the clinical trial. The two courses of action can thus be considered ethically equivalent in terms of patient risk.
> . . .
> [E]ven an opinion held with strong conviction is not a sufficient basis for ethical action; passionate opinion does not make an incorrect opinion into a correct one.

Id.

20. For a more detailed discussion, see Jay Katz, *Duty and Caring in the Age of Informed Consent and Medical Science: Unlocking Peabody's Secret*, 8 HUMANE MED. 187, 188-89 (1992) [hereinafter *Duty and Caring*].

21. The most significant difference between the common law doctrine of informed consent for therapy and the federal requirements for informed consent in research, resides in the "therapeutic privilege exception." It permits physicians to withhold information if it would "foreclose a rational decision, or complicate or hinder the treatment, or perhaps even pose psychological damage to the patient." Canterbury v. Spence, 464 F.2d 772, 789 (D.C. Cir. 1972).

14   SAINT LOUIS UNIVERSITY LAW JOURNAL   [Vol. 38:7

difference being that for research the informed consent process is subjected to review by IRBs. In application, however, disclosure and consent are taken all too lightly in both settings because physicians and physician-investigators do not consider patients and patient-subjects as equal partners in the decision-making process.

All the arguments about similarities between research and practice or complaints about inequitable burdens overlook an issue that speaks to the crucial importance of informed consent in research: In therapeutic encounters, unlike research encounters, physicians are expected to attend solely to the welfare of the individual patient before them. Throughout medical history this expectation has given physicians considerable discretion and authority to make decisions on behalf of patients. More recently, to be sure, such discretion and authority have been questioned on many grounds. I shall mention only two. First, since many of the diagnostic and therapeutic options now available allow patients to make choices that can have a decisive impact on the quality of future life, what a physician thinks is best may not necessarily comport with a patient's overall needs.[22] Second, because the available options may have

---

Courts in the past have construed the privilege not to disclose most liberally, but the *Canterbury* court cautioned that it must be "carefully circumscribed . . . for otherwise it might devour the disclosure rule itself. The privilege does not accept the paternalistic notion that the physician may remain silent simply because divulgence might prompt the patient to forego therapy the physician feels the patient really needs." *Id.* at 789. In a recent case, the Court of Appeals of California reduced the scope of the therapeutic privilege even further by requiring that in instances of hopeless prognosis (the most common situation in which the privilege has been invoked) the patient be provided with such information: "If not the physician's duty to disclose a terminal illness, then whose?" *Arato v. Avedon*, 11 Cal. Rptr. 2d 169, 181 n.19 (1992). The California Supreme Court reversed. *Arato v. Avedon*, 858 P.2d 598 (1993). Its opinion made too much of an issue raised by the plaintiffs which led the appellate court to hold that doctors must disclose "numerical life expectancy information." *Id.* at 604. To be sure, disclosure of statistical information is a complex issue, but in focusing on it, the supreme court's attention was diverted from a more important new disclosure obligation promulgated by the appellate court: the duty to inform patients of their dire prognosis. The supreme court did not comment on that obligation and, instead, reinforced the considerable leeway granted physicians to invoke the therapeutic privilege exception to full disclosure: "[W]e decline to intrude further, either on the subtleties of the physician-patient relationship or in the resolution of claims that the physician's duty to disclose was breached by requiring the disclosure of information that may or may not be indicated in a given treatment context." *Id.* at 607.

22. *See* THE SILENT WORLD, *supra* note 9, at 8.

The objectives of health and cure that supposedly unite physician and patient in a common pursuit can rarely be fully realized. Furthermore, these objectives can be pursued in a variety of ways, each with its own risks and benefits. The physician's personal and professional ethics and experience may dictate one course: the patient's needs, wishes and priorities, motivations, and expectations may indicate another one. Thus, health turns out to be an ambiguous state about which doctors and patients may have conflicting expectations . . . .

Id.

an impact on physicians' economic rewards, physicians' self-interests can readily influence their professional recommendations.[23]

Indeed, the doctrine of informed consent was promulgated in 1957 in response to both of these new realities.[24] Judges thought that the introduction of new powerful diagnostic and treatment modalities, which promised great benefits but could also inflict considerable harm, required that patients be given a greater voice in the medical decision-making process.[25] Yet, informed consent notwithstanding, the physician-patient encounter continues to be shaped by the belief, shared by doctors and patients, that in therapeutic settings doctors at least try to do their level best for the individual patient who seeks their help and, therefore, the doctor's recommendations can be trusted.

In clinical research, on the other hand, patient-subjects are also being used for the ends of science. One cannot dismiss with impunity the implications of this difference.[26] In these situations investigators are committed both to real, present patients and abstract, future patients. Individual patient-centered therapy gives way to a collective patient-centered endeavor in which the

---

23. *See, e.g.,* Arnold S. Relman, *Dealing with Conflict of Interest,* 313 NEW ENG. J. MED. 749 (1985); Bruce J. Hillman et al., *Frequency and Costs of Diagnostic Imaging in Office Practice—A Comparison of Self-Referring and Radiologist-Referring Physicians,* 323 NEW ENG. J. MED. 1604 (1990); Jean M. Mitchell & Elton Scott, *New Evidence of the Prevalence and Scope of Physician Joint Ventures,* 268 J.A.M.A. 80 (1992).

24. Salgo v. Leland Stanford Jr. University Board of Trustees, 317 P.2d 170 (1957). At the end of his opinion, Justice Bray introduced the doctrine of informed consent in a short, albeit confusing, paragraph. For a detailed analysis, see THE SILENT WORLD, *supra* note 9, at 60-65.

25. The situation in *Salgo, see supra* note 24, involved the use of a new diagnostic procedure to locate a block in the abdominal aorta. It required injection of a dye, sodium urokon. In 1954, aortography had not been performed in sufficient numbers in the San Francisco Bay area to constitute routine procedure. The doctors admitted that they had not disclosed to Martin Salgo the risk of the procedure which resulted in a permanent paralysis of his lower extremities. In Natanson v. Kline, 350 P.2d 1093 (1960), Irma Natanson suffered severe injuries from cobalt radiation, administered subsequent to a mastectomy for breast cancer. In 1955, cobalt radiation, instead of conventional x-ray treatment, had barely been introduced in Wichita, Kansas. Dr. Kline admitted that he had not informed his patient of the hazards of cobalt radiation or the availability of other post-operative treatment modalities. My reading of the two opinions suggests that the justices were astounded and troubled by the undisputed facts in both cases; that, without any disclosure, new technologies were employed which not only promised great benefits but also could expose patients to formidable and uncontrollable risks. *Natanson,* unlike *Salgo,* discussed the informed consent doctrine in some detail and it marked the true beginning of a new common law doctrine.

26. Consider the views of Foster Lindley:

I did not realize that decisions . . . regarding alternative therapies, have themselves become matters of life and death. That people die in the service of abstract, controversial, statistical proofs, I cannot accept. That they die at the hands of physicians who mistakenly prefer one therapy to another, I can accept. Some will see an inconsistency there; I do not.

Royall, *supra* note 19, at 74.

abstraction of the research question tends to objectify the person-patient.[27] It does so to a significantly greater extent than in therapeutic interactions, even though similar problems of objectification arise in therapeutic settings when doctors attend too much to the disease of the body in the bed and not to the person before them.[28]

The readiness with which clinical research continues to be viewed as an extension of clinical practice, both similarly grounded in the millennia-long Hippocratic commitment to the welfare of the individual patient, overlooks the transformation of medical practice since the age of medical science.[29] Throughout most of medical history, research was limited to careful bedside observation of the effects of innovative treatments, with the interests of the individual patient as a polestar. In today's world, on the other hand, the interests of patient-subjects may yield to varying extents to the interests of science. This revolutionary development has not been accompanied by a thoroughgoing re-examination of physicians' ethical obligations in a post-Hippocratic age.

Examples in point are the many cooperative clinical trials, generally randomized clinical trials (RCTs),[30] in which institutions throughout the

---

27. *See infra* note 66 and accompanying text.

28. In a conversation between a senior physician and a medical intern, the former asked how much the intern knew about "patients as human beings." The question led to a rather nonproductive exchange which the intern ended abruptly with the exasperated comment: "I cannot answer your questions. You're interested in patients. I'm interested in the disease in the body in the bed." RAYMOND S. DUFF & AUGUST B. HOLLINGSHEAD, SICKNESS AND SOCIETY 128 (1968).

29. Medical practice has become transformed in other ways as well which should have led to greater involvement of patients in the medical decision-making process:

Medicine's recent ascent from empiricism to science has brought forth spectacular technologic advances in the diagnosis and treatment of disease. Today the numerous options available for the treatment of many diseases allow patients greater choice. Moreover, the introduction into medicine of scientific reasoning, aided by the results of carefully conducted research, permits doctors to be more discriminating between knowledge, ignorance and conjecture in their recommendations for or against a treatment.

For the first time in medical history, it is possible, even medically and morally imperative, to give patients a voice in medical decision making; possible, because knowledge and ignorance can be better specified; medically imperative, because a variety of treatments are available, each of which can bestow benefits or inflict harm; morally imperative, because patients, depending on the lifestyle they wish [to lead] after treatment, must be given a choice.

Duty and Caring, supra note 20, at 189.

30. The randomized clinical trial (RCT) is generally regarded as the gold standard for the evaluation of therapeutic agents.

The RCT has four main elements. 1) It is "controlled," i.e., one part of the subject population receives a therapy that is being tested while another part, as similar as possible . . . , receives either another therapy or no therapy. . . . 2) The significance of its results is established through statistical analysis. . . . 3) When it is feasible, a double-blind

United States participate and which are designed to evaluate the effectiveness of various treatment modalities for breast cancer, coronary artery disease, prostate cancer and stroke. In the conduct of such clinical trials, conflicts between the interests of patients and science are ever-present and are all too readily swept aside by viewing patient-subjects less as subjects and more as patients who can only benefit from participation in such clinical trials. Convictions of therapeutic benefit thus shape decisively the informed consent dialogue in clinical research, aided and abetted by patients' belief that their doctors have their interest uppermost in mind.[31]

This belief is at best only partially warranted. Investigators have other personal and professional interests which can only be kept in check if both physician-investigators and patient-subjects fully appreciate that both are engaged in an enterprise in which patient-subjects are also being asked to serve as means for science's ends and that other therapeutic alternatives are often available which do not involve a research dimension.

From all I have said so far, it follows that a major problem which compromises the protection afforded to subjects of research resides in the obfuscation of the boundaries between clinical research and clinical practice. It is therefore imperative to view clinical research as a distinct category, sharply delineated from clinical practice.[32]

The need for such sharp distinctions may fade once physicians no longer exercise such sweeping authority over patients' medical fate. In *The Silent World of Doctor and Patient*, I not only questioned this authority but also argued that the doctrine of informed consent has insufficiently reduced this authority.[33] Thus, patients have not been provided with meaningful opportunities to make their own choices.[34] If the time ever comes when patients'

---

technique is employed. That is, neither the investigator nor the subject knows until the conclusion of the study who is in the treatment or control group. . . . 4) It is randomized, i.e., the therapies being compared are allocated among the subjects by chance.
ETHICS AND REGULATION, *supra* note 10, at 185. RCTs are frequently employed. "In 1975 there were over 750 separate protocols involving over 600,000 patient-subjects. These numbers are for NIH [National Institutes of Health] sponsored trials only; many additional RCTs are conducted or sponsored by drug companies or with funding from other sources." *Id.* at 186. For a complete account of the design and conduct of RCTs, see *id.* at 187-212.

31. Recently George J. Annas aptly noted: "Researchers tend to think that they do good, that they don't do bad. And patients feel the same way; they tend to minimize or totally downplay the risks." *Fatal Drug Trial, supra* note 12, at col. 2-3.

32. *See supra* note 21 and accompanying text.

33. *See* THE SILENT WORLD, *supra* note 9, at 85-103.

34. Alan Meisel said:
Instead of informed consent, what we usually find in the practice of medicine is what my colleague Loren Roth has called "informed compliance." Doctors make decisions about the treatment patients should have, and then they provide whatever information is necessary to get the patient to go along with the recommendation. Patients are not given information to facilitate their decision-making process. That patients "make" decisions

18   SAINT LOUIS UNIVERSITY LAW JOURNAL   [Vol. 38:7

rights to autonomy and self-determination are truly respected, the problem to which I now turn—the impact of the ideology of medical professionalism on clinical research—will be less pressing. It is this ideology which has given, and continues to give, physicians considerable latitude to decide for patients, in the belief that doctors can be trusted because their self-interest will yield to patients' interests. While I have already suggested that this is a questionable assumption for therapeutic settings, it surely is an untenable one for clinical research where physician-investigators have dual allegiances—to their patient-subjects and the research protocol.

III.   THE IDEOLOGY OF MEDICAL PROFESSIONALISM

The presumption of physician authority over the medical needs of their patients has been the bedrock of the ideology of professionalism. Throughout history, physicians have maintained that patients' needs are best served by following doctors' orders. As stated by the influential sociologist Talcott Parsons: "[The physician's] competence and specific judgments and measure cannot be competently judged by the layman. The latter must . . . take these judgments and measures on 'authority.' . . . The doctor-patient relationship has to be one involving an element of authority—we often speak of 'doctor's orders.'"[35] Physicians' insistence on complete authority over the needs of patients has been compellingly supported by another claim: that patients are incapable of understanding medicine's esoteric knowledge. As stated by Howard Becker:

> Professions . . . are occupations which possess a monopoly of some esoteric and difficult body of knowledge. [This knowledge] consists not of technical skills and the fruits of practical experience but, rather, of abstract principles arrived at by scientific research and logical analysis. This knowledge cannot be applied routinely but must be applied wisely and judiciously to each case.[36]

Most physician-investigators were first socialized as physicians and indoctrinated in the ideology of professionalism. While, in theory, it has yielded ground to the doctrine of informed consent, in practice, the impact of that ideology has, at best, only diminished. It is, therefore, not surprising that investigators continue to point to the esoteric knowledge problem. In addition, investigators maintain that this problem is compounded in clinical research

---

is a myth, at least as much (if not more) because they are not given an adequate opportunity to do so as because they are inherently unable to do so.

Alan Meisel, *Comments to T.M. Grundner, More on Making Consent Forms More Readable*, 4 IRB 9 (Jan. 1982).

35. TALCOTT PARSONS, THE SOCIAL SYSTEM 464, 465 (1954).

36. Howard Becker, *The Nature of a Profession, in* EXPERIMENTATION WITH HUMAN BEINGS 186-189 (1993).

because patient-subjects are even less capable of understanding the additional medical and scientific complexities which a clinical trial seeks to resolve. Thus, they argue that patient-subjects' consent, given on the basis of such disclosures, would be even more spurious than it is for therapy. Moreover, since they view subjects of research as patients, they also argue that full disclosure would do violence to the principle of beneficence,[37] which stresses the caring obligations of doctors toward their patients. Disclosure, they say, would reveal that customary treatments to which patients would be exposed if they were to decline to become subjects are beset by much uncertainty as to which treatment is best, effective, or harmful. All this can only make patients unduly frightened, cause them to lose hope in what medicine has to offer, and strip them of trust in their physicians.

For all these reasons, the argument goes, any respect for patient autonomy must be balanced against the principle of beneficence, of caring for the suffering patient who happens to be also a subject of research. In countless conversations with physician-investigators, I have heard paternalism and beneficence, and not respect for autonomy, defended as guiding principles for the conduct of research.

Thus, under the ideology of professionalism the autonomy of physicians is maintained at the expense of patients' autonomy. I have long believed that this ancient ideology no longer serves patients' interests well in an age of medical science and informed consent. Surely it cannot be transported into the research setting, where it is joined by the ideology of medical science, with its commitment to objectivity and search for ultimate answers that will benefit mankind. Such an unwarranted alliance has fateful consequences to persons who are not merely patients but also subjects.

---

37. For an extensive discussion of the principle of beneficence, *see* TOM L. BEAUCHAMP & JAMES F. CHILDRESS, PRINCIPLES OF BIOMEDICAL ETHICS 148-182 (2d ed. 1983).

Morality requires not only that we treat persons autonomously and that we refrain from harming them, but also that we contribute to their welfare, including their health . . . .

In its most general form, the principle of beneficence asserts the duty to help others further their important and legitimate interests. The duty to *confer* benefits and actively to prevent and remove harms is important in biomedical and behavioral contexts, but equally important is the duty to *balance* possible goods against the possible harms of an action.

Id. at 148-49.

Note that "the duty to *balance*" may require giving greater weight to beneficence than autonomy. While this may be necessary with incompetent patients and research subjects, such balancing is often carried on in interactions with competent patients and research subjects. This then leads to withholding crucial information from patients in order not "to distress" them. While even in therapeutic encounters with competent persons such "balancing" is questionable, it is inappropriate to balance possible goods against harms in the conduct of clinical research.

20   *SAINT LOUIS UNIVERSITY LAW JOURNAL*   [Vol. 38:7

The legal doctrine of informed consent has had little impact on moderating physician authority.[38] This is not surprising since the doctrine's underlying assumption, that patient autonomy deserves respect, has been foreign to physicians' thinking throughout medical history.[39] Though it is true that patients now receive more information about the risks and benefits of the recommended intervention than they did in earlier times, this change also obscures how little has changed. For such disclosures notwithstanding, the decision-making process continues to be under physician control.

Thus, the consequences of importing the ideology of medical professionalism into research settings are far-reaching. It permits, as I have already noted, viewing subjects as if they were patients. It permits physician-investigators to extend the invitation to participate in research with the same authority to which they have become accustomed as a result of their prior socialization as physicians. It permits not fully informing patient-subjects about uncertainties and risks inherent in clinical research on grounds of beneficence which physicians traditionally invoke for clinical practice. Any of these reasons, however questionable in therapeutic settings, are unwarranted justifications for non-disclosure in the context of research.

IV. RESPECT FOR AUTONOMY AND BODILY INVIOLABILITY

Twenty years ago, in the Introduction to my book *Experimentation with Human Beings*, I wrote:

> When human beings become the subjects of experimentation . . . tensions arise between two values basic to Western society: freedom of scientific inquiry and protection of individual inviolability. . . . At the heart of this [value] conflict

---

38. See the perceptive comments by Alan J. Weisbard on informed consent:

[I]n its attempt to translate the moral ideal of informed consent into a set of workable legal rules adapted to the technical requirements of the litigation process, the law has transformed that ideal into little more than a legal "duty to warn" of risks of medical treatment. This duty is measured not by the actual informational needs of the individual patient, but by the hypothetical needs of "reasonable patients" or by the prevailing norms of disclosure of the medical community. While purporting to assure respect for individual self-determination, the inaptly named law of informed consent has done little to "inform" the unique and sometimes idiosyncratic needs, concerns, and fears of individual patients on whose "consent" so much is said to rest. Indeed, one can plausibly maintain that the legal doctrine has done more to teach physicians how to practice medicine "defensively" (so as to minimize legal liability) than it has to foster physician-patient relationships that permit and encourage patients to participate actively and knowledgeably in decisions concerning their care.

Alan J. Weisbard, *Informed Consent: The Law's Uneasy Compromise with Ethical Theory*, 65 NEB. L. REV. 749, 751 (1986).

39. *See* THE SILENT WORLD, *supra* note 9, at 1-29. "The idea that patients may also be entitled to liberty, to sharing the burdens of decision with their doctors, was not [at least until recently] part of the ethos of medicine." *Id.* at 2.

lies an age-old question: When may a society, actively or by acquiescence, expose some of its members to harm in order to seek benefits for them, for others, or for society as a whole?[40]

My question assumed, at least implicitly, both the necessity of conducting human research and the inevitability of harm; it asked only when may society "expose some of its members to harm." I did not ask then as I shall do now: When, if ever, can it be justified to use human beings as means for the ends of others?

In now raising the question of justification, I do not wish to deny the morality of human experimentation. Ultimately it is necessary to conduct human trials in order to acquire the necessary knowledge to alleviate human suffering. I wish only to call attention to the fact that investigators' oft-invoked moral right to engage in human experimentation has left insufficiently considered the morality of how the invitation to participation in research must be extended so that the rights of subjects to be secure in their person and body remain sacrosanct.

Sir Isaiah Berlin addressed this fundamental issue in a different context when he asked: "In the name of what can [we] ever be justified in forcing men to do what they have not willed or consented to?"[41] His eloquent answer was this:

> [T]o manipulate [men], to propel them towards goals which [we] see, but they may not, is to deny their human essence, to treat them as objects without wills of their own, and therefore to degrade them. This is why to lie to men, or to deceive them, that is, to use them as means for [our], not their own, independently conceived ends, even if it is to their own benefit, is, in effect, to treat them as subhuman, to behave as if their ends are less ultimate and sacred than [our] own. . . . For if the essence of men is that they are autonomous beings—authors of values, of ends in themselves . . .—then nothing is worse than to treat them as if they were not autonomous but natural objects . . . whose choices can be manipulated . . . .[42]

Sir Isaiah speaks here to the importance of safeguarding the principle of autonomy. But in addition to this liberty interest, another human interest must be considered: the right to bodily integrity. John Locke encompassed both rights when he wrote that "every Man has *Property* in his own *Person*. This no Body has any Right to but himself."[43]

The United Nations' International Covenant on Civil and Political Rights in Article 7 juxtaposes the rights to autonomy and bodily integrity: "No one

---

40. JAY KATZ, EXPERIMENTATION WITH HUMAN BEINGS 1 (1972) [hereinafter EXPERIMENTA-TION WITH HUMAN BEINGS].
41. Isaiah Berlin, *Two Concepts of Liberty*, *in* FOUR ESSAYS ON LIBERTY 136-37 (1969).
42. *Id.*
43. JOHN LOCKE, TWO TREATISES ON GOVERNMENT 305 (Peter Laslett ed., 1960).

shall be subjected to torture or to cruel, inhuman, or degrading treatment or punishment. In particular, no one shall be subjected without his free consent to medical or scientific experimentation."[44] For years, I was puzzled by the inclusion of experimentation and torture within the same Article rather than giving each separate status as the Covenant does for the other rights it seeks to safeguard. I now see the connection. The drafters of the Covenant probably wished to convey that human experimentation "without his [or her] free consent" constitutes inhuman and degrading treatment akin to "torture," no matter what the motives of the investigator.[45] In the Western world we place a high value not only on autonomy but also on the inviolability of bodily integrity. Both make any unconsented invasions of subjects' bodies repugnant *even if* the physical risks are minimal.

Some commentators have suggested that too much is made of respect for autonomy in human research. While I do not share their views, I now want to add respect for bodily integrity, which is highly valued in our American jurisprudence,[46] as another reason for safeguarding citizens' rights to feel secure in their bodies. Since physicians have been given considerable discretion to inspect, touch and invade patients' bodies, it is easy to overlook that this privilege cannot be extended to research without a prior relentless

---

44. United Nations International Covenant on Civil and Political Rights, art. 7 (1966), *in* THE HUMAN RIGHTS READER (Walter Laqueur & Barry Rubin eds., 1979).

45. It could be argued that the juxtaposition of "scientific experimentation" and "torture" was solely a response to the sadistic ways in which the concentration camp research was carried out and, therefore, a prohibition only of such egregious conduct. If true, then I wish to broaden the implications of Article 7.

46. The United States Supreme Court first articulated the right to bodily integrity over a century ago, explicitly noting that such a right is fundamental to the common law: "No right is held more sacred, or is more carefully guarded, by the common law, than the right of every individual to the possession and control of his own person, free from all restraint or interference of others, unless by clear and unquestionable authority of law." Union Pacific Ry. v. Botsford, 141 U.S. 250 (1891) (refusing to order a plaintiff in a tort action to submit to a surgical examination). Since then, the Court has found a Fourth Amendment right to bodily integrity in the "right of the people to be secure in their *persons* . . . against unreasonable searches and seizures." Winston v. Lee, 470 U.S. 753, 759 (1985) (refusing to order a criminal suspect to undergo surgery to remove a bullet). Although this right is not absolute, the Court has stressed the importance of bodily integrity in strongly worded opinions: "Illegally breaking into the privacy of the petitioner, the struggle to open his mouth and remove what was there, the forcible extraction of his stomach contents . . . [, these] are methods too close to the rack and the screw to permit of constitutional differentiation." Rochin v. People of California, 342 U.S. 165, 171 (1952). More recently Justice Stevens in Planned Parenthood v. Casey, 112 S. Ct. 2791, 2840 (1991), citing *Rochin,* declared: "One aspect of [a woman's constitutional interest in liberty] is a right to bodily integrity, a right to control one's person." *See also* FRANCIS HILLIARD, 1 THE LAW OF TORTS 197 (2d ed. 1861) ("The plainest and simplest legal rights are those of the person. A man owns his body and limbs more unquestionably and unqualifiedly than his stock in trade or his farm. [One's body] belong[s] absolutely to the individual, and to him alone."). *Id.*

scrutiny about whether any State interest can be so compelling to override constitutional safeguards to both autonomy and bodily integrity.

Sir Isaiah's haunting question, raised in a different context, requires answers: Can manipulation of subjects of research, propelling them towards goals which we see but they may not, be justified in the name of medicine, science, and/or the State? I would answer: Not easily and, if at all, only under carefully circumscribed circumstances. The reasons for my answer are intertwined. First, it is difficult to defend the proposition that we can use human beings as means for others' ends, without their unequivocal consent unless authorized by a clear societal mandate, subsequent to a searching public debate; and second, medical research is by-and-large conducted with patients and by physicians under the aegis of medicine and physicians' primary Hippocratic commitment to the welfare of the individual. This commitment becomes tainted when, without a patient-subject's full knowledge, we allow the interests of science and society to intrude on the physician-patient relationship.

The historian Mario Biagioli in his essay on the Nazi concentration camp experiments pleaded that we need "to understand how [medical] science became (and could again become) implicated in [such a] tragedy."[47] It did become implicated because the contributions which science in its own right makes to the objectification of human beings, i.e., the transformation of persons into objects and data, was reinforced by the political ideology of the Nazi State, which totally objectified Jews and Gypsies by considering them "lives not worth living."[48] This unholy alliance led to the atrocities and sadism perpetuated against the subjects of research for the sake of medical science never before or since seen in the Western World. Yet, it would be a mistake to view the concentration camp experiments merely as a singular aberration rather than as an event which has much to teach us about research practices in the contemporary world. In Nazi Germany the State decreed that some "lives [are] not worth living,"[49] and medical scientists then seized the opportunity to pursue research in atrocious ways. While it is true that only with the active collaboration of the State can science produce an Auschwitz and Dachau, it is equally true that in contemporary research the claims of science invite a less perceptible, but nonetheless troublesome, disrespect for the person. Unless the greatest care is taken, medical science and physician-investigators are always trapped into making tragic choices for the sake of science and at the expense of the human beings who serve as subjects of

---

47. Mario Biagioli, *Science, Modernity, and the 'Final Solution,'* in PROBING THE LIMITS OF REPRESENTATION (Saul Friedlander ed., 1992).

48. *See infra* note 77 and accompanying text.

49. The idea that "lives not worth living" deserve to be eliminated gained wide currency in medicine during the 19th century. The debate focused on the merits of destroying the insane to relieve society of a terrible burden. For a detailed account, see ROBERT N. PROCTOR, RACIAL HYGIENE: MEDICINE UNDER THE NAZIS 177-222 (1988).

research. This is the eternal lesson to be learned from Auschwitz.

Respect for the person is the only counterweight to such tragedies. The judges at Nuremberg who passed judgment on the Nazi physicians recognized this and in uncompromising language spoke to the inviolability of research subjects. The Tribunal's first principle for the conduct of research—"the voluntary consent of the human subject [of research] is absolutely essential"[50]—eschewed any consideration of competing claims. This principle, soon after its promulgation, was attacked as being too visionary and too inhospitable to the advancement of science.[51] New codes and regulations for the conduct of research were then enacted which attempted to balance the claims of science and the inviolability of research subjects.[52] Balancing, however, necessitates discretion, and discretion invites physician-investigators to make tragic choices about future versus present lives.

The U.S. federal regulations on informed consent in research,[53] while protecting the rights of subjects better than had been the case in the past, do not go far enough in emphasizing the centrality of the inviolability of the human rights of research subjects, if not as an ethical obligation than surely as a societal obligation in a democracy. The drafters of the federal regulations needed to consider that their promulgations would confer on physicians a societal mandate to engage in clinical research and to use individuals for the good of society, a mandate not envisioned by the Hippocratic commandment to "use treatment to help the sick according to my ability and judgment."[54] A mandate to conduct research, on the other hand, is different in intent and implication and, therefore, the regulations on informed consent should have been formulated in a way that place considerable restrictions on the use of patient-subjects. To safeguard their autonomy would have required paying the most careful attention not only to the *criteria* for informed consent but also to the *process* of obtaining informed consent.

The drafters of the federal regulations should have explicitly insisted that taking informed consent seriously in research negotiations obligates physician-

---

50. TRIALS OF WAR CRIMINALS, *supra* note 2, at 181.

51. The critics were, of course, correct in pointing to the Nuremberg Code's lack of provisions for conducting research with children, the mentally disabled, and perhaps even with prisoners. Special provisions must be drafted for such vulnerable populations, and the extent of their participation in research should be precisely specified. The Code was limited, as are largely my comments throughout this article, to research with persons who have the capacity to consent.

52. *See Human Experimentation, Code of Ethics of the World Medical Association, Declaration of Helsinki*, 2 BRIT. MED. J. 177 (1964). For a discussion of this Declaration, see Jay Katz, *The Consent Principle of the Nuremberg Code: Its Significance Then and Now, in* THE NAZI DOCTORS AND THE NUREMBERG CODE, *supra* note 2, at 227-39. There I argued that in the Declaration of Helsinki, in contrast to the Nuremberg Code, "concerns over the advancement of science began to overshadow concerns over the integrity of person." *Id.* at 234.

53. 45 C.F.R. § 46 (1983) (providing for protection of human subjects).

54. HIPPOCRATES, I HIPPOCRATES 299-301 (W.H.S. Jones trans., Harvard Univ. Press 1972).

investigators to spend considerable time with prospective patient-subjects. They should have provided explicit instructions on the length to which investigators must go in explaining themselves and their intentions so that patient-subjects will not be misled. Respect for the subjects' human rights dictates that they know that the decision to participate in research entails making a gift for the sake of others.

The drafters of the federal regulations insufficiently cautioned physician-investigators against viewing clinical research as an extension of clinical practice. In not construing it more emphatically as a novel and distinctly separate activity, they contributed to importing the ideology of medical professionalism into the conduct of research.

Before promulgating the federal regulations, great pains should have been taken to alert Congress and the public that any societal mandate to conduct clinical research had to be sharply distinguished from the earlier societal mandate to superintend the health needs of citizen-patients, which was delegated to physicians at the turn of the 20th century.[55] That mandate cannot easily be transferred to medical research settings. At a minimum, it required a prior careful scrutiny and public debate about the limits to be imposed on the prerogatives of investigators to use human beings for scientists' and society's sake. Such a debate needed to be carried on with the same intensity as the one that has repeatedly taken place on the question as to whether it is preferable to rely on a military draft or a volunteer army to protect citizens' and society's interests.

V. THE TASK OF CLINICAL RESEARCH

The tasks of clinical practice and clinical research are different. Robert Levine has persuasively argued that the objectives of investigators and practitioners are not the same:

> The goal of research—the development of generalized knowledge—is advanced by working according to a detailed [relatively inflexible] protocol. . . . [Thus] an appropriate question might be: "What is the antihypertensive effect of administration of this thiazide diuretic in a specified dose range for six weeks to patients with moderately severe hypertension?" In medical practice a more appropriate question is: "What is the best way to control the [blood pressure] of this patient who not only has moderately severe hypertension but also has diabetes, congestive heart failure, and recently lost her job?"[56]

From this, Levine, on another occasion, drew a crucial conclusion:

> [T]he individualized dosage adjustments and changes in therapeutic modalities are less likely to occur in the context of a clinical trial than they are in the

---

55. *See* THE SILENT WORLD, *supra* note 9, at 39-42.

56. Robert J. Levine, *Informed Consent in Research and Practice: Similarities and Differences*, 143 AMA ARCHIVES OF INTERNAL MEDICINE 1229, 1231 (1982).

practice of medicine. This deprivation of the experimentation ordinarily done to enhance the well-being of a patient *is one of the burdens imposed on the patient-subject in a clinical trial.*[57]

In another article, Levine perceptively described an imaginary dialogue between a patient-subject and a physician-investigator about participation in a randomized, placebo controlled study on the effectiveness of a new antihypertensive agent:

> Do you mean to say you are asking me to spend six months taking either an inert substance or one that you have no cause to suspect is either better or worse than that inert substance when the risk of taking a placebo entails approximately a 28 percent chance per year of having a severe complication such as stroke, malignant hypertension, heart failure, or death? You offer me an invitation to participate in such an RCT when I could instead take any of the many antihypertensive drugs which are already approved by the FDA and which would reduce my risk of a major complication to 1.6 percent per year? Why would any rational person do that?[58]

Levine concluded "Why, indeed!"[59] It is difficult to believe that many patients will consent to participation in such a study if adequately informed about risks and alternatives. Levine's dialogue also highlights the formidable task which physician-investigators would face if they were to explain forthrightly to their patient-subjects what is currently known about the effectiveness of antihypertensive drugs; or if they were to alert patient-subjects in a placebo-controlled study that the purpose of the active agent is to mitigate aspects of the disease process that can lead to lethal or disabling complication and that the placebo will not protect them from such consequences; or if they were to alert patient-subjects that preliminary evidence in studies of the effectiveness of two different therapeutic agents has already accumulated on the superiority of one of the agents over the other in the treatment of disease.

Research is not entirely a voyage into the utterly unknown. When a clinical trial is contemplated, considerable information, though not yet scientifically validated, is generally available to suggest that experimental treatments may promise to be beneficial. Thus, in situations in which the experimental treatment is compared with existing standard therapy, all kinds of known or conjectured evidence has accumulated about their respective merits. Patient-subjects generally remain ignorant of most, if not all, of these complexities of knowledge and ignorance.[60] Instead, patient-subjects are told

---

57. ETHICS AND REGULATION OF CLINICAL RESEARCH, *supra* note 10, at 10.

58. Robert J. Levine, *Uncertainty in Clinical Research*, 16 L. MED. & HEALTH CARE 174, 178 (1988).

59. *Id.*

60. Levine states:

Quite commonly at the time a randomized clinical trial is begun, the investigators have available quite a bit of evidence about the agents to be tested. In the United States, for

that it is not yet known which treatment is best, but as Schafer observed, "this statement is misleading at best, deceptive at worst."[61] Very few patients are aware that by the phrase "scientifically validated knowledge" the physician-investigator only means "confirmed by a controlled trial."[62] Such statements conceal information from patient-subjects about alternative treatments whose effectiveness does not rise to a ninety-five percent level of confidence or that are based on clinical experiences or on more poorly designed earlier trials. All this suggests that informed consent does not just involve presenting scientific information to patient-subjects, but requires physician-investigators to translate that information into language relevant to subjects' life experiences and interests.

Investigators with whom I have talked confirm Schafer's observation. They admit that they know many things about risks and benefits, but they also insist that this information need not be communicated because they *really* do not know and will only know the true scientific state of affairs at the end of a rigorously conducted scientific study. Thus, to tell patients precious little is ethically justified. Moreover, even those who in principle are committed to obtaining their patient-subjects' consent will also admit that, in practice, their invitation to participation is affected by the belief that they have already carefully considered the project—its risks and benefits—and concluded that no undue physical harm will come to the subjects and, therefore, they can take some license with the informed consent process. In such conversations an old conviction ultimately surfaces; that subjects are better protected by the investigator being the "guarantor of [their] rights and safety"[63] than by their own consent which rarely is a "valid" one. Thus, in reality, the idea that the investigator is best situated to protect subjects of research continues to have a significant impact on the minds of investigators and the ways they extend their invitations.

VI.   THE NATURE OF THE INFORMED CONSENT PROCESS IN CLINICAL RESEARCH

If the tensions between the inviolability of research subjects and the advancement of knowledge are to be resolved in favor of respect for the

---

example, the results of extensive experience with new drugs obtained during clinical investigations or in medical practice in other countries are often available.

Robert J. Levine, *The Use of Placebos in Randomized Clinical Trials*, 7 IRB 112 (Mar.-Apr. 1985). Similar information is also available in clinical research studies other than randomized clinical trials.

61.   Arthur Schafer, *The Randomized Clinical Trial: For Whose Benefit?*, 7 IRB 4, 5 (Mar.-Apr. 1985).

62.   *Id.*

63.   G. Long et al., *Measurement of Anti-Arrhythmic Potency of Drugs in Man: Effects of Dehydrobenzperidal*, 28 ANESTHESIOLOGY 318-19 (1967).

human rights of the subjects, the mindset which investigators bring to the invitation of participation, the ethical principles which govern the invitation, and the conversations which physician-investigators and patient-subjects must engage in require re-examination. I shall take up each in turn.

A.   The Mindset of Physician-Investigators

Physician-investigators, *before* approaching a potential patient-subject, must first rid themselves of the customary attitudes which in the past shaped, if not determined, their invitation to patient-subjects.[64] A morally valid consent in research settings requires a radically new personal and professional commitment to the patient-subjects and the informed consent process: Physician-investigators must see themselves as scientists only and not as doctors. In conflating clinical trials and therapy, as well as patients and subjects, as if both were one and the same, physician-investigators unwittingly become double agents with conflicting loyalties. Only if they first know who they truly are can they begin to make the subject understand the burdens he or she is assuming when an invitation to participate in clinical trials is extended.

---

64. In *The Silent World* I drew attention to the "irrational and unconscious expectations [which] influence physicians' conduct." I noted that "[e]arly in his explorations, Freud recognized that doctors' unconscious has an impact on their relations with patients, and [that] he gave these manifestations the name 'countertransference.'" THE SILENT WORLD, *supra* note 9, at 147. I then argued that

> [a] broader definition of countertransference that encompasses not only physicians' personal conduct but also their deeply ingrained professional attitudes toward patients will move to center stage a re-examination of the impact on physician-patient interactions of a great many unquestioned professional attitudes. These attitudes include the need to appear authoritative, the importance of hiding uncertainties from patients, the need to view patients as incompetent to participate in decision making, and the belief that patients' welfare depends on patients' trusting doctors' capacities to know what is in patients' best interests.
>
> . . . My broader view of countertransference suggests that not only physicians' personal beliefs but also their professional beliefs are influenced by irrational and unconscious factors. Indeed, the most pernicious countertransference problem may turn out to be that in their professional interactions with patients, physicians view themselves as too rational and their patients as too irrational. A more realistic view of the balance between rationality and irrationality in both parties will itself improve decision making between physicians and patients. The projection of irrationalities originating within physicians onto patients is indeed one of the most pervasive and fateful countertransference reactions.

Id. at 149, 150.

I should mention, as I made clear in my book, that by "irrational" I only meant "not subjected to careful conscious reflection." Thus, in the context of this article I wanted to flag the *unexamined* countertransference reactions of investigators that are grounded in their commitment to advance knowledge but without sufficient reflection of the impact of these motives on the human rights of subjects of research.

Moreover, since loyalty to the research protocol will take precedence over faithfulness to the therapeutic mission, and since physician-investigators will tend to view the person before them as a patient and not as a subject, the tragic fact that human beings are used for the ends of others can readily become obliterated. It is then not surprising that physician-investigators, without fully knowing it, become confused about the nature of their task, as well as about their perceptions of themselves and their patient-subjects.

The investigators who appear before patient-subjects as physicians in white coats create confusion. Patients come to hospitals with the trusting expectation that their doctors will care for them.[65] They will view an invitation to participate in research as a professional recommendation that is intended to serve their individual treatment interests. It is that belief, that trust, which physician-investigators must vigorously challenge so that patient-subjects appreciate that in research, unlike therapy, the research question comes first. This takes time and is difficult to convey. It can be conveyed to patient-subjects only if physician-investigators are willing to challenge the misperceptions that many patients bring to the invitation.

B.   *The Primacy of Autonomy*

Physician-investigators must extend the invitation to participation in research with a thoroughgoing commitment to the principle of autonomy.[66]

---

65. *See infra* note 77 and accompanying text.

66. In their authoritative book *Principles of Biomedical Ethics*, Beauchamp and Childress define the concept of autonomy thusly: "Autonomy is a form of personal liberty of action where the individual determines his or her own course of action in accordance with a plan chosen by himself or herself. . . . A person's autonomy is his or her independence, self-reliance, and self-contained ability to decide." Tom L. BEAUCHAMP & JAMES F. CHILDRESS, PRINCIPLES OF BIOMEDICAL ETHICS 56 (1st ed. 1979). Beauchamp and Childress continue:

> It is one thing to be autonomous and to apprehend that others are acting autonomously, but quite another to be *respected* as an autonomous agent and to respect the autonomy of others. To respect autonomous agents is to recognize with due appreciation their own considered value judgments and outlooks even when it is believed that their judgments are mistaken. To respect them in this way is to acknowledge their right to their own views and the permissibility of their actions based on such beliefs. And to grant them this right is to say that they are entitled to such autonomous determination without limitations on their liberty being imposed by others.

Id. at 58. For purposes of this article I accept their formulation of autonomy. In *The Silent World* I offered a view of autonomy which is also based on psychoanalytic considerations but which does not disagree with their views on the respect to be accorded to autonomous choices:

> Respect for psychological autonomy requires that both parties pay caring attention to their capacities and incapacities for self-determination by supporting and enhancing their real, though precarious, endowment for reflective thought. In conversation with one another, patients may uncover mistaken notions [and] physicians may uncover [some of] their unconscious preferences and biases. . . . Without conversation, individual self-determination can become compromised by condemning physicians and patients to the isolation of

Edmund Pellegrino, in a recent article on the "Ethical Dilemmas in Clinical Research," explored the moral dilemmas faced by clinical investigators. He located them in the inevitable conflict among three values: "for science, it is truth; for medicine, it is beneficence toward the patient; and for the investigator as an individual, it is self-interest."[67] He concluded that

> [t]he safe rule in [clinical research] is to favor beneficence over scientific rigor when the two seem to be in conflict or when in doubt. The possible loss of knowledge cannot outweigh the possibility of harm to the subject even if the utilitarian calculus indicates great benefit to many and harm to only a few.[68]

He granted the scientist, however, "a certain latitude or 'discretionary space' in the pursuit of knowledge" which is difficult to define by rules and which "must be narrowly defined. Respect for persons and the imperative of beneficence take precedence over scientific curiosity."[69] Yet earlier he seemed to extend the discretionary space when he expressed the hope "that the investigator will judiciously *balance* the patient's interests and those of the scientific protocol."[70]

Pellegrino can be understood or misunderstood as giving considerable latitude to investigators, and for two reasons. First, he often moves from research with competent subjects to research with incompetent subjects without explicitly stating that entirely different considerations apply to both groups.[71]

---

solitary decision making, which can only contribute to abandoning patients prematurely to an ill-considered fate.

THE SILENT WORLD, *supra* note 9, at 128. Moreover:

> Even though choices are influenced by psychological considerations, it is one thing to appreciate that fact and quite another to interfere with choice on the basis of speculations, or even evidence, about underlying psychological reasons. . . . Short of substantial evidence of incompetence, choices deserve to be honored.

Id. at 112-13.

67. Edmund D. Pellegrino, *Beneficence, Scientific Autonomy, and Self-Interest: Ethical Dilemmas in Clinical Research*, GEO. MED. 21 (1991).

68. *Id.* at 27.

69. *Id.* at 26-27.

70. *Id.* at 22.

71. Similarly, the celebrated *Belmont Report* on principles and guidelines for human research is confusing by not making clear distinctions between the principles that should govern research with competent and incompetent persons. It considered three basic principles to be "particularly relevant to the ethics of research . . . : respect for persons, beneficence and justice." THE NATIONAL COMMISSION FOR THE PROTECTION OF HUMAN SUBJECTS OF BIOMEDICAL AND BEHAVIORAL RESEARCH, U.S. DEPARTMENT OF HEALTH AND HUMAN RESOURCES PUB. NO. (OS) 78-0012, THE BELMONT REPORT: ETHICAL PRINCIPLES AND GUIDELINES FOR THE PROTECTION OF HUMAN SUBJECTS OF RESEARCH 4 (1978). The report continues:

> 1. *Respect for Persons* . . . incorporates at least two ethical convictions: first that individuals should be treated as autonomous agents, and second, that persons with diminished autonomy are entitled to protection . . . .
>
> . . . .

Then one can readily overlook that he means to invoke the principle of beneficence only for research with incompetent subjects. He suggests that with competent subjects a "morally valid consent" is essential. Yet, later on he seems to modify his position when he writes: "It is the investigator who decides how much to tell the patient or family, what facts to emphasize, which to withhold, and how to present them."[72] Second, Pellegrino repeatedly shifts from issues germane to therapy to those that pertain to research without clearly distinguishing between the two settings. Thus, Pellegrino may be correct in saying that one of the value conflicts "for *medicine* . . . is beneficence toward the patient,"[73] but for clinical research with competent patients, respect for autonomy must be the guiding principle.

At times, Pellegrino seems to agree. He writes that

> [t]he intellectual autonomy of the scientist is autonomy held in trust, . . . [i.e.] the conscious acknowledgement by the investigator that he or she is allowed freedom to pursue rigorous scientific goals in human experimentation only if the welfare of the patient is always respected as primary and superior to the

---

To respect autonomy is to give weight to autonomous persons' considered opinions and choices while refraining from obstructing their actions unless they are clearly detrimental to others.

. . . .

In most cases of research involving human subjects, respect for persons demands that subjects enter into research voluntarily and with adequate information.

. . . .

2. *Beneficence.* Persons are treated in an ethical manner not only by respecting their decisions and protecting them from harm, but also by making efforts to secure their well-being.

. . . .

The obligations of beneficence affects both individual investigators and society at large, because they extend both to particular research projects and to the entire enterprise of research.

Id. at 4-7.

The examples given for justifying invocation of the principle of beneficence, however, address only vulnerable populations, e.g., children, prisoners, and the mentally ill. Yet, in setting forth three principles for the general conduct of research and then appealing to such vague terms of art as protection from "harm" and securing "well-being," for invoking the beneficence principle, can readily create the impression that with competent subjects too, autonomy may at unspecified times have to yield to beneficence. Respect for persons deserved a more unequivocal, or at least more precise, formulation.

For an interesting discussion of serious difficulties in the *Belmont Report*, see Ernest Marshall, *Does the Moral Philosophy of the Belmont Report Rest on a Mistake?*, 8 IRB 5-6 (Nov.-Dec. 1986). He notes, for example, that "the point of Kantian principles is precisely to say that certain things cannot be 'balanced out,' i.e., if certain actions are unjust or disrespectful of persons then they are wrong and therefore simply should not be done." *Id.* at 6.

72. Pellegrino, *supra* note 67, at 24.

73. *Id.* at 21.

values of science and self-interest.[74]

Pellegrino's use of the word "welfare" could suggest that it encompasses not only prevention of physical injury but also respect for subjects' autonomous choice. Welfare, however, is often used only to refer to preventing physical injury; therefore, it would have been better if he had emphasized that in clinical research with competent subjects it only pertains to respect for autonomy.

I raise these issues also because Pellegrino places so much faith in "the personal morality of the clinical investigator" whom he considers "the ultimate safeguard of the safety of the experimental human subject."[75] But his hybrid concept "autonomy held in trust," an amalgam of autonomy and benevolence, alienates the rights of subjects to be authors of their own fate. The implied idea that investigators are permitted to exercise a trusteeship over persons' autonomy is particularly problematic in today's world where respect for subjects' self-determination is not as abiding a motivating consideration in the conduct of research as is the advancement of science for the sake of mankind.[76]

Respect for autonomy imposes numerous burdens on the physician-investigator. First, he must not allow disclosures to be shaped by paternalistic or beneficent concerns that patient-subjects will make decisions which are not in their "best interests." Second, he or she must not allow disclosures to be shaped by concerns that patient-subjects will learn that the customary treatments which they may continue to take, should they decline the more promising experimental treatments, offer no hope for the alleviation of their suffering. Nor should disclosures be shaped by concerns that patient-subjects' trust in medicine will be undermined once they learn about the uncertainties inherent in all medical treatments, nor by concerns over upsetting hospitalized patients if they were to appreciate that they, too, are being asked to yield their individual interests to the interests of scientific investigations.

Moreover, physician-investigators must reflect on the fateful impact of their commitment to the ideology of medical science—its ethos to acquire knowledge for the sake of mankind—on the invitation to participation in research. Medical scientists share with their colleagues from the natural sciences a commitment to the pursuit of truth, objectivity, and the advancement

---

74. *Id.* at 26.

75. *Id.* at 21.

76. The personal morality of the investigator would not be impugned if he or she were to give greater weight to the advancement of science than to autonomy. Indeed, Pellegrino noted that an investigator "faces a difficult task of balancing and ordering the values of truth and beneficence against each other." *Id.* at 25. Thus, the question remains whether "autonomy-in-trust" permits such balancing with both competent and incompetent subjects. Since his recent paper is a major contribution to the ethics of research, I discussed it at some length. I can only hope that I interpreted him correctly.

of knowledge. The commitment to objectivity invites investigators' thought processes to become objectified and, in turn, to transform the human beings who are the subjects of research into data points to be plotted on a chart that will prove or disprove a research hypothesis.

Margaret Radin's observations about objectification illuminate this problem. In an article on women and people of color she noted that

> [o]bjectification comes about through *subordination* when one culture conceives of certain characteristics of persons ... as marks of lesser personhood. These marks license manipulation of those who bear the marks, and also license refusal to recognize in them rights and other indices of respect otherwise conceived of as universally applicable to persons.[77]

This license was usurped or conferred on physicians in clinical practice, and since the age of medical science has been extended to clinical research. Objectification begins with patients and becomes intensified when subordination is also affected by attitudes toward gender, color, religion, social and economic status and, of course, by the scientific imperative of clinical research.

Furthermore, human beings should not be used lightly and cheaply to serve as means for the ends of others, even though they are so readily available in large numbers. Prior to extending an invitation to subjects, physician-investigators must give thought to the minimal number of subjects required for obtaining satisfactory answers to a research question and must conduct a literature search of existing studies which will make a repetition of an experiment unnecessary. Science's commitment to truth and progress, particularly when human beings are needed for purposes of research, ought to disdain inquiries where the truth is already apparent and progress already a reality.

Finally, as I have already suggested, physician-investigators must go to considerable length in extending the invitation to participate in clinical research so that they can rest assured that patient-subjects understand the implications of their consent. Pellegrino, in his discussion of "valid consent," sensitively describes the difficulty patients experience in "[separating] the physician-scientist role from the physician-healer."[78] He further notes that "[t]he

---

77. Margaret J. Radin, *Reflections on Objectification*, 65 S. CAL. L. REV. 341, 346 (1991). Pellegrino is similarly concerned when he writes that "the values and standards [of science necessitate] a certain degree of objectivization of the subject under study. But in clinical investigations, the 'object' of study remains a human being." Thus, he cautions that "the canons of science may conflict with another set of values—those that define the endeavor of medicine." Pellegrino, *supra* note 67, at 22.

The objectification of patients is also illustrated by investigators' concerns in the outcome of a new treatment in terms of *longevity* while patients may be more concerned about the *quality* of life offered by one or the other treatment. For a detailed and sensitive discussion, see CHARLES FRIED, MEDICAL EXPERIMENTATION: PERSONAL INTEGRITY AND SOCIAL POLICY (1974).

78. Pellegrino, *supra* note 67, at 25.

34   SAINT LOUIS UNIVERSITY LAW JOURNAL   [Vol. 38:7

physician can easily obtain consent to an experimental protocol simply by emphasizing the hope of cure and downplaying the risk and the experimental nature of the treatment."[79] He cautions physicians that "[a] legally adequate consent form may not be morally valid [for a] morally valid consent aims at true 'con-sent,' an agreeing together."[80]

Only respect for persons' autonomy and self-determination can guarantee "true 'con-sent,' an agreeing together"; otherwise, the invitation subtly becomes a request or even a demand.   Invocation of the principle of beneficence, in the service of shielding patient-subjects from painful disclosures, can only mislead physician-investigators into "downplaying the risk and the experimental nature of the treatment."   Whenever beneficence suggests withholding of information, the better solution would be to exclude patient-subjects from participation in clinical research.

C.   The Conversation

To obtain a "morally valid consent [which] aims at true consent," is an inordinately difficult task. The physician-investigators must disclose to their subjects at least the following information: (1) that the subjects are not only patients and, to the extent to which they are patients, that their therapeutic interests, even if not incidental, will be subordinated to scientific interests; (2) that it is problematic and indeterminate whether their welfare will be better served by placing their medical fate in the hands of a physician rather than an investigator; (3) that in opting for the care of a physician they may be better or worse off and for such and such reasons; (4) that clinical research will allow doctors to penetrate the mysteries of medicine's uncertainties about which treatments are best, dangerous, or ineffective; (5) that clinical research may possibly be in the patient's immediate best interest, perhaps promise benefits in the future, or provide no benefit, particularly if the patient is assigned to a control (placebo) arm of a study; (6) that research is governed by a research protocol and a research question and, therefore, his or her interests and needs will yield to the claims of science; and (7) that physician-investigators will respect whatever decision the subject ultimately makes.

Conversing with patient-subjects in such a manner which will give them a clearer appreciation of the difference between clinical research and therapy is a daunting assignment.   I have on occasions been asked, "How will investigators know when to stop the conversation?" My response has been that they will know when to stop once they have learned to begin the conversation with a commitment to respect for personhood; for only then will they not shirk their responsibility to be utterly forthright in disclosing the research dimension of their work and the alternatives available to their patient-

---

79. *Id.*
80. *Id.* at 24.

subjects. It is the spirit in which the conversation begins which is the problem. If that problem is better resolved, the end will take care of itself.

Levine once wrote that in the current climate of extending the invitation to participation in research, "[the informed consent] requirement [serves] as a *pledge* made by researchers that in the pursuit of their salutary mission they will not exploit people; [or that i]ndividual persons will not be involved as research subjects without their awareness or approval."[81] If he meant by "pledge" a symbolic gesture "to secure and maintain public confidence in scientific research,"[82] rather than a true commitment, I would agree.

Guido Calabresi years ago expressed his doubts about informed consent serving as a "control system" for the value conflicts inherent in the conduct of research. He did not believe that it could in practice serve such a purpose. His argument was that "[c]onsent or its semblance keeps us from blatantly [destroying] the fabric of our commitment to human dignity."[83] I am not convinced that informed consent need only serve such a limited symbolic function once the idea of shared decision making becomes a guiding commitment. Levine's and Calabresi's observations, however, identify the mutual deceptions in which scientists and the public engage in order not to unduly impede scientific research. The public, propelled by its longings to benefit from the advancement of science, has made common cause with scientists' demand for freedom of inquiry by acquiescing to the human costs which research entails. The symbolic bow to informed consent then allows the public and scientists to have it both ways. Forcing a public debate on the morality of human experimentation may put an end to the all too silent evasion of confronting any tragic choices that must be made. To be sure, "public confidence in scientific research" is justified on the ground that physician-investigators will take great care in not exposing patient-subjects to unnecessary *physical* harm. But this is a different matter.

The disclosure obligations I have set forth so far emphasize the need to pay particular attention to explaining to patient-subjects how participation in research differs from how they would ordinarily be treated or would expect to be treated. Thus, the first task in extending the invitation is to be absolutely clear about the research dimension of the invitation, its implications and possible consequences. Such disclosures do not require patient-subjects to understand the esoteric knowledge of medicine and science. Indeed, at present, subjects are overwhelmed with unnecessary scientific information that clarifies little and serves more the purpose of obscuring the crucial information that

---

81. Robert J. Levine, *Deferred Consent*, 12 CONTROLLED CLINICAL TRIALS 546 (1991) (emphasis added).

82. *Id.*

83. Guido Calabresi, *Reflections on Medical Experimentation in Humans*, 98 DAEDALUS 387, 404 (1969).

they need to know,[84] such as the risks, benefits, alternatives, and uncertainties which patient-subjects face by their participation in clinical research, and the impact of participation, known and conjectured, on the quality of their future lives. Investigators have an obligation to translate scientific information into language which is relevant to patient-subjects' life and interests. Informed consent forms are so incomprehensible because they are written at a higher reading level than is appropriate for the intended population.[85] In addition, they include too much distracting technical information of little consequence to the decisions which patient-subjects must make. Put another way, current informed consent forms often provide IRBs rather than the subjects with a better understanding of investigators' intentions.

Physician-scientists will be reluctant to converse with patient-subjects in the spirit of the recommendation that I have outlined.[86] Such conversations take time, may have to extend over hours, perhaps even days, and must be continued until one is reasonably certain that the patient-subjects understand.

---

84. Alan Meisel has argued that the problem of the unreadability of informed consent forms is better resolved not "by improving [their] readability [but by abolishing them, even prohibiting] them by legal fiat if necessary." He then goes on to say that

> [t]he problem is not the unreadability of consent forms; that is merely symptomatic. The real problem is that physicians, for the most part, do not consider informed consent to be an important part of the practice of medicine. . . . Consent forms play no role in the informed consent process. Where used, they are intended merely to memorialize that in fact the informed consent process transpired.

Meisel, *supra* note 34.

Abolishing informed consent forms will not improve matters. As Meisel observed, physicians do not consider informed consent important and such attitudes will infect the oral informed consent process as well. Informed consent forms can be improved if their function were to truly inform patient-subjects about matters crucial to their decision. Too often they do not serve this purpose. *See infra* notes 117-124 and accompanying text.

85. Considerable literature exists on the "readability" of informed consent forms. For a recent article, see James R. Ogloff & Randy K. Otto, *Are Research Participants Truly Informed? Readability of Informed Consent Forms Used in Research*, 4 ETHICS AND BEHAVIOR 239-252 (1991).

86. Royall discusses some of the obstacles to informed consent:

> A more prosaic reason why informed consent is not a panacea is that in many cases it simply won't work. Sometimes too few patients will agree to participate in the study. And sometimes the consent process is simply too uncomfortable and time-consuming. Many physicians are reluctant to share their uncertainties with patients, and many patients do not want to hear about such uncertainties. Also, many patients know so little about research that to make them truly understand what they are being asked to do and why, to make their consent truly "informed," would require more time and effort than can reasonably be invested.

Royall, *supra* note 19, at 58. Since we have not had sufficient experience with an informed consent process as advocated in my article, we do not know whether it will work or not. Surely the process will require time and effort, but such a price must be paid if consent is to be taken seriously.

Of course, subjects may still make decisions which they later on will regret because they then believe, perhaps correctly so, that they had not given their participation the thought it deserved. This is inevitable, and physician-investigators must not allow that possibility to tailor their disclosures in order to avoid burdening subjects with guilt feelings over having made the wrong decision (another variant of beneficence) or that they will agree to what investigators believe to be in subjects' better interests. Autonomous persons must be held responsible for their own mistakes and must not be protected from making them by subterfuge. As Justice Stevens once put it when he spoke about a pregnant woman's distress in deciding whether or not to undergo an abortion. "[I]t is far better to permit some persons to make incorrect decisions than to deny all individuals the right to make decisions that have a profound effect upon their destiny."[87]

Thus, recruitment of subjects will prove to be more time consuming. Completion of research may also be delayed and, if too many patients refuse, selection bias will make some research impossible to conduct. Not only may scientific progress be impeded but physician-investigators' self-interests in recognition and advancement of their careers may be jeopardized.[88] Scientific discoveries do not occur in isolation and, more often than not, scientists in many centers are pursuing similar inquires. The imperative to publish first is of crucial personal significance, because so much depends on it in terms of recognition, fame, future grants and prospects. A commitment to disclosure and consent entails paying a great personal price which can be moderated, however, if the collectivity of physician-investigators embrace these responsibilities or find new ways of conducting research which will make forthright disclosures less of a burden.[89] It is also a great professional price to pay

---

87. Thornburgh v. American College of Obstetricians and Gynecologists, 106 S. Ct. 2169, 2189-90 (1986).

88. Pellegrino has given an excellent account of the impact on research practices of investigators' self-interests, be they advancement of careers, economic rewards, etc., or of their institutions' arrangements with pharmaceutical companies and other industries. Pellegrino, *supra* note 67, at 24-25. "[T]hey pose a potential danger to experimental subjects. They can compromise beneficence, the central value in medicine." *Id.* at 25.

89. Marcia Angell states:

I find it difficult to justify strategies to increase the accrual of patients if the result is that people do not act as they would if full and necessarily neutral information had been provided. It might be better in this situation to consider alternatives to randomized clinical trials. Several workers have emphasized that it is often scientifically adequate to use non-randomized controls in trials of treatments . . . . A final alternative, which deserves more attention, is better and more systematic analysis of available information; this might in some instances obviate the necessity for new studies.

Marcia Angell, *Patients' Preferences in Randomized Clinical Trials*, 310 NEW ENG. J. MED. 1385, 1386 (1984).

Science desires randomized clinical trials, it does not demand them. . . . [T]he importance of randomized trials is exaggerated by the false dichotomy that is implied when historical

38   *SAINT LOUIS UNIVERSITY LAW JOURNAL*   [Vol. 38:7

because physician-investigators come to research out of a deeply felt dissatisfaction with the current state of medical knowledge and out of a painful awareness of the suffering of their patients.

Insufficient attention has also been paid to the current reality which places physician-investigators at the mercy of the institutions in which they work and the private and public grant agencies which support their research. Medical research since World War II has become a research-industrial complex. Academic institutions rely on the revenues which accrue from the assessment of indirect costs to the providers of grants. Research proposals have to be generated and completed at a rapid rate to assure future grant support. Thus, investigators are under considerable pressure to recruit subjects as quickly as possible to support the institutions' buildings, laboratories, staff and salaries. With respect to career advancement and future grant support, physician-investigators are thus the victims of an institutional system (their own institutions and the National Institutes of Health) which penalizes them if in fulfillment of their ethical disclosure obligations toward patient-subjects, the pace of research would be slowed. Both at the national and local levels this problem deserves careful consideration and sustained discussion.[90]

VII. A NATIONAL HUMAN INVESTIGATION BOARD

The moral ambiguities inherent in the contemporary regulations of human research are also an inevitable consequence of policy makers' unwillingness to confront openly the lengths to which a democratic society like ours should go in protecting citizen-subjects' rights to autonomy and bodily integrity for

---

control trials are the only alternative discussed. In fact many of the weaknesses of historical controls can be avoided by using concurrent non-randomized controls. And of course comparing a treatment with both historical and concurrent controls can provide even stronger evidence about its efficacy.

Royall, *supra* note 19, at 60.

90. Pellegrino has commented on some of these problems:

Institutional pride or hubris is . . . a corrosive influence. The institution's drive to be "first" is a mixed motive; it can be effective in raising institutional morale and productivity, but it is also capable of submerging moral imperatives on grounds of exigency and "survival." In competition with other hospitals and universities, institutional pride can desensitize an institutional review board to certain dubious projects.

Pellegrino, *supra*, note 67, at 24.

The matter is further complicated when the health care industry enters long-term contractual arrangements with a university to support research. The usual proviso is that a company will support research facilities and personnel in return for privileged access and a share in the patenting rights to the products developed. These industry-university compacts are especially attractive today when governmental and philanthropic sources of research funding are insufficient. Some of our most prestigious universities have entered into what may well turn out to be Faustian compacts.

Id. at 25.

the sake of medical science. I have already suggested that whatever societal mandate exists for the conduct of human research has not been subjected to intensive congressional and public scrutiny as to the morality and legality of the enterprise. Instead, as Edmond Cahn once put it, we have been all too willing, in our longing to conquer disease and death, "to possess the end and yet not be responsible for the means, to grasp the fruit while disavowing the tree, to escape being told the cost, until someone else has paid it irrevocably."[91]

The policy questions underlying the tensions between the inviolability of subjects of research and advancing the frontiers of knowledge require more careful articulation and resolution than can be gleaned from the federal regulations so far enacted.[92] The concerns I have raised and the recommendations I have made need to be examined, debated and decided by a national regulatory body to which the IRBs can also turn for advice and guidance on difficult problems that require resolution.

The need for such a regulatory body, which I had already explored in *Experimentation With Human Beings*,[93] was supported by my colleagues who served with me on the Tuskegee Syphilis Study Ad Hoc Advisory Panel. We had been appointed by the Assistant Secretary for Health of the Department of Health, Education and Welfare "to investigate the circumstances surrounding the Tuskegee, Alabama, study of untreated syphilis in the male Negro initiated by the United States Public Health Service in 1932."[94] Our primary assignments were to make recommendations as to whether the Study should be terminated, to pass judgment on the ethics of the Study from its inception, and to make recommendations about necessary changes in "existing policies to protect the rights of patients participating in health research."[95]

Among the many recommendations we made with respect to the third assignment, one urged that Congress establish a permanent body, which we called the National Human Investigation Board (NHIB), with the authority to regulate at least all federally supported research involving human subjects. We suggested that

> [t]he primary responsibility of the National Human Investigation Board should be to *formulate research policies*, in much greater detail and with much more clarity than is presently the case. The Board [should also] promulgate detailed procedures to govern the implementation of its policies by institutional review committees. It [should] also promulgate procedures for the review of research decisions and their consequences. In particular, this Board should establish

---

91. Edmond Cahn, *Drug Experiments and the Public Conscience*, in DRUGS IN OUR SOCIETY 255, 260 (Paul Talalay ed. 1988).

92. See *supra* note 53 and accompanying text.

93. EXPERIMENTATION WITH HUMAN BEINGS, *supra* note 40, at 856-954.

94. TUSKEGEE SYPHILIS STUDY, *supra* note 3, at 2.

95. *Id.* at 1.

procedures for the publication of important institutional committee and Board decisions. Publication of such decisions would permit their intensive study both inside and outside the medical profession and would be a first step toward the case-by-case development of policies governing human experimentation. We [saw] such a development, analogous to the experience of the common law, as the best hope for ultimately providing workable standards for the regulation of the human experimentation process.[96]

Senator Edward Kennedy incorporated that proposal in a bill submitted to the Senate.[97] His bill was never enacted and I believe that a major reason was the Senate's reluctance to expose to public view the value conflicts inherent in the conduct of research. Had the Senate seriously debated the bill, it would have been forced to consider whether inadequately informed subjects should ever serve as means for society's and science's ends. Instead, by inaction, it left such painful decisions to the low visibility handiwork of local IRBs.

I believed then, as I do now, that the rejection of a National Human Investigation Board was a mistake for many reasons.[98] Most importantly, it precludes greater public visibility of the decisions made in the conduct of human experimentation. Current practices do not provide for either institutional review committees' publication of, or free access to, such decisions. This low level of visibility not only hampers efforts to evaluate and learn from attempts to resolve the complex problems of human research but also prevents the public at large from reacting to what is being done for the sake of the advancement of science.

Local IRBs cannot assume these and other functions that a National Human Investigation Board could serve, for yet another reason. As George Annas has observed, "IRBs as currently constituted do not protect research subjects but rather protect the institution and the institution's investigator."[99]

There is considerable truth to his allegation. The majority of IRB members are on the faculty of the institutions to which the investigators

---

96. *Id.* at 24.

97. S. 2072, 93d Cong., 1st Sess. (1973).

98. Such a Board, for example, should promulgate detailed regulations for research with vulnerable subjects. Moreover, it would have to address Ackerman's concerns that any absolute commitment to autonomy "suffers from fatal difficulties in an important range of situations. It is widely agreed that individuals have duties of beneficence to prevent substantial harm to other specific persons when doing so will involve no more than modest costs to their own interests." Terrence F. Ackerman, *Balancing Moral Principles in Federal Regulations on Human Research,* 14 IRB 4 (Jan.-Feb. 1992). If these concerns have merit, then the Board could consider Caplan's suggestion that a "general obligation [be imposed on persons] to participate in research." Arthur L. Caplan, *Is there a Duty to Serve as a Subject in Biomedical Research?,* 6 IRB at 1-5 (Sept.-Oct. 1984).

99. GEORGE J. ANNAS, JUDGING MEDICINE 331 (1988).

belong.[100] They not only share similar interests and objectives but they also know, when sitting in judgment of a research protocol, that their proposals may soon be subjected to similar scrutiny. Thus, particularly in the murky area of informed consent, it is unlikely that members of IRBs will hold investigators to a standard of disclosure and consent that would protect the subjects of research if doing so would place impediments on the conduct of research and, in turn, affect the well being of their colleagues in decisive ways.[101]

VIII.   A CASE EXAMPLE

A research study conducted at the Neuropsychiatric Institute of the University of California, Los Angles, (UCLA) which began in the early 1980s and is still in progress, illustrates the problems I have discussed. To orient the reader, I briefly summarize three facts about the design of the experiment and two facts about its aftermath that are of concern to me: (1) The study required schizophrenic patients who had recovered from their psychotic disorders to be withdrawn from medication even though "[i]t is generally accepted that maintenance antipsychotic medication will benefit a substantial proportion of chronic schizophrenics."[102]   (2) The study expected to produce a relapse (recurrence of symptomatology) in many patient-subjects in order to attain its objective to predict better relapse, particularly of those who would exhibit such severe symptoms as "bizarre behavior, self-neglect, hostility, depressive mood

---

100. For example, the IRB at Yale-New Haven Medical Center "currently consists of 26 members of whom 15 are full-time medical school faculty. . . . The other 11 committee members include [5 persons affiliated with the Medical Center], a psychological counselor who has . . . no [such] affiliation, 4 medical students . . . and 1 student from the School of Public Health." ETHICS AND REGULATION OF CLINICAL RESEARCH, *supra* note 57, at 330.

101. For a more critical assessment of IRBs, see ANNAS, *supra* note 99, at 331-33. For an opposing assessment, see ETHICS AND REGULATIONS OF CLINICAL RESEARCH, *supra* note 57, at 341-350.

102. Keith H. Nuechterlein & Michael Gitlin, Research Protocol for Developmental Processes in Schizophrenic Disorders Project: Protocol; Double Blind Crossover and Withdrawal of Neuroleptics in Remitted, Recent-Onset Schizophrenia, HSPC #86-07-336 1, 6 [hereinafter Protocol] (on file with author). In a 1988 article the investigators gave a clear account of these research objectives:

> The present study is a prospective examination of prodromal signs and symptoms of schizophrenic relapse, using a systematic and carefully controlled research design. One important improvement over the previous studies is that relapse was defined as the elevation of psychiatric symptoms to the severe or extremely severe level. Thus, minor symptom fluctuations that might often be inconsequential were not considered relapses. In contrast to the studies that defined the period of observation by the necessity to increase medication to avoid a possible relapse, we can be certain that any prodromal changes that we isolated actually did precede a clear relapse.

Kenneth L. Subotnik & Keith N. Nuechterlein, *Prodromal Signs and Symptoms in Schizophrenic Relapse*, 97 J. ABNORMAL PSYCHOLOGY 405, 406 (1988).

42   SAINT LOUIS UNIVERSITY LAW JOURNAL   [Vol. 38:7

and suicidability."[103]   (3) The informed consent form signed by the participants was inadequate in disclosing to the subjects the risks which their participation entailed.   (4) The IRB approved the research protocol and informed consent form without asking the investigators for clarifications that might have led the IRB to better protect the subjects of research.   (5) The subsequent response to the review of the study by the National Institutes of Health's Office for the Protection of Research Risks (OPRR) did not go far in remedying the problems which came to OPRR's attention.

I also want to emphasize at the outset that my analysis is limited to a review of one of the research protocols, including the informed consent form approved by UCLA's IRB, the action taken by the OPRR, once parents of one of the subjects had lodged a complaint about the study and a perusal of the psychiatric literature pertinent to the research project.[104]   I cannot address what might have been disclosed to the subjects in conversations between them and the investigators; about that I have no knowledge. I can only note that the data available from the protocol and the OPRR review hardly suggests that scrupulous attention was paid at any point to full disclosure and consent.

The UCLA experiment was designed to make an important contribution to a better understanding of the need for continuous medication following patients' recovery from a recent onset of schizophrenic disorder.   Thus, the research project sought to identify patients who can function without medication because antipsychotic medication can cause tardive dyskinesia, a syndrome consisting of involuntary and potentially irreversible movements for which no known treatment exists.[105]

All potential patient-subjects were being followed in UCLA's After Care Clinic.[106]   The study, according to the protocol, consisted of two sequential phases.[107]   In the first phase, lasting for twenty-four weeks, the patient-subjects were randomized, in a double-blind design,[108] to one of two groups. The first group received a standardized dose of 12.5 mgm of prolyxin decanoate, an antipsychotic medication, every two weeks, while the second was injected with a placebo, an inert, therapeutically ineffective substance. After twelve weeks, the injections given to members of each group were reversed so that those who had been receiving medication now received a

---

103. *Id.*

104. These and all other discussed unpublished documents are in the possession of the author and available upon request.

105. In some patients symptoms of tardive dyskinesia disappear within several months after antipsychotic drugs are withdrawn, but withdrawal of antipsychotic medication does not guarantee that symptoms will vanish. In some patients, symptoms may persist indefinitely. DORLAND'S ILLUSTRATED MEDICAL DICTIONARY 517-18 (27th ed. 1988).

106. *See infra* note 134 and accompanying text.

107. Protocol, *supra* note 102.

108. *See supra* note 30.

placebo, and vice versa. In the second phase, "all clinically appropriate patients" received no medication, i.e., those who were still on prolyxin were also deprived of the active drug.[109]

The patient-subjects were then followed for at least one year unless "1) the subject withdraws permission for the study or 2) clinical relapse or psychotic exacerbation occurs."[110] Criteria for psychotic relapse included "[high scores on test measures] for Hallucinations, Unusual Thought Content, or Conceptual Disorganization; [for] psychotic exacerbation [fairly severe recurrence of symptomatology; and] for relapse-other type, [high scores] on scales of *bizarre behavior, self-neglect, hostility, depressive mood, and suicidability.*"[111] Apparently the patient-subject's therapist was authorized in the first double-blind phase of the study to break the code for "clinical reasons" but the protocol contained no information, and therefore the IRB could not know, as to when the therapist might take such action. Clearly the intent was to tolerate severe recurrences in symptomatology. Once that had happened "the patient [would] be withdrawn from the study."[112]

The investigators noted in the protocol's section on "Potential Benefits" that since "no study shows 100% relapse in schizophrenics withdrawn from antipsychotics, unquestioned maintenance treatment may for any particular patient involve much risk and little benefit. At present, there is little consistent data regarding predictive factors for patients at low risk of relapse without pharmacotherapy."[113] In that section the investigators also stated

> that clinical relapse or psychotic exacerbation can be expected to occur in at least some of our patient subjects. *However, since most of our patients have been requesting drug withdrawal for months, and since our knowledge as to which acute schizophrenic patients will relapse following drug withdrawal is very meager, we feel this risk is justified, especially in view of the risk of tardive dyskinesia with long-term antipsychotic use.* Withdrawal from antipsychotic medication one year after the psychotic episode is not unusual in standard psychiatric practice for patients with acute, nonchronic schizophrenia, since little clear evidence exists regarding longer-term prophylactic effects for this nonchronic population.[114]

It is true that many schizophrenic patients complain about the side effects of anti-psychotic medication. However, therapists who believe that such treatment is clinically indicated generally do their level best to impress on patients the need for remaining on medication or to encourage its resumption as soon as symptoms recur. In the UCLA study, on the other hand, all patients

---

109. Protocol, *supra* note 102, at 4.
110. *Id.* at 6.
111. *Id.* (emphasis supplied).
112. *Id.*
113. *Id.* at 7.
114. Protocol, *supra* note 102, at 8.

werc withdrawn from medication, indeed required to do so, for research purposes until the needs of the study, and not those of the individual patient, had been satisfied.[115]   The expectation of relapse was an integral aspect of the research design; it was not an unfortunate consequence of treatment but one which the investigators deliberately induced.   This is particularly problematic because of the continuing controversy in psychiatric circles as to whether relapse leads to additional, at times irreversible, injury.[116]

The consent form submitted to the IRB for review and approval informed prospective patient-subjects that "the purpose of this study is to take people like me off medication in a way that will give the most information about the medication, its effects on me, on others and on the way the brain works."[117] It mentioned that an inactive substance (placebo) or an (active) medication would be randomly administered during the first phase and that then "all medication will be stopped and that I will continue to receive regular care at the UCLA After Care Clinic."[118]   Stating it in that way could only confuse potential subjects. In the same sentence they were told that medication would be stopped and that they would continue to receive regular care, without alerting them in most explicit language that "regular care" was compromised by the withdrawal of medication.[119]

---

115. The protocol does not make clear whether all the patient-subjects had been on medication for at least one year when enrolled in the study, which, according to the investigators, is the time when "in standard psychiatric practice" patients are often taken off medication. *Id.*

116. Although the issue is far from settled, many psychiatrists believe that relapse can be permanently harmful to patients: "[S]ome patients are left with a damaging residual if a psychosis is allowed to proceed unmitigated." Richard J. Wyatt, *Neuroleptics and the Natural Course of Schizophrenia*, 17 SCHIZOPHRENIA BULLETIN 325, 347 (1991). "[N]euroleptic drugs . . . if they fully control all acute episodes, may protect against the otherwise inevitable decline of mental function." R. Miller, *Schizophrenia as a Progressive Disorder: Relations to EEG, CT, Neuropathological and Other Evidence*, 33 PROGRESS NEUROBIOLOGY 17, 35 (1989).

117. Keith Nuechterlein, Informed Consent Agreement for Patients (Version 1): Double-Blind Drug Crossover and Withdrawal Project 1 (July 1988) [hereinafter Consent Agreement 1] (on file with author).

118. *Id.*

119. Being absolutely clear on this point was important since the subjects were recruited from the Continuing Care Program of The Neuropsychiatric Institute UCLA. The brochure, given to patients enrolled in this program, contained the following information:

THE CONTINUING CARE PROGRAM . . .

. . . is a specialty service combining treatment, research, and training in the care of the individual with psychotic symptoms. Jointly sponsored by NIMH, UCLA, Camarillo-NIP, and the Clinical Research Center, the Program offers continuing care to people who are experiencing their first psychotic episode.

The Program includes inpatient and outpatient treatment as well as an active follow-up evaluation of each person. Fully integrated with these services is a research project aimed at increasing understanding and knowledge of the factors that are related to relapse and remission.

PURPOSE

Moreover, the patient-subjects were not informed at the beginning of the study that already during the first phase they would not necessarily receive optimal individual treatment, but only a *standardized* dose of 12.5 mg of prolyxin. Such a standardized dose can itself lead either to a return of symptomatology or produce unnecessary side effects because it is known that the amount of prolyxin must be tailored to the individual needs of patients with some requiring larger or smaller amounts of medication.[120] The consent form then goes on to describe in considerable detail the psychological tests that would be administered to the patient-subject during the study period. That aspect of the research could have been presented in a more abbreviated fashion and surely, in light of other omissions, did not deserve the space it was given.

The goal of the Program is to assist persons in making a successful adaptation to life in the community and to improve their daily living and social skills. An equally important goal is to facilitate the family's coping skills for dealing with mental illness. Where appropriate, consultation with other community agencies and social support networks is provided.

. . . .

AFTERCARE CLINIC

A range of outpatient services are offered through the Aftercare Clinic at the UCLA Neuropsychiatric Institute. Following discharge, patients and their families are provided:

    Group Therapy: in small groups, patients learn problem-solving skills and interpersonal effectiveness.

    Family Education: counseling is aimed to upgrade the entire family's coping skills and understanding of the illness, and to facilitate use of resources both within the family and the community.

    Medication is administered at the lowest optimal dose to maximize coping with symptoms and stressors and to minimize side effects.

. . . .

PARTICIPATION

. . . is voluntary by patients and families in both the research and the clinical services. It is expected that a voluntary agreement to participate for a minimum of two years be made at the point a patient joins the Program.

UCLA Neuropsychiatric Institute, Continuing Care Program of the Mental Health Clinical Center 1-3 (on file with author). Since the Aftercare program serves dual objectives, treatment and research, any experimental interventions needed to be specified and differentiated from therapy with the greatest of care, particularly whenever the research component compromised therapeutic intentions.

120. *See* PHYSICIANS' DESK REFERENCE 619 (47th ed. 1993) ("Appropriate dosage of Prolyxin Decanoate (Fluphenazine Decanoate Injection) should be individualized for each patient. . . . The optimal amount of the drug and the frequency of administration must be determined for each patient, since dosage requirements have been found to vary with clinical circumstances as well as with individual response to the drug."); TEXTBOOK OF NEUROPSYCHIATRY 682 (Stuart C. Yudosky & Robert E. Hales eds., 2d ed. 1991) ("Blood levels vary widely in different patients given the same dose of a neuroleptic. . . . [T]here is no established correlation between serum concentration and clinical response."); Robert F. Asarnow & Stephen R. Marder, *Differential Effect of Low and Conventional Doses of Fluphenazine on Schizophrenic Outpatients with Good or Poor Information-Processing Abilities*, 45 ARCHIVE GEN. PSYCHIATRY 822 (1988).

46   *SAINT LOUIS UNIVERSITY LAW JOURNAL*   [Vol. 38:7

With respect to significant risks and benefits the following information was provided:

> I understand that during blood drawing, I may experience pain from the needle prick, a small amount of bleeding, infection or black and blue marks at the site of the needle mark which will disappear in about 10 days.
>
> I understand that because of the withdrawal of active medication, I may become worse during this study and that either a relapse of my initial symptoms or new symptoms may occur. I understand that I will not be charged for the active medication or the placebo that I am provided during this study. If I do show a significant return of symptoms, I understand the clinic staff will use active medication again to improve my condition. If I would require hospitalization during this study, although this is not likely, I understand that the clinic staff would help to arrange an appropriate hospitalization but the research project would not pay for the hospitalization.
>
> I understand that I may benefit from this study by being taken off medication in a careful way while under close medical supervision. The potential benefits to science in this study are that it will increase my doctor's knowledge of the relationship between the medication, its effect on people such as myself, and on the way the brain functions in certain forms of mental illness.
>
> I understand that my condition may improve, worsen or remain unchanged from participation in this study.[121]

No information was provided as to what constituted a "significant return of symptoms," that it could mean a return of hallucinations, conceptual disorganization, self-neglect, depressive mood, or suicidal ideation. Potential patient-subjects under the care of mental health professionals in an Aftercare Clinic might very well have believed that "significant" did not encompass such dire consequences. Moreover, while it was acknowledged that "I *may* become worse," the consent form of July 1988 did not state that at that time it was known that of those patient-subjects enrolled in the study so far, eighty-eight percent had suffered a relapse.[122]

In light of the high relapse rate it was misleading to aver "that my condition *may* improve, worsen or remain unchanged." The odds favoring

---

121. Consent Agreement 1, *supra* note 117, at 2.

122. Of the 24 patients who entered the drug withdrawal period, 21 have ultimately had psychotic exacerbations or relapses, ranging from 17 to 123 weeks after the last fluphenazine administration. For these 21 exacerbation/relapses plus the 3 psychotic exacerbations during the placebo phase of the crossover, the mean time to exacerbation/relapse is 33 weeks. Of these 24 patients who have developed an exacerbation/relapse after medication discontinuation, 5 exacerbation/relapses occurred after 60 or more weeks (21%), 6 after 40-59 weeks (25%), 7 after 20-39 weeks (29%), 4 after 10-19 weeks (17%), and 2 after less than 10 weeks (8%). Three more remain well after 104, 30 and 23 weeks. Keith H. Nuechterlein, Grant Application: Developmental Processes in Schizophrenic Disorders, RD 1 MH 37705-07, 1, 84 (Nov. 15, 1988) (on file with author).

relapse were far too great; few subjects would "improve" or "remain the same." Finally, it is not only ironic but also misleading that the risks of a needle prick were discussed in such exquisite detail. Such a forthcoming and honest acknowledgement could only leave patient-subjects with the impression that the investigators would disclose any other risks in similar detail and with similar candor.

The informed consent form should have highlighted in bold face that the primary objective of the study was to advance knowledge for the sake of future patients and, depending on outcome, only of value to some of the subjects' future well-being. The form, further, should have acknowledged that the study was not designed to attend to their *individual* therapeutic needs, and that the subjects exposed themselves to considerable risks. Moreover, the patient-subjects were not presented with any information about the merits of not joining the research project. They were deprived of considering that alternative. To be sure, the informed consent form must be supplemented by the oral informed consent process[123] and the latter may be more important than the former in providing patient-subjects with meaningful disclosures, particularly since the forms are generally written in such incomprehensible language. When, however, as in this instance, the written document provided incomplete information, and with insufficient candor, patient-subjects who are intent on reading it are deprived of crucial information. From a different perspective, the consent form, as written, cannot help but create concerns, though most difficult to substantiate, as to whether the oral informed consent was similarly flawed.[124]

---

123. UCLA claims to have presented much of the information required for informed consent to patient-subject's orally. Department of Health and Human Services (DHHS) regulations at 45 C.F.R. § 46.117 require, however, that the elements of legally effective Informed Consent (specified at 45 C.F.R. § 46.116 (1992)) be embodied in the *written* Informed Consent Document.

124. The special care that, I believe, must be given to the informed consent process whenever the research-therapy distinction, *see supra* text accompanying footnotes 19-34, is in danger of being compromised, is illustrated by a comment made by my respected colleague and friend Robert J. Levine who read an earlier draft of this paper:

> My perception of the investigators' motivation continues to be very different from yours. I see this as an instance of opportunistic research. The physician-investigators did not expose subjects to the risks of withdrawal from medication in order to do research. Rather, in the light of their reading of the results of observations published by others, they decided that it would be in the medical interests of these patients to have their medications withdrawn. Although they knew that some of them would develop symptoms, they could not predict which. What they planned to do was to keep a careful record of their observations of those who developed symptoms. They further made plans to remove patients from the study and treat them if certain specific criteria were met.

Letter from Robert J. Levine to Jay Katz (Sept. 24, 1993) (quoted by permission). Viewing the "motivation" of the investigators as "opportunistic research" in the service of the "medical interests of these patients" co-joins therapy and research. In the UCLA study the patient-subjects' medical interests were subordinated to the inflexibility of the research design. *See supra* text

After complaints about the study had come to OPRR's attention[125] and it had discussed the problem with UCLA, a letter from OPRR detailed "the agreed-upon actions" which UCLA would now take:

> [P]rovide (a) more detailed information regarding the risks associated with lengthy withdrawal of antipsychotic medication, including information regarding the likely rates of exacerbation or relapse and the consequences thereof; (b) an indication that, in the event of such exacerbation or relapse, it is likely that antipsychotic medication will need to be resumed; (c) a description of the risks associated with continued fixed dose medication treatment; and (d) a disclosure of alternative courses of treatment . . . .[126]
>
> . . . .
>
> The Continuing Care Brochure will be modified to ensure that it accurately reflects the parameters of the After Care Program's research protocols.[127]

In addition, OPRR required the following additional actions:

> (1) No new subjects should be enrolled in this research until the revised Informed Consent Documents have been reviewed and approved by the UCLA

---

accompanying notes 56-59. It is this fact that needed to be highlighted in the consent form, notwithstanding any accompanying therapeutic motivations of the investigators. Viewing research also as treatment, *see supra* text accompanying footnotes 28-34, invites confusion in the minds of all participants as to who they are: physicians or investigators, patients or subjects. In turn, it makes it easier for investigators to take license because of their "benevolent therapeutic intentions." Furthermore, the "specific criteria [for removal from the study]" noted by Levine included relapse to the severest level of psychosis, an unacceptable criterion for clinical practice. Long before that point is reached psychiatrists would urge their patients to resume taking medication. Thus, I would argue that the physician-investigators' conduct was motivated by their research interest, even though they might eventually also bestow benefits on their subjects or future patients. If I am correct, then the patient-subjects' medical interests are in this instance different from, and should not be conflated with, the investigators' research interests.

125. The complaint was lodged by Bob and Gloria Aller, parents of one of the subjects. The story of Greg's participation in, and gradual deterioration during, the study is graphically described in a recent article: Eventually, he not only dropped out of college, but also

> took out a carving knife, walked to the door of his mother's kitchen, [and thinking that] "my mom was possessed by the devil," . . . "[m]y plan was to scare the devil out of her literally." The Allers began barricading their bedroom door at night. [A few days later] he moved out, [and when he saw Nuechterlein's partner, Dr. Michael Gitlin, Greg kept this information from him, and thus Gitlin] noted "Moved out from parents. Says no symptoms present. Finishing the semester."

James Willwerth, *Tinkering with Madness*, 42 TIME 41-42 (Aug. 30, 1992). It took five more months, and the article describes what happened during that interval, before he was remedicated at UCLA. *Id.*

126. Letter from J. Thomas Puglisi, Acting Chief, Compliance Oversight Branch of the Office for Protection from Research Risks (OPRR) to Richard Sisson, Senior Vice Chancellor of Academic Affairs at the University of California Los Angeles 1 (Aug. 19, 1992) (on file with author).

127. *Id.* at 2.

Institutional Review Board (IRB).

(2) The revised IRB-approved Informed Consent Documents should be used to obtain renewed consent from all subjects currently participating in this research, including subjects for whom clinical monitoring constitutes the only research involvement.

(3) Copies of the revised IRB-approved Informed Consent Documents and of the revised Continuing Care Brochure should be forwarded to OPRR as soon as possible.

(4) UCLA should consider, and OPRR strongly recommends, contacting former research subjects in writing to provide them with the additional information included in the revised Informed Consent Documents. Copies of such communications with former subjects should be forwarded to OPRR as soon as they become available.[128]

OPRR did not insist that UCLA stop the research project immediately, or at least, that the patient-subjects be examined by independent psychiatrists in order to assess their individual treatment needs. In light of what already had transpired, such an opportunity would have made it easier for patient-subjects to decide whether they wished to continue in, or withdraw from, the study. Moreover, in light of the serious deficiencies in the informed consent form,[129] which is one of the prime responsibilities of IRBs to review,[130] OPRR did not institute a thorough investigation of the practices of UCLA's IRB. OPRR's evaluation was sufficiently critical of the IRB process to suggest that the IRB's review of other research proposals may be similarly flawed.[131] Undertaking such an investigation was even more pressing in this case since several subject-patients suffered severe schizophrenic relapses,[132] and one young man allegedly committed suicide.[133]

---

128. *Id.*

129. Even after modifying the consent forms initially used, UCLA continues to deny any wrongdoing and contends that the forms and process used to obtain initial consent were appropriate. *See* Letter from Richard Sisson, Senior Vice Chancellor of Academic Affairs at the University of California Los Angeles to J. Thomas Puglisi, Acting Chief, Compliance Oversight Branch of the OPRR 4-5 (Sept. 17, 1992) (on file with author).

130. Federal Regulations instruct IRBs to "determine that all of the following requirements are satisfied: . . . (4) Informed consent will be sought from each prospective subject . . . in accordance with, and to the extent required by § 46.117." 45 C.F.R. § 46.111(4) (1992).

131. The copy of the letter from OPRR to UCLA, made available to me through the Freedom of Information Act, excluded three paragraphs. They may have contained additional criticisms of UCLA's conduct in this case. See *supra* note 126.

132. Subotnik & Nuechterlein, *supra* note 102.

133. One participant in the UCLA project committed suicide on March 28, 1992, after being taken off psychotropic medication. Sandy Rovner, *Ethics Concerns Raised in Schizophrenia Study*, WASH. POST, Sept. 29, 1992, at H7. The Federal Regulations require that "[w]here appropriate, the research plan makes adequate provision for monitoring the data collected to insure the safety of subjects." 45 C.F.R. § 46.111(6) (1992). The protocol, however, did not describe in sufficient detail the special monitoring that would be provided, even though some of

50   *SAINT LOUIS UNIVERSITY LAW JOURNAL*   [Vol. 38:7

The revised informed consent form, while an improvement over the previous one, continues to leave patient-subjects uninformed, *inter alia*, about the *specific* severity of relapse which they might suffer, mentioning only "difficulties in relationship with others and problems with work or school"; or what specific "psychotic symptoms or severe symptoms" will lead to providing medication once again. It does not present in any meaningful detail the advantages and disadvantages of participating in the study or receiving customary treatment for their condition. The consent form did not state with sufficient clarity that the primary objective of the study was to conduct research for the sake of future patients, perhaps of benefit to those enrolled in this study *in the future*, and that it was not therapy for the subject's individual *present* needs. While the consent form now admits that "70-80% of patients who have entered this study in the past have experienced a psychotic exacerbation or relapse within one year" and that "I may become worse during the study," it says nothing about what subjects specifically should consider, and reflect on, before exposing themselves to these risks. On the other hand, with respect to benefits it is noted that withdrawal of medication will keep them from "developing tardive dyskinesia which involves abnormal movements of the face, hands, legs or trunk." And the form goes on to emphasize, "I may benefit from this study by being taken off medication in a careful way while under close medical supervision."[134] The risks deserved at least similar detailed explication and prominence.

What transpired in this study is not unique to UCLA; it is symptomatic of the flawed nature of current regulations and current practices protecting the human rights of research subjects. These flaws, as I have argued throughout this article, extend from the Federal Regulations themselves[135] to the supervision of projects by IRBs and OPRR. Thus, my analysis of UCLA's consent form should not be taken merely as a critique of the nature and depth

---

the research subjects could suffer a severe relapse. The protocol only stated that "a member of the clinic staff will meet regularly as needed" with the patient. See *supra* note 102.

134. Keith Nuechterlein, Informed Consent Agreement for Patients: Double-Blind Drug Crossover and Withdrawal Project 3 (Sept. 1992) (on file with author).

135. Shamoo and Irving recently noted that recommendations by various Federal Commissions to consider persons with mental illness as members of a vulnerable group who deserve special protection whenever they participate in research were not implemented. They learned that "[this] outcome was the result in large part of opposition from researchers on mental disorders who claimed that the population in question were no more vulnerable than most persons with severe medical disorders and that the suggested limitations would seriously restrict research on mental disorders." Shamoo and Irving concluded that "the issue of using persons with mental illness as human research subjects has been lost in the shuffle, due in part to the lobbying effort of some researchers on mental disorders." They also raise the important question, "what was the justification for delegating to local IRBs the essential responsibilities for affording protections for persons with mental illness ... ?" Adil E. Shamoo & Dianne N. Irving, *Accountability in Research Using Persons With Mental Illness* 1, 2 (1994) (forthcoming article, on file with author).

of the information that was or was not included in the written document, but, more importantly, as a critique of the entire informed consent process. The problems with this study, as with many others, are: (1) subject-patients' consent was manipulated; (2) trivial and non-trivial risks were insufficiently distinguished; (3) the severity of predictable risks was not highlighted nor was the incidence of their likelihood disclosed; and (4) the risks and benefits of non-participation were neither sufficiently disclosed nor satisfactorily discussed. Under these circumstances, patient-subjects were not offered a meaningful choice whether or not to participate in the study.[136]

IX. CONCLUSION

The history of experimentation with human beings testifies to physician-scientists' real and caring dedication to the alleviation of mankind's pain and suffering from the ravages of disease. It also testifies to the carelessness with which human beings have been recruited for participation in research, a carelessness that has been too readily obscured by the caring dimension of scientists' work. My colleague, the late Robert Cover, when writing about judicial sentencing reminded us that "judges deal pain and death."[137] He went on to say that "persons [he meant judges but he could have said the same about physician-scientists as well] act within social organizations that exercise authority violently without experiencing . . . the normal degree or inhibition which regulates the behavior of those who act autonomously."[138]

If informed consent is to fulfill its promise of protecting the rights of research subjects to autonomy and self-determination, we must ponder Hans Jonas' challenge:

> Let us not forget that progress is an optional goal, not an uncompromising commitment. [A] slower progress in the conquest of disease would not threaten society, grievous as it is to those who have to deplore that their particular disease be not yet conquered, but that society would indeed be threatened by the erosion of those moral values whose loss possibly caused by too ruthless a pursuit of scientific progress, would make its most dazzling triumphs not worth having.[139]

Jonas is concerned about the erosion of medicine's and society's moral integrity resulting from violations of the dignity of research subjects.

Some advances in medicine might have been slower in coming had physician-investigators pursued their clinical research less aggressively by not engineering consent. Would delay have been a price worth paying, even

---

136. See *supra* notes 32-34 and accompanying text.

137. Robert Cover, *Violence and the Word*, 95 YALE L.J. 1609 (1986).

138. *Id.* at 1615.

139. Hans Jonas, *Philosophical Reflections on Experimenting with Human Subjects*, 98 DAEDALUS 219, 245 (1969).

52   *SAINT LOUIS UNIVERSITY LAW JOURNAL*   [Vol. 38:7

though the suffering of future patients might have remained for a while longer without relief? Or is medical progress not an optional goal but one to which individual autonomy and self-determination must yield? Answers to these questions ultimately depend on one's vision of the future and the price our generation is willing to pay for the sake of medical progress at the expense of respect for the persons who are asked to make progress possible.

While in this article my personal views on these questions clearly emerge, my purpose in writing it has been less to advocate their implementation and more to draw attention to the fact that in the pursuit of scientific progress we have largely paid lip service to the subjects' rights to be fully informed. In setting forth the nature and quality of the conversations between physician-investigators and their patient-subjects, I wanted to highlight the wide chasm that separates contemporary rhetoric from practices in implementing human subjects' rights to make their own decisions about serving as means for others' ends.

In juxtaposing in the title of this article human rights and human experimentation, I appreciate that the contours of such rights are still ill-defined. The idea that human beings possess rights to inviolate dignity is of recent origin and in need of more precise construction and surely in need of a deeper commitment. However, it is an idea that since World War II has begun to capture the imagination of the world community, as attested by the many United Nations' resolutions on human rights.[140]

It is also an idea, in language of constitutional rights, that has captured the imagination of some of the Justices of the United States Supreme Court. In 1987, the Court was faced with the question of whether the constitutional rights of James Stanley, an army serviceman, were violated when in 1958, without his knowledge, LSD was administered to him in an army experiment to study the effects of this drug on human beings.[141] Stanley had sued the government under the Federal Tort Claims Act. The Court split five to four, and Justice Scalia, writing for the majority, concluded in a highly technical opinion that to allow Stanley to sue the army successfully would be a judicial intrusion upon military matters that "would call into question military discipline and decision making."[142] Justices O'Connor and Brennan wrote separate dissenting opinions, joined by Justice Marshall and, in part, by Justice Stevens. Justice Brennan began by arguing that the Court was wrong in holding

> that the Constitution provides him with no remedy, solely because his injuries were inflicted while he performed his duties in the Nation's Armed Forces.

---

140. See *supra* note 44 and accompanying text.

141. United States v. Stanley, 483 U.S. 669 (1987). For a more extended discussion of *Stanley*, see George J. Annas, *The Nuremberg Code in U.S. Courts: Ethics versus Expediency, in* THE NAZI DOCTORS AND THE NUREMBERG CODE, *supra* note 2, at 212-15.

142. *Stanley*, 483 U.S. at 682.

If our Constitution required this result, the Court's decision, though legally necessary, would expose a tragic flaw in that document. But in reality, the Court disregards the commands of our Constitution, and bows instead to the purported requirements of a different master, *military discipline*, declining to provide Stanley with a remedy because it finds "special factors counselling hesitation."[143]

He concluded his opinion with these words:

The subject of experimentation who has not volunteered is treated as an object, a sample. James Stanley will receive no compensation for this indignity. A test providing absolute immunity for intentional constitutional torts *only* when such immunity was essential to maintenance of military discipline would "take into account the special importance of defending our Nation without completely abandoning the freedoms that make it worth defending." But absent a showing that military discipline is concretely (not abstractly) implicated by Stanley's action, its talismanic invocation does not counsel hesitation in the face of an intentional constitutional tort, such as the Government's experimentation on an unknowing human subject. Soldiers ought not be asked *to defend a Constitution indifferent to their essential human dignity.*[144]

In a different context, my former colleague Charles L. Black, Jr. has eloquently advanced the proposition that our Constitution guarantees United States citizens universal human rights which can be asserted against the fifty local state governments. He found such guarantees in the Declaration of Independence, the Ninth Amendment, and the Privileges and Immunity Clause of the Fourteenth Amendment.[145] What particularly caught my eye were the concluding paragraphs of his article:

I want to add a word about the intentions and hopes that have guided the writing of this paper. First of all, it has seemed not to be generally understood that an amply developed human-rights system, good against the States, is absolutely essential to the moral unity and integrity of the whole nation. This is a thing so obvious that one ought not to have to write about it at all. But much exposure to public discourse has brought home to me that it does need to be written about. As many citizens as possible should be brought to realize that without such a corpus of national human rights law good against the States, we ought to stop saying, "One nation indivisible, with liberty and justice for all," and speak instead of, "One nation divisible and divided into fifty zones of political morality, with liberty and justice in such kind and measure as these good things may from time to time be granted by these fifty

---

143. *Id.* at 686.

144. *Id.* at 708 (quoting Goldman v. Weinberger, 475 U.S. 503, 530-532 (1986) (O'Connor, J., dissenting)).

145. Charles L. Black, Jr., *"One Nation Indivisible"; Unnamed Human Rights in the States,* 65 St. John's L. Rev. 17, 25 (1991).

54   *SAINT LOUIS UNIVERSITY LAW JOURNAL*   [Vol. 38:7

political subdivisions."[146]

The time may eventually come when violations of human rights, as in *Stanley*, will be afforded constitutional protection. Perhaps the recent revelations about radiation experiments conducted during the 1940s and 1950s with retarded boys, newborn infants, pregnant women, prisoners and hospitalized patients, more often than not without full disclosure and consent,[147] will lead to regulations of research which comport better with the human rights of subjects of research. This will only happen, however, if it is recognized that safeguarding such rights requires not only protection from physical harm but also, and equally important, a commitment to using human beings as means for our ends only with their voluntary consent.[148] Justice O'Connor put it well in *Stanley*: "I am prepared to say that our Constitution's promise of due process of law guarantees this much."[149] The dissenting Justices in *Stanley* and Charles Black point medicine in the right direction. In writing this article I wanted to add my voice to theirs by arguing that the caring dimension of medicine also requires taking most seriously the idea that research subjects possess human rights that are inviolate.

146. *Id.* at 55.
147. *See* Gary Lee, *U.S. Should Pay Victims, O'Leary Says 800 Were Deliberately Exposed to Radiation, Energy Chief Reveals*, WASH. POST, Dec. 29, 1993, at A1; Melissa Healy, *Payments Urged for Radiation Test Victims*, L.A. TIMES, Dec. 29, 1993, at A1; David Armstrong, *State Expects Further 1940s-50s Revelations*, BOSTON GLOBE, Dec. 29, 1993, at § 3, p.1; Associated Press, *Irradiated Deserve Aid, Energy Says*, CHICAGO TRIBUNE, Dec. 28, 1993, at 1.
148. Any new Presidential Commission or Ethics Advisory Board should also have the *authority* to formulate research policies that seek to resolve the inevitable tensions between the inviolability of subjects of research and the claims of science and society to advance knowledge. Such a Board's proposed policies should then be subjected to a relentless public debate and eventually approved by Congress. *See supra* notes 90-101 and accompanying text. Equally important, since biomedical research will continue to open up new frontiers in its quest to advance science, will be the Board's responsibility to promulgate guidelines for the conduct of research to which IRBs must adhere. Finally, such a Board should probably not be located within the Department of Health and Human Services. If it is, its relationship to, and independence from, the Department should be clearly specified. My major contention is this: The moral tensions inherent in human research have been debated at length. We do not need a Board that provides only advice but one that will resolve these tensions as best it can and with continuing authority to do so as we come face to face with new moral dilemmas in the conduct of human research.
149. *Stanley*, 483 U.S. at 710.

[14]

THE SOCIAL CONTROL OF HUMAN BIOMEDICAL RESEARCH: AN OVERVIEW AND REVIEW OF THE LITERATURE

PAUL R. BENSON

Department of Sociology, University of Massachusetts, Boston, MA 02125, U.S.A.

Abstract—Social control mechanisms have become an important element of human medical research in the United States. At first largely intraprofessional, controls over human experimentation have moved increasingly in the direction of externally developed, bureaucratically administered, and formally sanctioned rules. This paper examines intra- and extraprofessional methods of control over biomedical science and reviews available research assessing their effectiveness in promoting researcher adherence to high ethical standards concerning the use of human subjects. Research suggests that intraprofessional controls (including medical training, peer influence, ethical codes, and disciplinary boards), are, on their own, inadequate to ensure investigator ethicality. However, studies examining external controls over biomedical research (government regulations, institutional review boards, judicial and state law), also suggest that extraprofessional regulations are often ineffective. Further study of both forms of scientific social control is needed, as well as research examining their interactive effects on investigators' ethical attitudes and practices.

Key words—biomedical research, regulation, human subjects protection, social control

INTRODUCTION

One of the most prominent features of advanced industrial society is its reliance on specialized knowledge. As knowledge has accumulated and expanded, it has become the task of specialized 'professions' to store, apply, and extend this information. Predicated upon the belief that they possess unique expertise and are oriented primarily toward the public good, occupations such as medicine, law, and science have enjoyed significant autonomy [1–4].

Despite historically high levels of public support, medicine and science have, nonetheless, experienced significant problems during the past several decades. Specialization, bureaucratization, and commercialization have increased public disenchantment with medicine and the medical profession [5–7]. Public ambivalence toward science has also risen as technological and biomedical advances have outpaced society's ability to deal with the social, economic, and ethical dilemmas flowing from these discoveries [8–10]. Periodic media exposes of scientific fraud and the misuse of humans and animals in research have also led some to question the previously assumed altruism and ethical propriety of scientific investigators [11–13]. These concerns have resulted in calls for increased governmental control over the activities of physicians and scientists [14, 15].

Biomedical research constitutes a specialized field encompassing both medicine and science and, as such, presents unique problems of governance and control. In this paper, I examine social controls used to promote ethical conduct among biomedical researchers in the United States and review available research assessing the scope and effectiveness of these mechanisms [16]. While a number of areas of ethical concern might be fruitfully explored, I focus in this paper specifically upon investigators' use of human subjects.

Defined sociologically as the process by which a group induces and maintains conformity among its members [17, 18], social control may be internally or externally imposed through both formal and informal means. In this paper, four sources of control related to the promotion of ethical behavior among biomedical scientists are investigated:

(1) professional socialization and training;
(2) informal peer influence;
(3) intraprofessional norms and sanctions (professional codes of ethics and internal disciplinary procedures); and
(4) extraprofessional norms and sanctions (government regulations, external review mechanisms; judicial and legislative law).

As Swazey [19] has observed, relatively little attention has been given to specifying and assessing control mechanisms operating within the professions. Nevertheless, available research indicates that intraprofessional controls, by themselves, cannot ensure high ethical practices among biomedical investigators. As public and legislative confidence in the ability of biomedical science to regulate itself has waned, the use of extraprofessional (governmental) controls has increased. Some critics have disputed the effectiveness of current procedures and called for even stricter government controls over biomedical research [20–25]. Others have questioned whether government regulation is an effective means of ensuring subject protection and autonomy [26–29]. Hopefully, this paper, by reviewing what is known (and not known) about the social control of biomedical research, can aid in the development of sound policy

2   PAUL R. BENSON

and advance our understanding of the changing relationship between society and the professions.

INTRAPROFESSIONAL CONTROLS OVER BIOMEDICAL RESEARCH

Socialization and professional training

Medical education has been a major focus of sociological inquiry since the 1950s and the pioneering work of Becker *et al.* [30] and Fox [31–33]. Interestingly, the findings of these two studies differ markedly in their assessment of the effectiveness of professional training as a means of internal social control. Influenced by interactionism and sociological studies of work, Becker *et al.* stress immediate situational constraints as the primary determinants of medical students' actions. In contrast, Fox highlights the evolving self-directedness of student behavior, guided by professional values (detached concern, tolerance for uncertainty, and functional specificity) internalized during medical school training.

Despite Fox's emphasis on the internalization of physician ethicality through professional training, most sociological studies suggest that physicians are inadequately socialized in humanistic and ethical elements of patient care. Instead, empirical studies of undergraduate and advanced specialty training [34–40] indicate that medical education tends to produce physicians whose orientation is largely 'disease oriented' rather than 'patient oriented'. Speaking of British medical education in a manner highly applicable to its American counterpart, Meadow [41] has observed that:

... [V]ery many medical students are striving towards a sort of medicine that rarely exists—the isolated disease as a course of symptoms, illness always being associated with physical signs and acute problems uncomplicated by social and emotional factors.

Atkinson [42] has similarly suggested that Western medical education is geared toward 'training for certainty', based on clinical experience and an overly reductionistic view of biomedical science. As Maddison [43] has noted, such an orientation can be associated with 'massive disillusionment' decreased humanism, and increased cynicism on the part of physicians-in-training [44]. Thus in her study of undergraduate medical training, Carlton [45] concludes that students are "socialized into using the clinical perspective to resolve clinical problems with little or no regard for the ethical aspects of their professional behavior". Similarly, Mizrahi [40], in her study of internal medicine residents, found that primary emphasis was placed on the intellectual process of disease diagnosis rather than on patient care. In addition, Mizrahi found the residents she observed often learned to cope with problematic patients by dehumanizing them as 'gomers', 'dirtballs', and 'gorks' [46, 47].

Despite the strong biomedical orientation of contemporary medical education, the teaching of behavioral science and the medical humanities (including medical ethics) has become common in medical schools in the U.S. [48, 49]. While these courses vary greatly in their content, curriculum, pedagogical style, and timing [50, 51] most touch (at least briefly)

upon issues relating to research ethics. Unfortunately, very little is known about the effects of these courses upon the attitudes and behavior of student physicians [52, 53].

The professional socialization of physician-scientists differs significantly from that experienced by full-time clinicians. As such, it might be expected that the unique training of novice researchers would influence their subsequent ethical views and practices. Nonetheless, little research on the ethical socialization of biomedical scientists has been conducted. One exception is the work of Barber *et al.* [54], undertaken during the late 1960s. As part of a larger investigation of ethical controls in human experimentation, Barber and his co-workers interviewed 370 physician-investigators at two major U.S. research institutions. Respondents were asked to discuss when and how they had been made aware of ethical issues associated with biomedical research. Fifty-nine percent of the investigators interviewed reported experiences during their internship or residency that had sensitized them to research ethics in some new way. The bulk of these experiences stemmed from trainees' direct involvement in human experimentation as apprentice researchers. Ethical socialization was indirect, informal and largely unintended; none reported taking formal courses in medical ethics during their advanced training and only 6% reported that they had become more aware of ethical issues as the result of concerns raised directly by their teachers or mentors. Instead, respondents' heightened ethical sensitivity resulted, in some cases, from experiences where, as trainees, they had been asked by superiors to assist in research they believed to be ethically quesionable [55].

Sociologists have largely assumed that science operates on the basis of widely held moral norms: universalism, disinterestedness, organized skepticism, and communality [56–58]. Case studies of scientific activity, however, have indicated that these ideals are frequently not upheld in practice and that more pedestrian concerns, including status attainment and careerism, are commonplace [59–61]. It is well known that engaging in important research, obtaining grants, and publishing in top scientific journals are the keys to career advancement in science, especially for young investigators. Science is highly competitive and pressures to 'publish or perish' may promote deviant and unethical behavior on the part of some researchers [62, 63]. Barber *et al.* [54], for example, suggest that young scientists are routinely socialized to give unquestioned priority to their research activities, both as a means to advance knowledge and to promote their own careers. As research considerations gain ascendency, other issues, including ethical concerns for the protection of subjects, correspondingly decrease in importance.

Informal collegial control

Socialization promotes conformity through the internalization of group norms. However, as Barber notes, informal collegial (peer) influence is the first line of defense against overt deviant behavior:

These ... mechanisms ... occur in everyday, routine, working relationships among colleagues ... Sometimes by a

The social control of human biomedical research 3

word, sometimes in lengthier, more serious discussions, colleagues can set one another straight when they think they have violated some norms or are uncertain how to proceed in novel situations [64].

Freidson [65] has provided an extended analysis of informal collegial control in everyday medical practice. Examining a comprehensive prepaid medical group "deliberately set up to be as close as possible to the ideal of liberal medical reformers" [65, p. 14], Freidson uncovered scant evidence that physicians exert effective informal influence over one another's professional behavior. Physicians knew little about the clinical performance of their colleagues and acceptable standards of practice varied widely among individual group members. In addition, adherence to rules of professional etiquette discouraged physicians from critically assessing one another's activities. As a result, only the most severe professional deviations were collectively recognized and acted upon. Summarizing his findings, Freidson characterized the physicians he studied as a 'delinquent community', more concerned with defending their professional sovereignty than with promoting high standards of practice through collective self-regulation.

Employing sociometric data, Barber *et al.* [54] examined the impact of collegial influence on the ethical views and practices of their sample of 370 physician-investigators. Since 81% of the 424 medical studies conducted by Barber's respondents were collaborative in nature, collegial influence would appear to be a potentially important means of assuring ethical use of study subjects. However, when asked what characteristics they employed in selecting research collaborators, most investigators noted 'scientific ability' (86%), 'motivation to work hard' (45%), and 'intellectual honesty' (32%); few (6%) mentioned 'ethical concern for research subjects' as a relevant consideration. Investigators in the Barber *et al.* study also tended to enter into collaborative relationships with colleagues holding ethical positions similar to their own. Finally, senior investigators seldom provided effective supervision in projects on which they were collaborators. These results suggest that peer influence, in and of itself, is a largely ineffectual means of promoting and maintaining high ethical standards among biomedical researchers [66].

Codes of ethics and disciplinary procedures

Effective self-regulation (or at least its appearance) lies at the heart of any occupation's claim to professional status and sovereignty. As such, the ability of medicine and biomedical science to govern their own affairs through organized systems of control and discipline is an important indicator of their success as autonomous professional entities.

One important means by which professions attempt to regulate themselves is through the establishment of formal codes of ethical behavior. As Gass [67] has noted, the ethical codes of many (though not all) professional medical organizations are quite general, exhorting practitioners:

... to preserve human, to be good citizens, to prevent exploitation of patients, to promote the highest quality health care available, to perform their duties with objectivity and accuracy, to strive for professional excellence through

continuing education, to avoid discriminatory practices, to promote the highest ideals of the profession, to expose unethical or incompetent colleagues, to encourage public health through health-care education, to render service in times of public emergencies, to promote harmonious relations with other health care professions and to protect the welfare, dignity, and confidentiality of patients.

The most prominent professional organization in the U.S. with a formal code of medical ethics is the American Medical Association (AMA). Developed in 1847, the AMA Code of Ethics has undergone a number of major revisions. Beginning as a document of some 5600 words, by 1980, the code had evolved into a terse, 250-word statement expressing general ethical ideals such as compassion, respect for human dignity, skilled medical performance, obedience to law, advancement of scientific knowledge, free exercise of skills, and responsibility to patients, peers, and community [68]. The 'Principles of Medical Ethics' (as the code is now known), is periodically supplemented by a detailed set of interpretive 'Current Opinions' rendered by the AMA Council on Ethical and Judicial Affairs. The most recent of these 'Opinions' (published in 1986) includes the Council's views on a wide variety of subjects, including clinical investigation [69].

In some cases, codes of ethics are accompanied by formalized disciplinary procedures designed to enforce the code and discipline violators through censure, suspension, or in cases of especially heinous misconduct, expulsion from the professional organization. While imposition of these sanctions may prove detrimental to a practitioner's reputation (and thus indirectly to his or her career), rarely do they directly affect the offenders' right to practice. Few professional associations report code violations to their membership or to the public and none allow public access to disciplinary committee proceedings or deliberations. Due to the nonpublic character of their proceedings, very little is known about the disciplinary actions of professional organizations in medicine. However, available research indicates that intraprofessional disciplinary mechanisms are largely ineffective in policing physician misconduct [70].

Within organized medicine, the ethics committees of the American Psychiatric Association (APA) have probably been subjected to the greatest empirical scrutiny. Zitrin and Klein [71] investigated the performance of an ethics committee affiliated with an APA district branch and concluded that lack of funds and time, as well as the use of peers to judge alleged misconduct, made unbiased and thorough evaluations of complaints difficult. In addition, Zitrin and Klein noted committee reluctance to widen its investigations by referring complaints to state licensing bodies and other external regulatory agencies. In two additional studies, Moore [72, 73] examined the activities of all APA district ethics committees from 1950 to 1983, using compliant records filed by local committees with the association's central office. From 1950 to 1973, only 82 charges of unethical conduct were made against APA members; of these, 12 (15%) were found guilty of unethical conduct and six were expelled. A significant increase in ethics committee activity, however, was noted between 1974 and 1983, when 366 APA members were charged with unethical conduct. Of these, 86 (23%) were found guilty and 27 expelled. Marked variation was found in the levels of activity and findings of local disciplinary committees. Charges most frequently addressed by ethics committees involved patient exploitation (primarily sexual) and illegal conduct (primarily billing fraud); very few cases involved allegedly unethical research practices.

Within the American Medical Association, disciplinary cases are heard first at the district or state level. They may then be appealed to the Ethics and Judicial Council. No records of local or state disciplinary actions are maintained by the AMA, thus it is difficult to know the extent of disciplinary activity engaged in by county and state medical societies. No cases concerning alleged research misconduct have been addressed at the national level by the AMA during at least the past 20 years [74].

Finally, formal ethical standards promulgated by international medical and biomedical research organizations have also influenced the attitudes and activities of clinical investigators. The Nuremberg Code (1947) and the Helsinki Declaration of the World Medical Association (1964, revised in 1975 and 1983) are the most prominent of these ethical documents. They have been analyzed at length in other publications [12, 16, 75] and their content need not be detailed here. It is important to understand, however, that international ethical codes have no independent legal standing or enforcement provisions. Nevertheless, they often exert a major influence on bioethical thinking and on the development of enforceable national laws and regulations.

EXTRAPROFESSIONAL CONTROLS OVER BIOMEDICAL RESEARCH

The emergence of external controls in the United States

In the generation following World War 2, a series of untoward events prompted government officials in the United States to begin to question the long-held belief that researchers should be allowed to engage in human experimentation without external oversight. The horrors of Nazi 'medical research' on concentration camp inmates sensitized many to the potential for abuse in human subjects research, leading to worldwide concern and the development of the Nuremberg Code and other ethical declarations [76].

In 1962 the U.S. Congress passed the Kefauver–Harris amendments to the 1938 Food, Drug, and Cosmetic Act. Enacted largely in response to the Thalidomide tragedy, the amendments stiffened federal safety and efficacy requirements for the marketing of new medications. The amendments also required that pharmaceutical companies submit detailed statements to the U.S. Food and Drug Administration (FDA) outlining drug testing methods, investigator qualifications, and procedures used to secure test subjects' informed consent. The mandate concerning informed consent was added by Congress because no state at the time legally stipulated that physicians inform their patients when they were receiving an experimental drug [77].

In 1964 public attention was drawn to the Jewish Chronic Disease Hospital in New York where two physicians were charged with injecting live cancer cells into 22 elderly patients as part of a study partially funded by the National Institute of Health (NIH) [12]. Nor did it appear that this case was a totally isolated incident. In a 1966 article in the *New England Journal of Medicine*, Harvard University Professor, Henry K. Beecher, reviewed 22 cases of biomedical researcher containing serious ethical violations [78]. The 22 cases were taken from a larger pool of 50 ethically questionable studies collected by Beecher from leading American medical journals [79].

These events became even more troubling to federal officials when contrasted to the seeming complacency of biomedical research institutions. In a survey commissioned in 1962 by NIH and conducted by the Law-Medicine Research Institute of Boston University, 52 university departments of medicine responded to questionnaires assessing their use of procedural guidelines governing clinical research [80]. The survey indicated that few institutions had developed explicit research guidelines. Indeed, departments of medicine frequently objected to any form of institutional oversight, preferring instead to leave all aspects of the research, including its ethical elements, to investigators themselves.

By the mid 1960s, the accumulated weight of these findings had succeeded in convincing federal officials of the need for enforceable ethical guidelines and for procedures to ensure that human subjects were protected from possible misuse. As a result, in 1966, Surgeon General William Stewart announced that prior review by a panel of 'institutional associates' would be required for the approval of extramural research supported by the U.S. Public Health Service.

Between 1966 and 1981, federal research regulations were strengthened through a series of revisions. These modifications were prompted, in part, by further incidents of ethically problematic human experimentation, including the Tuskegee syphilis and Willowbrook State School studies [81]. In 1974, as a result of professional and public alarm concerning these incidents (as well as Congressional concern regarding abortion and fetal experimentation), the U.S. Congress created a major study group, the National Commission for the Protection of Human Subjects in Biomedical and Behavioral Research [82, 83]. In 1981, in response to the Commission's final recommendations, the U.S. Department of Health and Human Services [84] and the U.S. Food and Drug Administration [85] issued comprehensive research guidelines. It is under these two sets of federal regulations that most human subjects research in the United States is currently conducted [86].

The institutional review board

The cornerstone of regulatory control of human subjects research in the United States is the institutional review board or IRB. IRBs are local, institutionally sponsored panels whose purpose is to prospectively review, evaluate, and pass judgment on the ethics of proposed human subjects research. Specifically, federal regulations mandate that IRBs assess research with the aim of insuring that: (a) subjects' rights and welfare are adequately protected; (b) risks to subjects are minimized and are reasonable in relation to anticipated research benefits; and (c) subject informed consent is obtained by adequate and appropriate means. Federal regulations currently require that most federally funded biomedical research using human subjects receive IRB approval in order to proceed [87]. By 1980, over 560 research institutions in the U.S. had formally constituted IRBs reviewing human subjects research conducted under their auspices [86, app. 4.1].

IRBs constitute an innovative and distinctive method of professional control, blending elements of centralized government oversight and decentralized peer review [88]. Perhaps due to the special context in which IRBs operate, federal guidelines allow institutions great flexibility in the way review committees are designed and in the manner in which they evaluate and determine the ethical acceptability of proposed research. Both DHHS and FDA regulations require that IRBs include at least five members of varying backgrounds "able to ascertain the acceptability of research applications in terms of institutional commitments, applicable law, and professional standards" [84, p. 8388]. IRBs also cannot be composed entirely of members of either sex. In addition, federal regulations specify that review committees include at least one nonscientist and one member unaffiliated with the sponsoring institution (these two requirements may be met by the same individual).

Aside from these minimal standards, federal guidelines are silent concerning IRB size, structure, or other organizational features. Standing or *ad-hoc* IRB subcommittees are acceptable, as are multi-institutional 'supra-committees'. No minimum or maximum number of annual IRB meetings is required nor are uniform decision-making procedures (for example, whether board recommendations are arrived at by majority vote or general consensus).

The IRB system is, in sum, a decentralized system of institutionally controlled review boards. Under current regulations, local institutions retain significant discretion (within limits set by the federal government) over the structure, make-up, policies, and operations of individual IRBs. The broad discretionary power granted to institutions by federal guidelines is rooted in the belief that local review committees are best equipped to evaluate the ethics of research to be undertaken in that community. Despite this philosophy, empirical research on IRBs has raised a number of questions concerning the equity, efficiency, and efficacy of decision-making by local boards.

Empirical studies of IRBs

Despite their importance, surprisingly little research has been undertaken on IRBs. In addition, the two most extensive IRB studies completed to date were conducted over a decade ago. Nevertheless, these early studies offer an useful historical overview of IRB development and a glimpse at the system's continuing problems.

In 1969 Barber *et al.* [54] examined the activities of a national sample of IRBs associated with bio-medical research institutions. By that time, review committees were in place in nearly all surveyed institutions. Nonetheless, evidence gathered by the Barber group indicated that a significant amount of research never received IRB review. Furthermore, findings suggested that IRBs frequently had little impact on research proposals they did review. Of the 293 IRBs surveyed, 34% responded that they had *never* modified or rejected a research proposal (or had a proposal withdrawn in anticipation of IRB rejection).

A second major survey of IRBs was conducted in 1975 by the National Commission for the Protection of Subjects in Biomedical and Behavioral Research [89, 90]. Seventy-three IRBs from a representative national sample of 61 research institutions (conducting biomedical *and* behavioral research) were included in the study. From these institutions, a total of 810 IRB members, 2057 research investigators, and 1000 research subjects were interviewed.

Compared to the Barber study conducted 6 years before, the National Commission noted an marked increase in IRB activity and influence. Data provided by research investigators indicated that 40% of proposals underwent some modification as the result of IRB review. Most of these modifications, however, were minor. Most frequently, proposal alterations dealt with the langue used in informed consent forms. IRB-mandated modifications concerning other aspects of informed consent (including timing of the consent, who obtained the consent, and the setting in which consent was obtained) were seldom required. Changes in other important areas, such as subject selection, research risks, scientific design, and confidentiality were also rarely ordered by surveyed IRBs.

Given the age of the Barber *et al.* and National Commission studies, it is questionable whether their findings can be applied to current IRBs. Fortunately, more recent IRB studies are available. In a 1980 investigation, Goldman and Katz [91] examined the uniformity of IRB decision-making across 22 medical school IRBs. Three hypothetical research proposals, intentionally designed to raise ethical questions, were reviewed by each IRB [92]. While these 'studies' were rarely approved by participating IRBs, substantial inconsistencies were uncovered in the standards applied and rationales offered across committees in support of their decisions. More importantly, marked *internal* inconsistencies within IRBs were also noted in their treatment of the three mock proposals [93].

Another study examining IRB functioning was carried out in 1982 by the President's Commission for the Study of Ethical Problems in Medicine and Biomedical and Behavioral Research [94]. As part of that investigation, 12 IRBs were visited and evaluated by expert inspection teams. Following each visit, team members independently assessed IRB performance on a variety of criteria. Of the 12 IRBs evaluated, reviewers expressed serious reservations about the effectiveness of four committees and less serious concerns regarding five others. Significant problems encountered by IRB inspection teams included inadequate procedures for proposal review, an unclear understanding by some IRB members of their role and responsibilities, and minimal commitment and support by some institutions to IRB activities and goals.

6   PAUL R. BENSON

In a rare ethnographic study, Sackoff-Lambert [95] spent 8 months systematically observing the meetings of an IRB affiliated with a major university medical center. She found IRB discussion of research proposals to center primarily around technical, rather than ethical, issues. Committee decision-making was largely controlled by physician-scientists who comprised the vast majority of the board. Professional dominance within the IRB was also influenced by the committee's heavy reliance on preliminary proposal reviews by 'expert' members who were invariably physician-scientists. Input by nonprofessionals on the IRB was infrequent, leading Sackoff-Lambert to conclude that lay representation on the board was largely symbolic.

Ceci, Peters, and Plotkin [96] recently conducted an interesting experimental study of decision-making by IRBs reviewing nonmedical research. As part of the experiment, 157 university IRBs reviewed one of nine hypothetical research proposals. All nine proposals were substantively identical (all purportedly planned to investigate corporate hiring practices); however, each proposal differed in its level of sociopolitical sensitivity and ethical concern. 'Sociopolitically sensitive' proposals allegedly planned to investigate hiring differences by race and sex, while 'nonsensitive' proposals indicated that they would examine differences by weight and height. 'Ethical concern' (or lack thereof) was operationalized by the proposals' varying use of deception and subject debriefing.

Findings from the experiment suggest that IRB decision-making may at times inappropriately reflect board members' personal, sociopolitical values. Ethically nonproblematic and nonsensitive proposals nearly always received IRB approval. However, only 40–50% of ethically nonproblematic, *but socially sensitive*, proposals were likewise approved. In addition, proposals were significantly less likely to be approved when they indicated that they would test hypotheses related to 'reverse discrmination' by race or sex. IRB disapproval of these proposals were frequently justified by pointing to alleged methodological deficiencies (for example, inadequate sample size), while nonsensitive proposals rarely received such criticism. No study has yet attempted to replicate these disturbing findings employing IRBs reviewing biomedical research.

Lastly, several studies have assessed the economic costs of IRB review. The monetary issue is particularly of concern to research institutions in that the government makes no provision for the financial support of federally-mandated IRBs. One study, conducted in the late 1970s, examined annual IRB-related costs at the University of Texas Health Science Center in San Antonio [97]. Approximately 850 new or renewal applications were evaluated yearly by the IRB at the cost of $100,000 or about $100 per application. Federal regulations requiring ethical review have clearly added substantially to the indirect institutional costs of conducting human subjects research.

Case law

The influence of the courts in the development of legal controls governing human subjects research has generally been limited. As late as 1978, the U.S.

Department of Health, Education, and Welfare's official guidelines on human experimentation cited only one relevant decision by an appellate court. This 1965 Canadian case, *Halushka vs University of Saskatchewan*, involved a student volunteer who had agreed to test a new anesthetic after being informed that it was 'perfectly safe' [98]. While receiving the drug, he suffered a cardiac arrest. Finding that the subject had been inadequately informed of potential study risks, the Court upheld a lower court's ruling and awarded him $22,500 in damages.

Despite the general paucity of case law concerning human experimentation, court cases dealing with research have increased in recent years. Rising court involvement suggests that judicial social control may play a more prominent role in the future regulation of human subjects research than it has in the past. Predictions about the direction case law in this area may take, however, are premature. A brief look at three U.S. appellate court decisions concerning the use of human subjects illustrates both the diversity of judicial reasoning in this area and the complex issues these case often involve.

In a 1977 case, *Blanton vs United States* [99], the U.S. District Court for the District of Columbia awarded $15,000 to a woman who suffered numerous physical and emotional symptoms after she was informed that she had mistakenly been given an experimental drug in a study assessing different medications used to prevent harm to a future fetus from RH blood incapability. The plantiff had explicitly refused study participation, stating instead that she wished to receive the conventional drug for her condition. The court ruled that the hospital had violated its responsibility to the plaintiff in two respects: in failing to exercise 'due care' in the administration of the drug and in failing to inform her of the drug that was actually given (the plaintiff was not told of the medication error until several months after the fact). In its finding, the court emphasized the importance of informed consent in medical experimentation and cited federal human subjects regulations in support of its decision.

In a case stemming from the early 1950s, but decided in 1982 (*Burton vs Brooklyn Hospital*), the New York Supreme Court ruled that there had been insufficient consent when a physician's order to decrease the concentration of oxygen to a premature infant had been overturned by his superiors [100]. The infant was instead given increased oxygen concentration as part of a national research study being conducted to determine the possible role of oxygen in causing retrolental fibroplasia (a condition often leading to blindness). The infant subsequently became blind. Even though the standard of care for treating premature infants was unclear at the time of the study, the New York Court ruled that informed consent was necessary when exposing subjects to treatments suspected to constitute an unwarranted medical risk.

Lastly, in a 1985 case disturbingly reminiscent of the Tuskegee syphilis study (*Begay vs United States*), Navajo uranium miners participating in a long-term, epidemiological investigation sponsored by the U.S. Public Health Service (PHS) charged that they had been inadequately informed about research findings linking lung cancer to prolonged radiation exposure. During the study subjects were told only that it's purpose was to assess the health of uranium miners [101].

The plaintiffs' claims, however, were dismissed by the Ninth Circuit Court of Appeals, which ruled that the decision by the PHS not to warn the miners of radiation dangers (even after these were known) was within the 'discretionary function' exception of the Federal Tort Claims Act [102]. The exception states that the U.S. Government cannot be held liable for claims predicted on the actions of federal agencies exercising their proper regulatory authority.

The *Begay* case illustrates the dilemmas associated at times with the need to conduct vital research, while at the same time, attempting to provide maximum protection for the rights and welfare of human subjects. The study's scientific goal was laudable: to quantify long-term radiation risks so that federal safety levels could be set and occupational health regulations enacted. However, as the Court noted, "[I]n order to get the cooperation of the owners of the various mines and to retain the members of the cohort for study, PHS decided not to warn the miners of the possible radiation hazards associated with uranium mining" [101, p. 1064]. The *Begay* case also illustrates the limits of judicial involvement in redressing subjects' grievances stemming from research participation. The fact that a number of cases of subject misuse have been associated with research conducted under U.S. governmental auspices further underscores these limitations.

State law

Prior to the 1970s, state law protecting human research subjects was nonexistent. However, during the past decade and a half, a number of states have enacted human experimentation legislation, in many cases to close perceived gaps in federal regulations (which pertain only to research funded by the federal government). Statutory attention to human experimentation varies greatly by state, ranging from comprehensive and specific in a few (California, New York, and Virginia) to general in most [103]. Delaware, Missouri, New York, Virginia, and Wisconsin require that IRBs review and approve all research conducted within the state. In 1985 Illinois established an organ transplantation board to determine the eligibility of subjects for experimental transplant procedures. In California all drug studies employing human subjects must receive IRB approval. Legal statutes in other states may require that non-IRB bodies or agencies review research (human subjects research conducted in the District of Columbia, for example, must be approved by the U.S. Department of Health and Human Services).

Informed consent is an issue commonly covered in state law. California, New York, and Virginia have enacted legislation which specifically addresses informed consent in human experimentation and details what types of information must be provided to potential subjects by investigators. Louisiana and Florida have also passed legislation requiring that informed consent be obtained prior to performing research on human subjects. Neither state, however, provides guidance concerning what types of

information must be given to prospective subjects in order for 'legally effective' informed consent to be achieved. Some states (Michigan, Minnesota, Rhode Island, and Washington) require the informed consent of research subjects in their general patients' rights statutes, while others (Massachusetts, Nevada) note only that prospective subjects have the right to refuse research participation. Most states have not enacted legislation specifically addressing the use of informed consent in human experimentation; instead these issues are assumed to be covered in the state's general informed consent statutes.

Fetal research is also regulated by law in a number of states. Prior to the 1973 U.S. Supreme Court decision legalizing abortion, *Roe vs Wade*, fetal research was conducted with few, if any, state restrictions. What state law existed at the time was grounded in the Uniform Anatomical Gift Act (UAGA), which was passed by all 50 states between 1969 and 1973. UAGA provisions allow for the use of fetal remains for research or therapeutic purposes when the consent of either parent is granted.

Between 1973 and 1985, 25 states enacted statutes explicitly regulating fetal research. There is a high degree of diversity among these states in their statutory approach to fetal experimentation. Some states (South Dakota and Tennessee) permit fetal research of all kinds with maternal consent, while other states (including Arizona, Illinois, Indiana, Louisiana, Ohio, and Oklahoma) prohibit or place serious restrictions on the use of dead fetuses for research—thus undermining their own UAGA statutes. Perhaps the most restrictive state statute was passed by Arizona in 1975. That statute states:

A person shall not knowingly use any fetus or embryo, living or dead ... resulting from an induced abortion in any manner for any medical experimentation ... except as is strictly necessary to diagnose a disease or condition in the mother of the fetus or embryo and only where the abortion was performed because of such disease or condition [104].

The most detailed and comprehensive set of state statutes dealing specifically with human experimentation in general are those of California [105]. Enacted in 1978, the California law is based on the premise that international ethical standards are legally unenforceable and thus incapable of meeting "a growing need for protection of citizens of the state from unauthorized, needless, hazardous, or negligently performed medical experiments on human beings" [105, p. 8]. The statute contains an 'experimental subjects' bill of rights' and a detailed set of informed consent requirements. Criminal and civil penalties for violations of the law are also enumerated, including fines and, in some cases, possible imprisonment. These penalties apply to *all* medical studies conducted in California, whether or not they are conducted under federal sponsorship.

CONCLUSION

This paper has examined social control mechanisms used to develop, nurture and, in some cases, compel conformity by biomedical scientists to accepted norms of research ethics. Both intra- and extraprofessional controls were investigated. As

8   PAUL R. BENSON

the review indicates, internal controls have not been fully successful in promoting ethical propriety among researchers. As a result, the United States has moved increasingly toward a system of controls over science based on externally developed, bureaucratically administered, and formally sanctioned rules. Research, however, also suggests that the use of extraprofessional controls is far from problem free.

One area of continuing controversy concerns the role of institutional review boards as a regulatory device. As noted, empirical studies of IRBs have raised troubling questions about their effectiveness and fairness. A number of these problems are related to IRB decentralization, leading some to propose the creation of a national research review board [23, 24]. The precise organization, procedures, and goals of such a panel are unclear, although Katz [25] has suggested that the duties of a national board should include the promulgation of uniform procedural standards for IRBs and its use as a formal appeals board. The development of such a centralized decision-making body would almost certainly increase federal control over local IRBs, research institutions, and biomedical investigators.

In contrast, the emergence of AIDS as a major health crisis has recently served as the catalyst for a potentially significant relaxation of federal drug regulations. In May of 1987, the FDA promulgated new regulations allowing for the treatment use of certain investigational drugs before the end of their clinical trials, that is, before the drugs have been fully proven to be safe [106]. The basic intent of these new FDA regulations is to facilitate the availability of promising new drugs to individuals suffering from life-threatening illnesses (such as AIDS) where no comparable alternative therapy is available. Both the pharmaceutical manufacturer who intends to sponsor an investigational drug for treatment use and the physician who wishes to prescribe the drug to his or her patients must seek special FDA approval to do so. If approval is granted, pharmaceutical manufacturers may, under certain circumstances, charge for use of the drug when it is employed solely for treatment purposes.

The adoption of the new FDA regulations was lobbied for and strongly applauded by a variety of patient advocacy groups. Bioethicists and others, however, expressed concern over the potential abrogation of regulatory protections for human research subjects won over the previous decade. Critics were especially alarmed that, as originally proposed, the FDA regulations had indicated a willingness to waive IRB review for treatment protocols, noting that patients' rights would be adequately protected through informed consent. Following negative public comment, however, the plan to waive IRB review was dropped in the final regulations [107].

Clearly, social controls over human biomedical research in the United States is in a state of flux. If regulatory policy in this area is to be successful, it must be grounded on a solid informational base of well-designed empirical studies. Unfortunately, no such knowledge base presently exists.

Several different types of research are needed to construct such a base of information. In view of our highly rudimentary understanding of social controls

and their impact on researcher behavior, a particularly useful investigatory method at this point is ethnographic field-work [108]. These studies provide the essential descriptive grounding on which further research is based. While ethnographic studies have thoroughly examined medical education, no comparable studies have investigated the (ethical) socialization of physicians learning to become clinical scientists. Similarly, few studies have examined the way medical researchers choose their careers [109]. In addition, despite increased attention to ethnographic studies of the work of physical and natural scientists [101, 110], very little research has explored the day-to-day activities of medical investigators. Additional descriptive research also needs to be undertaken on IRBs. In particular, comparative studies are needed that examine the impact of different types of IRB organization, structure, and composition on board decision-making. Finally, ethnographic research is needed on professional disciplinary committees. Unfortunately, as in the case of IRBs, the study of these bodies is severely restricted by the general inability of ethnographers to achieve access to their deliberations.

There are a number of factors associated with the increased used of external controls over biomedical research. These include the specialization, bureaucratization, and impersonalization characteristic of modern industrial societies, dramatic advances in medical knowledge and technology, and high levels of governmental support for biomedical science. The development of extraprofessional controls is also clearly related to explicit examples of the unethical use of subjects and a historic unwillingness on the part of the medical research community to regulate itself. Given these considerations, governmental regulation of medical research is likely to continue. As Nelkin [111] notes: "The issue is no longer whether there will be public control over science but, rather, how restrictions should be applied and who should participate in establishing and implementing controls."

However, as necessary as they may be, in and of themselves, government regulations are ultimately of limited value. In the end, externally imposed procedures and restrictions cannot compel biomedical researchers, as a collectivity, to behave in an ethical manner. Only researchers themselves can do that. For this reason, an important set of questions concerns how, and under what circumstances, intraprofessional and extraprofessional controls impact upon one another. Unfortunately, we know almost nothing about these potentially important interactive influences. For example, is the ethical socialization of junior investigators strengthened (or weakened) through the presence of external controls? What is the impact of governmental regulations on investigators' attitudes toward ethical aspects of their work—for example, do they pay more (or less) attention to ethical considerations when they known an IRB will formally review their work? If sound regulatory policy is to be achieved, these questions (among many others) will need to be addressed and answered.

Acknowledgement—I wish to thank Loren H. Roth who provided helpful comments to an earlier draft of this article.

The social control of human biomedical research 9

REFERENCES

1. Carr-Saunders A. M. and Wilson P. M. *The Professions.* Claredon Press, Oxford, 1933.
2. Parsons T. The professions and social structure. In *Essays in Sociological Theory* (Edited by Parsons T.). Free Press, New York, 1964.
3. Friedson E. *The Profession of Medicine.* Dodd–Mead, New York, 1970.
4. Friedson E. *Professional Powers.* University of Chicago Press, Chicago, Ill., 1986.
5. Betz M. and O'Connell L. Changing doctor–patient relationships and the rise in concern for accountability. *Soc. Probl.* **31**, 84, 1983.
6. Haug M. and Lavin B. *Consumerism in Medicine: Challenging Physician Authority.* Sage, Beverly Hills, Calif., 1983.
7. Starr P. *The Social Transformation of Medicine.* Basic Books, New York, 1982.
8. Goggin M. The life sciences: is science too important to be left to the scientists? *Polit. Life Sci.* **3**, 28, 1984.
9. Pion G. M. and Lipsey M. W. Public attitudes toward science and technology: what have the surveys told us? *Publ. Opin. Q.* **45**, 305, 1981.
10. Miller J. D., Suchner R. W. and Voelker A. M. *Citizenship in the Age of Science: Changing Attitudes Among Young Adults.* Pergamon, New York, 1980.
11. Rowan A. N. and Rollin B. E. Animal research—for and against: a philosophical, social, and historical perspective. *Perspect. Biol. Med.* **27**, 1, 1983.
12. Katz J. *Experimentation with Human Beings.* Russell Sage, New York, 1972.
13. Swazey J. P. Protecting the "animal of necessity": limits to inquiry in clinical investigations. *Daedalus* **107**, 129, 1978.
14. Nelkin D. Social controls in the changing context of science. In *Social Controls and the Medical Profession* (Edited by Swazey J. P. and Scher S. R.). Oelgeschlager, Gunn & Hain, New York, 1985.
15. Goggin M. L. (Ed.) *Governing Science and Technology in a Democracy.* University of Tennessee Press, Knoxville, Tenn., 1986.
16. Public and quasi-public regulatory systems have developed in many other nations aside from the United States. Recent international developments in this area are discussed in Benson P. R. and Roth L. H., Trends in the social control of medical and psychiatric research. In *Law and Mental Health: International Perspectives*, Vol. 4. Pergamon, New York. In press.
17. Janowitz M. Sociological theory and social control. *Am. J. Sociol.* **81**, 82, 1975.
18. Bosk C. L. Social controls and physicians: the oscillation of cynicism and idealism in sociological theory. In *Social Control and the Medical Profession* (Edited by Swazy J. P. and Scher S. R.). Oelgeschlager, Gunn & Hain, New York, 1985.
19. Swazey J. P. Introduction. In *Social Control and the Medical Profession* (Edited by Swazy J. P. and Scher S. R.). Oelgeschlager, Gunn & Hain, New York, 1985.
20. Delgado R. and Leskovac H. Informed consent in human experimentation: bridging the gap between ethical thought and current practice. *UCLA Law Rev.* **34**, 67–130, 1986.
21. Woltjen M. Regulation of informed consent in human experimentation. *Loyola Univ. Law J.* **17**, 507–532, 1986.
22. McClellan F. M. Informed consent to medical therapy and experimentation: the case for invoking punitive damages to deter impingement of individual autonomy. *J. Legal Med.* **3**, 81, 1982.
23. Levine C. and Caplan A. L. Beyond localism: a proposal for a national research review board. *IRB: Rev. Human Subj. Res.* **8**, 7, 1986.
24. Annas G. J. Made in the U.S.A.: legal and ethical issues in artificial heart experimentation. *Law med. Hlth Care* **14**, 164, 1987.
25. Katz J. The regulation of human experimentation in the United States: a personal odyssey. *IRB: Rev. Human Subj. Res.* **9**, 1, 1987.
26. Cole J. O. Research barriers in psychopharmacology. *Am. J. Psychiat.* **134**, 896, 1977.
27. Garham J. C. Some observations on informed consent in non-therapeutic research. *J. Med. Ethics* **1**, 138, 1975.
28. Hamilton M. On informed consent. *Br. J. Psychiat.* **143**, 416–418, 1983.
29. Guze S. B. Federal regulation of psychiatric research: an editorial. *J. nerv. ment. Dis.* **167**, 265–266, 1979.
30. Becker H. S., Greer B., Hughes E. and Strauss A. *Boys in White: Student Culture in Medical School.* University of Chicago Press, Chicago, Ill., 1961.
31. Fox R. C. Training for uncertainty. In *The Student Physician* (Edited by Merton R. K., Reader G. and Kendall P.). Harvard University Press, Cambridge, Mass., 1957.
32. Fox R. C. The autopsy: its place in the attitude learning of second-year medical students. In *Essays in Medical Sociology* (Edited by Fox R. C.). Wiley, New York, 1979.
33. Fox R. C. and Lief H. Training for "detached concern" in medical students. In *The Psychological Basis of Medical Practice* (Edited by Lief H.). Harper & Row, New York, 1963.
34. Carlton W. *"In Our Professional Opinion...": The Primacy of Clinical Judgment Over Moral Choice.* University of Notre Dame Press, Notre Dame, Ind., 1978.
35. Coombs R. *Mastering Medicine: Professional Socialization in Medical School.* Free Press, New York, 1978.
36. Millman M. *The Unkindest Cut: Life in the Backrooms of Medicine.* Morrow, New York, 1976.
37. Bucher R. and Stelling J. *Becoming Professional.* Sage, Beverly Hills, Calif., 1977.
38. Burkett G. and Knafl K. Judgment and decision-making in a medical specialty. *Sociol. Work Occup.* **1**, 82, 1974.
39. Scully D. *Men Who Control Women's Health: The Miseducation of Obstetrician-Gynecologists.* Houghton-Mifflin, Boston, Mass., 1980.
40. Mizrahi T. *Getting Rid of Patients: Contradictions in the Socialization of Physicians.* Rutgers University Press, New Brunswick, N.J., 1986.
41. Meadow R. Student assessment of clinical training. *Guys Hosp. Rep.* **119**, 263, 1970.
42. Atkinson P. Training for certainty. *Soc. Sci. Med.* **19**, 949, 1984.
43. Maddison D. C. What's wrong with medical education? *Med. Educ.* **12**, 97, 1978.
44. For a general critique of the use of the biomedical model, see Engel G. The need for a new medical model: a challenge for biomedicine. *Science* **196**, 129, 1977.
45. Carlton W. *"In Our Professional Opinion...": The Primacy of Clinical Judgment Over Moral Choice*, p. 171. University of Notre Dame Press, Notre Dame Ind., 1978.
46. I am not arguing that a strict biomedical orientation alone causes physicians to become cynical concerning their work and detached from the emotional experiences of their patients. Certainly many other factors also contribute to this phenomena, including very high work loads during internship and residency, an increasing dependence on medical technology within hospitals, and perhaps predisposing personality factors as well. See Oratz R. Achieving aesthetic distance: education for an effective doctor–patient relationship.

In *Making Health Care Decisions.* Vol. 3: *Appendices.* Presidents Commission for the Study of Ethical Problems in Medicine and Biomedical and Behavioral Research. U.S. Government Printing Office, Washington, D.C., 1982.

47. Bosk found 'professional ethics' to be an important aspect of surgical training, with normative violations (lack of dedication, interest, and thoroughness) among the most serious mistakes a resident can make. Patient participation in treatment decision-making and informed consent, however, were not considered important ethical issues by either senior or resident surgeons studied by Bosk. See Bosk C. L. *Forgive and Remember: Managing Medical Failure.* University of Chicago, Chicago, Ill., 1979.

48. Rogers W. R. and Bernard D. (Eds) *Nourishing the Humanistic in Medicine: Interactions with the Social Sciences.* University of Pittsburgh Press, Pittsburgh, Penn., 1979.

49. Pellegrino E. D., Hart R. J., Henderson S. R. *et al.* Relevance and utility of courses in medical ethics: a survey of physicians' perceptions. *J. Am. med. Ass.* **253,** 49, 1985.

50. Loewy E. H. Teaching medical ethics to medical students. *J. Med. Educ.* **61,** 661, 1986.

51. Clouser K. D. *Teaching Bioethics: Strategies, Problems, and Resources.* Hastings Center Press, Hastings-on-Hudson, N.Y., 1980.

52. Presidents Commission for the Study of Ethical Problems in Medicine and Biomedical and Behavioral Research. Professional outlook and behavior. In *Making Health Care Decisions.* Vol. 1: *Report,* Chap. 6. U.S. Government Printing Office, Washington, D.C., 1982.

53. Kaufmann C. L. Medical education and physician-patient communication. In *Making Health Care Decisions.* Vol. 3: *Appendices.* Presidents Commission for the Study of Ethical Problems in Medicine and Biomedical and Behavioral Research. U.S. Government Printing Office, Washington, D.C., 1982.

54. Barber B., Lally J., Loughlin J. and Sullivan D. *Research on Human Subjects: Problems of Social Control in Medical Experimentation.* Transaction, New Brunswick, N.J., 1973.

55. Steven Miller in his participant-observation study of intern training at the Harvard Medical Unit at Boston City Hospital, noted that senior researchers often placed subtle pressure on their junior colleagues to help them identify and recruit potential study participants. As Miller comments: "I did not once see an intern refuse clinical investigators permission to use his patients. An intern occasionally complained that the clinical investigators were using his patients as guinea pigs, but he knew that his complaints would not influence those in authority." See Miller S. J. *Prescription for Leadership,* p. 154. Aldine, Chicago, Ill., 1970.

56. Merton R. K. Science and democratic social structure. In *Social Theory and Social Structure,* 2nd edn, Chap. 18. Free Press, New York, 1968.

57. Storer N. W. *The Social System of Science.* Holt, Rinehart & Winston, New York, 1966.

58. Zuckerman H. Deviant behavior and social control in science. In *Deviance and Social Change* (Edited by Sagarin E.). Sage, Beverly Hills, Calif., 1977.

59. Watson J. D. *The Double Helix.* New American Library, New York, 1968.

60. Mitroff I. I. *The Subjective Side of Science.* Elsevier, Amsterdam, 1974.

61. Knorr-Cetina K. and Mulkay M. (Eds) *Science Observed.* Sage, Beverly Hills, Calif., 1983.

62. Broad W. and Wade N. *Betrayers of Truth: Fraud and Deceit in the Halls of Science.* Simon & Schuster, New York, 1982.

63. Woolf P. Fraud in science. *Hastings Ctn. Rep.* **11,** 9, 1981.

64. Barber B. *Informed Consent in Medical Therapy and Research,* p. 129. Rutgers University Press, New Brunswick, N.J., 1980.

65. Freidson E. *Doctoring Together: A Study of Professional Social Control.* Elsevier, New York, 1975.

66. Some studies have suggested that researchers exert greater informal influence upon one another's behavior than is indicated by the work of Freidson and Barber. Using ethnographic methods, Renee Fox studied the interaction between physician-investigators and patient-subjects on a special metabolic unit during the early 1950s. She examined how investigators coped collectively with work stresses associated with uncertainty and therapeutic limitation, using techniques such as scientific magic, black humor, and probabilistic reasoning. Fox also noted close, personal, and almost collaborative relationships between the investigators and subjects on the research ward she studied. See Fox R. C. *Experiment Perilous.,* Free Press, Glencoe, Ill., 1959. Fox and Swazey also note the importance of informal collegial influence in their case studies of the 1928 clinical moratorium on mitral valve surgery and the 1969 moratorium on heart transplantation. See Swazey J. P. and Fox R. C. The clinical moratorium. In *Experimentation with Human Subjects.* Braziller, New York, 1970. Also see Fox R. C. and Swazey J. P. *The Courage to Fail.* University of Chicago Press, Chicago, Ill., 1974.

67. Gass R. S. Codes of the health care professions. In *Encyclopedia of Bioethics,* Vol. 4. Free Press, New York, 1975.

68. American Medical Association. *Principles of Medical Ethics.* AMA, Chicago, Ill., 1982.

69. American Medical Association. *Current Opinions of the Council on Ethical and Judicial Affairs of the American Medical Association.* AMA, Chicago, Ill., 1986. Council 'Opinions' were also published in 1982, 1983, and 1984.

70. The licensing and disciplining of physicians by state boards is also an important quasi-public form of medical regulation in the United States. While medical boards derive their regulatory powers from individual state legislatures, boards are almost always composed solely of physicians. Studies of state medical boards have generally shown them to be largely ineffective in policing medical practice. See, Derbyshire R. C. How effective is medical self-regulation? *Law & Human Behav.* **7,** 193, 1983. See also Dolan A. K. and Urban N. D. The determinants of the effectiveness of medical disciplinary boards, 1960–1977. *Law & Human Behav.* **7,** 203, 1983.

71. Zitrin A. and Klein H. Can psychiatry police itself effectively? The experience of one district branch. *Am. J. Psychiat.* **133,** 653, 1976.

72. Moore R. A. Ethics in the practice of psychiatry: origins, functions, models, and enforcement. *Am. J. Psychiat.* **135,** 157, 1978.

73. Moore R. A. Ethics in the practice of psychiatry: update on results of enforcement of the code. *Am. J. Psychiat.* **142,** 1043, 1985.

74. Personal communications: Mr William Tabor, staff person, Judicial and Ethical Council of the American Medical Association, August 1987.

75. Faden R. R. and Beauchamp T. C. *A History and Theory of Informed Consent.* Oxford University Press, New York, 1986.

76. Lifton R. J. *The Nazi Doctors: Medical Killing and the Psychology of Genocide.* Basic Books, New York, 1986.

77. Frenkel M. S. Public Health Service guidelines governing research involving human subjects: an analysis

of the policy-making process. George Washington University Program of Policy Studies of Science and Technology, Washington, D.C., 1972.

78. Beecher H. K. Ethics and clinical research. *New Engl. J. Med.* **274**, 1354, 1966.

79. In his article, Beecher noted that Maurice H. Pappworth was at the same time gathering information on over 500 cases of ethically problematic medical research in Britain. See Pappworth M. H. *Human Guinea Pigs*. Routledge & Kegan Paul, London, 1967.

80. Ladimer I. and Kennedy D. Clinical investigation in medicine: legal, ethical, and moral aspects. Law-Medicine Research Institute, Boston University, Boston, Mass., 1963.

81. The Tuskegee syphilis study involved a 40-year followup of 400 untreated, syphilitic, black males in order to observe the 'natural course' of the disease. Subjects (who were uniformly poor and uneducated) were informed only that they were receiving free treatment for 'bad blood'. The Willowbrook State School study was carried out for nearly 20 years and involved the deliberate infection of hospitalized mentally retarded children with hepatitis—partially on the assumption that they would contract the virus in the institution in any event. For a discussion of the Tuskegee syphilis study, see Jones J. H. *Bad Blood*. Free Press, New York, 1981. The Willowbrook State School study, is examined in Rothman D. J. and Rothman S. M. *The Willowbrook Wars: A Decade of Struggle for Social Justice*. Harper & Row, New York, 1984.

82. The role of the fetal research controversy in the creation of the National Commission is discussed in Maynard-Moody, S. Fetal research dispute. In *Controversy: Politics of Technical Decisions* (Edited by Nelkin D.). Sage, Beverly Hills, Calif., 1979.

83. Topics addressed by the 11-person Commission included informed consent, risks and benefits of research, selection of research subjects, and the use of fetuses, children, prisoners, and the mentally ill as research subjects, as well as psychosurgery and sterilization. When the Commission disbanded in 1978, after 4 years of work, it had published nine reports, each of which included a detailed set of legislative and regulatory recommendations, as well as extensive background materials.

84. U.S. Department of Health and Human Services. Final regulations amending basic NHS policy for the protection of human research subjects. *Fed. Registr.* **46**, 8386, 26 January, 1981.

85. U.S. Food and Drug Administration. Protection of human subjects; informed consent. *Fed. Registr.* **46**, 8942, 27 January, 1981.

86. While the research regulations of the Department of Health and Human Services and the Food and Drug Administration are nearly identical in most aspects, they are some differences. For a useful side-by-side comparison of HHS and FDA regulations governing human subjects research, see Maloney D. M. *Protection of Human Research Subjects: A Practical Guide to Federal Laws and Regulations*. Plenum Press, New York, 1984.

87. *All* federally funded human subjects research is subject to IRB oversight. However, some types of research, normally associated with the social sciences, are exempted from IRB review. These include most observational and survey studies, educational research, and investigations employing existing public documents or records. These exemptions are applicable only insofar as subject confidentiality is maintained; if subjects can be identified, IRB review of the research is required. The 1981 regulations also provide for 'expedited review' of certain biomedical investigations involving no more than minimal subject risk. Categories of

research for which expedited review is permitted include studies of human tissues which can be obtained through noninvasive means, voice recordings, moderate amounts of exercise by healthy volunteers, and the collection of modest amounts of blood by venipuncture. For detailed summaries of federal research regulations, see Ref. [86]; and Greenwald R. A., Ryan M. K. and Mulvihill J. E. *Human Subjects Research: A Handbook for Institutional Review Boards*. Plenum Press, New York, 1982.

88. Robertson J. A. The law of institutional review boards. *UCLA Law Rev.* **26**, 484, 1978. Also an interesting series of comparative IRB case studies is presented in DuVal B. S. The human subjects protection committee: an experiment in decentralized federal regulation. *Am. Bar Ass. Res. J.* **3**, 571–688, 1979.

89. Gray B. H., Cooke R. A. and Tannenbaum A. S. Research involving human subjects. *Science* **201**, 1094, 1978.

90. National Commission for the Protection of Human Subjects of Biomedical and Behavioral Research. *Appendix to Report and Recommendations: Institutional Review Boards*. U.S. Government Printing Office, Washington, D. C., 1978.

91. Goldman J. and Katz M. D. Inconsistency and institutional review boards. *J. Am. med. Ass.* **249**, 197, 1982.

92. It should be noted that IRB members were aware of the contrived nature of the proposals when making their assessments.

93. The Goldman and Katz study generated considerable controversy. Robert Levine (chairman of the IRB at Yale University Medical School), after noting what he viewed as the study's failure to approximate essential, interactive processes of 'real-life' IRB review, dismissed the study as misleading and inaccurate. Ethicist Robert Veatch, however, in a *J. Am. med. Ass.* editorial accompanying the Goldman and Katz article, noted: "For those of us who have served on IRBs over the years, their findings ring true." See Levine R. J. Inconsistency and IRBs: flaws in the Goldman–Katz study. *IRB: Rev. Human Subj. Res.* **6**, 4, 1984; also Veatch R. M. Problems with institutional review board inconsistency. *J. Am. med. Ass.* **248**, 178, 1982.

94. President's Commission for the Study of Ethical Problems in Medicine and Biomedical and Behavioral Research. IRB site visits: an exploratory assessment of a procedure for evaluating IRB performance. In *Implementing Human Research Regulations*, Chap. 4. U.S. Government Printing Office, Washington, D.C., 1983.

95. Sackoff-Lambert B. Institutional review boards: a sociological inquiry: protection for whom? Unpublished doctoral dissertation, Graduate Program in Sociology, School of Nursing, University of California, San Francisco, Calif., 1984.

96. Ceci S. J., Peters D. and Plotkin J. Human subjects review, personal values, and the regulation of social science research. *Am. Psychol.* **40**, 994, 1985.

97. Brown J. H. U., Schoenfeld L. S. and Allan P. W. The costs of an institutional review board. *J. Med. Educ.* **54**, 294, 1979.

98. *Halushka vs University of Saskatchewan*. 53 D.L.R. 2d 436, 437 (1965).

99. *Blanton vs United States*. 428 F. Supp. 360 (*Fed. Suppl.* **428**, 360 1977).

100. *Burton vs Brooklyn Doctors Hospital*. 452 N.Y.S.2d 875, N.Y. (1982).

101. *Begay vs United States*. 768 F.2d 1059 (*Fed. Report.* **768**, 1059, 1985).

102. 28 U.S.C. Section 2680, a.

103. For a detailed state-by-state overview of statutory law concerning human experimentation, see Ref. [21]. Other sources drawn upon for this section include:

Capron A. M. Human experimentation. In *BioLaw: A Legal and Ethical Reporter on Medicine, Health Care, and Bioengineering* (Edited by Childress J. F. *et al.*). University Press of America, Fredrick, Md; Rozovsky F. A. *Consent to Treatment: A Practical Guide*. Little, Brown, Boston, Mass., 1984; and Baron C. H. Fetal research: the question in the states. *Hastings Ctn. Rep.* **15**, 6, 1985.

104. Ariz. Rev. Stats. S 36-2302A.

105. California Laws, 1987, Chap 1.3, codified as California Health and Safety Code Sections 24170–24179.5 (*Deering's Health and Safety Code of the State of California*, 1987 pocket suppl. Bancroft–Whitey, San Francisco, Calif., 1987).

106. U.S. Food and Drug Administration. Investigational new drug, antibiotic, and biological drug product regulations; treatment use and sale; Final rule. *Fed. Regist.* **52**, 19,466–19,477, 22 May, 1987.

107. For a summary of the new FDA regulations and the events leading to their promulgation, see Maloney D. New rules proposed for protecting subjects of drug studies. *Human Res. Rep.* **2**, 1, May 1987; Maloney D. Research community wants and gets more protection for subjects. *Human Res. Rep.* **2**, 1, July 1987; and

Levine R. J. FDA's new rule on treatment use and sale of investigational drugs. *IRB: Rev. Human Subj. Res.* **9**, 1, 1987. For a general discussion of the ethnical dilemmas posed by research assessing the effectiveness of potential AIDS treatments, see Macklin R. and Friedland G. AIDS research: the ethics of clinical Trials. *Law Med. Hlth Care* **14**, 273, 1986.

108. Lofland J. and Lofland L. H. *Analyzing Social Settings: A Guide to Qualitative Observation and Analysis*. Wadsworth, Belmont, Calif. 1984.

109. The studies that have been conducted on scientists' career choice have largely been psychological, emphasizing the importance of personality, family background, educational experience, and occupation options. See Eiduson B. T. and Beckman L. (Eds) *Science as a Career Choice*. Russell Sage, New York, 1973.

110. Lynch M. *Art and Artifact in Laboratory Science*. Routlege & Kegan Paul, Boston, Mass., 1985.

111. Nelkin D. Value conflict and social controls over research. In *The Social Context of Medical Research* (Edited by Wechsler H., Lamont-Haven R. W. and Cahill G. F.), p. 24. Ballinger, Cambridge, Mass., 1981.

[15]

Goodbye to All That

The End of Moderate Protectionism in Human Subjects Research

by JONATHAN D. MORENO

Federal policies on human subjects research have undergone a progressive transformation. In the early decades of the twentieth century, federal policies largely relied on the discretion of investigators to decide when and how to conduct research. This approach gradually gave way to policies that augmented investigator discretion with externally imposed protections. We may now be entering an era of even more stringent external protections. Whether the new policies effectively absolve investigators of personal responsibility for conducting ethical research, and whether it is wise to do so, remains to be seen.

In May 2000 the Department of Health and Human Services announced new regulatory and legislative initiatives concerning federally sponsored research involving human subjects. In September, the Office for Protection from Research Risks was reconstituted as the Office for Human Research Protections and, with a new director, completed its transition to the Office of the Secretary at DHHS. In the months leading up to these changes, both the OPRR and the Food and Drug Administration had been increasingly active in levying sanctions against institutions whose ethics institutional review boards were malfunctioning or that had engaged in questionable research practices, especially in human genetics trials.

Weeks after DHHS secretary Donna Shalala's announcement, a bipartisan group of congressional sponsors led by Congresswoman Diane DeGette, Democrat from Colorado, introduced the Human Research Subjects Protections Act of 2000. Among other reforms, the act would extend informed consent and prior review requirements to all human subjects research, regardless of funding source. Senator Ted Kennedy, Democrat from Massachusetts, introduced a bill that would establish steep civil penalties for investigators and institutions that broke the rules. Leading up to all this activity, there had been since 1997 several congressional hearings on human subjects research as well as numerous reports and recom-

Jonathan D. Moreno, "Goodbye to All That: The End of Moderate Protectionism in Human Subjects Research," *Hastings Center Report* 31, no. 3 (2001): 9-17.

mendations by public and private panels concerning the state of the regulatory system.

All these hearings, bills, and reports had one thing in common: They all found or presupposed a need to strengthen the human subjects protections system. Although some individuals representing the community of scientific investigators raised their voices in objection to increased regulation—especially the psychiatric community in response to the National Bioethics Advisory Commission's recommendations concerning research involving persons with mental disorders—theirs were largely lonely voices. Protests that new measures would block important research seemed hard to sustain in light of two decades of remarkable advances under the current system, which at the time of its introduction was itself described as being so burdensome that it would threaten medical progress. Reservations about increased bureaucracy, or even the question whether the proposals being advanced would have avoided any actual patient or subject injuries, were overwhelmed by a historical tide that presages a new era in the history of human subjects regulations, an era that I call "strong protectionism."

A New World Order

The essence of strong protectionism is the minimization of clinical researchers' discretion in governing their conduct with regard to human subjects. Among the measures implied by strong protectionism are concurrent third party monitoring of consent and study procedures, disclosure of financial arrangements or other potential conflicts of interest, required training of investigators in research ethics and research regulations, and independent review of the decisionmaking capacity of potential subjects. All these and other measures have been proposed, and many may be implemented, in spite of the additional costs in time and money they represent, and regardless of the infer-

ence an observer may draw that clinical researchers are simply not to be trusted.

In this article my purpose is neither to challenge nor defend these early stirrings of what I believe to be a new era in the history of human subjects protections. It is, rather, to note how inured we have become to this grim view of investigator discretion, and how far we have traveled to reach this pass. The current transition to strong protectionism builds on two previous stages. During the first, singularly important period, lasting roughly from 1947 to 1981, the ancient tradition of weak protectionism, which granted enormous discretion to physician experimenters, began to break down. Following that was the era that is now passing away, a compromise between physician discretion and modest external oversight that I call moderate protectionism.

Perhaps it was inevitable that moderate protectionism could last only about twenty years. It was a compromise that combined substantial researcher discretion with rules enforced by a minimal bureaucracy. An important part of this compromise was that researchers for the most part had the prerogative of identifying potential conflicts of interest themselves, without external review. Researchers' use of human subjects was approved before and after it actually took place, and only very rarely was there third party observation of research activities themselves.

The moderately protectionist era might have lasted longer had the research environment not changed so much, had so much money not poured into research as the result of promising new areas for investigation and investment, had the proportion of private funding not increased so drastically, and had the number and complexity of studies not grown so rapidly. Together, these elements strained the twenty-year compromise and may have caused its collapse, even though it was a period little blemished by harms to persons, at

least as compared with the scandalous era that immediately preceded it.

Weak Protectionism: Virtue Has Its Day

Concerns about the involvement of human beings in research are at least a century old. In the nineteenth century, many institutionalized children in Europe and the United States were subjects in vaccine experiments, and by the 1890s antivivisectionists were calling for laws to protect children. At the turn of the century the Prussian government imposed research rules and Congress considered banning medical experiments for certain populations, such as pregnant women, in the District of Columbia. In the ensuing decades there were occasional well-publicized scandals, mostly involving child subjects, and the first attempt to test a polio vaccine was stopped after the American Public Health Association censured the program.[1]

Prior to World War II, however, medical researchers were largely inoculated against regulation by the nearly legendary status of the self-experimentation conducted by members of the Yellow Fever Commission, led by U.S. Army physician Walter Reed. One of the commissioners, Dr. Jesse Lezear, died after subjecting himself to the bite of the mosquito that transmits the disease. Lezear thereby helped to confirm the hypothesis of the disease's spread. A less celebrated but equally notable element of the Reed story is his use in Cuba of an early written contract for the Spanish workers who were among the commission's other subjects.[2]

For some reason, Reed himself was widely thought to have been one of the volunteer subjects, perhaps due to his untimely death only a few years later as a result of a colleague's error. This misconception added to the legend and to the model of medical researchers as having exceptional moral character, even to the point of martyrdom. The Reed myth became a singular reference point and justification for the self-regulation of medical science. During the 1960s, when researchers were coming under new scrutiny and weak protectionism was under attack, the distinguished physician-scientist Walsh McDermott referred to the Reed story to demonstrate the social importance of research and the high moral standing that went with it.[3]

By the early 1950s, there were gestures in the direction of a protectionist attitude toward human subjects, but they were in a fairly abstract, philosophical vein rather than in a robust set of institutionalized policies and procedures. An example is the Army's failure to implement a compensation program for prisoners injured in malaria or hepatitis studies when it was contemplated in the late 1940s.[4] The essential feature of the weak form of protectionism was its nearly wholesale reliance on the judgment and virtue of the individual researcher. Thus when the World Medical Association began deliberations in 1953 on the first Declaration of Helsinki, informed consent was made a far less prominent feature than it had been in the Nuremberg Code, which the medical community found unacceptably legalistic. Helsinki also introduced the notion of surrogate consent, permitting research when individuals are no longer competent to provide consent themselves. These moves place a substantial burden on the self-control of the individual researcher.[5]

To be sure, until the middle and later 1960s, and with the significant exception of the Nazi experience, to many there did not seem to be good reason to worry about human protections. The development of penicillin, the conquest of polio, and the emergence of new medical devices and procedures all bolstered the public prestige of biomedical research. There were only inklings of a continuing, low-intensity concern about the concentrated power of medical researchers even in the 1950s, exemplified perhaps in the gradual disappearance from professional discussions of

the term "human experiment" and its replacement with the more detached and reassuring "research."

On the whole, then, the world of clinical studies from the late 1940s up through the mid-1960s was one in which a weak form of protectionism prevailed, one defined by the placement of responsibility on the individual researcher. Obtaining written informed consent (through forms generally labeled "permits," "releases," or "waivers"), though apparently well-established in surgery and radiology, was not common in clinical research and cannot have provided more than a modicum of increased protection to human subjects. For example, whether a medical intervention was an "experiment" or not, and therefore whether it fell into a specific moral category that required an enhanced consent process, was a judgment largely left up to the researcher. Partly that judgment depended on whether the individual was a sick patient or a healthy volunteer. The former were likely to be considered wholly under the supervision of the treating doctor, even when the intervention was quite novel and unlikely to be of direct benefit. An individual might be asked to consent to surgery but might not be informed beyond some generalities about its experimental aspect.

There were some important exceptions. The Atomic Energy Commission established a set of conditions for the distribution of radioisotopes to be used with human subjects, including the creation of local committees to review proposals for radiation-related projects. Early institutional review boards were established in several hospitals (including Beth Israel in Boston

and the City of Hope in California) in order to provide prior group review for a variety of clinical studies. The Clinical Center of the National Institutes of Health in Bethesda, Maryland, which opened in 1953, appears to have been one of a handful of hospitals that required prospective review of clinical research proposals by a group of colleagues. Yet as advanced as the Clinical Center might have been, the prior group review process it established seems, at least at first, to have been confined to research with healthy, normal volunteers. That at least some sick patients who would probably not be helped by study par-

The world of clinical studies from the late 1940s up through the mid-1960s was one in which a weak form of protectionism prevailed, one defined by the placement of responsibility on the individual researcher.

ticipation were morally equivalent to normal subjects who would not be benefited (with the possible exception of those in vaccine studies) was apparently not appreciated.

Prior group review is essential to the transition beyond weak protectionism and was not common before the 1970s. Yet decades earlier there was a keen awareness of the psychological vulnerability inherent in the subject role, a vulnerability that could have argued for independent review of a research project. An extensive psychological literature, founded mainly on psychoanalytic theory, propounded a skeptical view of the underlying motivations of experiment volunteers as early as 1954. That year, Louis Lasagna and John M. von Felsinger reported in *Science* on the results of Rorschach studies and psychological interviews of fifty-six healthy young male volunteers in drug research. The authors concluded that the subjects exhibited "an unusually high incidence of severe psychological maladjustment." "There is little question," they wrote, "that most of the subjects . . . would qualify as deviant, regardless of the diagnostic label affixed to them by examining psychiatrists or clinical psychologists."[6] The authors theorized that the group might not be representative of the population from which it was drawn (college students), and that they might have been attracted to the study for various reasons having to do with their deviance, beyond financial reward.

I describe this study not to endorse its psychology or its conclusions, nor to imply that neurotic tendencies are either typical of research volunteers or a priori disqualifying conditions for decisionmaking capacity. The point is, rather, that thought was being given as early as 1954 to

lected from about 350 candidates. Although only 1,750 victims were named in the indictment, they were a handful of the thousands of prisoners used in a wide variety of vicious experiments, many in connection with the Nazi war effort. Some involved the treatment of battlefield injuries or prevention of the noxious effects of high altitude flight. Others, such as the sterilization experiments, were undertaken in the service of Nazi racial ideology, and still another category had to do with developing efficient methods of killing.

A strong defense mounted by the defendants' lawyers noted that the Allies had also engaged in medical experiments in the service of the war effort. As the prosecution's attempt to demonstrate that there were clear in-

Unlike the medical profession as a whole, some government agencies attempted to put the code to use, although with little success. In the early 1950s the Department of Defense adopted the Nuremberg Code, along with written and signed consent, as its policy for defensive research on atomic, biological, and chemical weapons. A 1975 report from the Army Inspector General pronounced that initiative a failure. In 1947 the new Atomic Energy Commission attempted to impose what it termed "informed consent" on its contractors as a condition for receiving radioisotopes for research purposes. It also established—or attempted to establish—a requirement of potential benefit for the subject. Both of these conditions were to apply to nonclassified research. This relatively protectionist attitude may not have been adopted with a great deal of appreciation of its implications. In any case, the AEC met with resistance among some of its physician contractors, but not its physician advisors. The agency's stance ultimately was not institutionalized, and the letters setting out the requirements seem to have been soon forgotten. (Indeed, the requirement of potential benefit seems incompatible with the research on trace-level radiation that the AEC sponsored shortly thereafter.)[8]

NAHC's seemingly innocent endorsement of "prior review by institutional associates" was the most significant single departure from the weakly protectionist tradition.

the question of the recruitment of subjects who might be vulnerable despite their healthy and normal appearance. The article was published in a major scientific journal. It would have been natural to ask further questions about the vulnerability of potential research subjects who are known to be seriously ill. Yet despite this psychological theorizing, which could be viewed as quite damning to the moral basis of the human research enterprise, protectionism was at best a weak force for years to come.

Doubts Triumphant

An occasion for the significant revision of this picture came at the end of the Second World War, when twenty-three Nazi doctors and medical bureaucrats were tried for crimes associated with vicious medical experiments on concentration camp prisoners. The defendants were se-

ternational rules governing human experimentation faltered, the judges decided to create their own set of rules, known to posterity as the Nuremberg Code, the first line of which is, "The voluntary consent of the human subject is absolutely essential." Although the court seemed to believe that protections were needed, it is not clear how intrusive they wished these protections to be in the operations of medical science. The judges declined, for example, to identify persons with mental disorders as requiring special provisions, although their medical expert urged them to do so. The very requirement of voluntary consent for all undermined the relevance of their code to experiments involving persons with diminished or limited competence, and the extreme circumstances that gave rise to the trial seemed quite distant from normal medical research.[7]

Historians of research ethics generally date the increasing vigor of protectionist sentiment among high-level research administrators, as well as the general public, to the series of events that began with the Thalidomide tragedy and continued with scandals such as the Brooklyn Jewish Chronic Disease Hospital Case and, later, the Willowbrook hepatitis research. These cases cast doubt on the wisdom of leaving judgments about research participation to the researchers' discretion. The Jewish Chronic Disease Hospital Case, in which elderly debilitated patients were injected with cancer cells, apparently without their knowledge or consent, attracted the attention and concern of James S. Shannon, director at that time of the NIH. Shannon's intervention, and the resistance from within his own staff, was an important and revealing moment in the history of human subjects protections.

In late 1963 Shannon appointed his associate chief for program development, Robert B. Livingston, as chair of a committee to review the standards for consent and requirements of NIH-funded centers concerning their procedures. The Livingston Committee affirmed the risks to public confidence in research that would result from more cases like that of the Jewish Chronic Disease Hospital. Nonetheless, in its 1964 report to Shannon the committee declined to recommend a code of standards for acceptable research at the NIH, on the grounds that such measures would "inhibit, delay, or distort the carrying out of clinical research." Deferring to investigator discretion, the Livingston Committee concluded that the NIH was "not in a position to shape the educational foundations of medical ethics" (pp. 99-100).

Disappointed but undeterred by the response of his committee, Shannon and Surgeon General Luther Terry proposed to the National Advisory Health Council that the NIH take responsibility for formal controls on investigators. The NAHC essentially endorsed the proposal and resolved that human subjects research should be supported by the Public Health Service only if "the judgment of the investigator is subject to prior review by his institutional associates to assure an independent determination of the protection of the rights and welfare of the individual or individuals involved, of the appropriateness of the methods used to secure informed consent, and of the risks and potential medical benefits of the investigation."[9] The following year Surgeon General Terry issued the first federal policy statement that required PHS-grantee research institutions to establish what were subsequently called research ethics committees.[10]

The seemingly innocent endorsement of "prior review by institutional associates" was the most significant single departure from the weakly protectionist tradition to a process that finally yielded the moderately protectionist system we have today.

The Surgeon General's policy was hardly typical of contemporary attitudes, however, and the practice it sought to implement is one we are still trying to effect. To appreciate the weakness of the form of protectionism that prevailed through the 1960s, it is useful to recall the dominant role that prison research once had in drug development in the United States. By 1974 the Pharmaceutical Manufacturers Association estimated that about 70 percent of approved drugs had been through prison research. Pharmaceutical companies literally built research hospitals on prison grounds. Although in retrospect we may think of limits on prison research as a triumph of protectionism (on the grounds that prisoners cannot give free consent), at the time it was a confluence of political and cultural forces that had little to do with actual abuses (though there certainly were some) and was resisted by prison advocates. Perhaps the most important public event that signaled the inevitable end of widespread prison research was the 1973 publication of "Experiments behind Bars" by Jessica Mitford in the *Atlantic Monthly*.[11]

Within the medical profession itself, then, weak protectionism remained the presumptive moral position well into the 1970s, if not later. Neither of the most important formal statements of research ethics, the Nuremberg Code and the Helsinki Declaration, had nearly as much effect on the profession as a 1966 *New England Journal of Medicine* paper by Harvard anesthesiologist Henry Beecher. The importance of timing is evident in the fact that Beecher had been calling attention to research ethics abuses since at least 1959, when he published a paper entitled "Experimentation in Man," but his 1966 publication "Ethics and Clini-

cal Research" attracted far more attention.[12] One important distinguishing feature of the latter work was Beecher's allusion to nearly two dozen cases of studies alleged to be unethical that had appeared in the published literature. By "naming names" Beecher had dramatically raised the stakes.

It would, however, be an error to conclude that Beecher himself favored external review of clinical trials that would remove them from medical discretion. To the contrary, Beecher was one among a large number of commentators who favored (and in some instances continue to favor) reliance primarily on the virtue of the investigator. Although he strongly defended the subject's right to voluntary consent, he argued in his 1959 paper that the best protection for the human subject would be obtained by ensuring that the investigator possessed "an understanding of the various aspects of the problem" being studied, and he was quite critical of the Nuremberg Code's dictum that the subjects themselves should have sufficient knowledge of the experiment before agreeing to participate. Nor was Beecher's attitude toward the Code's provisions limited to philosophical musings. In 1961 the Army attached a new provision to its standard research contract that essentially restated the Nuremberg Code. Along with other members of Harvard Medical School's Administrative Board, Beecher protested and persuaded the Army Surgeon General to insert into Harvard's research contracts a statement that its Article 51 offered "guidelines" rather than "rigid rules."[13]

Beecher's attitude was shared by many other distinguished commentators on research practices through the 1960s and 1970s. In 1967 Walsh McDermott expressed grave doubt that the "irreconcilable conflict" between the "individual good" and the "social good" to be derived from medical research could be resolved, and certainly not by "institutional forms" and "group effort"—apparently references to ethics codes and peer review. McDermott's comments were by way of introduction to a colloquium at the annual meetings of the American College of Physicians on "The Changing Mores of Biomedical Research." In his remarks McDermott alluded to the growing contribution of research to the control of disease, beginning with Walter Reed's yellow fever studies. Thus, he continued, "medicine has given to society the case for its rights in the continuation of clinical investigation," and "playing God" is an unavoidable responsibility, presumably one to be shouldered by clinical investigators.[14]

Another distinguished scientist who made no secret of his skepticism toward the notion that the investigator's discretion could be supplemented by third parties was Louis Lasagna. In 1971 Lasagna wondered "how many of medicine's greatest advances might have been delayed or prevented by the rigid application of some currently proposed principles to research at large."[15] Rather, "for the ethical, experienced investigator no laws are needed and for the unscrupulous incompetent no laws will help" (p. 109). Six years later, when the National Commission for the Protection of Human Subjects of Biomedical and Behavioral Research proposed a moratorium on prison research, Lasagna caustically editorialized that the recommendations "illustrate beautifully how well-intentioned desires to protect prisoners can lead otherwise intelligent people to destroy properly performed research that scrupulously involves informed consent and full explanation and avoids coercion to the satisfaction of all but the most tunnel-visioned doctrinaire."[16]

It is perhaps worth noting that both Beecher and Lasagna had good reason to reflect on the problem of research ethics. In 1994 Lasagna told interviewers for the Advisory Committee on Human Radiation Experiments that between 1952 and 1954 he was a research assistant in a secret, Army-sponsored project, directed by

Beecher, in which hallucinogens were administered to healthy volunteers without their full knowledge or consent. Lasagna said that he reflected "not with pride" on the episode.[17]

Weak Protectionism: The Death Knell

Among those who developed an interest in research ethics during the 1960s was Princeton theologian Paul Ramsey. Although Ramsey is today remembered as one who took a relatively hard line on research protections, and although he significantly advanced the intellectual respectability of a protectionist stance, in retrospect his position seems quite modest. In his landmark 1970 work, *The Patient as Person,* Ramsey declared that "No man is good enough to experiment upon another without his consent."[18] In order to avoid the morally untenable treatment of the person as a mere means, the human subject must be a partner in the research enterprise. However, Ramsey was prepared to accept nonconsented treatment in an emergency, including experimental treatment that might save life or limb. He also acceded to the view that children who cannot be helped by standard treatment may be experimental subjects if the research is related to their treatment and if a parent consents.

The emergence of modern bioethics at the end of the 1960s brought another nonphysician commentator onto the scene. While generally agreeing with the theologian Ramsey in advocating strict limits on professional discretion, the philosopher Hans Jonas struck a more passionate, even haunting tone: "We can never rest comfortably in the belief that the soil from which our satisfactions sprout is not watered with the blood of martyrs. But a troubled conscience compels us, the undeserving beneficiaries, to ask: Who is to be martyred? in the service of what cause? and by whose choice?"[19] In explicitly calling forth survivor guilt in the benefiting public, Jonas also

deepened the moral burden on the clinical investigator and called attention to the moral paradox of human experimentation.

By 1970 the notion that consent was ethically required was well established in principle (including surrogate consent for children and incompetents), however poorly executed in practice. Ramsey's contribution was in calling attention to the problem of nonbeneficial research participation, a decision that required at a minimum the human subject's active participation, while Jonas insisted on the inherent and unavoidable unfairness of human experimentation. As though to underline the point, only two years after Ramsey's and Jonas's writings, the Tuskegee Syphilis Study scandal broke into the open. Here was a case in which the subjects were clearly not informed participants in research and were obviously used as mere means to ends they did not share. The subsequent federal panel appointed to review the study, the Tuskegee Syphilis Study Ad Hoc Panel, concluded that penicillin therapy should have been made available to the participants by 1953. The panel also recommended that Congress create a federal panel to regulate federally sponsored research on human subjects, a move that foreshadowed and helped define the later transition from weak to moderate protectionism.

News of Tuskegee demolished the approach defended in the 1960s by McDermott and Lasagna. In the years immediately following Beecher's 1966 article it was still possible to argue that scientists should take responsibility to make what McDermott regarded as appropriately paternalistic decisions for the public good, decisions that recognize that societal interests sometimes take precedence over those of the individual. Although there are surely instances in which this general proposition is unobjectionable, following the syphilis study such an argument became much harder to endorse. In a word, the tide of history was turning against the physician commentators.

As the implications of Tuskegee became apparent, philosopher Alan Donagan published an essay on informed consent in 1977 that symbolized the altered attitude. Donagan's critique ventured well beyond those of Ramsey and Jonas. In Donagan's essay the invigorated informed consent requirement is taken as nearly a self-evident moral obligation in clinical medicine. In his discussion of informed consent in experimentation, Donagan explicitly compared the arguments of a Nazi defense attorney with those of McDermott and Lasagna, concluding that they are both versions of a familiar and (one infers) rather primitive form of utilitarianism. Donagan concluded that, by the lights of the medical profession itself, the utilitarian attitudes instanced in the Nazi experiments and the Brooklyn Jewish Chronic Diseases Hospital case cannot be justified. Perhaps still more telling is the mere fact that Donagan, a highly respected moral philosopher who could not be dismissed as a "zealot," could associate the arguments of Nazis with those of some of America's most highly regarded physicians. Donagan's essay underlined a leap in the evolution of protectionism through the Tuskegee experience, especially on the question of the balance between the subject's interests and those of science and the public, and on the subsequent discretion to be granted the lone investigator.[20]

Two Forms of Accessionism

To be sure, the story is not one of an inexorable march toward stronger protectionism. Although the tendency since the advent of the Nuremberg Code—greatly strengthened in the United States by the Belmont Report—has been to limit the scope of investigator discretion, there have been countervailing forces. One of these has been the Declaration of Helsinki, which has employed the concepts of therapeutic and nonther-

apeutic research, defining the former as "Medical Research Combined with Professional Care." According to the version of Helsinki drafted in 1989, "If the physician considers it essential not to obtain informed consent, the specific reasons for this proposal should be stated in the experimental protocol for transmission to the independent committee." Thus Helsinki continued to contemplate a relatively permissive attitude toward investigator discretion, as it has since the first version in 1954. Henry Beecher preferred Helsinki to Nuremberg precisely because the former is a "set of guides" while the latter "presents a set of legalistic demands."[21]

Another force counteracting the tendency to limit investigator discretion has been a movement on behalf of greater access to clinical trials. The most pronounced expression of this effort has occurred among AIDS activists, who in the later 1980s successfully insisted on the creation of alternative pathways for making unproven anti-AIDS drugs available. In the face of a disease that resisted treatment and struck down people just entering the prime of life, the determination to find solutions was understandable. The slogan embraced by ACT-UP (AIDS Coalition to Unleash Power), that "A Drug Trial is Health Care Too," was a political expression of confidence in the power of science. The slogan also depended on some assumptions about the benefits of research participation and the self-discipline of the medical research community. Further, it relied on the very protections it sought to shortcut. This movement has apparently already largely run its course; the activists who launched it have revised their attitude toward alternative pathways of access to nonvalidated med-

ications and have become more critical of their earlier position.

The ACT-UP slogan reflects what might be called "therapeutic accessionism." Another and much more durable movement could be described as "scientific accessionism." In the late 1980s female political leaders noted the paucity of women in clinical trials and finally brought about significant changes in NIH and FDA policies. Similar policy reforms have recently been introduced for children. Unlike therapeutic accessionism, this view is wholly consistent with strengthened protections for

> **H**elsinki continued to contemplate a relatively permissive attitude toward investigator discretion, as it has since the first version in 1954.

subjects. In fact, it could be said to follow from the principle of justice enclosed by the National Commission in *The Belmont Report*, since it attempts to further extend the benefits of research.

Beyond Moderation

Moderate protectionism was perhaps being dismantled as soon as it was born. In the early 1980s the later President's Commission for the Study of Ethical Problems in Medicine and Biomedical and Behavioral Research made recommendations on the evaluation and monitoring of institutional review boards[22] and endorsed the proposition that research-related injuries should be compensated.[23] The impact of the President's Commission's efforts to sustain the pressure brought to bear by the National Commission was muted, however, by a relatively (and uncharacteristically) scandal-free period in the history of human research ethics. Instead, the pressing need for anti-AIDS medications, and the accessionist movement that went with it, dominated the discussion of human subjects research for much of the 1980s and early 1990s.

The serenity was challenged in the 1990s by the revelations of cold war radiation experiments. Though the studies took place decades earlier, the story of human radiation experiments story provided an occasion for another look at the regulatory regime and how well it was working. Among the recommendations of the Advisory Committee on Human Radiation Experiments in 1995 were several that would strengthen human subject protections. For example, the ACHRE urged that regulations be established to cover the conduct of research with institutionalized children and that guidelines be developed to cover research involving adults with questionable competence. The ACHRE also recommended steps to improve existing protections for military personnel concerning human subject research. Substantial improvements were urged in the federal oversight of research involving human subjects: that outcomes and performance be evaluated beyond audits for cause and paperwork review, that sanctions for violations of human subjects protections be reviewed for their appropriateness in light of the seriousness of failures to respect the rights and welfare of human subjects, and that human subjects protections be extended to nonfederally funded research. The ACHRE also recommended the creation of a mechanism for compensating those injured in the course of participation as subjects of federally funded research.[24]

Within eighteen months of the ACHRE's final report, on 17 May 1997, the National Bioethics Advisory Commission unanimously adopted a resolution that "No person in the United States should be enrolled in research without the twin protections of informed consent by an authorized person and independent review of the risks and benefits of the research."[25] That same month President Clinton stated that "[w]e must never allow our citizens to be unwitting guinea pigs in scientific experiments that put

them at risk without their consent and full knowledge."[26]

At the end of 1998 NBAC recommended increased protections for persons with mental disorders that might affect their decisionmaking capacity, reminiscent of suggestions made by the National Commission twenty years before.[27] On the whole, two decades since its advent, moderate protectionism was on the run before a flurry of federal activity.

Whither Protectionism?

On the account I have presented, protectionism is the view that a duty is owed those who participate as subjects in medical research. The underlying problem is how to resolve the tension between individual interests and scientific progress, where the latter is justified in terms of benefits to future individuals. Weak protectionism is the view that this problem is best resolved through the judgment of virtuous scientists. Moderate protectionism accepts the importance of personal virtue but does not find it sufficient. Strong protectionism is disinclined to rely, to any substantial degree, on the virtue of scientific investigators for purposes of subject protection.

We are today so accustomed to moderate protectionism that we have nearly forgotten the struggle that led to its establishment. Where once it was considered radical, moderate protectionism is now embraced by the medical community. Consider, for example, the position exemplified in a recent essay on ethics in psychiatric research, in which the authors state that "the justification for research on human subjects is that society's benefit from the research sufficiently exceeds the risks to study participants." But then the authors continue, "potential risks and benefits must be effectively communicated so that potential subjects can make informed decisions about participation."[28] The current battleground, then, is not whether the subjects should in theory be full participants, or whether prior

review of experiment proposals should be required, but whether, or to what extent, subjects can take an active role in the clinical trials process. To the extent that such active participation can be achieved, the introduction of more strongly protectionist requirements may be forestalled.

Implicit in all discussions about the ethics of clinical trials has been the assumption that the investigator bears a significant degree of moral responsibility for the dignity and well being of the human subject, a responsibility that cannot be sloughed off and assigned to someone else. In the words of the first article of the Nuremberg Code, "The duty and responsibility for ascertaining the quality of the consent rest upon each individual who initiates, directs or engages in the experiment. It is a personal duty and responsibility which may not be delegated to another with impunity."

This sensibility has not wholly disappeared from our public discourse, even in the onslaught of calls for higher levels of subject protection by regulatory means. Rather, the dispute turns on how much we should rely on the moral virtue of the individual investigator. While he was still a medical school professor, the person who recently became the first director of the Office for Human Research Protections wrote a passage explicitly reminiscent of Beecher's sympathy for a system based on the scientist's virtue. "In truth," wrote Greg Koski in 1999, "investigators are much better positioned during the course of their studies to protect the interests of individual research subjects than are the IRBs. Paradoxically, the person most likely to do something to harm a subject, the investigator, is also the person most capable of preventing such harm. And so, as Beecher . . . concluded many years ago, the only true protection afforded research subjects comes from a well-trained, well-meaning investigator."[29]

Koski's admiration for Beecher (another Harvard anesthesiologist) is evident, but his peroration has an air of nostalgia about it. Since his assent to the OHRP directorship, Koski has emphasized the importance of research ethics training for investigators. It remains to be seen whether education alone can slow the historic march towards strong protectionism.

A Moral Hazard

I have argued that the march of history is resolute in its rejection of investigator discretion. There is nonetheless a moral hazard in the strong protectionism that aims to supplant the scientist's virtue.

It would be understandable, though of course not admirable, if the scientist's sense of personal responsibility for his subjects were to be undermined in a much more intensely regulated environment. Paradoxically, the research scientist's sense of personal moral responsibility might weaken as the official and continuous scrutiny of scientific work is strengthened. From the investigator's standpoint, the care of human subjects could come to be seen as a concern secondary to the efficient and careful execution of the scientific mission, especially when society has assigned to others the job of protecting subjects. The clinical researcher might then feel justified in taking what Josiah Royce called a "moral holiday," focusing only on the science and leaving the task of protecting human subjects to those whose charge it is.

In this way strong protectionism might inadvertently result in undermining physician investigators' sense of personal moral responsibility in the conduct of human experiments. For all the limitations of that virtue in the protection of human subjects, it is surely not one that we would want medical scientists to be without. No less an authority than the Nuremberg Code tells us so. But in spite of the stirring appeals it might still inspire, the code was a product of a long history of weak protectionism, and we shall not see that time again.

References

1. S.E. Lederer and M.A. Grodin, "Historical Overview: Pediatric Experimentation," in *Children as Research Subjects: Science, Ethics, and Law*, ed. M.A. Grodin and L.H. Glantz (New York: Oxford University Press, 1994).

2. S.E. Lederer, *Subjected to Science: Experimentation in America before the Second World War* (Baltimore: Johns Hopkins University Press, 1995).

3. W. McDermott, "Opening Comments on the Changing Mores of Biomedical Research," *Annals of Internal Medicine* 67, Supp. 7 (1967): 39-42.

4. Advisory Committee on Human Radiation Experiments, *The Human Radiation Experiments* (New York: Oxford University Press, 1996), p. 55-56.

5. R.R. Faden and T.L. Beauchamp, *A History and Theory of Informed Consent* (New York: Oxford University Press, 1986).

6. L.M. Lasagna and J.M. Von Felsinger, "The Volunteer Subject in Research," in *Experimentation with Human Beings*, ed. J. Katz (New York: Russell Sage Foundation, 1972), pp. 623-24, at p. 623.

7. J.D. Moreno, *Undue Risk: Secret State Experiments on Humans* (New York: W.H. Freeman, 1999).

8. See ref. 4, Advisory Committee Human Radiation Experiments, *The Human Radiation Experiments*, p. 63.

9. J.S. Reisman, Executive Secretary, NAHC, to J.A. Shannon, 6 December 1965 ("Resolution of Council").

10. W.J. Curran, "Governmental Regulation of the Use of Human Subjects in Medical Research: The Approach of Two Federal Agencies," in *Experimentation with Human Subjects*, ed. P.A. Freund (New York: George Braziller, 1970), pp. 402-54.

11. J. Mitford, "Experiments behind Bars: Doctors, Drug Companies, and Prisoners," *Atlantic Monthly* 23 (1973): 64-73.

12. H.K. Beecher, "Experimentation in Man," *JAMA* 169 (1959): 461-78; H.K. Beecher, "Ethics and Clinical Research," *NEJM* 274 (1966): 1354-60.

13. See ref. 4, Advisory Committee on Human Radiation Experiments, *The Human Radiation Experiments*, pp. 89-91.

14. See ref. 3, W. McDermott, "Opening Comments on the Changing Mores of Biomedical Research," pp. 39-42.

15. L. Lasagna, "Some Ethical Problems in Clinical Investigation," in *Human Aspects of Biomedical Innovation*, eds. E. Mendehlsohn, J.P. Swazey and I. Taviss, (Cambridge, Mass.: Harvard University Press, 1971), p. 105.

16. L. Lasagna, "Prisoner Subjects and Drug Testing," *Federation Proceedings* 36, no. 10 (1977): 2349.

17. L. Lasagna interview by J. M. Harkness and S. White-Junod (ACHRE), transcript of audio recording, 13 December 1994 (ACHRE Research Project Series, Interview Program File, Ethics Oral History Project), 5.

18. P. Ramsey, *The Patient as Person: Explorations in Medical Ethics* (New Haven, Conn.: Yale University Press, 1970), pp. 5-7.

19. H. Jonas, "Philosophical Reflections on Experimenting with Human Subjects," in *Experimentation with Human Beings*, ed. J. Katz. (New York: Russell Sage Foundation, 1972), p. 735.

20. A. Donagan, "Informed Consent in Therapy and Experimentation," *Journal of Medicine and Philosophy* 2 (1977): 318-29.

21. Sir W. Refshauge, "The Place for International Standards in Conducting Research for Humans," *Bulletin of the World Health Organization* 55 (1977), 133-35, quoting H. K. Beecher, "Research and the Individual," *Human Studies* 279 (1970).

22. President's Commission for the Study of Ethical Problems in Medicine and Biomedical and Behavioral Research, *Implementing Human Subject Regulations* (Washington, D.C.: Government Printing Office, 1983).

23. President's Commission for the Study of Ethical Problems in Medicine and Biomedical and Behavioral Research, *Compensating for Research Injuries: The Ethical and Legal Implications of Programs to Redress Injured Subjects*, Vol. I, *Report* (Washington, D.C.: Government Printing Office, June 1982).

24. Advisory Committee on Human Radiation Experiments, op. cit., pp. 527-28.

25. National Bioethics Advisory Commission, Full Commission Meeting, Arlington, Virginia, 17 May 1997.

26. W.J. Clinton, Morgan State University Commencement Address, 18 May 1997.

27. National Bioethics Advisory Commission, *Research Involving Persons With Mental Disorders That May Affect Decision-making Capacity* (Washington, DC, 1998).

28. J.A. Lieberman et al., "Issues in Clinical Research Design: Principles, Practices, and Controversies," in *Ethics in Psychiatric Research*, eds. H.A. Pincus, J.A. Lieberman, and S. Ferris (Washington, D.C.: American Psychiatric Association, 1999), pp. 25-26.

29. G. Koski, "Resolving Beecher's Paradox," *Accountability in Research* 7 (1999).

[16]

Is National, Independent Oversight Needed for the Protection of Human Subjects?

Alexander Morgan Capron

University Professor of Law and Medicine,
Co-Director, Pacific Center for Health Policy and Ethics,
University of Southern California, Los Angeles, CA 90089-0071

Science—which in this century has transformed our world and allowed us to probe everything from the heart of the atom to distant planets—proceeds not merely from theory but from experimentation. And when the object of science is to understand human beings, eventually humans become the experimental animal of necessity. Regrettably, this century has also taught that in the name of science, men and women—acting predominantly from a genuine desire to advance knowledge and, more particularly to develop means of preventing and curing disease, of lengthening life and relieving its burdens—have subjected one another to great harm and grievous wrongs.

The focus of this conference is on an area of research that has been marked by special problems, and it is tempting to think that it illustrates the need of vulnerable populations for special protections. Yet in the annals of research with human beings, the category of vulnerability seems almost limitless. Even putting aside the atrocities committed by the Nazi doctors on their concentration camp victims, the groups who have been harmed and wronged appear all-encompassing: pregnant women, children, students, farmers, prisoners, members of the public at large, and above all else, patients suffering from every sort of illness. Some have been knowing and willing collaborators in research; many others were more akin to victims.

The human costs of research have not gone unnoted but have provoked criticism, commentary, and action. While the judgment handed
down by the American tribunal at Nuremberg five decades ago was
not immediately translated into explicit expectations for American
researchers, by the mid-1960s federal officials had laid out the basic
framework that still governs research with human subjects. Their
actions seem to have been spurred partly by concerns for the welfare
of human subjects such as those articulated by a number of academics
(including physicians such as Henry Beecher and Jay Katz, philosophers like Hans Jonas, lawyers such as Paul Freund and Bill Curran,
to mention only a few of the pioneers) and partly by a desire to stay
ahead of those who would seize upon instances of harm or abuse as
reasons to impose outside controls over the scientific enterprise.

The framework first constructed some 35 years ago has evolved in
significant ways, but its core has been relatively constant, consisting
of five features: (1) *diffused authority* among the federal agencies
involved as sponsors of research or as regulators of the products of
research, (2) *delegated responsibility* from these federal agencies to
the institutions that carry on research, largely without anything
more than "paper oversight" of the adequacy of the institutions'
execution of their duties, (3) largely *individualized decisionmaking*
(one might even say *ad hoc*), based upon the limited guidance given
institutional review boards about how to carry out their functions,
the absence of any means of "appeal" or indeed any formal, regu-
larized method of developing "interpretations" based on case-
experience, and the absence of any means of ensuring that the same
committee reaches consistent decisions about similar protocols
much less that committees at different institutions are deciding consistently, (4) utilization of a *"peer-review" format*, in which not solely
the scientific but also the ethical adequacy of research protocols is
judged by a researcher's scientific colleagues, with what is typically
only a modest involvement of persons with more independent perspectives (either not affiliated with the research institution or at
least not from biomedical research), and (5) the *limitation of federal
rules* that results from their origin as contractual conditions
attached to federal support (and later to the need of certain research
sponsors to secure federal action, principally, approval of a new
drug or device by the Food and Drug Administration). I believe that
these features all need to be seriously examined because, despite the
evolution that has taken place regarding all of them, they effectively
constrain the effectiveness of our present structure for protecting

research subjects. The thesis of this paper is that the time has come for a paradigm shift, not simply evolutionary adjustments of the details of the regulations but a new way of developing, promulgating, monitoring, and revising the regulations. To effect a new paradigm, we need to consolidate authority in this field in a new, independent federal office, linked to but not controlled by research-sponsors.

Perhaps the simplest way to organize these remarks is to focus on what the National Bioethics Advisory Commission—which was established by Executive Order in October 1995 and appointed by President Clinton the following summer, and which held its first meeting just over two years ago—is up to regarding relocating the federal human subjects regulatory functions. I will begin by illustrating the need for change by describing the Commission's response to the last of the five factors I just set forth.

AN ILLUSTRATION: EXPANDING THE REACH OF HUMAN SUBJECT REGULATIONS

Early in its work, in discussing problems with the present regulations, the Commission focused on the fact that the federal rules are only binding for research that is supported by, or whose products need approval by, a federal agency. At the time, Senator John Glenn was preparing a bill that would extend the central protections provided by the present regulations to all persons including those enrolled in privately sponsored studies. The Commission agreed that everyone enrolled in research in this country should be afforded the basic protections of independent review and informed, voluntary consent. While still at work on how best to achieve such a result, the Commission formally approved this position in principle in the Spring of 1997 and incorporated it into the report on *Cloning Human Beings* which we sent to the President on June 9, 1997.[1]

---

[1] Recognizing that the ban on federal support for all forms of embryo research would mean that any attempt to apply to humans techniques like those that produced the famous sheep Dolly would take place in the private sector, we recommended a broad moratorium. But we also concluded that in the absence of a moratorium, any research trials of human cloning should be "governed by the twin protections of independent review and informed consent, consistent with existing norms of human subjects protection". CLONING HUMAN BEINGS: REPORT AND RECOMMENDATIONS OF THE NATIONAL BIOETHICS ADVISORY COMMISSION, Rockville, Maryland (June, 1997), at p. iv.

I supported this aspect of our report on human cloning, but it seemed to me that in order to mount a convincing case for the larger proposition, we needed a good deal of empirical support to establish that the present system of federal oversight of research actually provides effective protection for human subjects. After all, it is not enough to know that problems have arisen for subjects in privately sponsored research—a conclusion for which there is substantial anecdotal support. Rather, we need to be able to show that fewer problems have arisen in research conducted according to the dictates of the federal rules.

Yet, as the front page of the May 14, 1997 *New York Times* reported, the ability of the federal government's Division of Animal Care to account for "every cat, dog, hamster, guinea pig, chimpanzee, rabbit or farm animal used in a laboratory experiment [for the last 31 years] as well as any adverse effects that each animal suffered" stands in stark contrast to the absence of "comparable figures for people" who serve as research subjects.[2] While Gary B. Ellis, director of the Office for Protection from Research Risks (OPRR) at NIH took the opportunity of the *Times* article to highlight that an indeterminate amount of "unchecked human experimentation [is] taking place" in the private sector beyond the reach of the federal human-subjects rules, an underlying theme in the article was that OPRR could not supply data on research falling within its purview.

Yet, as I pointed out to the Commission in a memo shortly thereafter, the *New York Times* article was hardly "news." The government has known about (and apparently tolerated) this problem for many years. In fact, the President's Commission for the Study of Ethical Problems in Medicine and Biomedical and Behavioral Research drew attention to the need to remedy this problem in 1981. In its *First Biennial Report* on federal policies for the protection of research subjects, the President's Commission recommended that

All Federal departments and agencies that conduct or support research with human subjects should require principal investigators to submit, as part of their annual reports to the IRB and the funding agency, information

---

[2] Sheryl Gay Stolberg, "'Unchecked' Research on People Raises Concern on Medical Ethics," *NY Times*, 14 May 1997, at A1.

regarding the number of subjects who participated in each research project as well as the nature and frequency of adverse effects.[3]

This recommendation was prompted by the finding, which had been made when the Commission was preparing its earlier report on *Compensating for Research Injuries*, "that data on the number of human subjects who participate in Federally funded research are not routinely and systematically compiled. Data regarding the incidence and severity of injuries that occur in such research are also not collected."[4] IRB reporting standards, derived from the then existing Department of Health and Human Services (HHS) regulations, contributed to this lack of information.[5]

The absence of information on the number of research projects conducted in various categories (such as exempt, minimal risk, etc.) and the total number of subjects is particularly troubling for two reasons. First, as of 1981 the Director of OPRR reported that IRBs had interpreted the HHS regulation "to require reporting only adverse effects not anticipated by the investigator and thus not reflected in the research proposal and consent documents at the time of the initial review."[6] By simply expanding the catalogue of risks in advance, the President's Commission pointed out, researchers could greatly "reduce their obligation to report harm to subjects, even when some of the risks are so improbable that their manifestation would, in common sense terms, be 'unanticipated.'" Because of this practice, it was no surprise that under these standards, "only two adverse effects associated with HHS-supported research were apparently reported to OPRR by either IRBs or investigators from 1975 to 1980."[7]

The experience of the President's Commission is instructive on another score, namely, the slowness with which the federal bureaucracy effects change. The central recommendation that the Commission also made in the 1981 report—that all departments adopt a "common rule" for subject protection—took a decade to be implemented. The recommendation to collect data on the types of experiments

---

[3] President's Commission for the Study of Ethical Problems in Medicine and Biomedical and Behavioral Research, PROTECTING HUMAN SUBJECTS: THE ADEQUACY AND UNIFORMITY OF FEDERAL RULES AND THEIR IMPLEMENTATION, U.S. Government Printing Office, Washington, D.C. (1981) at p. 73.

[4] *Id.*

[5] 45 CFR § 46.6(d), 39 *Federal Register* 18914, 18918 (May 30, 1974).

[6] Protecting HUMAN SUBJECTS, *supra* note 2, at 50.

[7] *Id.*

and number of subjects still had not been addressed when the President's Commission published its second (and final) *Biennial Report* on research protections in March 1983, just as it was closing its doors. Indeed, as the President's Commission noted then, the hope it had expressed in 1981 that the reporting of adverse effects would be improved—based on ongoing efforts in the Veterans Administration—were dashed, as "definitional problems were so pervasive that the data collected during the first year of [the VA's] reporting requirement were not useful."[8] The President's Commission also noted that the FDA did not have a master list of Institutional Review Boards (IRBs), making it impossible to even select IRBs for routine systematic inspection, much less record the number of human subjects supposedly monitored by each IRB.[9]

This brief historical review should suggest the barriers that exist to extending the federal regulations to all research studies—not the least the huge delays that arise in trying to get agency agreement to modify the Common Rule. This reality—which I mentioned as the system's first factor—has been repeatedly emphasized in NBAC's deliberations. If we want to get something done, we'd better try for an "interpretation" of the terms of the Common Rule or for a separate "subpart," because it would take years to get the Common Rule modified since decisionmaking power is diffused among the nearly two dozen federal departments or agencies that conduct or fund research with human beings.

PROBLEMS WITH DELEGATION, PEER REVIEW, AND AD HOC DECISIONMAKING

Having mentioned the first and last of the five factors, I turn now to the middle three as they relate to the topic at hand. The second factor—the delegation of responsibility for ensuring regulatory compliance to the institutions that are carrying on the research—may have been well intentioned when adopted but it is rife with conflicts of interest. This delegation not only makes it hard for OPRR and its

---

[8] President's Commission for the Study of Ethical Problems in Medicine and Biomedical and Behavioral Research, IMPLEMENTING HUMAN RESEARCH REGULATIONS: THE ADEQUACY AND UNIFORMITY OF FEDERAL RULES AND OF THEIR IMPLEMENTATION, U.S. Government Printing Office: Washington, D.C. (1983) at p. 23.
[9] *Id.* at 57.

counterparts in other federal agencies to know what is going on but also reinforces the third factor: the *ad hoc* nature of decisions about protocols, which are made with only minimal guidance from the federal regulators and without any formal structure either for higher review of individual institution's decisions or for sharing (and building on) deliberations at other institutions.[10] Finally, the format for protocol review by Institutional Review Boards (as prescribed by the 1974 National Research Act) grew out of the peer-review process used for in-house research at the NIH. Despite the presence of some non-affiliated members (whose number but not proportion is specified in the Common Rule), IRBs not only have all the deficiencies identified in the recent Inspector General's report—including too much work and too few resources—but conflicts of interest based not only on the inevitable personal and professional ties between the IRB and the researchers whose protocols are up for evaluation but also on the interest most IRB members have in their institution's success in garnering research dollars.

While some of these problems would probably inhere in any system, the failure to address them and to seek solutions for those that would be most easily soluble—such as having adequate data on research participation and injuries, aiming for greater communication to and among IRBs, providing means to make their decisions more consistent and visible, and introducing more objectivity and independence into the review process—this failure is noteworthy in itself. And it is here that the strands come together, for—as I argued to my fellow Commissioners at our June 1997 meeting—this failure results not merely from the diffusion of authority among the federal agencies that sponsor research but from the very assignment of responsibility to research sponsors in the first place. In light of experience with other federal agencies—such as the Atomic Energy Commission—it is hardly surprising that those charged with

---

[10]Under § 491 of the Health Research Extension Act of 1985, which updates provisions first enacted in the National Research Act of 1974 (including the requirements of prior IRB review and approval of protocols), the Secretary of HHS is required to have a "program ... under which requests for clarification and guidance with respects to the ethical issues raised in connection with ... research involving human subjects are responded to promptly and appropriately." OPRR has not used this provision to establish a system of "appellate jurisprudence" or even publication of decisions about difficult or controversial protocols, which would foster a more nuanced and detailed understanding of the meaning and application of the Common Rule. OPRR has, from time to time, sponsored educational programs nationally and regionally.

promoting a field do not make the best guardians against problems and abuses. With this in mind, NBAC voted to undertake a study of the desirability and feasibility of moving the regulatory functions now played by OPRR (and its counterparts) out of the agencies that conduct or sponsor research and into a less conflicted setting.

THE NBAC STUDY AND A PROPOSAL FOR CHANGE

As an aid to this study, we commissioned three papers: two by bio-ethicists with substantial experience at the NIH and one providing an outside analysis (namely from an academic administrator who is very knowledgeable about the regulation of human subjects research). The first two papers were intended to take opposing views on the question of whether the oversight function should be moved, so it is all the more significant that Charles McCarthy, the long-time director of OPRR, and John Fletcher, who was the first in-house ethicist for the NIH Clinical Center, largely agreed on their diagnosis of the problem and differed only in how far away from NIH they thought the oversight function needed to be moved. Indeed, the tale that McCarthy tells from an insider's perspective about just how resistant NIH has been to the whole process—to the point of being non-compliant with the very rules that were being applied to the outside investigators it was funding—makes clear that concerns about conflicts of interest are not mere academic speculation. Furthermore, even when OPRR can cleverly overcome the handicaps inherent in its organizational placement (within the NIH directorate), it faces other bureaucratic weaknesses, such as trying to carry out regulatory functions in an institution (NIH) that sees itself as non-regulatory, or attempting to get cooperation (much less compliance) from other subunits of its own department (Health and Human Services) that resist recognizing its authority.

McCarthy and Fletcher differ principally as to where this authority ought to be lodged if not with OPRR. McCarthy recommends creating an Office of Research Ethics (ORE)[11] who would have government-wide jurisdiction but answer directly to the HHS Secretary,

---

[11]In addition to a Human Subjects Protection Division, ORE would also have divisions dealing with laboratory animals and with scientific integrity; my discussion focuses solely on the first, which McCarthy divides into two branches, Education and Compliance.

whereas Fletcher would create an independent agency. The argument in favor of the first view is that the human subjects office would be better protected from bureaucratic and Congressional interference if it were under the wing of a powerful Cabinet secretary; on the other hand, placing the office in a single department—albeit the one with the largest human subjects research budget—is likely to cause problems when the office needs to get involved with research sponsored by other departments or agencies. Moreover, while McCarthy would ensure that the head of the human subjects division would have a separate budget and reporting authority, the office would still be a part of HHS, and should the office's activities offend NIH, CDC, or other research sponsors, the HHS secretary might, understandably, be inclined to give their concerns great weight.

The advantages of Fletcher's recommendation to establish a National Office of Human Subjects Research (NOHSR) are that it would give more visibility to human subjects protection and ensure that the agency was independent of the federal agencies that sponsor research. The disadvantages are primarily political: that in an era of "smaller government," Congress would be unwilling to create a new agency and that such an agency once created would be vulnerable to pressure (such as threats of being discontinued if its actions discomfitted a research institution in the district of a powerful Representative or Senator). This is a risk that exists for all independent agencies. Some protection could be expected to result from the existence of a board of commissioners (drawn from outside government) who would serve as the policymaking council for NOHSR; such individuals could defend the Office in the sort of public fashion that is more difficult for federal employees.

Plainly, such a government-wide Office could overcome the problems of diffuse responsibility (with the attendant difficulties of making changes in regulations in a timely fashion), and it would also be better positioned to draw together the process of interpreting the regulations and developing means to allow a sort of "common law" to help local review boards in applying the Common Rule. I believe that by avoiding conflicts of interest within the federal government, the Office would also be better positioned to find solutions to the conflicts that inhere in the use of the institution- and peer-based IRB process. Finally, the creation of such an Office does not mean that research sponsors would abolish their own human subjects protection offices (such as OPRR), which would continue to apply the uniform rules to the intra- and extramural research sponsored or conducted by their agency, just as each department now has its own ethics office, which operates under the umbrella of the government-wide ethics office. By serving this function of providing on-going independent oversight, NOHSR would not only check the work of the agency offices (just as the National Transportation Safety Board checks the work of the FAA) but could also support and buttress the agency offices in their internal struggles with the agencies in which they are lodged, which may understandably sometimes regard them as irritants.[12]

I hope that the National Bioethics Advisory Commission will, in the coming year, officially endorse the idea of a new government-wide office on human subjects research, for all the reasons I have surveyed here.

---

[12] On 8 July 1999 (after this article was in press) HHS Secretary Donna E. Shalala accepted the recommendation made to her on 3 June 1999 by the Advisory Committee to the Director, NIH, based on the report of the Office for Protection of Research Risks Review Panel, that OPRR be relocated in the Office of the Secretary. She also accepted the committee's recommendation that an independent advisory committee be established to provide scientific and ethical guidance to OPRR in its oversight role. Secretary Shalala also directed that the position of OPRR director be upgrade to Senior Executive Service level and that the resource needs of the office be reviewed as part of the relocation. *See* HHS Fact Sheet, protecting Research Subjects, U.S. Department of Health and Human Services, July 8, 1999.

[17]

National, Independent Oversight: Reinforcing the Safety Net for Human Subjects Research*

*Anna C. Mastroianni***

School of Law and Public Health Genetics Program, University of Washington, 608 Condon Hall, Box 354600, 1100 NE Campus Parkway, Seattle, WA 98105-6617

National, independent oversight is vital to resolve the problems and inconsistencies in oversight of human subjects research. Three key functions that must be considered in any proposal for such a mechanism are (1) issue spotting, (2) guidance on identified issues, and (3) sampling and follow-up. The 1998 report and recommendations of the National Bioethics Advisory Commission concerning research involving persons with mental disorders that may affect decisionmaking capacity address these functions in part, but application is limited to a small segment of the research population. Incorporation of these three key functions in a formal, national, independent oversight process is necessary in order to ensure accountability and maintain public trust in research.

Keywords: Ethics; human subjects research; oversight; regulation; NBAC; government

---

*This paper was originally presented at the 2nd National Ethics Conference on Research Involving Persons with Mental Disorders that may Affect Decisionmaking Capacity in Baltimore, MD, November 15, 1998. It has been modified in light of the subsequent finalization of the NBAC report, "Research Involving Persons With Mental Disorders That May Affect Decisionmaking Capacity" to accurately reflect the final recommendations contained therein.

**Corresponding author: Tel.: (206) 616-3482. Fax: (206) 616-3480. E-mail: amastroi@u.washington.edu.

The report and recommendations of the National Bioethics Advisory Commission (NBAC) concerning research involving persons with mental disorders that may affect decisionmaking capacity (NBAC, 1998) have engendered public debate and interest among a widely diverse set of interests—patients, subjects and their families, investigators, IRBs, institutions, and funders. The report and this debate have highlighted issues that need to be addressed not only in subjects with mental disorders, but also throughout human subjects research generally. More specifically, they point to a need for an integrated plan for addressing new and recurring issues in the ethics of human subject research.

Problems with the current system of oversight of human subjects research have been well described by many, and include scholars (Annas 1994, 1998; Capron, this journal issue; Edgar and Rothman, 1995; Katz, 1993; 1995; Phillips, 1996), government commissions (Advisory Committee on Human Radiation Experiments, 1996), the Inspector General of the Department of Health and Human Services (DHHS-IG, 1998), the U.S. Government Accounting Office (GAO, 1996), and Congressional bills and hearings (U.S. Congress, 1997a; 1997b; 1998). These commentators, the government, and NBAC have all recognized the need to strike the appropriate balance between adequate protection of research subjects and the advancement of biomedical research. They have implicitly or explicitly recognized a corresponding need for responsibility and accountability at every level of the research enterprise. Dating back to the early 1970s, a range of solutions have been proposed to address this need, which include the establishment of national, independent oversight body. (Advisory Committee on Human Radiation Experiments, 1996; Annas, 1994; 1998; Edgar and Rothman, 1995; Katz, 1972; 1993; 1995; U.S. Department of Health, Education and Welfare, 1973).

Capron (in this issue) in this issue does an excellent job of highlighting the history and current rationale for a national and independent oversight mechanism. I add my voice to the chorus of those advocating such a mechanism. In this article, I will briefly outline some additional reasons why creation of such a body would benefit efforts to promote the protection of human subjects research. Specifically, I will advocate for consideration of three broad, but key, functions that should be addressed in the development and operation of such a mechanism: (1) issue spotting, (2) guidance on identified issues, and (3) sampling and follow-up.

ISSUE SPOTTING

The first key function that should be required of national, independent oversight is *issue spotting*. In our fast paced world where new techno-logical advances are reported every day in the national media, there is clearly a need for consideration of complex social, ethical and legal implications of such research—in advance, and in-depth, and with expert and public participation. At the same time, there are recurring issues and gaps in research policy that have real, everyday repercussions, but that do not incite high level debate and may not be recognized as problems that are more widespread. For example, empirical research performed by the Advisory Committee on Human Radiation Experi-ments (1996) provided evidence of the persisting need to address central issues in human subjects protection. These issues included: the quality of informed consent; the confusion by patient-subjects and investigators regarding the distinction between research and therapy; therapeutic misconception by researchers and patient-subjects; blur-ring roles of physician-investigators; as well as issues related to par-ticular subject populations, such as those with cognitive impairments.

Institutional review boards (IRBs) are on the front lines of research protection and are in a position to recognize issues in need of prompt and ongoing attention, and to share their successes and failures in addressing them. The topics covered in agendas at national conferences sponsored by the federal Office of Protection from Research Risks and the professional organization focused on IRB issues (PRIMR— Public Responsibility in Medicine and Research), and the email cor-respondence on MCWIRB (a national listserv for IRB administrators and others interested in human subjects research ethics issues) show that to be true. But no formal, routine mechanism exists to facilitate such sharing of information and resolution of difficult issues.

Indeed, under our current system of human subjects protections, an efficient means does not exist for identifying, reporting and accessing this type of information—a process of issue spotting. One of NBAC's recommendations partially accomplishes this goal, but only in a responsive way, and with a specific focus on research on sub-jects with impaired decision-making capacity. In Recommenda-tion 2, NBAC asks that the U.S. Department of Health and Human Services (DHHS) establish a special standing panel on research involving persons with mental disorders that may affect decision-making capacity. The stated tasks of the panel would be to review certain problematic protocols forwarded by IRBs, and to promulgate guidelines for local IRBs. Thus, NBAC relies solely on a referral mechanism originating in IRBs to identify difficult protocols for resolution in this limited area of research. In addition, the proposed panel would be housed in the DHHS, raising a potential conflict of interest issue about the location of the current Office of Protection from Research Risks (OPRR) (GAO, 1996). A national, independent oversight body with wider scope could address these concerns and fulfill this coordinated issue spotting function.

GUIDANCE ON IDENTIFIED ISSUES

The second key function that should be required of national, independent oversight is *guidance on identified issues*. It is vital that we as a community arrive at a shared understanding about ethical approaches to research with human subjects. In order for guidance to have credibility, it is essential that identified issues are discussed and deliberated in the sunshine, and with the advice of experts (i.e., investigators, IRB members, and scholars), as well as advocates, potential subjects and interested members of the public. For consistency of process and focus, it is essential that guidance ultimately be delivered from a recognized source that is independent from any funding mechanism. A vehicle for national, independent oversight could address these needs for both credibility and consistency. In NBAC's Recommendation 2, one of the functions of the special standing panel located at DHHS would be to promulgate guidelines in response to the difficult issues identified, and NBAC provides an example of how a constituted body might function. But, as stated above, it is too narrowly focused to be of general applicability to human subjects research issues.

Guidance will not be successful without dissemination. Some mechanisms for dissemination include email lists of IRB chairs, web-based publication, and periodic reports. Moreover, guidances are insufficient without education and training for current and future researchers. As of now, the only governmental requirement for training or education in ethics of human subjects research affects only a very small proportion of future investigators (Mastroianni and Kahn, 1998, in press). The roles of national, independent oversight should include acting as a resource for institutional efforts to educate researchers, students and trainees in the ethics of human subjects research.

Another issue that needs to be resolved is whether the status of the oversight body's advice is guidance only or whether it has some regulatory force. It should be recognized that systematic identification of issues, discussed above, would create impetus for guidances that are responsive to the needs of the research community. A credible and consistent process will help to ensure a willing acceptance of guidance. Repeated failure to follow guidances is either an indication that they are not properly formulated or may indicate a need for requirements in the form of regulations. Only follow-up will indicate whether this is the case. The challenge then becomes how to ensure successful implementation of guidances, as addressed below.

SAMPLING AND FOLLOW-UP

The third key function that should be required of national, independent oversight is *sampling and follow-up*. While implementation of guidances must take place at the local level, there is a need to assess its quality. It is physically impossible for national, independent oversight to monitor all implementation of guidances at the level of every research project. Targeted, routine sampling at both the IRB and subject level is a mechanism that has been recommended by the Advisory Committee on Human Radiation Experiments (1996) and by Edgar and Rothman as well (1995). In addition, sampling would also support the issue spotting function mentioned earlier. Indeed, NBAC recognized the value of sampling: it undertook limited form of protocol sampling for issue spotting purposes in the context of their report (the Protocol Project, NBAC, 1998, p. 13), and suggested that interviews of potential subjects for their perspectives on research would be beneficial to the work of the standing panel it proposed (NBAC, 1998, Recommendation 19). Even more importantly, sampling inserts a level of accountability on the part of investigators, IRBs and institutions. There also may be a role for pilot studies to assess the practical aspects of implementation, before guidances or regulations are put into place.

PRACTICAL ISSUES

I would like to suggest that consideration of the three key functions briefly introduced here would help ensure attention to ethical issues arising in the conduct of human subjects research. They also raise practical questions in need of attention.

First, should we separate the issue spotting, guidance, sampling and follow-up functions from enforcement of human subjects protections? An oversight body with enforcement authority offers the benefit of greater influence in research policy, but it risks being viewed as just another layer in bureaucracy, perhaps reducing its credibility.

Second, any effort to improve human subjects protection will fail without sufficient funding. The NBAC report acknowledges this, and simply recommends that public, private and academic research sponsors arrive at a solution to this problem (NBAC, 1998, Recommendation 21). Funding could be obtained through direct or indirect costs supported by public and private sponsors, the President could tax executive branch agencies, since most if not all, engage in human subjects research, or Congress could allocate necessary resources. The latter two approaches are less desirable, because they are subject to the vagaries of politics. There must be a constant, predictable, reliable source of funding for any such effort to succeed.

And finally, there are numerous procedural issues that need to be addressed that are beyond the scope of this brief paper. They include consideration of how to ensure that such an entity would not become another layer of bureaucracy that risks becoming unresponsive to the community it is designed to serve. Also, there needs to be a way to include within its purview research across both the public and private spheres.

To conclude, trust is key to balancing the tension between protecting research subjects and fostering advances in biomedical research. To ensure this trust, we need accountability at every level of the research enterprise combined with a system of checks and balances. NBAC has attempted to do this within the limited context of one subpopulation of potential research subjects. A mechanism for national, independent oversight, that includes the three key functions outlined here, would be an important step in ensuring that this trust is maintained.

REFERENCES

Advisory Committee on Human Radiation Experiments (1996). *The Human Radiation Experiments: Final Report of the Advisory Committee.* New York, Oxford: Oxford University Press.

Annas, G. (1994). Will the real bioethics (commission) please stand up? *Hastings Center Report* 24(1): 19–21.

Annas, G.J. (1998). Human cloning: a choice or an echo? *University of Dayton Law Review* 23(2): 248–275.

DHHS-IG (Department of Health and Human Services-Inspector General) (1998). *Institutional Review Boards: A Time for Reform,* Testimony before the Committee on Government Reform and Oversight, Subcommittee on Human Resources, U.S. House of Representatives, 11 June (Washington, D.C.: DHHS-IG). Available at http://www.hhs.gov/progorg/oig/. Accessed 2/7/99.

Edgar, H. and Rothman, D.J. (1995). The institutional review board and beyond: future challenges to the ethics of human experimentation. *The Milbank Quarterly* 73(4): 489–506.

GAO (Government Accounting Office) (1996). *Scientific Research: Continued Vigilance Critical to Protecting Human Subjects,* Report to the Ranking Minority Member, Committee on Governmental Affairs, U.S. Senate, GAO/HEHS-96-72 (Washington, D.C.: Government Accounting Office) Available at http://www.gao.gov/reports.htm. Accessed 2/5/99.

Katz, J. (1972). *Experimentation With Human Beings: The Authority of the Investigator, Subject, Professions, and State in the Human Experimentation Process.* New York, Russell Sage Foundation.

Katz, J. (1993). Human experimentation and human rights. *St. Louis University Law Journal* 38(1): 7–54.

Katz, J. (1995). Do we need another advisory commission on human experimentation? *Hastings Center Report* 25(1): 29–31.

Mastroianni A. and Kahn J. (1998). The importance of expanding current training in responsible conduct of research. *Academic Medicine* 73(12): 1249–1254.

Mastroianni A. and Kahn J. (in press). Encouraging accountability in research: a pilot assessment of training efforts. *Accountability in Research* xx(xx): xx–xx.

Moreno, J.D. (1998). IRBs under the microscope. *Kennedy Institute of Ethics Journal* 8(3): 329–337.

NBAC (National Bioethics Advisory Commission) (1998). *Research Involving Persons With Mental Disorders That May Affect Decisionmaking Capacity: Report and Recommendations of the National Bioethics Advisory Commission,* Vol. I. Available at http://bioethics.gov/nbac.html.

Phillips, D.F. (1996). Institutional review boards under stress: will they explode or change? *JAMA* 276(20): 1623–1626.

U.S. Congress (1997a). Human Research Subject Protection Act of 1997, Senate Bill 193, 105th Congress.

U.S. Congress (1997b). *Oversight of NIH and FDA: Bioethics and the Adequacy of Informed Consent: Hearings Before the House Comm. on Gov't Reform and Oversight,*105th Congress.

U.S. Congress (1998). *Institutional Review Boards (IRBS): A System in Jeopardy? Hearing before the Subcomm. on Human Resources of the House Comm. on Government Reform and Oversight,* 105th Congress Federal News Service transcript available in LEXIS, News Library, Script file.

U.S. Department of Health, Education and Welfare, Public Health Service (1973). *Final Report of the Tuskegee Syphilis Study Ad Hoc Advisory Panel.* Washington, D.C.: U.S. Government Printing Office.

[18]

Regulating Research for the Decisionally Impaired: Implications for Mental Health Professionals

Marshall B. Kapp[1]

Mental health professionals, in fulfilling their different roles, often become involved with research protocols involving decisionally impaired current or prospective human subjects, many of whom are elderly. The opening section of this paper briefly describes the present regulatory environment regarding human subjects research, followed by an overview of the Institutional Review Board (IRB) process. There then ensues an enumeration of some of the general criticisms of the current regulatory scheme that have been enunciated recently. Particular concerns concerning decisionally impaired persons as research subjects are then addressed, referring when applicable to the recommendations made by the National Bioethics Advisory Commission (NBAC) in its 1998 report on this subject and the implications of those recommendations for mental health professionals.

KEY WORDS: regulation; research; law; ethics.

Underscoring its importance as a current subject of vital national concern for older persons and their professional and personal caregivers, "Assessing Research Risks and Potential Benefits When the Subjects Are Incapable of Informed Consent" was the topic chosen for attention by the 1999 Congress of Clinical Societies sponsored by the American Geriatrics Society. There are a variety of contexts in which mental health professionals may come into contact with the constellation of legal and ethical issues raised by biomedical and behavioral research protocols proposing to use decisionally impaired persons, many of whom are older, as human subjects. Mental health professionals may need to deal with these issues in their varied roles as researchers, treating clinicians, consultants hired to evaluate decisional capacity, Institutional Review Board (IRB) members, public or agency policy makers (or both), administrators, funders or reviewers of grant proposals, patient advocates, and intermediate consumers or users of research results.

This paper attempts to provide guidance to mental health professionals who, while fulfilling these often distinct but sometimes conflicting roles (Marquis, 1999; Rabins, 1998), become involved with research protocols involving decisionally impaired actual or prospective human subjects, with particular emphasis on the elderly. The next section briefly describes the present regulatory environment regarding human subjects research, followed

[1]Departments of Community Health and Psychiatry, Wright State University School of Medicine, Dayton, Ohio 45401-0927; e-mail: marshall.kapp@wright.edu.

by an overview of the IRB process. Next, there is an enumeration of some of the general criticisms of the current regulatory scheme that have been enunciated recently. Particular concerns regarding decisionally impaired persons as research subjects are then addressed, referring when applicable to the recommendations made in the National Bioethics Advisory Commission's report on this subject and to the implications of these recommendations for mental health professionals (NBAC, 1998).

REGULATORY ENVIRONMENT

Background and General Provisions

The historical developments leading up to the current state (Destro, 1997) of government command and control regulation of biomedical and behavioral research involving human subjects in the United States have been amply chronicled (Jonsen, 1998; Rothman, 1991; Wolpe *et al.*, 1999). Beginning with the Nuremberg Code, adopted in 1947 for use in Nazi war crimes trials in which defendant physicians tried to justify their inhumane treatment of human beings under the guise of scientific experimentation (Annas and Grodin, 1992), principles determining the proper conduct of human experimentation have been formalized into over 30 different international guidelines and ethical codes (Brody, 1998).

In the United States, federal government involvement in the regulation of research began in 1966. Officials at the U.S. Public Health Service (PHS) became concerned about the increasing frequency with which human subjects were being used in research. Formulation of a formal PHS policy was initiated, and resulting guidelines were eventually released in May, 1969. These guidelines served as a model for the development of a Department of Health, Education, and Welfare (DHEW; now Department of Health and Human Services [DHHS])—wide policy announced in April, 1971. This policy retained the institutional review process initiated by PHS; that is, the administrative review machinery was adjusted to cope with the rising tide of research being conducted with human subjects by switching from the prior centrally conducted, grant-by-grant review procedure to a model of individual institutional responsibility for compliance with ethical standards. The DHEW policy also included more specific requirements for obtaining informed consent than did the PHS guidelines.

In 1974, the DHEW policy was translated into enforceable regulations. These regulations formalized IRBs by withholding DHEW financial research support from institutions unless they had established an organizational review committee that was scrutinized and approved by DHEW. It became incumbent on these internal review committees to provide both general and special assurances of subject protection, as well as documentation of informed consent.

The next significant step was Congressional enactment of Public Law No. 93-348 on July 12, 1974. This statute, commonly known as the National Research Act, established the National Commission for the Protection of Human Subjects in Biomedical and Behavioral Research (the Belmont Commission). This body was charged to (1) conduct a comprehensive study to identify the basic ethical principles that should underlie the conduct of biomedical and behavioral research involving human subjects and (2) recommend research guidelines and administrative actions for the implementation of those guidelines. The accelerating public concern with the protection of subjects thought to be at special risk can be seen in Congress' specific directive to the Commission to investigate the ethics of research on, among other enumerated groups, the institutionalized mentally infirm (delineated as those "mentally retarded, emotionally disturbed, psychotic, or senile" persons who reside as patients in health care institutions). After extensive hearings, meetings, and deliberations, the Commission issued a series of reports and recommendations between 1975 and 1977.

The Commission followed the thrust of earlier federal pronouncements by recommending (1) that all research involving human subjects conducted at an institution that receives federal funding be reviewed by an IRB before it is begun and (2) that there be prior informed consent by the subject involved. Final regulations resulting from these recommendations were issued January 26, 1981, became effective July 27 of that year, and are codified at 45 Code of Federal Regulations, part 46.

These regulations originally applied on their face only to research involving human subjects that was conducted by the DHHS itself or was funded in whole or part by DHHS. However, most institutions conducting research have voluntarily agreed to apply the federal regulations to all of their research protocols regardless of the funding source for a particular study. Additionally, other federal agencies have adopted a Common Rule for human subjects protection in any research protocol that they sponsor, 45 Code of Federal Regulations, part 46, subpart A. Research involving testing of investigational drugs or medical devices are concurrently regulated by the federal Food and Drug Administration (FDA; Merrill, 1997).

Some states have also passed their own laws concerning conditions for human experimentation, requiring some manner of prior review and supervision. The precise content of these state statutes vary significantly, and particularly represent a (no pun intended) crazy quilt in terms of requirements for research involving decisionally impaired human subjects (Hoffmann and Schwartz, 1998).

In addition, private civil lawsuits may be brought by individual participants against researchers and protocol sponsors for violation of common law tort standards in the conduct of human subjects research. Further, constitutional protections predicated on an individual's Fourteenth Amendment right to due process and equal protection of the laws and the Eighth Amendment's prohibition against cruel and unusual punishment may be applicable to potential subjects of research conducted or sponsored by government agencies (Weiner, 1985).

The Institutional Review Board (IRB) Role

Research to which the federal Common Rule applies must be reviewed and approved by a local IRB and is thereafter subject to continuing IRB review. IRB approval is necessary initially and at least annually afterwards (Wichman, 1998). To approve a protocol, the IRB must determine that each of the following requirements is satisfied:

- Physical and psychological risks to subjects are minimized;
- Physical and psychological risks to subjects are reasonable in relation to anticipated benefits to those subjects and to the importance of the general knowledge that may reasonably be expected to result. This is arguably, and intentionally, an exercise in paternalism, the IRB deciding *for* individuals what is in their best interests (Ferenz, 1997);
- Selection of subjects is equitable;
- Informed consent will be obtained;

- Informed consent will be appropriately documented;
- Where appropriate, the research plan makes adequate provisions for monitoring the data collected to ensure the safety of subjects;
- Where appropriate, there are adequate provisions to protect the privacy of subjects and maintain the confidentiality of data.

The IRB must police the requirement that no human subject is involved in research unless legally effective informed consent has been obtained and "only under circumstances that provide the prospective subject . . . sufficient opportunity to consider whether or not to participate and that minimize the possibility of coercion or undue influence." The regulatory provisions for informed consent in research are basically a codification and extension of the common law that was developed in the therapeutic setting (Faden and Beauchamp, 1986).

Local IRBs themselves are monitored by the former Office of Protection from Research Risks (OPRR; McCarthy, 1995), which was recently moved from the National Institutes of Health to the Office of the Secretary, DHHS (Marwick, 1999) and renamed the office for Human Research Protections. OHRP may award an IRB either a Single Project Assurance that allows the IRB to review a single study or a Multiple Project Assurance that allows that IRB to review any number of studies over a 5-year period (Campbell, 1999a).

CRITICISMS OF THE CURRENT REGULATORY SCHEME

The effectiveness of the current regulatory scheme and the performance of IRBs in enforcing legal and ethical requirements have been harshly criticized lately from a number of directions, fueled largely by reports of abuses of subjects' rights. For example, in October 1995, the President's Advisory Committee on Human Radiation Experiments recommended continuous interpretation and application of ethical rules and principles for human subjects research in an open forum, and public debate and resolution on the appropriate guidelines for research with adults of questionable decisional capacity (Advisory Committee on Human Radiation Experiments, 1996; Faden, 1996). Studies commissioned for that Committee found that potential subjects regularly misunderstand the likely benefits and risks of participating in a particular protocol, and that the quality of local IRB reviews is far from consistent (Kass and Sugarman, 1996).

On June 11, 1998, the DHHS's Office of Inspector General (OIG) issued four reports on human subjects research and IRBs (Office of Inspector General, U.S. Department of Health and Human Services, 1998a,b,c,d). Among the concerns noted in these reports were: overburdened IRBs with insufficient time and resources to properly conduct initial and (especially) continuing reviews; ineffective monitoring of and response to adverse events happening to subjects; insufficient ethics training for researchers and IRB members; inadequate attention to evaluation of IRB effectiveness; and conflicts of interest between IRBs and the institutions of which they are a part, especially as research funds become more scarce (Dresser, 1998). Also in June 1998, the National Institutes of Health Office of Extramural Research released a contractor's report (James Bell Associates, 1998) which, although considerably less critical than the OIG reports, concluded that protection of human subjects could be improved by fine-tuning IRB procedures and providing increased education and training to researchers as well as to IRB members and staff. The OIG and NIH reports were accompanied by well-publicized Congressional hearings before the Subcommittee on Human Resources of the House Committee on Government Reform and Oversight.

In 1999, the National Institute of Mental Health (NIMH) announced creation of a new review panel to screen high risk intramural and extramural studies funded by the Institute and other initiatives driven "by a desire to make sure that the science in NIMH studies is good enough to justify the use of human subjects" (Marshall, 1999). Typically, IRBs have essentially taken a "hands-off" approach to review of the scientific merits of research protocols, ignoring the logical link between the quality of the science and the justification for allowing any risk to volunteers.

Amidst these critical activities, a small number of recent disciplinary actions against specific institutions have been imposed. For example, in the fall of 1998, OPRR temporarily suspended human subjects studies at Rush-Presbyterian-St. Luke's Medical Center, finding that some research projects there had enrolled ineligible persons, badgered patients into participating, and failed to obtain adequate consent (Manier, 1998). In 1999, OPRR temporarily suspended federally funded research at the West Los Angeles Veterans Affairs Medical Center and at Duke University, and faulted Mount Sinai School of Medicine and Queens College for putting children at unacceptable risk during psychiatric experiments that involved administering a controversial diet drug (Campbell, 1999b). In the same year, OPRR instructed the University of Illinois at Chicago to temporarily halt enrollment of new subjects in all federally supported human research because of informed consent irregularities. Citing administrative deficinecies, OPRR also shut down most human subjects research at the University of Colorado Health Sciences Center and its major affiliated institutions. In a preemptive move, the University of Rochester now requires all of its researchers who perform tests on human subjects to pass a written examination on pertinent safety and ethical issues (Carnevale, 1999).

Several particular types of biomedical and behavioral research studies, disproportionately utilizing mentally impaired individuals as research subjects, have been the target of specific ethical scrutiny. Regardless of the potential subjects' decisional capacity, but especially when they are unusually psychologically vulnerable, there is special concern about the necessity and safety of: placebo controlled clinical trials, wherein subjects may be denied, by virtue of random assignment to the placebo control group, the chance to receive a direct benefit from a proven treatment (Baer, 1996; Farlow, 1998; Hellman and Hellman, 1991; Karlawish and Whitehouse, 1998; Knopman et al., 1998; McCarthy, 1998; Rothman and Michels, 1994; Weijer, 1999); medication washout studies, in which effective medication for the subject's specific medical or mental problem is taken away from the subject so that the medication's effects do not confound the results obtained by the subject receiving an experimental intervention; and symptom provocation (challenge) experiments, in which subjects are given increasingly higher doses of the study intervention until certain undesirable symptoms have been activated (Abelson et al., 1994; Janowsky and Overstreet, 1995; Mohs et al., 1985).

PARTICULAR CONCERNS AND RECOMMENDATIONS REGARDING THE DECISIONALLY IMPAIRED

No Specific Regulations

The Belmont Commission recommended in 1978 that, at least for individuals institutionalized as mentally disabled, the federal government should promulgate distinct regulations controlling human subjects research. Although proposed regulations were published, these were never made final (i.e., legally binding). Among the explanations for this purposeful inaction, beyond a vague admonition in the Common Rule that IRBs should be "particularly cognizant" of the needs of all vulnerable subjects and should require "additional safeguards" when such populations are included in a study, 42 Code of Federal Regulations sec. 46.111 (b), are (1) the objections of the mental health research community that specially targeted requirements would be cumbersome and stifle scientific progress and (2) acceleration of the trend toward deinstitutionalization of the mentally ill and developmentally disabled in the late 1970s and into the 1980s (Childress, 1998).

Neither has action been taken in response to subsequent calls for specific research regulations targeting the decisionally impaired. Recommendations in this vein have emanated from, among other sources, a National Institute on Aging (NIA)-sponsored study group that convened in the early 1980s to discuss the use of demented persons in research (Melnick and Dubler, 1985; Melnick *et al.*, 1984) and the President's Commission for the Study of Ethical Problems in Medicine and Biomedical and Behavioral Research (1983, pp. 54–56).

Lately, however, special protections for the decisionally impaired, both within institutions and the community, have become a renewed item of interest (Levine, 1996). The national Alzheimer's Association (1997, p. 3) has called "upon state and federal authorities to clarify existing laws and regulations as they relate to people with cognitive impairments." Among the other organizations that have developed and adopted relevant research guidelines in this sphere are the American College of Physicians (1989), the Council for International Organizations of Medical Sciences (1993, in collaboration with the World Health Organization), Council of Europe (de Wachter, 1997), and the British Medical Research Council (Medical Research Council Working Party on Research on the Mentally Incapacitated, 1991). The American Psychiatric Association has organized a work group for the purpose of formulating ethical guidelines for psychiatric researchers dealing with the decisionally impaired. Several scholars, laboring individually and within groups, also have weighed in with comprehensive policy proposals in the area (Dresser, 1996; High *et al.*, 1994; Keyserlingk *et al.*, 1995).

On December 2–3, 1997, the National Institutes of Health sponsored an Inter-Institute Conference on Research Involving Individuals With Questionable Capacity to Consent: Ethical Issues and Practical Considerations for IRBs. The latest significant foray into this arena was launched with the release of the NBAC (1998) report entitled "Research Involving Persons With Mental Disorders That May Affect Decisionmaking Capacity."

Why Use Decisionally Impaired Persons in Research?

One possible regulatory response to the ethical and legal quandaries that will be discussed below might be an outright ban on the use of decisionally impaired individuals in any research protocol. This is the threshold question confronting each of the groups and individuals involved in or recommending policy and practice in this subject area: Why ought decisionally impaired persons be even considered as potential human research subjects in the first place?

There are several reasons why a prohibitory approach would be unconscionable. First, such an approach would thwart any chance for achieving further scientific progress in diagnosing, preventing, curing, or caring for precisely those persons afflicted with dementia, schizophrenia, and other disorders jeopardizing decisional capacity (Hertzman, 1997). As put straightforwardly by one geropsychiatrist (Rabins, 1998, p. 26):

> If the important research questions could be answered by studying individuals with intact capacity to consent, then decisionally incapacitated subjects should not be included. However, most of the important research questions about dementia require the participation of individuals who have dementia. They cannot be answered by studying cognitively intact individuals or by studying animal models.

In accordance with this view is the American Geriatrics Society, Ethics Committee (1998, p. 1308):

> Research on the causes and treatments of dementia, management of the complications of dementia, or health services research related to problems experienced by people with dementia certainly warrant conducting research on subjects with dementia. Examples of research on conditions commonly associated with dementia include studies on pressure sores and urinary incontinence. People with dementia living in long-term care settings are appropriate subjects for research and should be selected on scientific and clinical grounds.

Conversely, NBAC (1998) would require IRBs to disapprove any research proposal seeking to use mentally impaired subjects if nonmentally impaired subjects could be used in the study instead.

Second, as stated by the Belmont Commission (National Commission for the Protection of Human Subjects of Biomedical and Behavioral Research, 1978, p. 58), "[P]rohibiting such research might harm the class of mentally infirm persons as a whole by depriving them of benefits they could have received if the research had proceeded." According to leaders of the National Alliance for the Mentally Ill (NAMI), "The existence of a hard and fast rule prohibiting research using decisionally incapacitated individuals as subjects would have the effect of barring those who are most severely ill from participating in research which may alleviate their suffering and provide them with significant benefits. This, in our opinion, would be unjust and unnecessary" (Flynn and Honberg, 1998, p. 181). Some of the most promising interventions may be available only on an investigational basis through participation in a research trial (Hall and Flynn, 1999). Moreover, while outcomes of a research protocol that might benefit a particular participant directly are possible, it is more likely that the knowledge gained will primarily benefit others similar to the protocol participants at some time in the future; the decisionally impaired, it may be argued, should not be deprived of the opportunity to practice altruism by voluntarily contributing to a future benefit that will be enjoyed by others.

At the same time, society must strike the proper balance between promoting appropriate research that moves the scientific frontiers forward, on one hand, and protecting individuals from being taken advantage of because of their vulnerability, on the other. Since "[i]n general, people who cannot provide their own informed consent deserve protection from exploitation," "enrolling subjects with dementia in research must be justified on scientific, clinical, and ethical grounds" (American Geriatrics Society, Ethics Committee, 1998, p. 1308). In other words, mental health professionals are obliged to ensure that decisionally impaired persons are enrolled in research studies only when they are needed, and not as a matter of convenience to or as a captive population for the investigator. One prominent set of ethics experts has recommended that federal regulations be amended to "include a requirement that principal investigators proposing research with human subjects who are cognitively impaired or who are at foreseeable risk of becoming cognitively impaired during the research process include a written section in the protocol that addresses the importance of the research and an assessment of the risks and benefits for the subject" (Moreno *et al.*, 1998, p. 1953).

Voluntariness

To be legally and ethically valid, a person's consent to participate as a human research subject must be given voluntarily, free from coercion (Weiner, 1985). Because voluntariness in this regard may be influenced by physical setting and the potential subject's dependency on others and susceptibility to suggestion and manipulation, assuring the presence of this element of consent may be problematic in the case of the decisionally impaired (Destro, 1997). Institutionalized individuals may be especially vulnerable to subtle or direct pressure to "volunteer" their participation in a research study.

Mental health professionals, functioning in their various roles, should work to minimize as much as possible those factors that might *unduly* exert influence or coercive effect on potential subjects. For example, many individuals who are asked to participate in research protocols agree to do so based on the misperception that the experimental intervention is likely to, and indeed is expected and intended to, provide them with direct benefit, rather than being expected and intended to generate generalizable data for future use, with any benefit to the particular subject welcome but only incidental to the research endeavor. Individuals with decisional impairments may be particularly vulnerable to the coercive influence of the therapeutic misconception (Appelbaum *et al.*, 1982), especially in light of the "sense of desperation" that many mentally disabled persons experience due to the personal disruption of their lives caused by their illnesses and the limited effectiveness of available treatments (Capron, 1999; Tanouye, 1999). By working to overcome misunderstandings among potential subjects about reasonably anticipated risks and benefits, and fostering the effective disclosure of accurate information (McEvoy and Keefe, 1999; Morin, 1998), mental health professionals can improve the level of voluntariness within the actual subject cohort.

Capacity

To understand such concepts as the difference between research and therapeutic interventions, a prospective human research subject must have the mental capacity to engage in a rational decision making process; individuals cannot autonomously, authentically volunteer to take part in research protocols if they are not able to comprehend material information about respective risks and benefits (Berg and Appelbaum, 1999). This requirement of decisional capacity poses substantial ethical and legal difficulties regarding the research participation of many mental health professionals' patients.

Some mentally disabled individuals lack sufficient decisional capacity to validly volunteer for research participation at the time enrollment is requested, while some who are capable of giving autonomous consent to participate at the inception of the protocol may subsequently become unable to give valid consent to continue that participation (Lieberman *et al.*, 1999). Importantly, however, mental disability per se does not necessarily equal decisional incapacity, which must be assessed on a decision-specific rather than a global basis (American Geriatrics Society, Ethics Committee, 1998), with a focus on function rather than clinical diagnosis (Michels, 1999). Many individuals with various forms of mental disability, including early dementia (Rabins, 1998) and schizophrenia (Pinals *et al.*, 1998; Stephenson, 1999), are nonetheless sufficiently able to consent on their own behalf to research participation if the disability is not too severe. NBAC (1998) has recommended that capable subjects' own consent be accepted as sufficient for enrollment even in protocols entailing greater than minimal risk with no prospect of direct benefit to the subject.

Ethicist Baruch Brody (1998) has suggested that better explanations of information may frequently "cure" what at first appears to be a decisional incapacity situation. Forensic psychiatrist Paul Appelbaum (1998) has chided his mental health colleagues for being too quick to discount the decisional capacity of many mental patients, urging that educational and other interventional efforts ought to be directed instead toward enhancing the decisional participation of those individuals. This position has been adopted by the American Psychiatric Association (1998, p. 1650):

> The identification of some degree of decision-making impairment in potential subjects need not result in their automatic exclusion from research participation. Many cognitively impaired subjects can give adequate consents when additional efforts are made to educate them about the nature and consequences of study participation.

IRBs have been roundly criticized for devoting too much attention to the minute parsing of the wording of written consent forms submitted as part of the research protocols being reviewed, while spending little if any time and resources monitoring the actual process of obtaining informed consent from human subjects (or their surrogates; Appelbaum, 1996). Of particular concern has been the virtual absence of IRB or other external oversight regarding identification of who should be assessing the present (let alone future) decisional capacity of prospective subjects and the standards and methods used to carry out the capacity assessment (Derrickson, 1997). Several recommendations concerning the capacity assessment process have emerged recently.

NBAC (1998; Capron, 1999) advocated the promulgation of regulation mandating that, for any human subjects research protocol involving greater than minimal risk, there be an independent assessment of each potential subject's decisional capacity. This is consistent with NAMI's position (Flynn and Honberg, 1998), which recognizes possible risks of error, in either direction, in the way that subjects' capacity assessment ordinarily is handled today:

> [T]here may, in some instances, be incentives for researchers not to be vigilant in monitoring the capacity of vulnerable research participants or in failing to determine that certain individuals lack capacity, if such determinations will delay or interfere with the course of the research protocol. On the opposite side of the spectrum, ... [there may be] incentives for potential subjects to be found lacking in decisional capacity, ... [since] "Once a patient is deemed incapable, his or her ability to have an objection of continued participation honored is severely ... curtailed by provisions allowing for override of the objection." (quoting T.D. v. New York State Office of Mental Health, 1996, p. 187.)

The British Medical Research Council's Working Party on Research on the Mentally Incapacitated (1991) recommended that the determination of decisional capacity be made by the potential subject's physician if the physician is not involved in the research protocol; otherwise, it should be made by an independent party acceptable to the committee that reviews and approves the research protocol. Neither NBAC, NAMI, nor the British Working Party have gone so far as the New York State Court of Appeals in T.D. v. New York State Office of Mental Health (OMH; 1996), which compelled a formal judicial assessment of incompetency for every potential research subject receiving services in a facility operated or licensed by the OMH.

NBAC also recommended that IRBs require that, in each protocol involving greater than minimal risk, the investigator explicitly describe to the IRB the process to be used to assess the decisional capacity of potential human subjects. Moreno *et al.* (1998), too, would command researchers to explain how capacity will be evaluated, both at the start of a protocol and as capacity changes during the course of the research. The American Psychiatric Association (1998) has issued guidelines regarding both procedures and standards for assessing decision making capacities. Although numerous commentators (Appelbaum, 1997; DeRenzo *et al.*, 1998) have endorsed development of standardized written instruments for assessing capacity to decide about research participation (as well as to decide about other matters), this author elsewhere has cautioned against placing too much weight on the quantitative results of testing with such instruments (Kapp and Mossman, 1996).

Surrogate Decision Making

When a prospective research subject lacks mental capacity to personally consent to or refuse participation in a research protocol, the investigator ordinarily looks to a surrogate decision maker to act on behalf of the incapacitated potential subject. Who qualifies as a surrogate for this purpose has, in theory, depended on individual states' laws pertaining to guardianship/conservatorship, the permissible scope of advance medical directives, and family surrogacy in the medical sphere. In practice, even in the absence of clearly delineated legal authority, investigators normally rely on available "next of kin" as a matter of longstanding custom to decide about research participation. Among the problems noted regarding the current surrogate decision making practice are possible conflicts of interest between surrogate and subject, discordance of preferences between surrogate and subject (e.g., because possible benefits like "improvement in the quality of life" often are very subjective [Hertzman, 1997, p. 19]), the cumbersomeness of relying on surrogates, and in an increasing number of situations the unavailability of a capable and willing person to act as a conscientious and timely surrogate (Baskin *et al.*, 1998).

In 1964, the Declaration of Helsinki softened the previous absolute ban on surrogate consent to research participation by allowing the legal guardians of incompetent persons to provide consent on their behalf, at least for protocols offering a realistic likelihood of direct benefit to the individual subjects (Michels, 1999). NBAC (1998) in its recommendations distinguishes among different categories of research.

For protocols involving only minimal risk, NBAC would permit subject enrollment if:

- Consent is waived by the IRB per current regulations; or
- A capable subject gives consent; or
- The subject has given Prospective Authorization (PA) and the Legally Authorized Representative (LAR) consents; or
- The subject's LAR gives permission.

For protocols presenting greater than minimal risk but offering a prospect of direct benefit to subjects, NBAC would allow subject enrollment when:

- The subject gives consent; or
- The subject has given PA and the LAR consents; or
- The subject's LAR consents.

For research protocols involving greater than minimal risk and no prospect of direct benefit to that study's human subjects, a category into which most research seeking to enroll the mentally impaired probably falls, NBAC, as well as the American Geriatrics Society, Ethics Committee (1998), would permit subjects to be enrolled only under the following conditions:

- A capable subject consents; or
- The subject has given PA and the LAR consents; or
- The protocol is approved by a new national IRB that NBAC suggests be created as the DHHS Special Standing Panel, or under special IRB guidelines established by the Panel, and the subject's LAR consents.

Central to these recommendations are the concepts of PA and the LAR. Under the NBAC proposal, a capable person may give PA to future research participation. PA may be either of the instruction (e.g., living will) or the proxy (e.g., durable power of attorney) type. For an instruction type of PA to be valid, NBAC would require that the risks and benefits of the specific class of research involved must have been explained to the prospective subject while he or she was still decisionally capable; moreover, the greater the risk of the research, the more specific PA should be.

In the NBAC formulation, an LAR may enroll a subject in a research protocol after the subject has become decisionally incapacitated, provided:

- The LAR uses substituted judgment (i.e., makes the choice that the subject would have made if currently able to make and express his or her own autonomous decision about research participation);
- The LAR monitors the subject's recruitment for, participation in, and withdrawal from the study; and
- The LAR is chosen by the subject or is a relative or friend.

According to NBAC, the LAR for research purposes should be the same friend or relative of the prospective subject who is recognized under state law for purposes of clinical, therapeutic decision making.

The NBAC recommendations in many respects represent a proposed codification of ideas that are widely promoted already. Regarding recognition of a proxy type of PA for research purposes, for example, Moreno *et al.* (1998, p. 1953) have argued:

> The possibility of enrollment of an incompetent subject in research involving interventions that are potentially beneficial to the individual patient-subject and in research that involves minimal incremental risk should be part of the durable power of attorney for health care authority for several reasons: it is an expression of patient autonomy, it is an opportunity for the surrogate to act for the potential benefit of the now incompetent subject, and it might benefit future patients and therefore society in general.

Others support this idea as well (Dukoff and Sunderland, 1997; Sunderland and Dukoff, 1996), with the American Geriatrics Society, Ethics Committee (1998, p. 1309) agreeing with NBAC that "[s]urrogates should be allowed to refuse to enroll potential subjects or to withdraw a subject from an ongoing trial on the basis that the surrogate believes that the research protocol is not in the best interests of the subject or is not what the subject intended, even if that decision would conflict with the subject's advance directive."

On another note, NBAC's recommendation 7, that "Any potential or actual subject's objection to enrollment or to continued participation in a research protocol must be heeded in all circumstances," that is, guaranteeing to even incapacitated persons the right to veto their LAR's consent to research participation, embodies the prevailing ethical consensus (British Medical Research Council, Working Party on Research on the Mentally Incapacitated, 1991; Flynn and Honberg, 1998, pp. 184–185). According to the American Geriatrics Society, Ethics Committee (1998, p. 1309), "In general, the refusal of a (potential) subject, even if that subject has lost decision-making capacity, should be followed."

However, despite a vigorous defense by most NBAC members (Capron, 1999; Charo, 1999), some of that body's majority recommendations have been criticized. NBAC member Bernard Lo filed a partial dissent (NBAC, 1998), saying that he would permit surrogate consent to enroll decisionally incapacitated persons in protocols involving a small increase over minimal risk if there were the meaningful possibility of significant benefit to the public in the future. The Alzheimer's Association (1997) position on dementia research, while largely consistent with the NBAC report, would permit, for greater than minimal risk research when there is no reasonable chance for benefit to the individual, enrollment of those persons who are capable of giving their own informed consent or have executed a research specific advance directive, and who have a proxy available to monitor the individual's involvement in the protocol.

At least one prominent psychiatrist (Michels, 1999) has attacked NBAC's recommended requirement of both IRB and national review panel approval for research involving more than minimal risk with no real probability of benefit when the subject cannot personally consent, saying that "This represents an extraordinary shift of authority from the community in which the research is being conducted to a central body distant from both the subjects and the researchers." The same critic (Michels, 1999, p. 1428) opines that, regarding NBAC's recommendation for independent assessment of potential subjects' decisional capacity for all research involving more than minimal risk, "Many psychiatric researchers consider these recommended procedures expensive, cumbersome, and clinically insensitive to the experience of impaired subjects, and some patient advocates fear that the implied mistrust of care givers may have a negative effect on the doctor–patient relationship." The American Psychiatric Association has expressed agreement with these sentiments, adding that regulations singling out persons with mental disorders for special attention risks unfairly stigmatizing those individuals (News and Notes, 1999).

On another point, NBAC essentially left empowerment of LARs for research purposes up to state law, through statutes pertaining to guardianship/conservatorship and durable powers of attorney. Support has been expressed for recognizing the authority of family members to function in the surrogate role, even absent a formal transfer of power by a court or the decisionally capable potential subject, at least for protocols reasonably holding out the possibility of direct benefit (American College of Physicians, 1989; American Geriatrics Society, Ethics Committee, 1998; Flynn and Honberg, 1998; Rabins, 1998).

Some would place more stringent limitations on surrogate consent in the research context than those contained in the NBAC report. The then-Chairperson of the New York State Commission on Quality of Care for the Mentally Disabled would disallow any nontherapeutic research that exposes decisionally incapacitated human subjects to more than minimal risk, unless the person had explicitly authorized a proxy to consent to the specific type of research protocol involved.

> While competent adults are free to make martyrs of themselves in the cause of science, they do not have the license to make martyrs of other people by volunteering them for experiments that

expose them to significant risks, especially when those experiments cannot do them any good. The authorization for such research must reliably and authentically find its source in the exercise of free will by the subject when competent. (Sundram, 1998, p. 62.)

In a 1996 decision (T.D. v. New York State Office of Mental Health) that has been soundly condemned as erecting an enormously unnecessary and unwise barrier to the conduct of useful research on problems encountered by mentally disabled persons (Haimowitz *et al.*, 1997; Oldham *et al.*, 1998), the New York Court of Appeals effectively precluded the conduct of biomedical and behavioral research, regardless of funding source, using any person residing in facilities either owned or licensed by OMH. In reaction to this judicial overreaction to perceived ethical abuses in the preexisting research enterprise, the New York State Department of Health established an Advisory Work Group on Human Subject Research Involving the Protected Classes, which in early 1999 proposed, with adequate safeguards, allowing the conduct of research involving more than minimal risk on decisionally incapacitated subjects even in the absence of likely benefit to the subjects themselves (Birnbaum, 1999).

CONCLUSION AND IMPLICATIONS FOR MENTAL HEALTH PROFESSIONALS

The regulation of biomedical and behavioral research using mentally impaired persons as human subjects is in a dynamic state. Numerous recommendations for protecting vulnerable individuals while promoting medical progress have been suggested by commentators and official entities, such as NBAC. Although some of these recommendations would just explicitly codify current practice in the field, at the time this paper was being written none of the recommendations for changing the status quo had yet achieved legal status and the fate of these recommendations was difficult to predict.

Nevertheless, mental health professionals should draw some important guidance from the flurry of debate that has emerged in this arena, while awaiting the regulatory outcome. Some suggestions to mental health professionals have been interspersed throughout this paper already, while a few others are offered here.

First, extensive efforts should be exerted to prevent the sorts of abuses and dangers to the rights and well-being of mentally impaired individuals that have inspired some of the more radical recommendations for expanding the scope of external intrusion into the ethical conduct of research. In the T.D. case (1996), for example, the court based its overreaching decision in large measure on its perception that many biomedical and behavioral researchers routinely and unethically exploit and abuse vulnerable, dependent, indeed often helpless, mental patients for their own personal and professional gain; mental health professionals must dispel this perception and any reality that underlies it.

Second, mental health professionals must understand that, no matter how sincerely researchers attempt to respect and enhance subject autonomy by meeting and even exceeding regulatory mandates to explicitly set out information about risks, benefits, and conflicts of interest, ultimately most people—perhaps especially including those with mental impairments—will still trust and rely on their treating clinicians to tell them what to do. A treating clinician merely mentioning the possibility of enrollment in a research study more frequently than not is interpreted by the patient as irresistibly endorsing both the study and that patient's personal participation in it (Kass *et al.*, 1996). Consequently, mental health professionals working in the treating clinician role must be extremely sensitive to the power of persuasion they yield.

Third, because many recommendations would draw regulatory distinctions among different research protocols on the basis of reasonably anticipated risks and benefits, mental health researchers need to assiduously work to design studies so as to minimize risks to subjects and maximize potential benefits (i.e., useful knowledge gained) to society and, when possible, individual participants. Additionally, use of mentally impaired persons as research subjects must be justified at the time the protocol is designed, with alternative subject populations carefully considered.

Fourth, mental health professionals must continue to hone procedures and standards for assessing potential subjects' capacity to make autonomous decisions about research participation. For persons determined to possess sufficient present decisional capacity, mental health professionals should discuss the opportunity to anticipate subsequent incapacity by timely executing written advance directives either expressing the individual's wishes regarding participation in research protocols in the future or appointing a surrogate to make those decisions on the incapacitated person's behalf. Once enrollment of subjects has occurred, involved mental health professionals have a legal, ethical, and scientific responsibility to closely monitor, and initiate appropriate responses to, the risks and benefits that actually materialize for particular subjects.

Mental health professionals should be thoroughly conversant with existing, as well as credible proposed, statutes, administrative rules, and judicial decisions pertaining to research involving mentally impaired human subjects. In the final analysis, though, no set of regulations can take the place of the commitment to ethical conduct that ought to permeate the research enterprise and all of the professionals who play a part—direct or indirect—in that enterprise. "One danger of excessive regulations is that they can actually undermine researchers' sense of moral responsibility as their attention shifts from their obligation to research subjects to their compliance with the regulations" (Michels, 1999, p. 1429). The most significant contribution that mental health professionals, acting in their various roles and functions, can make to the welfare of present mentally impaired persons and to future generations is to guard against that danger.

REFERENCES

Abelson, J. L., Nesse, R. M., and Vinik, A. I. (1994). Pentagastrin infusions in patients with panic disorder, II: Neuroendocrinology. *Biol. Psychiatry* 36: 84–96.

Advisory Committee on Human Radiation Experiments. (1996). *The Human Radiation Experiments*, Oxford University Press, New York.

Alzheimer's Association. (1997, May 18). *Ethical Issues in Dementia Research: Position of the Alzheimer's Association*, Chicago.

American College of Physicians. (1989). Cognitively impaired subjects. *Annals Intern. Med.* 111: 843–848.

American Geriatrics Society, Ethics Committee. (1998). Informed consent for research on human subjects with dementia. *J. Am. Geriatr. Soc.* 46: 1308–1310.

American Psychiatric Association. (1998). Guidelines for assessing the decision-making capacities of potential research subjects with cognitive impairment. *Am. J. Psychiatry* 155: 1649–1650.

Annas, G. J., and Grodin, M. A. (eds.). (1992). *The Nazi Doctors and the Nuremberg Code: Human Rights in Human Experimentation*, Oxford University Press, New York.

Appelbaum, P. S. (1996). Examining the ethics of human subjects research. *Kennedy Inst. Ethics J.* 6: 283–287.

Appelbaum, P. S. (1997). Patients' competence to consent to neurobiological research. In Shamoo, A. E. (ed.), *Ethics in Neurobiological Research With Human Subjects*, Gordon and Breach, Amsterdam, The Netherlands, pp. 253–263.

Appelbaum, P. S. (1998). Missing the boat: Competence and consent in psychiatric research. *Am. J. Psychiatry* 155: 1486–1488.

Appelbaum, P. S., Roth, L. H., and Lidz, C. W. (1982). The therapeutic misconception: Informed consent in psychiatric research. *Int. J. Law Psychiatry* 5: 319–329.

Baer, N. (1996). Debate about placebos points to issue surrounded by many shades of grey. *Can. Med. Assn. J.* 155: 1475–1476.

Baskin, S. A., Morris, J., Ahronheim, J. C., Meier, D. E., and Morrison, R. S. (1998). Barriers to obtaining consent in dementia research: Implications for surrogate decision-making. *J. Am. Geriatr. Soc.* 46: 287–290.

Berg, J. W., and Appelbaum, P. S. (1999). Subjects' capacity to consent to neurobiological research. In Pincus, H. A., Lieberman, J. A., and Ferris, S. (eds.), *Ethics in Psychiatric Research: A Resource Manual for Human Subjects Protection*, American Psychiatric Association, Washington, DC, pp. 81–106.

Birnbaum, G. (1999, Jan. 17). State eyes 'no consent' medical testing. *The New York Post*, p. 5.

British Medical Research Council, Working Party on Research on the Mentally Incapacitated. (1991). *The Ethical Conduct of Research on the Mentally Incapacitated*, London, UK.

Brody, B. A. (1998). *The Ethics of Biomedical Research: An International Perspective*, Oxford University Press, New York.

Campbell, P. W. (1999a, May 28). Government restores Duke U's right to conduct research on humans. *Chron. Higher Educ.* A30.

Campbell, P. W. (1999b, June 25). Federal officials fault 2 New York institutions for research risks to children. *Chron. Higher Educ.* A43.

Capron, A. M. (1999). Ethical and human-rights issues in research on mental disorders that may affect decision-making capacity. *N. Eng. J. Med.* 340: 1430–1434.

Carnevale, D. (1999, July 23). Rochester requires test on research on humans. *Chron. Higher Educ.* A59.

Charo, R. A. (1999, March 26). Academe should support new guidelines to protect mentally ill research subjects. *Chron. Higher Educ.* B9.

Childress, J. F. (1998). The National Bioethics Advisory Commission: Bridging the gaps in human subjects research protection. *J. Health Care Law Policy* 1: 105–122.

Council for International Organizations of Medical Sciences. (1993). *International Ethical Guidelines for Biomedical Research Involving Human Subjects*, Geneva, Switzerland.

DeRenzo, E. G., Conley, R. R., and Love, R. (1998). Assessment of capacity to give consent to research participation: State-of-the-art and beyond. *J. Health Care Law Policy* 1: 66–87.

Derrickson, D. (1997). Informed consent to human subject research: Improving the process of obtaining informed consent from mentally ill persons. *Fordham Urb. Law J.* XXV: 143–165.

Destro, R. A. (1997). Government oversight. In Shamoo, A. E. (ed.), *Ethics in Neurobiological Research With Human Subjects*, Gordon and Breach, Amsterdam, The Netherlands, pp. 81–99.

de Wachter, M. A. M. (1997). The European convention in bioethics. *Hastings Cent. Rep.* 27: 13–23.

Dresser, R. (1998). Time for new rules on human subjects research? *Hastings Cent. Rep.* 28: 23–24.

Dresser, R. (1996). Mentally disabled research subjects. *JAMA* 276: 67–72.

Dukoff, R., and Sunderland, T. (1997). Durable power of attorney and informed consent with Alzheimer's disease patients: A clinical study. *Am. J. Psychiatry* 154: 1070–1075.

Faden, R. R. (1996). The Advisory Committee on Human Radiation Experiments: Reflections on a Presidential commission. *Hastings Cent. Rep.* 26: 5–10.

Faden, R. R., and Beauchamp, T. (1986). *A History and Theory of Informed Consent*, Oxford University Press, New York.

Farlow, M. R. (1998). New treatments in Alzheimer disease and the continued need for placebo-controlled trials. *Arch. Neurol.* 55: 1396–1398.

Ferenz, L. (1997). Ethical considerations of federal guidelines and models of moral responsibility governing neuropharmacologic research. In Hertzman, M., and Feltner, D. E. (eds.), *The Handbook of Psychopharmacology Trials: An Overview of Scientific, Political, and Ethical Concerns*, New York University Press, New York, pp. 23–45.

Flynn, L. M., and Honberg, R. S. (1998). Achieving proper balance in research with decisionally-incapacitated subjects. *J. Health Care Law Policy* 1: 174–192.

Haimowitz, S., Delano, S. J., and Oldham, J. M. (1997). Uninformed decisionmaking: The case of surrogate research consent. *Hastings Cent. Rep.* 27: 9–16.

Hall, L. L., and Flynn, L. (1999). Consumer and family concerns about research involving human subjects. In Pincus, H. A., Lieberman, J. A., and Ferris, S. (eds.), *Ethics in Psychiatric Research: A Resource Manual for Human Subjects Protection*, American Psychiatric Association, Washington, DC, pp. 219–238.

Hellman, S., and Hellman, D. S. (1991). Of mice but not men: Problems of the randomized clinical trial. *N. Eng. J. Med.* 324: 1585–1589.

Hertzman, M. (1997). The importance of clinical trials for central nervous system treatments. In Hertzman, M., and Feltner, D. E. (eds.), *The Handbook of Psychopharmacology Trials: An Overview of Scientific, Political, and Ethical Concerns*. New York University Press, New York, pp. 3–20.

High, D. M., Whitehouse, P. J., Post, S. G., and Berg, L. (1994). Guidelines for addressing ethical and legal issues in Alzheimer disease research: A position paper. *Alzheimer Dis. Assoc. Disord.* 8(suppl. 4): 66–74.

Hoffmann, D., and Schwartz, J. (1998). Proxy consent to participation of the decisionally impaired in medical research—Maryland's policy initiative. *J. Health Care Law Policy* 1: 123–153.

James Bell Associates. (1998, June 15). *Evaluation of NIH Implementation of Section 491 of the Public Health Service Act, Mandating a Program of Protection for Research Subjects*, NIH Contract No. N01-OD-2-2109.

Janowsky, D. S., and Overstreet, D. H. (1995). The role of acetylcholine mechanisms in the affective disorders. In Bloom, F. E., and Kupfer, D. J. (eds.), *Psychopharmacology: The Fourth Generation of Progress*, Raven, New York, pp. 945–956.

Jonsen, A. R. (1998). *The Birth of Bioethics*, Oxford University Press, New York.

Kapp, M. B., and Mossman, D. (1996). Measuring decisional capacity: Cautions on the construction of a 'capacimeter.' *Psychol. Pub. Policy Law* 2: 73–95.

Karlawish, J. H. T., and Whitehouse, P. J. (1998). Is the placebo control obsolete in a world after donepezil and Vitamin E? *Arch. Neurol.* 55: 1420–1424.

Kass, N. E., and Sugarman, J. (1996). Are research subjects adequately protected? A review and discussion of studies conducted by the Advisory Committee on Human Radiation Experiments. *Kennedy Inst. Ethics J.* 6: 271–282.

Kass, N. E., Sugarman, J., Faden, R., and Schoch-Spana, M. (1996). Trust: The fragile foundation of contemporary biomedical research. *Hastings Cent. Rep.* 26: 25–29.

Keyserlingk, E. W., Glass, K., Kogan, S., and Gauthier, S. (1995). Proposed guidelines for the participation of persons with dementia as research subjects. *Perspec. Biol. Med.* 38: 319–361.

Knopman, D., Kahn, J., and Miles, S. (1998). Clinical research designs for emerging treatments for Alzheimer disease: Moving beyond placebo-controlled trials. *Arch. Neurol.* 55: 1425–1429.

Levine, R. J. (1996). Proposed regulations for research involving those institutionalized as mentally infirm: A consideration of their relevance in 1995. *Accountab. Res.* 4: 177–186.

Lieberman, J. A., Stroup, S., Laska, E., Volavka, J., Gelenberg, A., Rush, A. J., Shear, K., and Carpenter, W. (1999). Issues in clinical research design: Principles, practices, and controversies. In Pincus, H. A., Lieberman, J. A., and Ferris, S. (eds.), *Ethics in Psychiatric Research: A Resource Manual for Human Subjects Protection*, American Psychiatric Association, Washington, DC, pp. 23–60.

Manier, J. (1998, Nov. 19). Rush is told why studies were halted. *Chicago Trib.* 1–1.

Marquis, D. (1999). How to resolve and ethical dilemma concerning randomized clinical trials. *N. Eng. J. Med.* 341: 691–693.

Marshall, E. (1999). NIMH to screen studies for science and human risks. *Science* 283: 464–465.

Marwick, C. (1999). Protecting subjects of clinical research. *JAMA* 282: 516–517.

McCarthy, C. (1995). When OPRR comes calling: Enforcing federal research regulations. *Kennedy Inst. Ethics J.* 5: 51–55.

McCarthy, J. (1998). Letter, placebo in research on schizophrenia. *Psychiatric Serv.* 49: 699.

McEvoy, J. P., and Keefe, R. S. E. (1999). Informing subjects of risks and benefits. In Pincus, H. A., Lieberman, J. A., and Ferris, S. (eds.), *Ethics in Psychiatric Research: A Resource Manual for Human Subjects Protection*, American Psychiatric Association, Washington, DC, pp. 129–157.

Medical Research Council Working Party on Research on the Mentally Incapacitated. (1991). *The Ethical Conduct of Research on the Mentally Incapacitated*, London, UK.

Melnick, V. L., and Dubler, N. N. (eds.). (1985). *Contemporary Issues in Biomedicine, Ethics, and Society*, Humana Press, Clifton, NJ.

Melnick, V. L., Dubler, N. N., Weisbard, A., and Butler, R. N. (1984). Clinical research in senile dementia of the Alzheimer type: Suggested guidelines addressing the ethical and legal issues. *J. Am. Geriatr. Soc.* 32: 531–536.

Merrill, R. A. (1997). FDA regulation of clinical drug trials. In Hertzman, M., and Feltner, D. E. (eds.), *The Handbook of Psychopharmacology Trials: An Overview of Scientific, Political, and Ethical Concerns*, New York University Press, New York, pp. 61–99.

Michels, R. (1999). Are research ethics bad for our mental health? *N. Eng. J. Med.* 340: 1427–1430.

Mohs, R. C., Davis, B. M., Greenwald, B. S., Mathe, A. A., Johns, C. A., Horvath, T. B., and Davis, K. L. (1985). Clinical studies of the cholinergic deficit in Alzheimer's disease, II: Psychopharmacologic studies. *J. Am. Geriatr. Soc.* 33: 749–757.

Moreno, J., Caplan, A. L., Wolpe, P. R., and the Members of the Project on Informed Consent, Human Research Ethics Group. (1998). Updating protections for human subjects involved in research. *JAMA* 280: 1951–1958.

Morin, K. (1998). The standard of disclosure in human subject experimentation. *J. Legal Med.* 19: 157–221.

National Bioethics Advisory Commission. (1998 Dec.). *Research Involving Persons with Mental Disorders That May Affect Decisionmaking Capacity*, Washington, DC.

National Commission for the Protection of Human Subjects of Biomedical and Behavioral Research. (1978). *Report and Recommendations: Research Involving Those Institutionalized As Mentally Infirm*, U.S. Government Printing Office, Washington, DC.

News and Notes. (1999). Research guidelines issued for persons with mental disorders and impaired capacity to make decisions. *Psychiatric Serv.* 50: 128–129.

Office of Inspector General, U.S. Department of Health and Human Services. (1998a). *Institutional Review Boards: Their Role in Reviewing Approved Research*, OEI-01-97-000190, Washington, DC.

Office of Inspector General, U.S. Department of Health and Human Services. (1998b). *Institutional Review Boards: Promising Approaches*, OEI-01-97-000191, Washington, DC.

Office of Inspector General, U.S. Department of Health and Human Services. (1998c). *Institutional Review Boards: The Emergence of Independent Boards*, OEI-01-97-000192, Washington, DC.

Office of Inspector General, U.S. Department of Health and Human Services. (1998d). *Institutional Review Boards: A Time for Reform*, OEI-01–97–000193, Washington, DC.

Oldham, J. M., Haimowitz, S., and Delano, S. J. (1998). Regulating research with vulnerable populations: Litigation gone awry. *J. Health Care Law Policy* 1: 154–173.

Pinals, D. A., Malhotra, A. K., Breier, A., and Pickar, D. (1998). Letter, Informed consent in schizophrenia research. *Psychiatric Serv.* 49: 244.

President's Commission for the Study of Ethical Problems in Medicine and Biomedical and Behavioral Research. (1983). *Summing Up*, U.S. Government Printing Office, Washington, DC.

Rabins, P. V. (1998). Issues raised by research using persons suffering from dementia who have impaired decisional capacity. *J. Health Care Law Policy* 1: 22–35.

Rothman, D. J. (1991). *Strangers at the Bedside*, Basic Books, New York.

Rothman, K. J., and Michels, K. B. (1994). The continuing unethical use of placebo controls. *N. Eng. J. Med.* 331: 394–398.

Stephenson, J. (1999). Probing informed consent in schizophrenia research. *JAMA* 281: 2273–2274.

Sunderland, T., and Dukoff, R. (1996). Informed consent with cognitively impaired patients: An NIMH perspective on the durable power of attorney. *Accountab. Res.* 4: 217–226.

Sundram, C. J. (1998). In harm's way; Research subjects who are decisionally impaired. *J. Health Care Law Policy* 1: 36–65.

Tanouye, E. (1999, Aug. 25). To avoid his brother's illness, a young man tries a risky experiment. *Wall Street J.* B1.

T. D. v. New York State Office of Mental Health, 650 N.Y.S.2d 173 (N.Y. App. Div. 1996).

Weijer, C. (1999). Placebo-controlled trials in schizophrenia: Are they ethical? *Schizophr. Res.* 35: 211–218.

Weiner, B. A. (1985). Rights of institutionalized persons. In Brakel, S. J., Parry, J., and Weiner, B. A. (eds.), *The Mentally Disabled and the Law* (3rd edn.), American Bar Foundation, Chicago.

Wichman, A. (1998). Protecting vulnerable research subjects: Practical realities of institutional review board review and approval. *J. Health Care Law Policy* 1: 88–104.

Wolpe, P. R., Moreno, J., and Caplan, A. L. (1999). Ethical principles and history. In Pincus, H. A., Lieberman, J. A., and Ferris, S. (eds.), *Ethics in Psychiatric Research: A Resource Manual for Human Subjects Protection*, American Psychiatric Association, Washington, DC, pp. 1–10.

[19]

ARE RESEARCH ETHICS BAD FOR OUR MENTAL HEALTH?

ROBERT MICHELS

PATIENTS with mental illness are much better off now than they were only a few decades ago. Diagnostic methods are more reliable, and treatments are more effective. Only a minority of psychiatric patients require long-term hospitalization, and the practice of psychiatry is now more like the practice of other medical specialties. At the same time, the prevalence of psychiatric disease is more clearly recognized. Five of the world's 10 leading causes of disability are psychiatric: depression, alcohol abuse, bipolar mood disorder, schizophrenia, and obsessive–compulsive disorder.[1] Each of these disorders has important genetic determinants and biologic correlates. In the past 40 years, specific effective treatments for each have replaced nonspecific concern and support.[2] We have developed pharmacologic agents for depression, mania, psychosis, obsessions, and panic, as well as agents that block the craving for drugs of abuse, calm hyperactive children, and slow the progress of Alzheimer's dementia. We have also developed psychological treatments for depression and methods of psychosocial management for patients with schizophrenia. This progress has been based on the immense growth of both basic and clinical psychiatric research. By 1995, academic departments of psychiatry were second only to departments of medicine in terms of funding for research.[3]

However, there has been concern about the ethical aspects of psychiatric research. Are mentally ill subjects especially vulnerable to exploitation? Are they competent to give informed consent? Are psychiatric research methods particularly dangerous? Are special procedures or regulations needed for such research? There have been attacks and defenses of psychiatric research in the courts, in the media, and in statements made by groups that advocate for the rights of the mentally ill.

Perhaps the most vexing ethical problem has concerned mentally ill patients who have a diminished capacity to consent to participate in research. The Nuremberg Code, formulated in 1947 as a result of the trial of Nazi physicians who had experimented on unwilling subjects, stated that "the voluntary consent of the human subject is absolutely essential."[4] Henry Beecher, a pioneer of research ethics, wrote in 1959 that this principle would "effectively cripple if not eliminate most research in the field of mental disease."[5] Society has struggled with this ethical dilemma ever since. There is agreement that research on human subjects requires informed consent but that, at the same time, we must learn as much as possible in order to improve the care of those who suffer from diseases that impair their capacity to provide informed consent. How do we proceed when these goals are in conflict, when conducting research on those who cannot themselves consent to participate in it is the route to improving their care?

In 1964, the Declaration of Helsinki softened the absolute ban of the Nuremberg Code by allowing the legal guardians of incompetent persons to provide consent on their behalf, at least for "therapeutic" research.[6] In 1974, the National Commission for the Protection of Human Subjects of Biomedical and Behavioral Research, which was created after the revelation of the exploitation of subjects in the Tuskegee study of syphilis, discussed the special problem of the use of vulnerable groups as research subjects. Its recommendations moved beyond both the Nuremberg Code and the Declaration of Helsinki. The commission argued that "prohibiting such research might harm the class of mentally infirm persons as a whole by depriving them of benefits they could have received if the research had proceeded."[7]

The commission suggested special regulations to govern research on "persons institutionalized as mentally infirm," but these regulations were viewed as overly burdensome and were never adopted. However, the commission's general comments paved the way for the so-called common rule. This is an executive order, first proposed in 1986 and issued in 1991, that governs the basic structure of regulations for research on human subjects conducted by the federal government or in facilities receiving federal funds.[8] The common rule recognizes the special problems of "vulnerable populations," including the mentally disabled. It requires that institutional review boards (IRBs) include additional safeguards to protect the rights of such groups[9] but provides no specific guidelines as to how IRBs should do so.

The National Bioethics Advisory Commission (NBAC) is the latest federal panel to address the issue. Its 17 members were appointed by President Bill Clinton in 1995 to advise the government on bioethical issues, and especially to "consider the problem of the rights and welfare of human research subjects." Its report was released in 1998.[10]

The NBAC reviewed judicial and public concerns about research on the mentally ill, including a 1992 lawsuit against the University of California at Los Angeles alleging that a research protocol involving a drug "washout" aggravated a patient's schizophrenic illness and led to his suicide.[11] (The university won in court, but its procedures were subsequently criticized by the Office for Protection from Research Risks of the National Institutes of Health. The patient's family has not permitted disclosure of the clinical data.) The NBAC also reviewed the series of judicial decisions in New York State that challenged regulations governing participation in research by persons who lack the capacity to give informed con-

The New England Journal of Medicine

sent,[12] and it reviewed media exposés (such as a recent series of articles in the *Boston Globe*[13]). The commission concluded that there were three justifications for its work: first, the perceived regulatory gap since the rejection of the recommendations of the earlier commission (although it did not find evidence that the current regulations governing IRBs are not effective); second, the apparently inadequate protection of human subjects in some cases (although the NBAC did not itself investigate such cases and did not find evidence of a "broken system"); and finally, the need to ensure public confidence in the research enterprise.

The ethical problems of research on the mentally ill seem somewhat different today from the way they did in the 1970s. The proposals rejected at that time referred to "persons institutionalized as mentally infirm," but today, clinical psychiatric research is performed largely in the outpatient setting. In the past, mentally ill persons were often viewed as broadly incompetent. Because of that view, their civil liberties were curtailed, and involuntary treatment was common. Today, there are few patients who are hospitalized against their will. Even those who are retain their rights, including their right to refuse treatment. Empirical studies suggest that impaired decision-making capacity may be less common among psychiatric patients (it is estimated to be present in about 52 percent of hospitalized patients with schizophrenia) and more common among those with serious medical illnesses (about 12 percent) than previously believed.[14,15] For example, a survey of patients with medical disorders found that 6 percent of those who believed they had never participated in medical research had actually done so, and 7 percent of those who had participated in research did not understand that they had the right to withdraw from it.[16]

The NBAC considered some of these changes, but nevertheless made the fundamental and highly controversial decision to focus its report on persons with mental disorders that may affect the capacity to make decisions rather than on all potential research subjects with actual or probable impaired capacity. In my view, this focus reflects the persistence of outmoded stereotypes. Psychiatric patients and psychiatric research are fundamentally similar to medical patients and medical research, respectively, and psychiatric patients should have the same rights, governed by the same safeguards and regulations, as those of medical patients. Regulations should be based on functional characteristics such as decision-making capacity rather than on diagnostic categories, particularly categories, such as mental illness, that have been subject to stigma.

The traditional definition of the capacity to consent to research requires that the subject understand the difference between treatment and research, the nature of the research being conducted, its risks and benefits, available alternatives, and the fact that he or she is making a decision and that the decision can be changed. The subject must not be swayed by a pathologic affective state, a false belief, or a dependent relationship that might interfere with the decision or with his or her autonomy and must be capable of making a stable, reasoned choice and communicating it. The NBAC agrees with this definition. Its most controversial recommendations concern the process of assessing the capacity to consent to research, the arrangements for surrogate decision making if this capacity is impaired, and the evaluation of the risks and benefits of research.

Currently, the capacity to consent to research is assessed in much the same way as the more familiar capacity to consent to treatment — that is, by the health care professionals and care givers who are closest to the patient. The NBAC would change this approach for all research involving more than minimal risk. The category of "more than minimal risk" is quite broad. It includes, for example, noninvasive magnetic resonance imaging (MRI) of the brain (because the noise, confinement, and apparatus could be distressing to a subject) or explicit questions about sexual preferences (which might upset a subject). Such research would require an assessment by an "independent qualified professional"; even the treating clinician would be disqualified from judging the capacity to consent to research if he or she were either participating in the research or employed by the institution conducting it. The NBAC considers the present system for evaluating a patient's capacity to consent to dangerous treatment inadequate even to assess the capacity to consent to MRI for research purposes. A similar proposal to use independent monitors of consent was a major factor in the rejection of the 1978 recommendations. Many psychiatric researchers consider these recommended procedures expensive, cumbersome, and clinically insensitive to the experience of impaired subjects, and some patient advocates fear that the implied mistrust of care givers may have a negative effect on the doctor–patient relationship.

For subjects found to have an impaired capacity to make decisions, the NBAC recommended acceptance of surrogate consent by legally authorized representatives, but with strict limits on their authority. Surrogate consent for research involving more than minimal risk (again, this includes brain imaging) would require approval of the protocol by a federal review panel, not just the IRB. This represents an extraordinary shift of authority from the community in which the research is being conducted to a central body distant from both the subjects and the researchers.

There are two problems with this suggestion. The first concerns what might seem to be a detail but turns out to be crucial. Similar regulations concerning children specify three levels of risk: "minimal risk," "minor increase over minimal risk," and "greater than minor increase over minimal risk." The middle category allows flexibility; there might not be the same concern about an MRI or probing questions about sexual behavior (examples of a minor increase over minimal risk) that there would be about a muscle biopsy (an example of a greater than minor increase). The requirement that a federal panel review research involving only a minor increase over minimal risk will be a serious barrier to research that has been free of ethical difficulties, such as studies of psychosocial interventions designed to reduce high-risk sexual behavior in psychotic patients or to determine the value of brain imaging in elucidating the mechanism of action of psychotropic drugs.

The second problem relates to the NBAC's view not only that mental patients and psychiatric researchers are different from medical patients and medical researchers, but also that psychiatric research methods themselves entail special risks. The commission cites three such methods: challenge studies (such as the administration of ketamine, which causes transient increases in psychotic symptoms, to patients with schizophrenia), drug washouts or holidays (periods when drugs are withdrawn), and studies in which some patients receive placebos. The NBAC ignored the extensive literature on the actual risks of these research strategies (although in the week before its report was released to the public, the commission added a recommendation that the Institute of Medicine study the issue), but it nevertheless concluded that they "require special attention." Yet cardiac stress tests and glucose-tolerance tests are also challenge studies, drug-withdrawal strategies are commonly used in nonpsychiatric pharmacologic research, and placebo studies are often required by the Food and Drug Administration for drug approval. The risks of research may be small or large and it may be difficult to evaluate them, but there is nothing special about the evaluation of risk in psychiatric research as compared with other types of medical research.

The NBAC has made some excellent suggestions. One is that a federal panel collect data on the risks of various research interventions and the views of potential subjects. This will allow future guidelines to be based on facts rather than speculation and impressions. Another good suggestion is that funds be provided to cover the additional expenditures that the commission's recommendations would require. Oddly, the commission ignores the practical and ethical questions of who should provide these funds and what might have to be given up to make them available. Many psychiatrists and advocates for the mentally ill fear that the most likely result of adopting this recommendation will be a reduction in psychiatric research.

Finally, the NBAC suggests that IRBs that consider proposals involving persons with mental disorders should include members who represent the interests of the group being studied. This is a good principle. Unfortunately, it was not followed in the creation of the NBAC itself. Its 17 members include ethicists, scientists, physicians, patient advocates, and even an

executive of a pharmaceutical company, but neither clinicians nor researchers in the fields of psychiatry or neurology. The New York[17] and Maryland[18] working groups that were studying the same issues at the same time made far less intrusive recommendations, each working group included at least 4 psychiatrists among its 13 or 17 members. The participation of psychiatrists might have ensured that the NBAC had a fuller understanding of contemporary psychiatric practice and research. Herbert Pardes, the psychiatrist who was chairman of the New York working group, has stated that as they stand, the NBAC recommendations would "set us back twenty years."[19]

The NBAC saw the absence of special guidelines for research involving mentally ill persons with impaired decision-making capacity as a "regulatory vacuum" and rushed to fill it. The absence of special regulations, however, does not necessarily define a vacuum, and providing additional regulations is not the best solution to all problems. The NBAC recognized that "unless individual investigators understand their ethical responsibilities no regulatory system will function properly" and quoted Henry Beecher, who observed that for human research subjects, "there is the more reliable safeguard provided by the presence of an intelligent, informed, conscientious, compassionate, responsible investigator."[20] One danger of excessive regulations is that they can actually undermine researchers' sense of moral responsibility as their attention shifts from their obligation to research subjects to their compliance with the regulations.

The NBAC also justified its efforts by alluding to cases in which the protection of research subjects appeared to be inadequate. This is, of course, the most important justification; if protection has been inadequate in some cases, this problem should receive the highest priority. However, the commission did not determine whether research subjects have had inadequate protection. It would have been wise to find out how the current system is working and what problems exist before recommending new regulations to correct them — that is, to establish a diagnosis before prescribing a treatment.

Finally, the commission wanted to enhance public confidence in the psychiatric research enterprise. Singling out research on the mentally ill for special regulatory oversight, particularly in the context of media attention to unevaluated and unconfirmed allegations of abuse, is not likely to enhance public confidence.

Mentally ill persons with impaired decision-making capacity do not have one problem in regard to research ethics; they have two. The focus of the NBAC report is that the inability of such persons to provide full informed consent may leave them vulnerable to exploitation. The greater problem is that too little research is conducted on their behalf. Psychiatric research is burdened by a long history of public fear of mental illness, prejudice against the mentally ill, and distrust of those who treat or study

The New England Journal of Medicine

them. The methodologic problems of studying the brain and behavior and the clinical burdens of working with psychiatric patients have contributed to this problem in the past but are abating at present. It would be unfortunate if the NBAC's attempts to address the problem of impaired capacity not only were incomplete and ineffective but also had the unintended effect of impeding research on mental illness.

If the mentally ill are different in a way that raises questions about their civil liberties and prevents them from participating in research, and if psychiatric research is dangerous and researchers are not to be trusted, the strategy recommended by the NBAC has merit. On the other hand, if persons with psychiatric disorders are as able and entitled as those without such disorders to take part in and benefit from research, if creative researchers can design valuable, yet safe studies, if clinicians and researchers regularly place their research subjects' interests first, and if the public, patients, ethicists, researchers, and clinicians all share a common goal, then it is time to expand the dialogue and collect data about the strengths and weaknesses of the current system. We should search for solutions that will protect all persons who have impaired decision-making capacity without further stigmatizing the mentally ill, undermining the research agenda for mental illness, or diluting the moral responsibility of researchers.

ROBERT MICHELS, M.D.

Cornell University Medical College
New York, NY 10021

REFERENCES

1. World Health Organization. The global burden of disease. Cambridge, Mass.: Harvard University Press, 1997.
2. Michels R, Marzuk PM. Progress in psychiatry. N Engl J Med 1993; 329:552-60, 628-38.
3. Datagram: NIH extramural support to institutions of higher education by department. Psychiatr Rep 1995;10(2):19.
4. Trials of war criminals before the Nuremberg Military Tribunals under Control Council Law No. 10, Nuremberg, October 1946–April 1949. Vol. 2. Washington, D.C.: Government Printing Office, 1949:181-2.
5. Beecher HK. Experimentation in man. American lecture series publication no. 52. Springfield, Ill.: Charles C Thomas, 1959.
6. World Medical Association. Declaration of Helsinki: recommendations guiding physicians in biomedical research involving human subjects. JAMA 1997;277:925-6.
7. National Commission for the Protection of Human Subjects of Biomedical and Behavioral Research. Report and recommendations: research involving those institutionalized as mentally infirm. Washington, D.C.: Government Printing Office, 1978:58.
8. Wolpe PR, Moreno J, Caplan AL. Ethical principles and history. In: Pincus HA, Lieberman JA, Ferris S, eds. Ethics in psychiatric research. Washington, D.C.: American Psychiatriac Association, 1999:11.
9. Protection of human subjects. In: Pincus HA, Lieberman JA, Ferris S, eds. Ethics in psychiatric research. Washington, D.C.: American Psychiatric Association, 1999:282.
10. Research involving persons with mental disorders that may affect decisionmaking capacity. Rockville, Md.: National Bioethics Advisory Commission, 1998.
11. Evaluation of human subject protections in schizophrenia research conducted by the University of California, Los Angeles, 1994. Bethesda, Md.: Office for Protection from Research Risks, 1994.
12. T.D., et al. v. New York State Office of Mental Health, et al., 626 N.Y.S. 2d 1015 (N.Y. Sup. Ct. 1995).
13. Kong D, Whitaker R. Doing harm: research on the mentally ill. Boston Globe. November 15–18, 1998:A1.
14. Appelbaum PS. Rethinking the conduct of psychiatric research. Arch Gen Psychiatry 1997;54:117-20.
15. Grisso T, Appelbaum PS. The MacArthur Treatment Competence Study. III. Abilities of patients to consent to psychiatric and medical treatments. Law Hum Behav 1995;19:149-74.
16. Sugarman J, Kass NE, Goodman SN, Perentesis P, Fernandes P, Faden RR. What patients say about medical research. IRB 1998;20(4):1-7.
17. New York State Department of Health Advisory Work Group on Human Subject Research Involving the Protected Classes. Recommendations on the oversight of human subject research involving the protected classes. Albany: New York State Department of Health, 1998.
18. Final report of the Attorney General's Working Group on Research Involving Decisionally Incapacitated Subjects. Baltimore: Office of the Maryland Attorney General, 1998.
19. Marshall E. Panel tightens rules on mental disorders. Science 1998; 282:1617.
20. Beecher HK. Ethics and clinical research. N Engl J Med 1966;274: 1354-60.

[20]

The Reform of Adult Guardianship Laws:

The Case of Non-Therapeutic Experimentation

George F. Tomossy* and David N. Weisstub**

Introduction

It is a well-established ethical and legal principle that experiments should not be conducted without first obtaining a subject's free and informed consent. In the case of cognitively impaired adults, however, meeting this standard is difficult, if not impossible, as such persons often lack the requisite mental capacity to make autonomous and contemporaneous decisions with respect to their personal welfare. The need for concern is heightened when involving research that is non-therapeutic, that is, provides no direct medical benefit to the subject. A simple solution would be to ban such experiments entirely; however, scientific progress in the understanding and treatment of conditions specific to special populations is of great social utility, and an absolute prohibition would be an excessive paternalistic response. Understandably, attempts to accommodate this social incentive raise difficult ethical and legal dilemmas.

The doctrine of informed consent, although serving well the interests of fully competent persons, falls short when applied in the context of individuals with compromised decision-making ability. Viable alternative methods for obtaining a subject's consent, such as the use of advance directives and substituted decisions, must therefore be considered. Neither of these options is currently available (in the context of research) in Canada's English-speaking provinces, where guardianship statutes, and also the common law, fail to provide a satisfactory solution. This concern was expressed recently by the *Enquiry on Research Ethics,*[1] which examined the legal and ethical issues raised by the use of members of vulnerable populations, including cognitively im-

*Research Associate, Chaire de psychiatrie légale et d'éthique biomédicale Philippe Pinel, Faculté de médecine, Université de Montréal, C.P. 6128, Succ. Centre-ville, Montréal, Québec H3C 3J7, Canada.

**Philippe Pinel Professor of Legal Psychiatry and Biomedical Ethics, Faculté de médecine, Université de Montréal C.P. 6128, Succ. Centre-ville, Montréal, Quebec H3C 3J7, Canada.

[1]*Enquiry on Research Ethics: Final Report* (Chairman: David N. Weisstub, Submitted to the Hon. Jim Wilson, Minister of Health of Ontario, Aug. 28, 1995). [hereinafter *Enquiry on Research Ethics*]

paired adults, as experimental subjects. The *Enquiry* delineated the boundaries of ethically permissible research, recommended that certain principles be
enshrined in a statutory regime, and advised the Province of Ontario to create
a quasi-judicial regulatory authority with the ability to promulgate official
guidelines and regulations.

It is our intention to develop further the *Enquiry's* conclusions by exposing
the deficiencies in the present legal order, canvassing various issues raised by
the use of advance directives and of substituted decisions to enroll cognitively
impaired adults in non-therapeutic biomedical experiments, and suggesting
much-needed reforms in existing adult guardianship laws.

Definitions

We must first define certain key terms that will be used throughout the discussion. *Research* and *experiment*, employed interchangeably in the literature,
are distinguished from *treatment* by the respective absence or presence of a
benefit accruing to the subject/patient. This benefit is calculated by applying
predictions made in accordance with established standards of medical practice. The descriptors *therapeutic* and *non-therapeutic* can be rationalized in a
similar fashion.[2] As antonymous labels, reflecting the often puristic nature of
definitions, these terms are somewhat artificial, given that a research protocol
is described most appropriately as falling along a spectrum between two poles,
therapy and non-therapy.[3] Indeed, it is this element of uncertainty that has
contributed to the evolution of a confusing array of terms, including *innovative therapy* and *therapeutic research*, the use of which should be discontinued.[4]
Nevertheless, being able to categorize an experiment is vital, despite its seeming arbitrariness, because the duties and responsibilities owed by the re-

---

[2]The presence or absence of a benefit to the subject forms the core of this categorization and should be
assessed on the basis of "immediacy of application" as substantiated by acceptable scientific data. A high
standard should be applied, with "possible," "hypothetical," or "speculative" therapeutic results being
deemed insufficient to assign a *therapeutic* label; rather, the proffered benefit should be "likely,"
"probable," or even "reasonably foreseeable." Otherwise, the research should be classified as *non-
therapeutic*. See *ibid.* at 54.

[3]See e.g. C. Fried, *Medical Experimentation: Personal Integrity and Social Policy* (New York: American
Elsevier Publishing, 1974) at 25–26. Annas, although acknowledging the continuum from experiment to
treatment, assumes a more rigid stance, stating that "few interventions are in the gray zone and [that] an
objective distinction can almost always be made between an experimental intervention and a treatment,"
See G. J. Annas, "Questing for Grails: Duplicity, Betrayal and Self-Deception in Postmodern Medical
Research" (1996) 12 Journal of Contemporary Health Law and Policy 297 at 321.

[4]The term *therapeutic research* has been described as a tool used to facilitate self-deception in the research
process, allowing a researcher to assume the mantle of a physician, thereby confusing subjects who may, as
patients, submit to research with the expectation of a benefit that in fact does not exist. Hence, *therapeutic
research* constitutes a doublethink "used to disguise the true nature of experimental protocols and to
obscure the ideology of science (which follows a protocol to test a hypothesis) with the ideology of medicine
(which uses treatments in the best interests of individual patients)." [footnotes omitted] See Annas, *ibid.* at
314. The Law Reform Commission of Canada recommended that this term be dropped from the medical
lexicon. See Law Reform Commission of Canada, *Working Paper No. 61: Biomedical Experimentation
Involving Human Subjects* (Ottawa: Law Reform Commission, 1989) at 5.

searcher to the subject will be determined largely by the nature of their relationship, that is, whether it is therapeutic or not. Our present discussion will be restricted to research that is categorized as *non-therapeutic*,[5] meaning that the protocol is *primarily* non-therapeutic, based on an objective appraisal of the experiment as a whole rather than on the stated intent of the researcher.[6]

Cognitively impaired adults refers to a heterogeneous group of individuals, including those with mental disorders and developmental disabilities, such as dementing or psychotic disorders and mental retardation, and persons suffering from sudden physical or mental traumas.[7] Cognitive impairment may vary in degree and in kind, potentially arising suddenly, developing over a period of time, fluctuating from day to day, or having existed prior to reaching adulthood. The common feature shared by all members of this diverse group is a diminished capacity to make decisions, or in the present context, the inability to understand properly, make choices about, or communicate decisions regarding participation in research.[8] This definition takes into account the modern trend in competency assessment, which requires that mental incapacity be determined on a functional basis, that is, with respect to the specific matter in question.[9] Incapacity in one area of decision making does not automatically imply incapacity in another; for although belonging to the class of cognitively impaired adults, a person cannot be presumed to be incapable of making the decision of whether or not to become a subject in an experiment. Consequently, and because of the heterogeneity of the population, any protective legal regime must be sufficiently flexible to accommodate the different needs of indi-

---

[5]The discussion will also generally be confined to clinical research, although some aspects will certainly bear relevance to research in the social sciences.

[6]It is important to consider an experiment as the sum of its component parts, which may individually have therapeutic or non-therapeutic applications. For example, in the administration of a known treatment, repeated incidental and diagnostic procedures may preclude the classification of the protocol as a whole as *therapeutic*. Also, the researcher/physician has an inherent conflict of interest between his loyalty to the therapeutic needs of the subject/patient and the scientific integrity of the experiment. As such, it is important that an objective assessment be conducted, independent of the stated intent of the researcher. See also J. Katz, "Human Experimentation and Human Rights" (1993) 38 Saint Louis University Law Journal 7; and more generally, *Enquiry on Research Ethics, supra* note 1 at 51–55, 57–59. A clear-cut classification is difficult when considering randomized clinical trials (RCTs), where claims of a therapeutic objective may be confounded by the element of randomization and the use of placebos. The literature on this specific topic is extensive and will not be addressed here. Although such trials should generally be classified as *non-therapeutic*, this may not always be the case, such as where non-therapeutic elements are minimized and treatment options of participants are not compromised. See generally *Enquiry on Research Ethics, supra* note 1 at 55–57. The Law Commission (UK) stated that RCTs should be labeled as *therapeutic* only where it is genuinely impossible to identify whether an old treatment, no treatment, or new treatment is preferable, and therefore all three may equally be in the best interests of a patient. See The Law Commission, *Mental Incapacity* (London: HMSO, 1995) at para. 6.28.

[7]The definition is derived from technical definitions of mental disorder and mental retardation. See American Psychiatric Association, *Diagnostic and Statistical Manual of Mental Disorders*, 4th ed. (Washington, D.C.: A.P.A., 1994) at xxi–xxii, 39–42.

[8]American College of Physicians, "Position Paper on Cognitively Impaired Subjects" (1989) 111 Annals of Internal Medicine 843 at 843.

[9]D. N. Weisstub, *Enquiry on Mental Competency: Final Report* (Toronto: Queen's Printer, 1990).

viduals that may vary not only from group to group, such as persons with mental disorders as opposed to the developmentally disabled, but also within a group, where needs may vary on a case by case basis.

Justifications and Incentives

If we decide, as a society, that we are justified in exposing vulnerable persons to risks inherent in non-therapeutic research, however minute, for benefits to be reaped by others, then we must avoid the pitfalls of legal and moral fictions that may result from our efforts to appease our collective moral conscience. An appeal to a sacrificial ethic that presumes a person's desire (and perhaps consent) to participate in the research endeavour, if given the opportunity, would be a valiant model for citizenship. However, such a model would in fact be immoral if applied to persons who, because of their inability to act as autonomous agents, can neither affirm nor deny such a presumption. To speak in terms of a "duty" to accept the role of experimental subject would likewise be inappropriate.[10]

There is also the issue of a right to participate in biomedical experiments. Such a "right" is supported by arguments that hold that a person should not be paternalistically restrained from risk-taking.[11] Individuals have always enjoyed the freedom to participate in activities that do not provide any direct benefits other than moral or personal satisfaction and which may even expose them to substantial risks of harm.[12] Although control over our bodies is a fundamental value insofar as it reflects our interest in preserving individual autonomy, this right cannot be without limits. Indeed, the principle of personal inviolability

---

[10]An attempt to rationalize the inclusion in research of persons whose rationality is at issue, relies upon the view that " . . . if it is morally elevating for persons of normal intelligence to participate in research beneficial to others, we should elevate persons of limited capacity by taking them into this world of beneficial exchanges." The danger in promoting such a view is clear: "By such a rationale, and indeed fiction, we can decide to ask handicapped persons to give their organs to siblings in need, thereby making whole as moral beings persons who for other purposes have been given lesser evaluations with respect to their worth in the social system." It is therefore unacceptable that a presumption of implied consent, even if couched in terms of a social duty, be rooted in such moral fictions. See D. N. Weisstub, "Roles and Fictions in Clinical and Research Ethics" (1996) 4 Health Law Journal [in press].

[11]A second argument in support of a right to participate in research stems from the principle of beneficence, whereby persons should not be prevented from access to benefits of research, including certain drugs or therapies. See M. L. Elks, "The Right to Participate in Research Studies" (1993) 122 Journal of Laboratory & Clinical Medicine 130 at 131. Although arguments favouring a right to participate in research may be justified when concerning persons who are fully competent, such as in cases involving innovative treatments where no other options are available, they are difficult to apply in the context of non-therapeutic research involving cognitively impaired adults whose ability to make autonomous decisions is diminished, or perhaps even nonexistent. The notion of a *right* becomes relevant, however, in those cases where it is possible to express choices prior to the point at which autonomous behaviour is no longer possible.

[12]In Canada, discrimination on the basis of mental disability runs contrary to s. 15(1) of the *Canadian Charter of Rights and Freedoms*, Being Part I of the *Constitution Act, 1982*, being Schedule B to the Canada Act, 1982, c. 11. However, it is doubtful that the infringement of a "right to participate in non-therapeutic research," if in fact it could be demonstrated that such a right exists, would actually attract the censure of the courts.

must at times supersede that of autonomy, including in the context of research.[13] This limitation becomes all the more relevant in the case of a person whose ability to make decisions is compromised. Someone with a serious developmental disability, for example, may lack the life experiences necessary to formulate certain moral choices. The decision of whether or not to expose oneself to risks for the benefit of others is very much a matter of morality. To appeal to a "right" in such cases as a basis for justifying participation would lead us to embark upon a "pathway of fictionalizing the moral enhancements of vulnerable populations,"[14] which could in fact lend credence to slippery slope arguments favouring a ban on all research involving vulnerable persons.

We must therefore acknowledge that any decision to condone experiments involving cognitively impaired adults has at its root a societal need, rather than imagined altruistic motivations of mentally incompetent subjects, which we could not, in all fairness, attribute to ourselves in all cases.

The decision to permit non-therapeutic research is not merely a question of morality or social policy, but one of necessity. Researchers studying cognitive disorders, including Alzheimer's dementia, are faced with a lack of alternative animal models, and consequently must employ human subjects.[15] Also, as a result of the changing demographics of our population, the importance of such research is increasing; and in fact, the growing number of elderly persons has created an important therapeutic market.[16] A decision *not* to conduct relevant research would be neglectful of the special needs of this population.[17] However, these necessities have not been recognized consistently. Both the *Nuremberg Code*[18] and the *International Covenant on Civil and Political Rights*[19] effectively prohibit non-therapeutic experimentation with persons who are unable to provide consent. This stance is maintained by the United Nations Human Rights Committee[20] and is an understandable reaction to his-

---

[13]The principle of inviolability is predicated on the notion that "the State has a legitimate interest in protecting its citizens not only from external threats to their physical integrity, but also from their own choices where there is an unjustified risk of injury or death." See S. N. Verdun-Jones & D. N. Weisstub, "Consent to Human Experimentation in Québec: The Application of the Civil Law Principle of Personal Inviolability to Protect Special Populations" (1995) 18 International Journal of Law & Psychiatry 163 at 166–167.

[14]See Weisstub (1996), *supra* note 10.

[15]E.W. Keyserlingk *et al.*, "Proposed Guidelines for the Participation of Persons with Dementia as Research Subjects" (1995) 38 Perspectives in Biology & Medicine 319 at 319.

[16]See e.g. Health and Welfare Canada, *Fact Book on Aging in Canada* (Ottawa: Minister of Supply and Services, 1983) at 14, 25. The population aging phenomenon is one of Canada's major social issues, having as its implication an increasing demand for health care and other social services. See R. M. Gordon & S. N. Verdun-Jones, *Adult Guardianship Law in Canada*, Rel. 2 (Scarborough: Carswell, 1995) at 1-12-1-13.

[17]See e.g. C. G. Swift, "Ethical Aspects of Clinical Research with the Elderly" (1988) 40 British Medical Journal of Hospital Medicine 370.

[18]The *Nuremberg Code* constituted part of the judgment resulting from *U.S.* v. *Karl Brandt et al., Trials of War Criminals Before the Nuremberg Military Tribunal Under Control Council Law No. 10.* (October 1946–April 1949).

[19]G. A. Res. 2200 (XXI), 999 U.N.T.S. 171 (1966), art. 7.

[20]Human Rights Committee, 53rd Sess., 1413 Mtg., CCPR/C/SR. 1413, (6 April 1995), paras. 21, 35.

toric incidents of scientific misconduct that include, in addition to the horrendous abuses of World War II, the infamous Tuskegee Syphilis Study,[21] the Willowbrook Hepatitis Experiments,[22] the American Radiation Studies,[23] and the Cameron Affair.[24]

A further justification for restricting research is founded upon slippery slope arguments, which hold that procedural safeguards can never suffice to forestall the potential harms that can occur as a result of making what may seem at the outset to be a minor moral concession. This position, however, can be countered on two grounds. Firstly, the populations, if not the individuals, to be called upon to assume risks would also be the beneficiaries.[25]

Secondly, our tools for surveillance and protection, if carefully harnessed, can indeed provide the requisite monitors and safeguards, assuming that the actors, including political ones, are not acting in bad faith.[26] An absolute ban, therefore, should not be the chosen course of action. Rather, there should be a balancing of society's interest in conducting important and promising research with the interests of the potential subject.[27] The social incentive to expand scientific knowledge, even at the cost of exposing individuals with impaired decision-making capacity to risks of harm, cannot be without bounds.[28] Over the years, the extended dialogue on this topic has yielded an international consensus that condones experimentation involving vulnerable populations, provided that appropriate safeguards are introduced, and that also recognizes the social utility in increasing our understanding of illness and disease. This view is

---

[21]J. H. Jones, *Bad Blood* (New York: Free Press, 1981).

[22]See H. Beecher, "Ethics and Clinical Research" (1966) 274 New England Journal of Medicine 1354; M. A. Grodin & J. J. Alpert, "Children as Participants in Medical Research" (1988) 35 Pediatric Clinics of North America 1389.

[23]Advisory Committee on Human Radiation Experiments, *Final Report* (Washington, D.C.: U.S. Government Printing Office, 1995).

[24]See Government of Canada, *New Release: Background Information—Depatterning at the Allan Memorial Institute* (Ottawa: Department of Justice, 17 November 1992); G. Cooper, *Opinion of George Cooper, Q..C., Regarding Canadian Government Funding of the Allan Memorial Institute in the 1950's and 1960's* (Ottawa: Supply and Services Canada, 1986).

[25]The need for action is heightened further by pressures to develop more efficient tools for low-cost health protection for these special populations.

[26]This, in any event, is never ultimately guaranteed in any civil society, including democratic ones. In attaining these standards of surveillance, the position taken here is that self-regulation or highly discretionary decision making is unacceptable.

[27]See also V. L. Melnick *et al.*, "Clinical Research in Senile Dementia of the Alzheimer Type: Suggested Guidelines Addressing the Ethical and Legal Issues" (1984) 32 Journal of the American Geriatric Society 531 at 535.

[28]The *Declaration of Helsinki* clearly states that "[i]n research on man, the interest of science and society should never take precedence over considerations related to the well-being of the subject." See Medical Association, *Declaration of Helsinki*, Adopted at the 18th World Medical Assembly in Helsinki in June 1964. Amended at the 19th World Medical Assembly in Tokyo in October 1975; the 35th World Medical Assembly in Venice in October 1983; and the 41st World Medical Assembly in Hong Kong in September 1989.

upheld by the *Declaration of Helsinki*[29] and by the recent *International Ethical Guidelines for Biomedical Research Involving Human Subjects* promulgated by the Council for International Organizations of Medical Science in collaboration with the World Health Organization.[30]

Regulating Research

The historical record supports the unfortunate conclusion that members of certain populations, including cognitively impaired adults, may always be prone to exploitation and abuse in the research setting. Society must remain forever vigilant in order to protect its vulnerable members. This can be accomplished only by enforcing well-defined standards of ethical conduct. The question that lies before us is whether this goal can best be realized through internal or external regulatory mechanisms. Although a moot point in France, given its extensive legislation governing the area,[31] the question remains a source of contention in Canada where, with the exception of Québec, experimentation has been "regulated" only through the use of ethical guidelines, such as those promulgated by the Medical Research Council of Canada.[32] Although professional self-regulation and medical education both play an important role in instilling ethical behaviour, the mere availability of ethical guidelines, from a legal perspective, is of limited worth as a regulatory authority.[33] They are insufficient in establishing a uniform set of rules that are legally binding, "unless buttressed by overarching political and social institutions."[34] This point is illustrated by a recent Canadian case in which both the researcher and the university-affiliated hospital (for its research ethics committee) were held to be liable for the death of a subject in a non-therapeutic experiment.[35] The case turned on the failure of the researcher to disclose certain risks to the subject and did nothing to clarify the legal status of professional guidelines as sources for defining standards of conduct, which if adhered to would absolve researchers and their affiliated institutions from liability. Although the case

---

[29]See *Declaration of Helsinki, supra* note 28.

[30]Council for International Organizations of Medical Science, in collaboration with the World Health Organization, *International Ethical Guidelines for Biomedical Research Involving Human Subjects* (Geneva: CIOMS, 1993). [hereinafter *CIOMS Guidelines*]

[31]C. Huriet, "La loi francaise relative à la protection des personnes qui se prêtent à des recherches biomédicales; origine et histoire" (1992) 43 Recueil International de Législation Sanitaire 414.

[32]Medical Research Council of Canada, *Guidelines on Research Involving Human Subjects* (Ottawa: Supply & Services Canada, 1987). These guidelines are currently under revision. See Tri-Council Working Group, *Code of Conduct for Research Involving Humans (Draft Document)* (Ottawa: Supply & Services Canada, 1996).

[33]P. R. Benson, "The Social Control of Human Biomedical Research: An Overview and Review of the Literature" (1989) 29 Social Sciences & Medicine 1,

[34]P. R. Benson & L. H. Roth, "Trends in the Social Control of Medical and Psychiatric Research" in D. N. Weisstub, ed., *Law and Mental Health: International Perspectives, Volume 4* (New York: Pergamon Press, 1988) 1 at 5.

[35]*Weiss v. Solomon* [1989] R.J.Q. 731 (S.C.).

Human Experimentation and Research

G. F. TOMOSSY and D. N. WEISSTUB

refers to the *Declaration of Helsinki*,[36] there is no mention of the 1978 Medical Research Council of Canada Guidelines, which were being followed at the time the events took place. The judgment was therefore criticized on the basis that, in establishing a legal standard of professional conduct, a court should begin by examining the practice of the profession, regardless of whether this proves inconclusive or deficient.[37] However, even if professional guidelines are followed, they will not automatically provide legal protection in negligence actions. As in the United Kingdom, decisions by research ethics committees do not make researchers' actions lawful.[38] The Medical Research Council of Canada is a corporation created by a federal statute,[39] and committees adhering to its guidelines lack the power to authorize conduct that is not otherwise sanctioned by law. Therefore, it is in the interests of subjects, researchers, and their institutions, that a statutory basis prescribing ethical and legal conduct in biomedical research be established.

It comes as no surprise, therefore, that the tendency in many countries has been to enact legislation or to promulgate official regulations, with prominent examples including the Department of Health and Human Services Regulations in the United States[40] and amendments to the French *Code de la santé publique*.[41] This trend is further reflected in recent law reform initiatives in Canada,[42] the United Kingdom,[43] Australia[44] and the Netherlands.[45] Consistent with this international tenor of reform, the *Enquiry on Research Ethics* recommended that the Province of Ontario enact legislation delineating the criteria for ethical conduct in research and establish a statutory body with the authority to promulgate additional regulations.[46]

---

[36]*Ibid.* at 741.

[37]B. Freedman & K. C. Glass, "*Weiss* v. *Solomon: A Case Study in Institutional Responsibility for Clinical Research*" (1990) 18 Law, Medicine & Health Care 395 at 401–402.

[38]See The Law Commission, *supra* note 6 at paras. 6.29–6.33. This view is shared by the Queensland Law Reform Commission. See Queensland Law Reform Commission, *Assisted and Substituted Decisions: Decision-making by and for People with a Decision-Making Disability, Vol. 1* (Brisbane: Queensland Law Reform Commission, 1996) at 64.

[39]*Medical Research Council Act*, R.S.C. 1985, c. M-9.

[40]Title 45 Code of Federal Regulations Part 46 (18 June 1991).

[41]*Loi No. 88-1138 du 20 décembre 1988* (J.O. December 22, 1988); *Loi 90-86 du 23 janvier 1990, (J.O. 25 January 1990); Loi 90-549 du 2 juillet 1990,* (J.O. 5 July 1990); *Loi 91-73 du 18 janvier 1991,* (J.O. 20 January 1991); *Loi 94-630 du 25 juillet 1994,* (J.O. 27 July 1994).

[42]Law Reform Commission of Canada (1989), *supra* note 4; Law Reform Commission of Canada, *Toward a Canadian Advisory Board on Biomedical Ethics* (Ottawa: Law Reform Commission of Canada, 1990).

[43]See The Law Commission, *supra* note 6.

[44]See Queensland Law Reform Commission, *supra* note 38.

[45]A "Medical Experimentation Bill" was introduced to the Second Chamber of Parliament on April 18, 1992; however, the new Minister of Health, Welfare, and Sports withdrew the bill from further discussion on March 16, 1995, because she and the Minister of Justice were planning to "formulate a definitive regulation on scientific research of human embryos and sex-cells." [Personal communication from G. Dekker, Chief Inspector of Health Care for the Netherlands (6 July 1995).]

[46]*Enquiry on Research Ethics, supra* note 1 at 106.

Legal Necessity

As mentioned earlier, Québec is the only Canadian jurisdiction that specifically regulates human experimentation.[47] In the rest of Canada, neither existing adult guardianship statutes nor the common law provide a satisfactory solution. Before discussing much-needed reforms, it is important to identify the deficiencies of the present legal order, beginning with the failure of the doctrine of informed consent as a protective regime for vulnerable adults.

The Doctrine of Informed Consent

Informed consent is one of the great canons of medical law, which includes the law on human experimentation. Indeed, the duty of disclosure of potential risks, irrespective of how remote they may appear, is greater in the context of research than of treatment[48]; this principle is clearly enunciated in Canadian case law.[49] Because individuals who submit to non-therapeutic experiments are exposed to risks without the promise of receiving any complementary benefits, other than perhaps a sense of satisfaction, participation must never result from consent that is not genuine, or worse yet, is coerced. What remains to be seen is whether the doctrine of informed consent can satisfy this directive fully when applied to adults with diminished cognitive capacities.

The exercise of empowering rights, those that promote an individual's right to self-determination, relies upon the ability to communicate choices effectively, which involves the capacity to understand properly all relevant factors that may influence a given decision. A cognitively impaired adult may be unable to satisfy this requirement.[50] The doctrine of informed consent, which appeals to the principle of autonomy, "can only be employed as a means of protecting a *competent* person from exploitation and abuse,"[51] and hence can

---

[47]Arts. 20-26 C.C.Q. It is worthwhile to note that, despite the existence of the *Civil Code* articles governing research, current regulatory models in Québec were criticised as being inconsistent and inadequate in protecting research subjects while at the same time maintaining scientific integrity. It was recommended, therefore, that a more elaborate regime be developed, one which properly takes into consideration the ethical, scientific, and financial aspects of research, and that a permanent regulatory authority be created. See Comité d'experts sur l'évaluation des mécanismes de contrôle en matière de recherche clinique, *Rapport sur l'évaluation des mécanismes de contrôle en matière de recherche clinique au Québec*, (Chairman: Pierre Deschamps, Submitted to the Hon. Jean Rochon, Minister of Health and Social Services, Province of Québec, June 9, 1995).

[48]See e.g. R. Delago & H. Leskovac, "Informed Consent in Human Experimentation: Bridging the Gap Between Ethical Thought and Current Practice" (1986) 34 UCLA Law Review 67; K. C. Glass, "Informed Decision-Making and Vulnerable Persons: Meeting the Needs of the Competent Elderly Patient or Research Subject" (1993) 18 Queen's Law Journal 191.

[49]See *Halushka* v. *University of Saskatchewan* (1965), 52 W.W.R. 608 (Sask. C.A.); and *Weiss* v. *Solomon, supra* note 35.

[50]It is important to reiterate that a cognitively impaired adult's inability to make meaningful decisions in the experimentation context must not be presumed, but rather, as discussed in our definition above, determined on a functional basis.

[51]See Verdun-Jones & Weisstub, *supra* note 13 at 166–167.

serve the interests only of those who are able to fend for themselves without assistance or intervention by others.[52] Total reliance upon autonomy-based principles would therefore be unwise in the context of research involving persons with impaired decision-making abilities. Perhaps a more appropriate basis for the development of legal protections would be the principle of personal inviolability, which can be equated to an aspect of the ethical maxim of respect for persons.[53] This course was adopted in the recently revised *Civil Code of Québec*, which restricted the participation of even fully competent adults in non-therapeutic research.[54] Legal reform in common law jurisdictions should reflect, at least in part, this protectionist approach.[55] However, the ideal foundation for developing legal safeguards should be a middle ground between these two positions, that is, one that seeks to maximize decision-making capacity while proscribing behaviour that could compromise an individual's mental and bodily integrity.

The doctrine of informed consent has been criticized for its inability to reconcile personal values and beliefs, which leads to its failure to elicit truly meaningful responses.[56] Also, from a practical perspective, the usefulness of the doctrine has been questioned in the light of the lack of a proper allocation of the resources necessary to fulfill its mandate effectively.[57] Nevertheless, informed consent should not be abandoned in its entirety. Indeed, the impetus behind the historical evolution of the doctrine, the reaction against paternalistic patterns of behaviour in the doctor/patient relationship that became unac-

---

[52]See M. A. Somerville, "Label versus Contents: Variations Between Philosophy, Psychiatry and Law in Concepts Governing Decision-Making" (1994) 39 McGill L.J. 179 at 193, who state that ". . . there is danger in promoting the adoption of autonomy as a factor relevant to legal rights in relation to personal decision-making, because this could result in the invasion of the human rights of, a lack of interest for, and wrongful discrimination against, persons characterized as non-autonomous." An alternative view is to treat informed consent as a "gatekeeping" device, which can be used to distinguish those persons who are capable of making their own decisions from those who require additional protection. See R. R. Faden & T. L. Beauchamp, *A History and Theory of Informed Consent* (Oxford: Oxford University Press, 1986).

[53]*Respect for persons* calls not only for the promotion of self-determinative rights, but for the protection of persons with an impaired decision-making capacity. See *CIOMS Guidelines, supra* note 30 at 10. See also Verdun-Jones & Weisstub, *supra* note 13.

[54]"A person of full age who is capable of giving his consent may submit to an experiment provided that the risk incurred is not disproportionate to the benefit that can reasonably be anticipated." Art. 20 C.C.Q.

[55]Ethical research involving vulnerable populations should fall within clearly stated boundaries of permissible behaviour, whereby the actions of both prospective subjects and persons acting on their behalf (*i.e.* legal guardians) are carefully circumscribed. In particular, restrictions should be placed on acceptable levels of risk, and there should be a mandatory relationship between the purpose of the research and the condition or circumstances of the subject of special population to which the subject belongs. The latter requirement necessarily implies that research not be conducted on vulnerable persons where alternative methods, treatments, or subjects are available. See D. N. Weisstub, J. Arbodeda-Florez & G. F. Tomossy, "Establishing the Boundaries of Ethically Permissible Research with Special Populations" (1996) Health Law in Canada [in press].

[56]R. M. Veatch, "Abandoning Informed Consent" (1995) 25:5 Hastings Center Report 5.

[57]J. Katz, "Informed Consent—Must it Remain a Fairy Tale?" (1994) 10 Journal of Contemporary Health Law & Policy 69. See also P. H. Schuck, "Rethinking Informed Consent" (1994) 103 Yale Law Journal 899.

ceptable in an increasingly sophisticated and litigious culture of health care consumers, is equally relevant, if not more so, in the research context. We must forestall the abuse and exploitation of vulnerable persons by researchers who, whether well-meaning or for unscrupulous designs, may take advantage of their positions of trust and/or authority in order to expedite a preferred decision. This goal can be realized by first obtaining a free and informed consent to participate, a choice which, as mandated by the doctrine of informed consent, must be reached through a dialogic exchange of information. Traditionally, the burden of this decision would fall upon the prospective subject, and therein lies the insufficiency of the doctrine as a protective regime when applied to non-autonomous persons. Indeed, blind reliance upon a notion of informed consent, without properly accommodating the special needs of incapable subjects, such as providing for the legal intervention of a guardian or advocate, can jeopardize the ethical and legal integrity of research. A solution to the problems raised by non-therapeutic experimentation with cognitively impaired adults cannot therefore be founded solely upon the doctrine of informed consent, regardless of its importance in the course of making decisions, without the support of complementary legal institutions.

Adult Guardianship Law

The principal objective of adult guardianship law is to provide assistance to adults who cannot act for themselves. It governs many aspects of daily life, and can be broadly divided into two categories: the management of property and of the person, with the latter being concerned primarily with health matters.[58] The issue of participation in research is either specifically excluded, not mentioned at all, or if referred to, dealt with in an ambiguous manner.[59] Indeed, existing guardianship laws are generally poorly suited to resolving questions that cannot be answered easily through the application of a "best-interests" calculation.[60] Non-therapeutic experimentation, and indeed any other activity that does not lead to a concrete benefit for the subject, throws the proverbial wrench into the machinery of substitute decision making. It is difficult enough for guardians, and also for the judiciary, to rationalize exposing an incompetent adult to risks, however minute, for a hypothetical treatment or cure, let alone in those cases where the benefits will never accrue to the subject, but

---

[58]See generally Gordon & Verdun-Jones, *supra* note 16.

[59]For example, in Ontario it is stated specifically that "nothing in this Act affects the law relating to giving or refusing consent on another person's behalf to a procedure whose primary purpose is research." See *Substitute Decisions Act, 1992*, S.O. 1992, c. 30, s. 66(13). British Columbia is the only province where guardians might be able to make decisions relating to research, insofar as the definition of *health care* includes "participation in a medical research program approved by an ethics committee designated by regulation." See *Health Care (Consent) and Care Facility (Admission) Act*, S.B.C. 1993, c. 48, s. 1. [not yet in force]

[60]As will be discussed below, a "substituted judgment" test is also inappropriate. Rather, a hybrid of both standards should be applied in consideration of each particular situation.

rather to others with the same affliction or disability. This effort is frustrated further because it entails placing the interests of society ahead of those of the subject, which may constitute a breach of the guardian's cardinal duty to protect his ward.[61] Therefore, if we agree that we are justified in exposing incompetent members of our population to carefully controlled risks for the benefit of others, then we must provide in our legal system for exceptional situations in which guardians may act for reasons that do not produce tangible benefits for their dependents. Granted, such an allowance raises a host of ethical and legal concerns; these will be discussed further below. For the present, we will restrict ourselves to identifying the deficiencies of current guardianship laws, as applied to the research context.

One substantial criticism relates to the "all or nothing" approach,[62] which is reflected in "the plenary nature of most guardianship orders and the requirement that a guardian be appointed only when there is evidence of total mental incompetency or incapacity."[63] This state of affairs runs contrary to the view that "incompetence is not to be understood in any global sense, but rather as reflecting incapacities with respect to specific decisions or areas of decision."[64] The modern model requires a functional assessment of competency, which would allow for a finding of partial incapacity and an award of corresponding powers to the guardian.[65] The rigidity of plenary guardianship appointments can be mitigated when appointing personal guardians; however, the courts appear to be unwilling to implement this option where not expressly authorized by statute.[66] Although the courts' *parens patriae* jurisdiction can be used to fill in gaps in legislation and thus act to restrict the authority of guardians,[67] this common law power, at least in Canadian jurisprudence, is not likely to prove useful in the context of experimentation.[68]

The problem of inflexibility impacts directly upon the research endeavour. The abandonment of the plenary approach is only the first step. Each class of cognitive impairment requires a different level and kind of intervention, depending upon whether incapacity increases or fluctuates over a period of time, arises suddenly, or is the result of a developmental disability. With the latter two cases, there is often no alternative other than to rely upon a substitute decision maker; however, guardians are not presently empowered by statute to make such decisions. In all other situations where a person can anticipate future incapacity, that individual may conceivably, while still competent, prepare an advance directive for research. Although legislation governing the use of enduring powers of attorney was enacted in all provinces, only some prov-

---

[61]See e.g., *Re Leeming,* [1985] 1 W.W.R. 368 (B.C.S.C.).

[62]G. B. Robertson, *Mental Disability and the Law in Canada,* 2d. ed. (Toronto: Carswell, 1994) at 118.

[63]See Gordon & Verdun-Jones, *supra* note 16 at 1-16–1-19.

[64]See Weisstub (1990), *supra* note 9 at 35.

[65]See e.g. *Substitute Decisions Act, 1992,* S.O. 1992, c. 30, and also text at note 114.

[66]See Robertson, *supra* note 62 at 119.

[67]*Ibid.* at 170–171.

[68]A critique of the common law will follow.

inces provide for the creation of *health care* directives.[69] Even so, with the possible future exception of British Columbia, the specific application of advance directives for research is not presently supported in Canada's common law provinces.

If non-therapeutic research is to be facilitated, various elements of existing guardianship statutes will require modification, the extent and substance of which will depend upon their respective levels of sophistication. These areas include the manner by which guardians are appointed, the nature and scope of their powers, the criteria upon which they are required to base their decisions, provisions for research directives, the degree to which participation of the subject in the consent process is facilitated, termination of guardianship, and various other factors, including mental competency assessment, the confidentiality and accessibility of written directives, and the review of decisions made by either the subject or the guardian. Current guardianship laws are generally lacking in one or more of these respects.

The Common Law

In Canada, in the absence of guiding legislation, the *parens patriae* jurisdiction empowers the superior courts, when necessary, to protect those who cannot care for themselves. It is well established that such interventions must be based upon a "best interest" or "welfare" standard, for the benefit of the person concerned and not others.[70] The leading case, *Eve*, addressed the issue of whether the courts could approve the "non-therapeutic" sterilization of a mentally retarded women who was incapable of giving an informed consent to the procedure. The request, made by Eve's mother, was denied on the grounds that non-therapeutic sterilization constituted a highly invasive procedure that would cause irreversible physical damage while providing questionable advantages and led the court to conclude that "it can never safely be determined that such a procedure is for the benefit of that person."[71] In so doing, the court chose to apply a narrowly interpreted best-interests standard and declined to adopt a substituted judgment test. This decision, although supported by some,[72] was criticized by others for various reasons. For example, the court prioritized the "privilege" of procreation over other factors, such as "the freedom to form satisfying human relations and experience sexuality without risking pregnancy or paternity,"[73] and effectively restricted legally permissible

---

[69]See Robertson, *supra* note 62 at 177–178; Gordon & Verdun-Jones, *supra* note 16 at 3–129. The provinces that provide for health care directives include Manitoba, Nova Scotia, Ontario, and Newfoundland, with legislation coming into force in British Columbia and in preparation in P.E.I.

[70]*E. (Mrs.)* v. *Eve*, [1986] 2 S.C.R. 388 at 426,427. [hereinafter *Eve*]

[71]*Ibid.* at 431.

[72]See e.g., M. D. A. Freeman, "Sterilising the Mentally Handicapped" in M. D. A. Freeman, ed. *Medicine, Ethics and the Law: Current Legal Problems* (London: Stevens, 1988) 55.

[73]M. A. Shone, "Mental Health—Sterilization of Mentally Retarded Persons—*Parens Patriae* Power: *Re Eve*" (1987) 66 Canadian Bar Review 635 at 640. See also Manitoba Law Reform Commission, *Report on Sterilization and Legal Incompetence* (Winnipeg: Law Reform Commission, 1992).

medical interventions (at least within the context of sterilization) to those that provide a clear therapeutic benefit. The House of Lords, distinguishing both *Eve* and an earlier decision,[74] arrived at a different conclusion, choosing instead to adopt the substitute judgment test, and to reject both the non-therapeutic/therapeutic distinction and the conclusion that sterilizations should never be authorized for "non-therapeutic" purposes.[75] These cases, with their conflicting results, demonstrate the difficulty faced by the judiciary in arriving at consistent decisions when applying discretionary powers, including the *parens patriae* jurisdiction, in morally troubling cases.

The analysis in *Eve*, if applied to the context of non-therapeutic research, could lead to a similar conclusion, although the outcome would likely depend upon the level of risk involved. The Court stated that the *parens patriae* jurisdiction "must at all times be exercised with great caution, a caution that must be redoubled as the seriousness of the matter increases."[76] *Eve* focused on the irreversibility and certainty of physical harm. It is therefore possible that experiments with low or negligible risks would not attract the censure of the courts. After all, parents, when exercising their common law authority as the natural guardians of their children, are not prevented from involving them in sports activities, some of which may give rise to risks that are in fact quite substantial.

It is also conceivable that in the case of a person who was previously competent in life, such as someone suffering from Alzheimer's dementia, a substitute judgment test could be adopted and legitimate a guardian's decision to enroll a dependent in non-therapeutic research. This would call for the guardian to

---

[74]In an earlier case involving a minor, the House of Lords decided not to authorize a non-therapeutic sterilization under the *parens patriae* jurisdiction. See *In Re D (A Minor) (Wardship: Sterilisation)*, [1976] 1 All ER 326 (H.L.). Although acknowledged by subsequent cases to have been correctly decided on its facts, this decision was not upheld. See e.g. *In Re B (A Minor)(R, [1987] 2 All E.R. 206 (H.L.) [hereinafter In Re B]*. In Australia, however, it was recently decided that neither the *parens patriae* power nor existing legislation dealing with decision making for persons with impaired capacity could authorize parents to consent to a non-therapeutic sterilization of their child. See *Secretary, Department of Health and Community Services v. J.W.B. and S.M.B. (Marion's Case)* (1992), 175 C.L.R. 218.

[75]This English case involved a minor and is of interest as it involved the application of the *parens patriae* power to authorize a non-therapeutic sterilization. However, in his criticism of La Forest J in *Eve*, Lord Hailsham of St. Marylebone was also censured for his statement that "[t]o talk of the "basic right" to reproduce for an individual who is not capable of knowing the causal connection between intercourse and childbirth, the nature of pregnancy, what is involved in delivery, unable to form maternal instincts or to care for a child appears to me wholly to part company with reality." The unfortunate inference that can be drawn from such an assertion is that a person who is incapable of understanding or expressing a right may not be entitled to it. See *In Re B, ibid.* at 213. In another case, this time involving an adult, the House of Lords applied the common law concept of necessity, as the *parens patriae* jurisdiction could at that time no longer be applied to adults in England. See *F. v. West Berkshire Health Authority* (1989), 2 All E.R. 545 (H.L.). The application of this approach was criticized as tenuous, given that "necessity" should apply only in cases of genuine need, with non-therapeutic sterilization being a dubious example. For a detailed discussion of these cases and the points mentioned above, see D. Tomkin & P. Hanafin, *Irish Medical Law* (Dublin: Betaprint, 1995) at 192–200.

[76]See *Eve, supra* note 70 at 423.

believe that the now incompetent ward would have consented if competent.[77] Such an opinion would be based on knowledge of the values, views, and beliefs previously held by the incapable subject. Thus, mental incompetence itself would not preclude the use of the substitute judgment test.[78] *Eve*, however, involved a person with a serious mental disability who was never able to express views, values, or beliefs. As such, a substitute judgment test would have been meaningless and purely speculative, and the Supreme Court was correct in rejecting it.

It is possible that subsequent cases could distinguish *Eve* either on the basis of the nature of cognitive impairment or on the relative level of risk or harm, thereby not forcing a superior court to invoke its *parens patriae* powers to invalidate a guardian's decision to enroll a dependent in non-therapeutic research. However, it is difficult to predict the judicial outcome of such fact-specific case, which rely so strongly on the court's discretion. In fact, because of the emphasis on "necessity" and "benefit" in determining whether or not to invoke the *parens patriae* power, which should be applied only in favour of the individual concerned and not for the sake of others, it is more likely than not that Canadian courts would refuse to sanction a guardian's decision to submit a ward to an experiment.[79] Indeed, the Supreme Court forthrightly rejected the invitation to formulate social policy (at least in the context of sterilization), preferring to concern itself with the immediate interests of the incompetent person.[80] Given that our motivation to enroll incapable adults in non-therapeutic research is socially driven, it is likely that the courts would choose to prohibit the practice in order to encourage a legislative resolution.

We must also question whether the judiciary is the appropriate arbiter in such cases,[81] given that the review of research protocols requires multidisciplinary expertise, which would therefore require the participation of persons trained in the health sciences and legal medicine. There may be a place for the judiciary in the approval process; however, a specialized tribunal with quasi-judicial powers would likely be more effective.[82] The position taken here is

---

[77]See B. M. Dickens, "Substitute Consent to Participation of Persons with Alzheimer's Disease in Medical Research: Legal Issues," in J. M. Berg, H. Karlingky & F. H. Lowy, eds., *Alzheimer's Disease Research: Ethical and Legal Issues* (Toronto: Thomson Professional Publishing, 1991) 60. The additional requirement added by Dickens is that there would have to be no risks associated with the research.

[78]See *Eve, supra* note 70 at 425.

[79]The view that the *parens patriae* jurisdiction is unlikely to permit the authorization of non-therapeutic experimentation is shared by the Queensland Law Reform Commission, *supra* note 38 at 64.

[80]See *Eve, supra* note 70 at 427.

[81]*Ibid.*

[82]The Queensland Law Reform Commission and The Law Commission (UK) concurred with this view, recommending that non-therapeutic research with mentally incapacitated adults be authorized only by a specialized statutory authority. The UK Commission, however, makes the additional requirement of either court approval, the consent of an attorney or manager, a certificate from a doctor not involved in the research that the participation of the person is appropriate, or designation of the research as not involving contact. See Queensland Law Reform Commission, *supra* note 38 at 393; The Law Commission, *supra* note 6 at paras. 6.33, 6.37.

that a centralized statutory body should be established in each province, possessing the investigative powers necessary to review the decisions of local research ethics committees[83] and also the power to promulgate regulations that would carry the force of law, with the corresponding ability to impose sanctions. Conduct authorized under such a regime, such as the use of substituted consent, would thus become lawful. The central body could also serve a consultative role or act in a quasi-judicial capacity to resolve difficult cases or situations of conflict.[84] A supervisory/regulatory emphasis is preferred for two reasons: firstly, the desire to create a system that will ensure the observance of minimal requirements for ethical conduct while leaving research ethics committees considerable discretion for their application in the light of local conditions and current developments in science and medical technology; and secondly, for reasons of administrative efficiency. Therefore, the decision to enroll a cognitively impaired adult in research, and the experiment itself, would require the approval of a research ethics committee that would ultimately be responsible to the central board. Making the initial decision with regard to participation, however, preferably based on the prior wishes of the subject, should be entrusted in the legal guardian, who is presumably in the best situation to assess the desires and needs of the incapable subject. The duties of guardians would therefore have to be defined clearly, not through inconsistent rulings by the courts or according to standards of uncertain legal merit as described in professional guidelines, but through detailed legislation. Otherwise, researchers, their institutions, and guardians who enroll cognitively impaired adults in non-therapeutic biomedical experiments, may be open to liability.[85] Legal reform in common law Canada is thus necessary in order to clarify the existing situation and to establish a viable legal regime that is compatible with the research endeavour.

The Elements of Reform

We must first adopt an appropriate philosophical approach, one that requires us to abandon the exclusive reliance on benign paternalism that lies at the root of early (and many existing) adult guardianship laws.[86] Such laws are problematic in that they rely upon the assumption that, owing to their incapacity, cognitively impaired adults are to be treated like children and "are either denied or lose most of the powers and fundamental rights and freedoms en-

---

[83]Local research ethics committees should be formally constituted, certified, and subject to review by a central statutory authority. The composition of committees should include not only persons with scientific and legal training, but on an *ad hoc* basis, representatives of the subject or the class to which the subject belongs. The committee would be required to apply scientific and official guidelines, and be free of institutional and personal bias. See *Enquiry on Research Ethics, supra* note 1.

[84]The central board would also reserve an exclusive right to make certain decisions, such as with regard to research involving substantial risks.

[85]H. Sava, P. T. Matlow & M. J. Sole, "Legal Liability of Physicians in Medical Research" (1994) 17 Clinical & Investigative Medicine 148 at 165.

[86]This generalization, although currently applicable to many of Canada's common law provinces, no longer applies to current Australasian models, nor indeed to many jurisdictions elsewhere in North America.

joyed by others."[87] This perception is no longer compatible with our modern culture of rights and entitlements, which requires not only the preservation of personal autonomy, but of a right to the least restrictive and intrusive forms of assistance and protection.[88]

In order to further this ideal, we must entrench in legislation various fundamental presumptions. The first relates to mental competence. Upon attaining the age of adulthood, a person normally acquires full legal rights to manage personal affairs and to make decisions related to health and welfare. Adults should therefore be presumed to be competent unless proven otherwise. Secondly, it is well acknowledged that incompetence in one area of decision making does not necessarily extend to another.[89] Thus, a person's inability to consent to participate in experiments should not be presumed, despite the presence of a mental disorder or disability. The presumption of competence, however, does not discharge the obligation to conduct a functional assessment of capacity when there is a reason to do so.[90] Finally, acceptance should not be assumed; and neither "assent" nor the lack of an objection, although important prerequisites to participation in research, should be sufficient to imply consent.[91]

It is also important that certain fundamental conditions defining the parameters of permissible experimentation be satisfied.[92] First and foremost is a requirement for the review and approval of all research protocols by a research ethics committee.[93] Briefly, a committee must be satisfied that an experiment is scientifically valid, of significant value, and involves an acceptable level of risk that is proportionate to the potential benefits. The use of cognitively impaired adults must not only be justified by the experimental design, but essential to its stated objective.[94] Finally, the committee must ensure that a valid consent to participate was given, either by the subject or by the legal guardian where the former is impossible to obtain.[95]

---

[87]See Gordon & Verdun-Jones, *supra* note 16 at 1–28.

[88]*Ibid.* at 1–29; See also Robertson, *supra* note 62 at 118–123.

[89]To take a classic example, a person may lack testamentary capacity, but may be sufficiently competent to marry.

[90]For an in depth discussion of mental competency and its assessments, see Weisstub (1990), *supra* note 9.

[91]See for example Title 45 Code of Federal Regulations 46 (18 June 1991) § 46.402 (b), 46.408 (a).

[92]See e.g. Queensland Law Reform Commission, *supra* note 38 at 391–393; The Law Commission, *supra* note 6 at para. 6.34.

[93]This process should involve a review of the scientific and ethical merits of the proposed research.

[94]In other words, no alternative (less vulnerable) pool of subjects can be available. Furthermore, non-therapeutic research involving cognitively impaired adults must be restricted to a condition or circumstance affecting the subject or the class of subjects to which the person belongs. The decision to enroll an individual in non-therapeutic experiments must not be based solely on the availability of the person nor on the inability of that person to object, but rather on the genuine social need to conduct the research in question. See Weisstub, Arboleda-Florez & Tomossy, *supra* note 55.

[95]The list presented is by no means complete. Additional considerations include the issues of confidentiality, conflict of interest, risk assessment, and various obligations of researchers and ethics committees, prior to, during, and subsequent to the completion of an experiment, particularly with respect to minimization of risks. For further discussion, see Weisstub, Arboleda-Florez & Tomossy, *supra* note 55, where general safeguards are presented based on a synthesis of the various codes, guidelines, legislation, and regulations promulgated to date.

On this note, legislative reform must also be geared towards developing a regime that is flexible enough to accommodate the different classes and degrees of cognitive impairment. Alternative modes for obtaining a legal consent must be provided for. We refer of course to decisions made in advance or by a substitute. Although the latter can be applied to any situation of incapacity, use of the former is preferred.[96] There will of course always be cases where the only option is to elicit the consent of a surrogate, particularly in cases of serious unforeseen or developmental disabilities. Therefore, reforms must proceed along both lines. However, in providing mechanisms for maximizing personal autonomy, such as through the availability of research directives, it is important that bases for intervention, such as by a guardian, be available to protect individuals even if contrary to wishes made contemporaneously or in advance. Hence, safeguards founded on the principle of personal inviolability must complement those promoting individual autonomy.

Research Directives

Advance directives provide a means for individuals, while mentally competent, to document and project their will into a future time where they anticipate a state of impaired decision-making ability. These devices yield an opportunity for persons to preserve their dignity by ensuring that the manner in which they will be treated is consistent with their wishes. Likewise, research directives would allow someone with decreasing or fluctuating cognitive capacity to provide an advance consent or refusal to participate in non-therapeutic experimentation. Guardianship statutes should be amended to include specifically research among the array of options available to the authors of health care directives. Those jurisdictions that do not yet provide for health care directives must enact corresponding reforms. It is not our intention here to provide an exhaustive review of ethical and legal considerations relating to the use of research directives, as this area has been dealt with in detail elsewhere.[97] Rather, specific ethical and legal concerns will be addressed insofar as they impact on the reform of guardianship laws in general and on the decision-making process of guardians in particular.

---

[96]The Alberta Law Reform Institute and the Newfoundland Law Reform Commission each went one step further in proposing that guardians should not be permitted to enroll their dependents in non-therapeutic research unless authorized through a valid advance directive. It is our view that, at least for the present, and until the use and application of research directives becomes sufficiently widespread, this requirement would unduly inhibit research. See Alberta Law Reform Institute, *Advance Directives and Substitute Decision-Making in Personal Health Care* (Edmonton: Alberta Law Reform Institute, 1993) at 41; Newfoundland Law Reform Commission, *Discussion Paper on Advance Health Care Directives and Attorneys for Health Care* (St. John's: Newfoundland Law Reform Commission, 1988) at 51.

[97]See A. Moorhouse & D. N. Weisstub, "Advance Directives for Research: Ethical Problems and Responses" (1996) 19 International Journal of Law & Psychiatry 107. The authors discussed the social utility of research directives, balancing their pros and cons from an ethical perspective, and outlined various recommendations with respect to their preparation, including the requisite threshold of mental capacity, their durability and execution, and fundamental restrictions on their implementation.

Research directives should be in writing, and witnessed and should provide sufficient details to present an accurate portrayal of the individual's wishes, values, and beliefs. Hence, detailed instructions providing an enumeration of acceptable procedures and levels of risk should be complemented by statements of principle that indicate general preferences. The prospective guardian should also be named. Since the goal is to ensure that one's wishes will be observed, specificity should be favoured over generality. Indeed, research directives ought to be read in a restrictive manner, and ambiguous instructions subsequently disregarded unless they can be clarified by a research ethics committee in consultation with the legal guardian. A person should not be enrolled as a subject in the absence of an explicit indication of the desire to participate in *non-therapeutic* research. Likewise, a failure to enumerate or classify acceptable risks should invoke the assumption that the subject wishes to participate only in research without risks. Standard forms should be made available, directives should be updated often to avoid becoming obsolete, and a system for their registration should be considered.[98]

All research directives would have to be reviewed by research ethics committees prior to their endorsement, ensuring that both legal and ethical requirements are satisfied. If the directive fails under examination, it becomes void. An important consideration would be to ensure that the person possessed the requisite level of capacity for preparing a research directive. Evidence of the author's consultation with family members, a legal advisor, the treating physician, or the proposed guardian would assist in this determination. The cause of concern is based on the fact that, unlike treatment, research is unlikely to yield an immediate medical benefit for the subject.[99] Moreover, a person in anticipation of diminished autonomy may act out of despair, lacking the frame of mind to make sensible choices or to formulate a sincere altruistic intent. Hence, the threshold for the capacity to prepare a research directive

---

[98]However, registration of research directives should not be onerous. In fact, the Alberta Law Reform Institute recommended against the requirement that all advance directives be registered, fearing that a complicated bureaucratic system would discourage individuals from preparing directives. See Alberta Law Reform Institute, *supra* note 96 at 17. The Queensland Law Reform Commission concurred with this perception, rejecting many arguments in favour of registration and reaching the conclusion that enduring powers of attorney for decisions other than financial matters should not be registrable. With respect to standard forms, the Commission recommended against the imposition by legislation of a prescribed form, owing to problems of inflexibility and potential invalidation on technical grounds, but rather that forms be developed by professional organizations in collaboration with consumer groups for use as guides. See Queensland Law Reform Commission, *supra* note 38 at 148–159, 355–356. The UK Law Commission, on the other hand, recommended that, in order to be valid, a continuing power of attorney should be registered after its execution. See The Law Commission, *supra* note 6 at para. 7.28–7.31. The position held here is that registration should be required upon the invocation of a research directive. The process should bear no cost to prospective subjects and should be streamlined to avoid administrative delays. Of course, there would be the corresponding onus of confidentiality placed on the registering authority, which could by delegation be the research ethics committee itself. See also Moorhouse & Weisstub, *supra* note 97 at 129–131.

[99]Review committees must also ensure that guardians are free from bias and that the advance consent was not obtained in a coercive or misleading fashion, resulting from the undue influence of a family member, treating physician, or researcher. Institutionalized persons might be particularly vulnerable in this regard.

should be greater than that required for testamentary instruments or health care directives generally.[100] In Ontario, a person giving a health care directive is not required to possess the capacity to make personal care decisions, only to have sufficient competence to give a power of attorney.[101] Lowering the threshold in such a way for the preparation of research directives can be justified only upon satisfying one of the following two conditions: the individual was already enrolled in a research protocol to which he had previously consented while fully competent; or the person had clearly expressed the desire to participate in non-therapeutic experiments on an earlier occasion, and the decision to give a research directive is consistent with those earlier wishes.

Naturally, there would be the requirement of a complete disclosure of all known risks and elements of the research in question, as required by the doctrine of informed consent, and also of an individual's full understanding of the nature and consequences of preparing the directive, including in particular the fact that choices will be acted upon at a time when the individual is no longer competent.[102] Special care must also be taken in order to avoid confusing claimed comprehension with true understanding, especially when dealing with persons with fluctuating mental capacities.[103]

Research directives cannot authorize the enrollment of an incompetent person in experiments that run counter to general principles of ethical permissibility, namely the restriction of such research to conditions or circumstances directly affecting the subject or the class of cognitively impaired adults to which the subject belongs.[104] Research directives also require limitations with respect to their scope, meaning that generally protocols with high levels of risk should not be condoned. Even fully competent adults are so restricted under Québec law.[105] It would be unusual therefore to allow a person to consent to high levels of risk, pain, or discomfort through a research directive that would be invoked when the person lacked the capacity to appreciate the consequences of the decision. It has been argued that an exception should be made in the case of persons who could give evidence of having previously experienced comparable conditions.[106] However, there is the difficulty of accurately quantifying "risk," "pain," and "discomfort."[107] Also, such a policy would be

---

[100]The concept of a threshold for capacity reflects the need to consider situational parameters affecting decisions, including increased complexity of information and the level of significance. This has been referred to as a "contextual" sliding scale and in no way interferes with a functional assessment of capacity, which requires that a determination be made on the ability to understand and appreciate both the reasons for and consequences of a specific decision while taking into account the vulnerabilities and special characteristics of the individual in the light of cultural and social factors. See Weisstub (1990), *supra* note 9.

[101]See *Substitute Decisions Act, 1992, supra* note 65, s. 47(2).

[102]See also Moorhouse & Weisstub, *supra* note 97 at 131–133.

[103]See e.g. M. Irwin *et al.*, "Psychotic Patients' Understanding of Informed Consent" (1985) 142 American Journal of Psychiatry 1351.

[104]See Weisstub, Arboleda-Florez & Tomossy, *supra* note 55.

[105]Art. 20 C.C.Q.

[106]See Keyserlingk *et al.,.supra* note 15 at 351.

[107]See the discussion on "risk" in Weisstub, Arboleda-Florez & Tomossy, *supra* note 55.

prejudicial against those persons who are fortunate enough *not* to have previously experienced high levels of the aforementioned. An inquiry into a subject's medical history could prove useful; although it would be preferable to adopt a policy that permits high levels of risk only in exceptional circumstances and only with the approval of the legal guardian, the research ethics committee, and a judicial or quasi-judicial authority.[108] A related issue involves the use of Ulysses Contracts,[109] which should be permitted but only for research that does not involve substantial risks of harm, pain, or discomfort.[110]

The requirement for consent exists not only prior to enrollment in an experiment, but throughout its duration.[111] This principle is mirrored by the right to withdraw from a protocol at any time without fear of reprisal.[112] Thus, it should be possible to revoke research directives at any time, even when a subject is mentally incompetent. The exception would be in the case of a valid "Ulysses" directive with low or negligible risks. The right to withdraw must be protected for other reasons, including the need for flexibility in the light of changing conditions, or perhaps owing to an underestimation of the actual pain and discomfort involved.[113] This is not to say that each objection should lead automatically to a termination of research. For example, individuals in a delusional state may resist or object to participation. Although a presumption should lie in favour of the subject who is at risk, the assessment of whether an objection is genuine might be in order. If either the guardian or research ethics committee reaches the conclusion that to continue to obey a directive would

---

[108]For example, the *Enquiry on Research Ethics* recommended that both the legal guardian and the proposed Provincial Ethics Review Board approve research directives consenting to participation in experiments with a substantial level of risk. See *Enquiry on Research Ethics, supra* note 1 at 92. See also Moorhouse & Weisstub, *supra* note 97 at 135–136. An onerous approval process in cases involving a substantial risk should contribute to a system that is in effect self-regulating, whereby, in order to avoid such an arduous review process, researchers would have an added incentive to minimize potential risks of harm, pain or discomfort.

[109]"Ulysses Contracts," referring to the Greek hero in the *Odyssey*, involve decisions made by patients in the context of treatment whereby instructions issued in advance are to be carried out despite any protest to the contrary made while incompetent. See A. Macklin, "Bound to Freedom: The Ulysses Contract and the Psychiatric Will" (1987) 45 University of Toronto Faculty Law Review 37.

[110]The justification for the use of Ulysses Contracts, although valid with respect to treatment, are not commutable to the context of research and should be permitted only when involving negligible or minimal risks. See Moorhouse & Weisstub, *supra* note 97 at 136. All requirements stated earlier for research directives in general should also apply to the specific cases of Ulysses Contracts, particularly the needs for specificity and a restrictive interpretation of ambiguous instructions. A guardian or research ethics committee should be able to withdraw the subject in the event where a protocol exceeds or compromises the terms specified in the Ulysses Contract.

[111]Certain authorities have suggested the adoption of a "consent monitor" to ensure that consent is preserved throughout the entire research process. See Melnick *et al., supra* note 27 at 534; Office for Protection of Research Risks, National Institutes of Health, *Protecting Human Subjects: Institutional Review Board Guidebook* (Washington, D.C.: U.S. Government Printing Office, 1993) at 6–30.

[112]See Weisstub, Arboleda-Florez & Tomossy, *supra* note 55.

[113]In fact, a researcher should be required to notify immediately both the guardian and research ethics committee for any change in the conditions of the experiment, health of the subject, or indication by the subject of a desire to withdraw.

be unethical, then they should be able to withdraw the subject from the experiment. Otherwise, once a valid research directive has been invoked, in the absence of special intervening circumstances, it should be followed without deviation.

The Guardian for Research

Research directives provide an ethical solution to the dilemma of consensual research involving cognitively impaired adults only in those situations where the adult was previously competent. Otherwise, such as with adults who possess severe mental disabilities and are therefore unable to express wishes in advance, the only alternative is to obtain the consent of a substitute decision maker. Guardianship laws should therefore be amended in order to provide for this alternative.

The powers of guardians should be granted only in accordance with a functional determination of incapacity.[114] Specifically, a finding of incompetence would be based on evidence of an inability to understand and make decisions in respect of participation in experimentation. It is important to reiterate that such choices belong in a special class of decisions that is distinct from those normally made in relation to personal health and welfare. This brings us back to the original therapy/non-therapy dilemma: treatment provides a benefit; non-therapeutic research does not. To condone the latter forces us to entertain an area of decision making that is for the most part alien to traditional notions of guardianship.[115] It is therefore necessary that, along with appropriate safeguards and restrictions, special provisions allowing for the appointment of a "guardian for research" be incorporated into adult guardianship laws.

The guardian of choice should be the person identified by the cognitively impaired adult, ideally through a research directive containing additional instructions to assist the guardian. Failing such, a close family member or friend should be appointed. The prospective guardian should be familiar with the individual and should understand and agree to respect the dependent's wishes, values, and beliefs. However, a close family member may not always be the best choice. For example, the inheritability of certain cognitive disorders such as Alzheimer's dementia may lead to a conflict of interest.[116] Care must also

---

[114]This approach would be consistent with a "least restrictive and intrusive" means of protection, which was supported most recently by the Law Commission of the United Kingdom, *supra* note 6 at para. 3.14. See also Weisstub (1990), *supra* note 9. A practical example can be found in Ontario, where:

> "A person is incapable of personal care if the person is not able to understand information that is relevant to making a decision concerning his or her own health care, nutrition, shelter, clothing, hygiene or safety, or is not able to appreciate the reasonably foreseeable consequences of a decision or lack of decision."

See *Substitute Decisions Act, 1992, supra* note 65, s. 45. Full guardianship is awarded only if there is an incapacity in all of the areas listed above. Otherwise, partial powers will be granted (ss. 59(1), 60(1)).

[115]An exception to this rule includes the occasional need for a guardian to order the commitment of a dependent for the protection of others.

[116]Children might have a personal stake in the outcome of research to be conducted on their elderly parents and would therefore be unsuitable guardians in this respect.

be taken in situations where participation in research would require institutionalization throughout the course of an experiment. The promise of a reward for the guardian or of special treatment for the dependent in exchange for participation in research is unethical and should not be allowed. Indeed, before accepting the role, all guardians must declare that they are free from bias and conflict of interest. As an additional precaution, the decision by a guardian to enroll a dependent in an experiment should be subject to the scrutiny of a research ethics committee, which would address the individual concerns raised by family members, the treating physicians, the dependent (even if incompetent), and independent third parties (such as advocate groups).[117] If the guardian breaches his fundamental obligations to his dependent, steps should be taken, which could be through an appeal to a judicial or quasi-judicial authority for the termination of guardianship.

Guardians for research should be empowered not only to enroll their dependents in research protocols, but to withdraw them as well. The latter should be exercised without fear of reprisal for either the guardian or the dependent and should not be overruled. Irrespective of the existence of a research directive, withdrawal from an experiment is justified in the event of unforeseen risks, the availability of new treatments, or a change in the nature of the experiment. In so doing, the guardian fulfills his obligation to act in the dependent's best interests. This duty, which is the primary responsibility of all guardians, should not be interpreted restrictively. It includes the duty to honour and respect the subject's known wishes, values, and beliefs, even if incompatible with those of the guardian. This charge can be rationalized through a prioritized system of substitute decision making.

A person's wishes would be given the first priority, including the instructions contained within a research directive and others expressed previously. When this is not possible, the guardian must act in the person's best interests, which involves taking into consideration current wishes (if they can be ascertained) and the values and beliefs known to have been held by the person when competent, which it is believed would still be acted upon if he or she were capable.[118] At all times, the guardian must strive to maximize the depen-

---

[117]The guardian for research would not, therefore, be operating in a vacuum and without accountability. Moreover, as indicated earlier, research ethics committees would also be subject to review by a central statutory authority. See note 83 and accompanying text.

[118]Although specifically excluded from application to the context of research, this approach is embraced by the current legislation in Ontario. See *Substitute Decisions Act, 1992, supra* note 65, ss. 66(3–4):

> (3) The guardian shall make decisions on the incapable person's behalf to which the *Health Care Consent Act, 1996* does not apply in accordance with the following principles:
>
> 1. If the guardian knows of a wish or instruction applicable to the circumstances that the incapable person expressed while capable, the guardian shall make the decision in accordance with the wish or instruction.
> 2. The guardian shall use reasonable diligence in ascertaining whether there are such wishes or instructions.

dent's role, even if incompetent, in the decision-making process. This approach effectively incorporates advance instructions into a hybrid model of best interests and substituted-judgment decision making. For each of these principles, although individually attractive in theory, apply poorly in real-life situations.[119] The discomfort faced by the Supreme Court in *Eve* illustrates this point well. There are obvious problems in applying either standard on its own, given that, in the application of each, one is forced to rely, at least in part, upon elements of the other. For how can we balance benefits that are instinctively calculated on a subjective plane, such as the right to procreate *versus* the freedom to experience sexuality without fear of pregnancy, and claim that we have arrived at an objective determination of another person's best interests? In deciding that one option outweighs another (and therefore lies in the person's best interests), are we not in effect making a substituted judgment? Indeed, we can no more readily divorce ourselves from our personal values and moralities than guess those of another. What, then is the difference between a "substituted judgment" and a decision made in a person's "best interests"?[120]

The Court in *Eve* was concerned about the irreversibility and non-necessity of the sterilization procedure and thus chose to err on the side of caution by

---

      3. A later wish or instruction expressed while capable prevails over an earlier wish or instruction.

      4. If the guardian does not know of a wish or instruction applicable to the circumstances that the incapable person expressed while capable, or if it is impossible to make the decision in accordance with the wish or instruction, the guardian shall make the decision in the incapable person's best interests.

   (4) In deciding what the person's best interests are for the purpose of subsection (3), the guardian shall take into consideration,

     (a) the values and beliefs that the guardian knows the person held when capable and believes the person would still act on if capable;

     (b) the person's current wishes, if they can be ascertained; and

     (c) the following factors:

        1. Whether the guardian's decision is likely to,

          i. improve the quality of the person's life,

          ii. prevent the quality of the person's life from deteriorating, or

          iii. reduce the extent to which, or the rate at which, the quality of the person's life is likely to deteriorate.

        2. Whether the benefit the person is expected to obtain from the decision outweighs the risk of harm to the person from an alternative decision.

[119]We refer to the advance directive principle, the substituted judgment principle, and the best interests principle. It is important to recognize that surrogates will use a combination of these standards in their reasoning. The degree to which advance directives will influence decision making will depend upon the evidentiary weight of the person's expressed wishes: as the level increases, one approaches a substituted judgment; as the level decreases, one must rely on a calculation of best interests. See D. W. Brock, "Good Decision-making for Incompetent Patients" (1994) 24:6 Hastings Center Report Supplement S8 at S9.

[120]Indeed, this observation was made in response to a series of American cases involving the application of the substituted judgment test in treatment-related decisions for cognitively impaired persons. See T. G. Gutheil & P. S. Appelbaum, "Substituted Judgment: Best Interests in Disguise" (1983) 13(3) Hastings Center Report 8 at 11.

disallowing it. But was this decision truly in Eve's best interests? Could she not have been exposed to even greater risks of harm resulting from an un-planned pregnancy with the associated psychological trauma.[121] A best-inter-ests decision, especially when superimposed upon a person's previously ex-pressed wishes, is therefore nothing more than benign paternalism. Furthermore, both the best-interests and substituted judgment standards rely intrinsically on value judgments made by a person other than the incompetent adult for whom the decision is being made. The former involves an external assessment and balancing of interests, while the latter requires the decision maker to "stand in the shoes" of the incompetent person, an act that is in fact rooted in fantasy.[122] The difference is purely semantic, and in reality, any decision made for a men-tally incompetent person will inevitably rely on a combination of the two pat-terns of decision making. In other words, a true substituted decision would logically be in the individual's best interests from that person's perspective. Conversely, any attempt to make a best-interests decision can be accom-plished only by emulating the person's unique style of decision making, which is in effect a substituted decision. We must therefore abandon any attempts to effect an idealized "best-interests" or "substituted judgment" model, prefer-ring instead to adopt the system advocated above.[123]

In the course of performing their duties, guardians may find themselves in conflict with the various participants in the research process. For example, the treating physician may seek to intervene if participation in an experiment would interfere with the subject's treatment plan, researchers may wish to dis-courage a guardian from withdrawing the dependent once committed, or the now incompetent subject may have consented in advance to participate in an experiment that has taken an unexpected turn but does not wish to withdraw. The overriding responsibility of a guardian for research in all cases must be to protect the interests of the dependent, which entails balancing various obliga-tions:

- to act in the dependent's best interests, which includes carrying out previ-ously expressed wishes, such as instructions found in research directives;
- to remain informed of the progress of an experiment and to be prepared to withdraw the subject;
- to assist and support the dependent in whatever manner required, includ-ing the maximization of the ward's participation in the consent process, both prior to and throughout the experiment;

---

[121]See also Shone, *supra* note 73.

[122]As a "construct of imagination," the doctrine of substituted judgment in fact constitutes a dangerous legal fiction, whereby an assumption can easily lead one to forget the underlying reality of decisions made in such a manner: that one person is rational and therefore in a position of control, while the other, because of mental incapacity, is neither. See L. Harmon, "Falling Off the Vine: Legal Fictions and the Doctrine of Substituted Judgment" (1990) 100 Yale Law Journal 1 at 70–71.

[123]Indeed, the Law Commission of the UK decided upon a "best interests" criterion that included an element of "substituted judgment." The exception, of course, is where it is impossible to ascertain a person's prior wishes, in which case, one must rely upon a best-interests determination. See The Law Commission, *supra* note 6 at para. 3.24–3.28.

- to interact with family members, public advocates, the researcher and the treating physician in order to ensure that the dependent's wishes are properly observed and that the person is not exposed to unreasonable risks; and
- to remain free of conflicts of interest, and to refrain from permitting personal values and beliefs to supersede those of the dependent.

Finally, it is important to bear in mind that experiments are by nature fraught with uncertainty and always possess an element of risk. Guardians who act to fulfill their duties towards their dependents in good faith should be exempt from liability for unfortunate accidents or harms befalling their dependents despite their efforts. This protection, and all others discussed here, should be guaranteed by statute.

Conclusion

The conduct of non-therapeutic biomedical experimentation involving cognitively impaired adults raises fundamental ethical, moral, and legal concerns. At the root of these issues lies the dilemma in resolving the conflict between the social incentive to advance scientific knowledge and the need to protect vulnerable persons from exploitation. Indeed, the historical record on abuses in research warrants caution in developing any policy that deviates from an outright prohibition. The problem is further compounded by the fact that non-therapeutic research, by definition, yields no benefit for the person who is placed at risk for the sake of others, a situation that is even more troubling when involving non-autonomous subjects. Nevertheless, the international consensus shows that biomedical research involving this population is both necessary and desirable. Extensively debated models defining the boundaries of ethical permissibility are available to assist us in developing a sound policy towards the regulation of research. Two goals must form the heart of any such initiative: to protect subjects, and to facilitate the research endeavour.

The law on experimentation requires that researchers meet a high standard of disclosure when recruiting subjects. Cognitively impaired adults, however, may be unable to understand properly, make choices, or communicate decisions about participation in research and therefore be unable to provide a direct and contemporaneous consent. The doctrine of informed consent, as a tool designed to preserve self-determinative rights, is insufficient in protecting non-autonomous persons, including adults who possess diminished, fluctuating, or non-existent decision-making capacities. Alternative means of obtaining a valid consent to participate in research must be made available to researchers. These include decisions made in advance or by a substitute.

Unfortunately, for example, in Canada, neither existing adult guardianship laws nor the common law provide a satisfactory solution. Not all provinces provide for health care directives, and no province explicitly includes research among the decisions that can be made by guardians or authors of directives. The common law on the subject is unclear, having adopted a restrictive interpretation of the best-interests principle in the context of non-therapeutic sterilization. Although it is possible that the court's *parens patriae* jurisdiction may be used to validate a decision to enroll an incompetent person in low-risk research or where the desire to serve as a subject had been expressed in advance, reliance upon the common law will not deliver a positive response in all cases, particularly where the prospective subject was never previously able to formulate wishes, values, or beliefs.

Consequently, adult guardianship laws require extensive reform in order to accommodate this special category of guardianship powers. Appropriate safeguards and regulatory mechanisms must be established in order to protect subjects; to govern the activities of researchers, including the review of all elements of the research process; and to provide regulations concerning the use of research directives and the behaviour of substitute decision makers. Reforms must be flexible so as to provide for an array of cognitive impairments, endeavouring to sustain an approach not based on benign paternalism, but rather one that respects individuals rights and entitlements.

· In adopting provisions for the use of research directives, it is necessary to establish formal requirements for their creation, limitations on their scope, and rules governing their review, implementation, and revocation. These include the notions of a restrictive interpretation of ambiguous instructions; a prohibition of the use of directives for consenting a high-risk procedures, especially in the context of Ulysses directives; and a requisite threshold of competence for their preparations that is in general higher than that required for consent to treatment. Adult guardianship laws must abandon archaic models that fail to recognize the notions of functional incapacity and thus allow for the appointment of a "guardian for research," whose authority would apply to the experimentation context. Guardians for research must be free of conflicts of interest and act in the best interests of their wards, applying a prioritized system of decision making that includes in their calculation the previously expressed wishes, values, and beliefs held by their dependents. They must therefore respect the instructions contained in research directives, but always be concerned with the safety of their dependents and prepared to withdraw them from an experiment if circumstances so require. Finally, guardians who fulfill their obligations in good faith should be absolved of all liability in the event of unforeseen mishaps.

Only in keeping with these guiding principles, and through the application of strictly enforced ethical and legal requirements, can society, in good conscience, benefit from the use of cognitively impaired adults as subjects in nontherapeutic biomedical experimentation.

Part III
Risk and Responsibility

[21]

The Ethical Analysis of Risk

Charles Weijer

T he institutional review board (IRB) is the social-oversight mechanism charged with protecting research subjects. Performing this task competently requires that the IRB scrutinize informed-consent procedures, the balance of risks and potential benefits, and subject-selection procedures in research protocols. Unfortunately, it may be said that IRBs are spending too much time editing informed-consent forms and too little time analyzing the risks and potential benefits posed by research.[1] This time mismanagement is clearly reflected in the research ethics literature. A review of articles published between 1979 and 1990 in *IRB: A Review of Human Subjects Research*, for example, reveals a large number of articles on informed consent and confidentiality (142 articles) and considerably fewer on the assessment of risks and potential harms (40), study design (20), and subject-selection procedures (5).[2]

The obligation to ensure that study participation presents a favorable balance of potential benefits and risks to subjects is central to upholding the ethical principle of beneficence and fulfilling the IRB's protective function.[3] Some believe it to be the single most important determination made by the IRB. It ensures that potential research subjects — be they sick or well, young or old, capable or not — are presented with the option of entering a research study only when agreeing to do so would be a *reasonable choice*. Accordingly, the Common Rule requires that the IRB ensure that:

(1) Risks to subjects are minimized:
    (i) by using procedures which are consistent with sound research design and which do not unnecessarily expose subjects to risk, and

Journal of Law, Medicine & Ethics, 28 (2000): 344–361.

    (ii) whenever appropriate, by using procedures already being performed on the subjects for diagnostic or treatment purposes.
(2) Risks to subjects are reasonable in relation to anticipated benefits, if any, to subjects, and the importance of the knowledge that may reasonably be expected to result. In evaluating risks and benefits, the IRB should consider only those risks and benefits that may result from the research (as distinguished from risks and benefits of therapies subjects would receive even if not participating in the research). The IRB should not consider possible long-range effects of applying knowledge gained in the research (for example, the possible effects of the research on public policy) as among those research risks that fall within the purview of its responsibility.[4]

The moral analysis of risk is neither obvious nor intuitive. Rules, including those of the Common Rule, are not self-interpreting. They must be situated within a conceptual framework that facilitates their interpretation by the IRB. The articulation of a conceptual framework for the ethical analysis of risk might therefore be a project assisting IRBs in fulfilling their mandate — the protection of research subjects.

Regarding the analysis of risk in research, the authors of *The Belmont Report* observed that "[i]t is commonly said that benefits and risks must be 'balanced' and shown to be 'in a favorable ratio.' The metaphorical character of these terms draws attention to the difficulty of making precise judgments."[5] Unpacking these metaphors for the sake of

The Journal of Law, Medicine & Ethics

enabling more precise judgments will occupy the bulk of this paper. What are the risks and potential benefits of research? How was the ethical analysis of risk understood by the members of the U.S. National Commission for the Protection of Human Subjects of Biomedical and Behavioral Research (hereafter the "National Commission")? What can be learned about the conceptual foundations of current regulation? What conceptual framework should guide the ethical analysis of risk? What changes to U.S. regulations would the implementation of such a framework require?

My work on this paper was commissioned by the U.S. National Bioethics Advisory Commission (NBAC) as a part of its project "Ethical and Policy Issues in the Oversight of Human Research in the United States." It is fitting, therefore, that the work of an earlier commission, the National Commission for the Protection of Human Subjects of Biomedical and Behavioral Research, receives special consideration in this paper. No other ethics body has had as much influence on the development of research ethics and regulation. As we shall see, pivotal conceptual advances in the moral analysis of risks and potential benefits can be traced back to the National Commission.

There have been considerable refinements in our understanding of the ethical analysis of risk in the last twenty-five years. Nonetheless, this paper relies heavily of the solid intellectual work that precedes this period. All of the work of the National Commission is a source for learning and much of it ought to be preserved in our current understanding and regulation. Two papers of Robert J. Levine, a staff member and consultant to the National Commission, remain foundational in research ethics: "The Boundaries Between Biomedical or Behavioral Research and the Accepted and Routine Practice of Medicine" and "The Role of Assessment of Risk Benefit Criteria in the Determination of the Appropriateness of Research Involving Human Subjects." This paper will assume familiarity with them.[6]

RISKS AND POTENTIAL BENEFITS IN RESEARCH

Risk is a multidimensional concept involving both the *probability* and *magnitude* of harms to research participants.[7] All too often, risk is equated with the magnitude of the outcome (e.g., death or serious disability). The proper ethical analysis of risk requires that both the magnitude of the harm and its probability of occurring be considered. A one-in-a-million risk of death is properly treated differently from a one-in-ten risk of death. Benefit, on the other hand, is the magnitude of a positive outcome without reference to its probability. In the comparison of harms to benefits, reference is often made to the need to consider the "risk-benefit ratio" presented by study participation. But this is not a parallel construction and, hence, it is strictly speaking incorrect. One speaks accurately of "harms and benefits" or "risks and potential benefits."

Research subjects may be exposed to a broad array of risks and potential benefits as a result of study participation. Risk is not a concept exclusive to biomedical research; social science studies also present risks to participants. Indeed, there is a surprising degree of overlap between the kinds of risks presented in biomedical and social science research. As study methodologies continue to cross conventional disciplinary boundaries, we can expect increasing convergence in the risks and potential benefits involved in biomedical and social science studies. We will thus need to consider whether the moral calculi involved in risk assessment suffice for the assessment of risks in research in a variety of disciplines. Consider the risks to participants in the following four case studies.

Study A: Placebo-controlled trial of a drug for people with acutely symptomatic schizophrenia

The study involves schizophrenic patients who are newly hospitalized with acute symptoms of their disease.[8] Despite the existence of an effective treatment for such symptoms, patients are randomly assigned to take a new antipsychotic drug, a standard drug, or a placebo. Patients are treated in a hospital for four weeks, where they are assessed with a variety of psychometric scales. Risks to subjects include the possibility that the new medication may have serious adverse effects, some of which may be irreversible; patients assigned to the placebo will be deprived of needed treatment for a month; patients may suffer from continuing hallucinations or paranoia; they may be at increased risk of suicide; and, finally, they may pose a risk to others. The ethics of placebo-controlled trials in schizophrenia is discussed in detail elsewhere.[9]

Study B: Hypnotic induction of partial deafness to see whether paranoid symptoms result

Several hypnotically suggestible, but otherwise healthy college students are randomly selected to receive one of three hypnotic suggestions: partial deafness without awareness of the cause; partial deafness with awareness of the cause; and no deafness but an ear itch.[10]

The hypothesis is that persons in the first group, as compared with those in the other two groups, will demonstrate more symptoms of paranoia. Subjects are assessed with a variety of measures, including psychometric scales and a scoring of observed behavior. After being evaluated, the subjects are hypnotized again, debriefed at the end of the study, and reassessed after one month. The study poses a variety of risks to participants, including the distress associated with paranoia and hearing loss, risk of suicide, the possibility of harm to others, and uncertain sequelae from hypnosis. Some of the ethical issues raised by this study are discussed elsewhere.[11]

Volume 28:4, Winter 2000

Study C: Questionnaire examining high school students about their sexual practices

The study involves the administration of a pencil-and-paper questionnaire to 400 Minneapolis high school students during regularly scheduled health classes.[12] The survey seeks to document attitudes and behaviors related to HIV prevention. Accordingly, the adolescent participants are asked whether they are sexually active, what types of sexual activity they have experienced (e.g., oral, vaginal, or anal intercourse), and the sex(es) of their partners. Various risks are presented by this study to participants: teachers or parents may become aware of undisclosed sexual activity; others may become aware of same-sex relationships; and participants might become aware that they are at risk of developing HIV. The ethical issues raised by this study are thoroughly reviewed elsewhere.[13]

Study D: Genetic epidemiology of BRCA1 and BRCA2 mutations in Ashkenazi Jews

The BRCA1 and BRCA2 mutations are known to be associated with an increased risk of breast and ovarian cancer. The study seeks to determine what proportion of Ashkenazi Jews (i.e., Jews of middle, northern, or eastern Europe or those of such ancestry) carry the mutations in question and what risk is conferred by them in a non-high-risk population.[14] Participants who respond to advertisements will be asked to give a blood sample and fill out an epidemiological survey, including questions on health, family history of cancer, and family members who might also be willing to participate. Personal identifiers will be destroyed before genetic tests are conducted and test results will not be disclosed to participants. The risks to participants are the risks of venipuncture, anxiety provoked by answering questions related to family history of cancer, and the risks of genetic testing, including unwanted disclosure of risk, discrimination, and stigmatization. A review of the ethical issues in genetic epidemiology studies may be found elsewhere.[15]

Four categories of risk

As illustrated by these four examples, research participation may expose the study participant to a wide spectrum of risks. Levine divides risks into four categories: physical, psychological, social, and economic.[16] Let us consider each briefly:

- *Physical risks*: The research subject may suffer bodily harm — minor or serious, temporary or permanent, immediate or delayed — as a result of his or her participation in the study.
- *Psychological risks*: Study participation may af-

fect the research subject's perception of self, cause emotional suffering (e.g., anxiety or shame), or may induce aberrations in thought or behavior.
- *Social risks*: Research findings, or even study participation itself, may expose subjects to the possibility of insurance or employment discrimination, or other forms of social stigmatization.
- *Economic risks*: Research subjects may directly or indirectly bear financial costs related to research participation.

So defined, risk is an inherently inclusive concept. As demonstrated by the above examples, a given study may present a variety of types of risk. For example, Study C (the sexual practices questionnaire) poses both psychological and social risks. Furthermore, no category of risk is exclusive to medical or social science studies: Study B (deafness and paranoia) — a social science study — presents physical risks, and Study A (schizophrenia trial) and Study D (breast cancer genes) — medical studies — generate psychological risks. Despite the diverse research settings and issues involved, all four of the study examples pose non-trivial risk to research subjects.

Levine provides a comprehensive description of particular potential benefits and risks presented to research subjects and society by biomedical and social science research and the listing will not be repeated here.[17]

ANALYSIS BY THE NATIONAL COMMISSION

How was the ethical analysis of risk understood by the members of the National Commission for the Protection of Human Subjects of Biomedical and Behavioral Research? What can be gleaned from their reports about the conceptual foundation of current regulations?

The National Commission sat from 1975 to 1978 and issued ten reports on human subjects research. The National Commission's work represents the first sustained, in-depth exploration of the moral analysis of risk in research. As such, it has had a lasting influence on research ethics scholarship and federal regulation. Little recognized is that the National Commission's views on risk analysis evolved over its four-year term. Three distinct views on the ethical analysis of risks and potential benefits in research can be found in the National Commission's opus: analysis of entire protocols; analysis of protocols with particular components; and analysis of components. In turn, each underlies an aspect of current federal regulations on human subjects research.

Six reports of the National Commission were selected for analysis based on their impact on public policy and the perception of the National Commission staff on the par-

The Journal of Law, Medicine & Ethics

ticular report's overall success.[18] These reports are *Research on the Fetus* (1975); *Research Involving Prisoners* (1976); *Research Involving Children* (1977); *Research Involving Those Institutionalized as Mentally Infirm* (1977); *Institutional Review Boards* (1977); and *The Belmont Report* (1978).[19] What follows is a critical review of the ethical analysis found in each report.

Ethical analysis according to entire protocols

Research on the Fetus was the first of the National Commission's reports. It was produced under several constraints.[20] Congress required that the report be completed in only four months and it imposed a moratorium on fetal research pending the completion of the report. Thus, Levine observes:

> As a consequence of these time constraints, the Commission completed its report, *Research on the Fetus*, before it had the opportunity to address the general conceptual issues in its mandate. If the conceptual clarifications ... had preceded the report, it is likely that the Commission would have developed substantially different recommendations.

In the report, the National Commission defines research as "the systematic collection of data or observations in accordance with a designed protocol."[21] The schema for risk analysis presented in *Research on the Fetus* relies on separating whole research proposals into two types, therapeutic research and non-therapeutic research. Therapeutic research is that which is "designed to improve the health condition of the research subject by prophylactic, diagnostic, or treatment methods that depart from standard medical practice but hold out a reasonable expectation of success."[22] Non-therapeutic research, on the other hand, is "not designed to improve the health condition of the research subject by prophylactic, diagnostic, or treatment methods."[23]

Separate recommendations are presented for each type of study. Recommendation (1) addresses therapeutic research directed toward the fetus. Under this provision,

> *Therapeutic research directed toward the fetus* may be conducted or supported, and should be encouraged, by the Secretary, DHEW [Department of Health, Education, and Welfare], provided such research (a) conforms to appropriate medical standards, (b) has received the informed consent of the mother, the father not dissenting, and (c) has been approved by existing review procedures with adequate provision for the monitoring of the consent process.[24]

Recommendation (4) outlines ethical criteria for the assessment of non-therapeutic research. It states:

> *Nontherapeutic research directed towards the fetus in utero* (other than research in anticipation of, or during, abortion) may be conducted or supported by the Secretary, DHEW, provided (a) the purpose of such research is the development of important biomedical knowledge that cannot be obtained by alternative means, (b) investigation on pertinent animal models and non-pregnant humans has preceded such research, (c) minimal or no risk to the well-being of the fetus will be imposed by the research, (d) the research has been approved by existing review procedures with adequate provision for the monitoring of the consent process, (e) the informed consent of the mother has been obtained, and (f) the father has not objected to the research.[25]

While there is intuitive appeal in categorizing studies as a whole, the validity of this approach has been criticized. Levine points out that this categorization invariably leads to deep conceptual problems. This is illustrated by inserting the National Commission's definition of research into its definition of therapeutic research. Levine argues:

> There is, of course, no such thing as a "systematic collection of data or observations ... designed to improve the health condition of a research subject ... that departs from standard medical practice." Thus, the Commission developed recommendations for the conduct of a nonexistent set of activities ....[26]

A further problem exists with this approach. The inclusion of one or more therapeutic procedures in a study leads to it being identified as therapeutic research. Once this categorization has taken place, there is no limit to the number of procedures without therapeutic intent that might be presented to research subjects as therapeutic. Thus, this approach not only leads to confusion, it leaves research subjects without adequate protection.

Despite its shortcomings, this approach is found in the current U.S. Department of Health and Human Services (DHHS) regulations on the protection of fetuses in research. The regulations divide research on the fetus into two categories: research "to meet the health needs of the particular fetus," i.e., therapeutic research; and research for "the development of important biomedical knowledge," i.e., nontherapeutic research.[27] As this approach to the ethical analysis of risk is not found elsewhere in the federal Common Rule or DHHS regulations, it may be a historical artifact of *Research on the Fetus* in the current regulations.

Volume 28:4, Winter 2000

Ethical analysis according to whole protocols with particular components

Recognizing the problems arising from the distinction of therapeutic versus non-therapeutic, the National Commission largely abandoned the use of these terms in subsequent reports. In the preface to *Research Involving Prisoners*, it states: "The Commission recognizes problems with employing the terms 'therapeutic' and 'nontherapeutic' research, notwithstanding their common usage, because they convey a misleading impression."[28]

In *Research Involving Prisoners*, the category of therapeutic research is replaced with "research on practices which have the intent and reasonable probability of improving the health and well-being of the subject."[29] While cumbersome, this manner of speaking at least avoids the conceptual confusion pointed to by Levine *supra*. In creating this new means of analyzing risk, the National Commission recognized that:

> additional interventions over and above those necessary for therapy may need to be done, e.g., randomization, blood drawing, catheterization; these interventions may not be "therapeutic" for the individual. Some of these interventions may themselves present risk to the individual — risk unrelated to the therapy of the subject.[30]

Despite this recognition, the report fails to advise the acceptable level of non-therapeutic risks. Indeed, in this regard, Recommendation (4) merely states:

> All research involving prisoners should be reviewed by at least one human subjects review committee or Institutional Review Board .... [T]he committee or board [IRB] should consider at least the following: the risks involved ....[31]

Clearly, IRBs require more detailed guidance on the ethical analysis of risks and potential benefits in research than is provided in *Research Involving Prisoners*.

The report does contain early ruminations about the notion of "minimal risk." Minimal risk is referred to nominally in *Research on the Fetus*, but only in *Research Involving Prisoners* do we see recognizable beginnings of what would become a central concept in the moral analysis of risk. First, a standard similar to that of minimal risk is articulated for research without therapeutic procedures:

> Research designed to determine the effects on general health of institutional diets and restricted activity, and similar studies that do not manipulate bodily conditions (except innocuously, e.g., obtaining blood samples) but merely monitor or analyze such conditions, also present little physi-

cal risk and are necessary to gain some knowledge of the effects of imprisonment.[32]

Second, there is an explicit recognition that in determining which risks ought to be acceptable, a comparison should be made between the risks of research and those of daily life — in this case, the daily lives of persons who are not incarcerated:

> The risks involved in research involving prisoners should be commensurate with risks that would be accepted by non-prisoner volunteers. If it is questionable whether a particular project is offered to prisoners because of the risk involved, the review committee might require that non-prisoners be included in the same project.[33]

Both of these standards find expression in current Department of Health and Human Services regulations.[34]

The concept of minimal risk is first fully expressed in the National Commission's report *Research Involving Children*.[35] It is natural that the most detailed recommendations regarding the analysis of risks and potential benefits are found in this report. Levine explains that:

> because infants and very young children have no autonomy, there is no obligation to respond to it through the usual devices of informed consent. Rather, respect for infants and very small children requires that we protect them from harm. No discernable risk seemed to the commission to be virtually impossible; therefore, they stipulated a definition of "minimal risk" as the amount that would be acceptable without unusual standards for justification.[36]

The National Commission defines minimal risk as "the probability and magnitude of physical or psychological harm that is normally encountered in the daily lives, or in the routine medical or psychological examination, of healthy children."[37] This definition differs from the one found in the DHHS regulations in its stipulation of *healthy* children; DHHS does not so limit minimal risk.[38] The National Commission provides a number of *prima facie* examples of procedures that pose no more than minimal risk, including "*routine immunization*, modest changes in diet or schedule, physical examination, obtaining blood and urine specimens, and developmental assessments" (emphasis added).[39] Again, this differs from the DHHS regulations in its inclusion of a procedure — routine immunization — administered with therapeutic intent.

The concept of minimal risk is central to the schema for risk analysis presented in *Research Involving Children*. Recommendation (2) requires that the IRB ensure that "[r]isks are minimized by using the safest procedures consistent with sound research design and by using procedures performed for diagnostic or treatment purposes whenever feasible."[40] Thus, if a blood sample is needed from a child, one ought, whenever possible, to use blood left over from a venipuncture done for therapeutic purposes. If the research does not involve therapeutic or non-therapeutic procedures that present more than minimal risk, it may be approved provided the above condition is fulfilled. Recommendation (3) states:

> Research that does not involve greater than minimal risk to children may be conducted or supported provided that an Institutional Review Board has determined that: (A) the conditions of Recommendation (2) are met; and (B) adequate provisions are made for assent of the children and permission of their parents or guardians, as set forth in Recommendations (7) and (8).[41]

Separate recommendations, as follows, apply to research involving therapeutic or non-therapeutic interventions that exceed the minimal risk threshold.

If research involving a therapeutic intervention poses more than minimal risk, the IRB must ensure that the balance of potential benefits and risks is at least as favorable as alternatives. Recommendation (4) states:

> Research in which more than minimal risk to children is presented by an intervention that holds out the prospect of direct benefit for the individual subjects, or by a monitoring procedure required for the well-being of the subjects, may be conducted or supported provided that an Institutional Review Board has determined that:
>
> (A) such risk is justified by the anticipated benefit to the subjects;
> (B) the relation of anticipated benefit to such risk is at least as favorable to the subjects as that presented by available alternative approaches;
> (C) the conditions of Recommendation (2) are met; and
> (D) adequate provisions are made for assent of the children and permission of their parents or guardians, as set forth in Recommendations (7) and (8).[42]

In short, the IRB should evaluate such interventions in the same way they are evaluated in clinical practice:

> [The IRB] should compare the risk and anticipated benefit of the intervention under investigation (including the monitoring procedures necessary for the care of the child) with those of available alternative methods for achieving the same goal, and should also consider the risk and possible benefit of attempting no intervention whatsoever.[43]

If, on the other hand, the research involves a non-therapeutic intervention that poses more than minimal risk, the provisions of Recommendation (5) apply:

> Research in which more than minimal risk to children is presented by an intervention that does not hold out the prospect of direct benefit for the individual subjects, or by a monitoring procedure not required for the well-being of the subjects, may be conducted or supported provided an Institutional Review Board has determined that:
>
> (A) such risk represents a minor increase over minimal risk;
> (B) such intervention or procedure presents experiences to subjects that are reasonably commensurate with those inherent in their actual or expected medical, psychological or social situations, and is likely to yield generalizable knowledge about the subject's disorder or condition;
> (C) the anticipated knowledge is of vital importance for understanding or amelioration of the subject's disorder or condition;
> (D) the conditions of Recommendation (2) are met; and
> (E) adequate provisions are made for assent of the children and permission of their parents or guardians, as set forth in Recommendations (7) and (8).[44]

Risks presented by non-therapeutic procedures are justified, therefore, in part by the importance of the knowledge to be gained from the research study as a whole. However important the knowledge, risks associated with the non-therapeutic interventions are effectively limited to "a minor increase over minimal risk." Risks exceeding this threshold require the approval of a national ethics advisory board and the secretary of the responsible federal agency (Recommendation (6)). The majority of the members of the National Commission defend this threshold for permissible risk as posing no significant threat to the child's health. The added requirement that such risks be commensurate to the child's experience ensures that such risks will be familiar. "Such activities, then, would be considered normal for these children."[45] Importantly, if the research

Volume 28:4, Winter 2000

Table 1. Applying the Recommendations from *Research Involving Children* in a Mixed Clincial Study.

NON-THERAPEUTIC PROCEDURE	THERAPEUTIC PROCEDURE	
	No more than minimal risk	More than minimal risk
No more than minimal risk	Recommendation (3) only	Recommendations (3) and (4)
More than minimal risk	Recommendations (3) and (5)	Recommendations (4) and (5)

involves both a therapeutic intervention and a non-therapeutic intervention that exceed minimal risk, then *both* Recommendations (4) and (5) are to be applied by the IRB.

This provision (Recommendation (5)) was the subject of the most enduring disagreement among members of the National Commission. Commission member Robert Turtle dissented from the provision, arguing that it should be impermissible to expose children to non-therapeutic procedures that pose more than minimal risk. He objected strenuously to the suggestion that sick children might be exposed to greater non-therapeutic research risk than healthy children would be:

> Children, who through no fault or choice of their own, are subjected to greater risks incident to their condition or treatment, cannot ethically be assumed to qualify for additional increments of risk. To do so, is to add to the potential burdens that result, directly or indirectly, from the child's illness.[46]

It scarcely needs to be observed that these provisions for the moral analysis of risk are complex. The recognition that a study may involve therapeutic procedures, non-therapeutic procedures, *or both* is a substantial leap forward over the schema for risk analysis found in *Research on the Fetus*. In *Research Involving Children*, the members of the National Commission solved both of the shortcomings associated with attempting to classify research as therapeutic or non-therapeutic (i.e., confusion and leaving research subjects without adequate protection) discussed *supra*.[47] The solution nonetheless created problems of its own.

First, the concept of minimal risk is applied to both therapeutic and non-therapeutic procedures in the examples provided in Recommendation (3). It is unclear in what meaningful way minimal risk can apply to therapeutic procedures. According to Recommendation (4), therapeutic procedures that involve more than minimal risk are justified, just as they are in clinical practice. In other words, there is no limit to the risk that may be posed by such procedures as long as they are reasonable in relation to potential benefits. Only non-therapeutic procedures should be subject to a threshold for permissible risk, such as "a minor increase over minimal risk."

Second, the National Commission's use of minimal risk in the recommendations seems at odds with its definition of "minimal risk." Recall that the National Commission defined "minimal risk" as risk commensurate with the risks of daily life of *healthy* children. Fixing the standard to the daily lives of healthy children seems designed to protect sick children from being exposed to more non-therapeutic research risks than healthy children. This presumed intention is contradicted by Recommendation (5), which allows non-therapeutic risks that are a "minor increase over minimal risk" as long as "such intervention of procedure presents experiences to subjects that are reasonably commensurate" with their experience.[48] Thus, a spinal tap done purely for research purposes may be permissible in a child with a neurological disorder for which such procedures are common, but not in a healthy child. The definition of "minimal risk" would be consistent with its use in Recommendation (5) if there were no reference to healthy children, as is the case in the current DHHS regulations.[49]

Third, little guidance is provided for the analysis of risks and potential benefits for procedures that pose no more than minimal risk (Recommendation (3)). Recommendation (2) requires that risks be "minimized by using the safest procedures consistent with sound research design."[50] This cannot, however, sensibly apply to risks posed by therapeutic procedures, since considerations of research design are largely irrelevant to them. One might reasonably ask: What ethical test ought the IRB apply to research involving a therapeutic procedure posing no more than minimal risk? From this report, no answer is forthcoming.

Fourth, research may involve both therapeutic and non-therapeutic procedures. Indeed, it is fair to say that this is often the case in clinical research. If a study involves a therapeutic intervention and a non-therapeutic intervention, then multiple recommendations may apply. The various possibilities are summarized in Table 1. If both procedures present only minimal risk, then only Recommendation (3) applies. If the therapeutic procedure presents more than minimal risk, but the non-therapeutic procedure presents minimal risk, then Recommendations (3) and (4) apply. If the reverse is the case, then Recommendations (3) and (5) apply. If both procedures present more than minimal risk, then Recommendations (4) and (5) apply. Since each of the recommendations refers to whether the research study as a whole involves a particular type of intervention, it is unclear how multiple recommendations are to be applied to a

The Journal of Law, Medicine & Ethics

particular study. Without doubt, it is a cumbersome approach and it may easily lead to confusion or conflict.

Despite these difficulties, the model for risk assessment found in *Research Involving Children* is clearly reflected in the current DHHS regulations for the protection of children in research. Indeed, there is a one-to-one correspondence between certain regulations and Recommendations made by the National Commission. More specifically, 45 C.F.R. § 46.404, "Research not involving greater than minimal risk," corresponds to Recommendation (3); § 46.405, "Research involving greater than minimal risk but presenting the prospect of direct benefit to the individual subjects," corresponds to Recommendation (4); § 46.406, "Research involving greater than minimal risk and no prospect of direct benefit to individual subjects, but likely to yield generalizable knowledge about the subject's disorder or condition," corresponds to Recommendation (5); and § 46.407, "Research not otherwise approvable which presents an opportunity to understand, prevent, or alleviate a serious problem affecting the health or welfare of children," corresponds to Recommendation (6). Note that the conceptual model for risk analysis underlying 45 C.F.R. §§ 46.404–407 differs from that underlying protections for the fetus noted *supra*.

The schema for the analysis of risks and potential benefits of research found in *Research Involving Those Institutionalized as Mentally Infirm* is essentially identical to that found within *Research Involving Children*.[51] Accordingly, I will add only a few comments at this point. The report refers primarily to persons who are both incapable of providing informed consent and institutionalized. It addresses the problems of including such persons in research by incorporating elements of *Research Involving Prisoners* and *Research Involving Children*. The definition of "minimal risk" refers to the "risk ... normally encountered in the daily lives ... of normal persons."[52] Thus, the risks associated with institutionalization may not be used to justify exposing subjects to greater research risks. Recommendations (1) through (5) track with Recommendations (2) through (6) from *Research Involving Children* and they will not be further elaborated here.

Ethical analysis according to a study's components

The final reports by the National Commission support an ethical analysis of the risks and potential benefits of a study according to its components, be they therapeutic interventions or non-therapeutic interventions.

The previous reports of the National Commission focused on risk analysis for particular vulnerable populations. In *Institutional Review Boards*, members of the National Commission articulated for the first time ethical standards to apply to the review of all human subjects research. The report explicitly acknowledges that a protocol may contain therapeutic procedures, non-therapeutic procedures, or both:

> A research project is described in a protocol that sets forth explicit objectives and formal procedures designed to reach those objectives. The protocol may include therapeutic and other activities intended to benefit the subjects, as well as procedures to evaluate such activities.[53]

According to *Institutional Review Boards*, risks must be analyzed systematically and should involve a procedure-by-procedure review of risks, benefits, and alternatives. In the words of the National Commission, "[t]his evaluation should include an array of alternatives to the procedures under review and the possible harms and benefits associated with each alternative."[54] The risks associated with particular procedures are acceptable only if "risks to subjects are minimized by using the safest procedures consistent with sound research design and, wherever appropriate, by using procedures being performed for diagnostic or treatment purposes; [and] risks to subjects are reasonable in relation to anticipated benefits to subjects and importance of knowledge to be gained ...."[55]

The Belmont Report provides little additional detail with regard to this model of ethical analysis. It famously articulates three ethical principles to guide the conduct of clinical research: respect for persons, beneficence, and justice. Beneficence demands that one do no harm *and* maximize possible benefits while minimizing risks.[56] Translating this principle into practice requires that the IRB ensure that research participation presents subjects with a favorable balance of possible benefits and risks. *The Belmont Report* once again emphasizes that this is to be done in a systematic and rigorous manner:

> ... The idea of systematic, nonarbitrary analysis of risks and benefits should be emulated insofar as possible. This ideal requires those making decisions about the justifiability of research to be thorough in the accumulation and assessment of information about all aspects of the research, and to consider alternatives systematically. This procedure renders the assessment of research more rigorous and precise, while making communication between review board members and investigators less subject to misinterpretation, misinformation and conflicting judgments.[57]

Levine renders the thinking of the National Commission somewhat clearer in two papers contained in the appendix of *The Belmont Report*. In the first, "The Boundaries Between Biomedical or Behavioral Research and the Accepted and Routine Practice of Medicine," Levine rec-

Volume 28:4, Winter 2000

ognizes the existence of "complex activities."[58] Such activities involve procedures administered with different intents. Some interventions may be administered for therapeutic purposes, while others solely to answer a scientific question. It is this difference in intent that drives the ensuing moral analysis according to the components of a research study.

The recognition of "complex activities" is further elucidated by Levine in *Ethics and Regulation of Clinical Research*, the seminal text in research ethics. He states:

> ... the Commission calls for an analysis of the various components of the research protocol. Procedures that are designed solely to benefit society or the class of children of which the particular child-subject is representative are to be considered as the research component. Judgments about the justification of the risks imposed by such procedures are to be made in accord with other recommendations. For example, if the risk is minimal, the research may be conducted as described in Recommendations (3) and (7) [of *Research Involving Children*], no matter what the risks are of the therapeutic components. The components of the protocol "that hold out the prospect of direct benefit for the individual subjects" are to be considered precisely as they are in the practice of medicine.[59]

Levine's description is clearly at variance with the actual text of *Research Involving Children*. The passage is significant as an account of Levine's own views on the ethical analysis of risk, developed for the National Commission. It may also be an accurate description of the view of the National Commission itself, as reflected in *Institutional Review Boards* and *The Belmont Report*.

It is this last model of risk assessment, "component analysis," that serves as the conceptual framework for the analysis of risk found in the Common Rule. Risks associated with non-therapeutic procedures must be minimized and "reasonable in relation to ... the importance of the knowledge that may reasonably be expected to result."[60] Risks associated with therapeutic procedures must be "reasonable in relation to anticipated benefits ... to subjects."[61]

Our historical analysis of the National Commission reports reveals that differing aspects of the current DHHS regulations are, in fact, supported by differing, and mutually incompatible, conceptual frameworks for the moral analysis of risk. The following is a summary of these differing frameworks.

- Regulations for the protection of fetuses in research reflect a "whole protocol" approach to risk analysis, which requires that protocols be classified as either "therapeutic" or "non-therapeutic" research.[62]

- Regulations for the protection of children in research reflect a "protocols with particular components" approach. This approach defines separate standards for protocols with either therapeutic or non-therapeutic components. Recognizing that a given study may contain both a therapeutic and non-therapeutic procedure, it allows for both standards to apply simultaneously to a given study.[63]

- The Common Rule, outlining general protections for research subjects, relies on the "component" approach to risk analysis. Procedures administered with therapeutic intent are justified when the benefits to subjects outweigh the risks. Procedures administered without such a warrant — so-called non-therapeutic procedures — are justified only if they are minimized and if the risks are reasonable in relation to the knowledge to be gained.[64]

The existence of incompatible frameworks underlying the current regulations is obviously problematic. It has surely led to ambiguity in enforcement and confusion among IRBs attempting to implement the regulations in a consistent manner. One conceptual framework ought to guide the moral analysis of risks and potential benefits in research.

Towards a Comprehensive Approach

The ethical analysis of the various "components" in a research study presents a number of advantages:

- It acknowledges that clinical research often contains a mixture of procedures, some administered with therapeutic intent and others that answer the research question.
- Therapeutic procedures and non-therapeutic procedures are, by definition, administered with differing intents. This difference is morally relevant.
- Therapeutic procedures are justified by their potential to benefit the subject, while non-therapeutic procedures are justified by their potential to generate knowledge. These two benefits are largely incommensurable.
- A rigorous separation of the moral calculi for therapeutic and non-therapeutic procedures protects research subjects better than any other approach. This separation prevents the justification of risky non-therapeutic procedures by the benefits that may flow from therapeutic procedures.

The Journal of Law, Medicine & Ethics

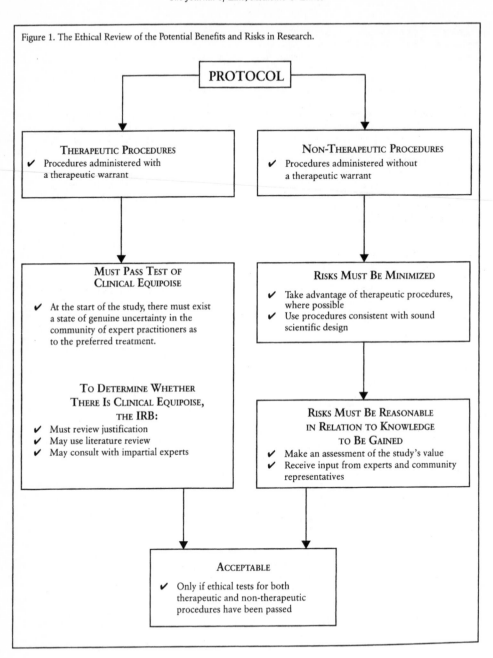

Figure 1. The Ethical Review of the Potential Benefits and Risks in Research.

PROTOCOL

THERAPEUTIC PROCEDURES
✔ Procedures administered with
  a therapeutic warrant

NON-THERAPEUTIC PROCEDURES
✔ Procedures administered without
  a therapeutic warrant

MUST PASS TEST OF CLINICAL EQUIPOISE

✔ At the start of the study, there must exist
  a state of genuine uncertainty in the
  community of expert practitioners as
  to the preferred treatment.

TO DETERMINE WHETHER THERE IS CLINICAL EQUIPOISE, THE IRB:
✔ Must review justification
✔ May use literature review
✔ May consult with impartial experts

RISKS MUST BE MINIMIZED
✔ Take advantage of therapeutic procedures,
  where possible
✔ Use procedures consistent with sound
  scientific design

RISKS MUST BE REASONABLE IN RELATION TO KNOWLEDGE TO BE GAINED
✔ Make an assessment of the study's value
✔ Receive input from experts and community
  representatives

ACCEPTABLE
✔ Only if ethical tests for both
  therapeutic and non-therapeutic
  procedures have been passed

Volume 28:4, Winter 2000

- It is a more parsimonious model for analysis than other alternatives, and it therefore avoids confusion and conflict.

Freedman and colleagues were the first to formalize a "component" approach to the ethical analysis of research risk.[65] This approach is summarized in Figure 1. Three main topics will be discussed here: the moral analysis of potential benefits and risks presented by therapeutic procedures; the moral analysis of potential benefits and risks presented by non-therapeutic procedures; and the role of the concept of minimal risk in the protection of vulnerable research subjects.

Therapeutic procedures

Therapeutic procedures are those interventions in research — drugs, surgical procedures, devices, or psychological procedures — administered with therapeutic intent (Figure 1). This category also encompasses monitoring procedures that would reflect ideal practice, even if these procedures are not routinely used in clinical practice. Consider what procedures might be considered therapeutic in the four case studies presented at the beginning of the paper.

- In Study A, a novel antipsychotic drug is compared with placebo. Both of these procedures are therapeutic interventions. The use of psychometric scales may be therapeutic if they are used routinely in clinical practice to guide treatment or if their use would reflect ideal practice. We do not have enough information to make this judgment, so we will assume that they are non-therapeutic.
- In Study B, hypnosis is used to implant one of three suggestions related to deafness. Hypnosis is used therapeutically in certain circumstances, but in this case, the use is non-therapeutic. The study population is not in need of any treatment. They are healthy college students and are participating solely for the purpose of testing a hypothesis.
- In Study C, a questionnaire related to sexual activity is administered to high school students. This is not a therapeutic intervention.
- In Study D, an epidemiological survey is administered and genetic tests for mutations associated with breast cancer are done on blood samples. The study is directed at all adult members of a community, not merely those who may require a detailed work-up for a genetic predisposition to breast cancer. Furthermore, results will not be given to participants. These interventions are, therefore, non-therapeutic.

Having determined which procedures are administered with a therapeutic warrant, how do we determine whether they are morally acceptable? Therapeutic procedures must pass the test of clinical equipoise (see Figure 1).[66] A major competing notion — the uncertainty principle — has recently been shown to be inferior to clinical equipoise.[67] Clinical equipoise is a norm developed in response to the question: When may the ethical physician offer trial participation to his or her patient? Competent medical practice requires that the physician exercise a standard of care — that is, practice accepted by at least a respectable minority of expert practitioners. The innovation of clinical equipoise is the recognition that study treatments — whether they be the experimental or control treatments — must be consistent with this standard of care. Thus, a physician, in keeping with his or her duty of care to the patient, may offer trial enrollment when "[t]here exists ... an honest, professional disagreement among expert clinicians about the preferred treatment."[68]

A state of clinical equipoise may arise in a number of ways. Evidence may emerge from early clinical studies that a new treatment offers advantages over standard treatment. Alternatively, there may be a split within the clinical community, with some physicians preferring one treatment and other physicians preferring another. This scenario is well documented in the literature and calls for a randomized controlled trial (RCT) to settle which is the better treatment.[69] Clinical equipoise permits these important randomized controlled trials. It would have physicians respect the fact that "their less favored treatment is preferred by colleagues whom they consider to be responsible and competent."[70]

When evaluating a study containing one or more therapeutic procedure, the IRB must take reasonable steps to assure itself that a state of clinical equipoise exists. This will involve a critical evaluation of the study's justification. In selected cases, it may also require a search of the medical literature or consultation with relevant experts who have no connection with the study or its sponsor. A variety of treatment-related factors are also likely to contribute to this determination: the efficacy of the treatment; side effects, both reversible and irreversible; ease of administration; patient compliance; and perhaps even cost. It is important to recognize that clinical equipoise does not require a numeric equality of treatment risks (or benefits, for that matter). It is more accurate to say that equipoise requires approximate equality in treatments' therapeutic index — a compendious measure of potential benefits, risks, and uncertainty. Thus, a novel treatment may pose considerably more risk to subjects as long as it also offers the prospect of considerably greater benefit. With novel interventions, the uncertainty associated with the intervention's side effects will almost always be greater than the uncertainty associated with the treatments currently used in clinical practice.

Study A is the only one of our four case studies that involves the use of therapeutic procedures. The IRB must ask itself whether a state of clinical equipoise exists among the new antipsychotic drug, the placebo, and the alternatives available in clinical practice? It follows from clinical equipoise that placebo controls will generally only be permissible for first-generation treatments — that is, when no standard treatment is available. Once effective treatment exists, new interventions must be tested against the best available standard treatment.[71] This standard is consistent with that found in the most recent revision of the *Declaration of Helsinki*.[72]

Because effective treatment exists for the treatment of schizophrenia, the use of a placebo in this case is impermissible.[73] The IRB must not approve the study unless either the placebo control is replaced with an active control or the patient population is restricted to those who have had no response to standard therapy, including any routinely used second-line or third-line agents. A detailed rebuttal of scientific arguments made in favor of the routine use of placebo controls can be found elsewhere.[74]

Non-therapeutic procedures

The remaining procedures administered in a clinical study are, by definition, not administered with a therapeutic warrant and are properly referred to as "non-therapeutic procedures" (see Figure 1). Such procedures are administered solely for scientific purposes — to answer the research question at hand. As all research is a "systematic investigation ... designed to develop or contribute to generalizable knowledge," it is difficult to imagine a study that does not include a non-therapeutic procedure.[75] A non-therapeutic procedure may be as simple — and innocuous — as randomization, chart review, filling out a questionnaire, an interview, or recording data in some other manner; it may, however, be invasive or otherwise fraught with risk, as with genetic testing, organ biopsy, or collection of information related to illegal practices. All four of our case studies include non-therapeutic procedures.

- Study A (trial of new medication in schizophrenia) proposes to test subjects regularly with psychometric scales. Filling out such forms is time consuming and potentially upsetting, and may expose subjects to the risk of discrimination.
- Study B (hypnosis and deafness) involves a number of non-therapeutic procedures. Subjects will be hypnotized and given a hypnotic suggestion solely for research purposes. Subjects will be observed, fill out psychometric scales, and be hypnotized again to remove the hypnotic suggestion. Distress and paranoia may result from the hypnosis; the effect of the hypnotic sugges-

tions is uncertain; and there are risks associated with the administration of psychometric tests.
- Study C (adolescent sexual practices) also involves only non-therapeutic procedures. The questionnaire addresses a number of sensitive areas of inquiry, including sexuality and practices that predispose the subject to the transmission of HIV. Subjects may find the questions anxiety-provoking and authority figures in the subjects' lives may learn of what the subjects' said, leading to stigmatization.
- Study D (breast cancer genes) also involves only non-therapeutic procedures. The epidemiological survey and genetic tests may generate information that is anxiety-provoking or indeed may lead to workplace or insurance discrimination. Beyond risks to the individual study participants, the Jewish community as a whole may be wrongly labeled as "cancer-prone" and subjected to discrimination and stigmatization.

By definition, risks associated with non-therapeutic procedures cannot be justified by the prospect of benefits to individual research subjects. Hence, a risk-benefit calculus is inappropriate to assessing the acceptability of these risks. The IRB must first ensure that the risks associated with non-therapeutic procedures are minimized "by using procedures which are consistent with sound research design and which do not unnecessarily expose subjects to risk, and whenever appropriate, by using procedures already being performed on the subjects for diagnostic or treatment purposes" (see Figure 1).[76] Second, the IRB must ascertain that the risks of such procedures are reasonable in relation to the knowledge to be gained (see Figure 1).[77] Thus, the ethical analysis of risks associated with non-therapeutic procedures involves a risk-knowledge calculus. The knowledge that may result from a study is essentially its scientific value. Freedman has argued that the proper assessment of the scientific value of a study requires not only the opinion of experts from relevant disciplines, but also the opinion of representatives from the community at large.[78]

In Study A, the IRB should ensure that all of the tests being administered are required and consider whether psychometric tests that are routinely administered might provide equivalent information. In Study B, hypnosis and hypnotic suggestion present worrisome risks. Can the information be gained in another way — for example, by studying those who are already deaf? Can the risks associated with hypnosis be minimized? Study C also presents non-trivial risk, in part because the questionnaire is administered in a high-school setting. Paying careful attention to maintaining anonymity, allowing students to unobtrusively opt out of the questionnaire or certain questions, and seating stu-

Volume 28:4, Winter 2000

dents so they cannot see each other's answers will minimize risk. In Study D, destroying subject identifiers and not informing participants of the results of the genetic testing considerably alleviate some of the risks to subjects. In all of the case studies, the risks of these procedures must be reasonable in relation to the knowledge to be gained.

Study D poses one category of risk that is not dealt with by this model — risks of discrimination and stigmatization to the Jewish community. The protection of communities in research is a novel area of inquiry in research ethics. Another paper commissioned by the NBAC argues for a new ethical principle of respect for communities.[79] Subsequent work has detailed possible protections for communities in research.[80] Most recently, a rational schema for mapping appropriate protections onto specific communities, such as Ashkenazi Jews, has been reported.[81] More work is required to determine how the ethical analysis of risk for communities in research ought to proceed.

Minimal risk

Minimal risk is a widely used concept in the regulation of research internationally. It can be found in the present-day laws or guidelines of Australia, Canada, the Council for International Organizations of Medical Sciences, the Council of Europe, the United Kingdom, and the United States.[82] That a research study poses minimal risk means that "the risks of harm anticipated in the proposed research are not greater, considering probability and magnitude, than those ordinarily encountered in daily life or during the performance of routine physical or psychological examinations or tests."[83]

Minimal risk has been the subject of considerable debate and confusion in the literature. As we have seen, the concept of minimal risk was applied to both research with a therapeutic procedure and research with a non-therapeutic procedure in *Research Involving Children*. In the context of our schema for the ethical analysis of risk, this makes little sense. If a state of clinical equipoise exists, it follows that the therapeutic indices of the various study treatments (and the alternatives available in clinical practice) are roughly equivalent. Thus, when considering the limit of risk to which research subjects may be exposed, we must focus on non-therapeutic risks. The risks of non-therapeutic procedures are the incremental risks associated with participation in a study.

Freedman and colleagues have argued that the definition of "minimal risk" in the Common Rule is best understood as a core definition with examples.[84] Minimal risk refers to risks "ordinarily encountered in daily life" — or, shorter, risks of daily life.[85] The second part of the definition provides two examples of minimal risk, both of them being procedures encountered "during the performance of routine physical or psychological examinations or tests."[86]

This definition has been criticized on the grounds that it is difficult to know what counts as risks of daily life and that the quantification of such risks is elusive.[87]

Freedman and colleagues concluded that the first claim is untrue and the second irrelevant.[88] Minimal risk does not refer to *any risk* encountered by *any person*, as some individuals engage in hazardous professions and pastimes and others never leave their house. Rather, it refers to the risks that are common to us all — driving to work, crossing the street, exchanging information over the Internet, or getting a blood test at the doctor's office. While it may be difficult to quantify the precise probability of given outcomes associated with each of these activities, we can nonetheless easily identify them as risks of daily life. As Freedman and colleagues observe: "We are, by definition, ... acquainted with them; and, almost by definition, if we are unsure whether they belong within the set of common tasks then they don't."[89] The assessment of whether a procedure presents a minimal risk is not primarily a quantitative determination; rather, it is a qualitative or categorical judgment made by the IRB. Research interventions may be determined to be of minimal risk because either the procedure is in fact encountered in daily life or it is sufficiently similar to those routinely encountered.

The threshold of "a minor increase over minimal risk" corresponds to the custodial duty that parents have for their children. Responsible parents make decisions regarding new activities for their child based on the child's daily life ("minimal risk") and make allowances for the importance of new experiences ("a minor increase over"). Thus, the threshold of a "minor increase above minimal risk" corresponds to the decisions made by responsible parents. This does not speak to the motivation of parents in enrolling their child in research; rather, it demonstrates that enrollment may be consistent with the norms of the parents' custodial duty to their child. While the majority of researchers and parents are scrupulous, some are not. The IRB acts *in loco parentis* by evaluating non-therapeutic risks as a responsible parent would, thereby ensuring that parents, scrupulous or not, will only have an opportunity to enroll a child in a study that passes such a test.

The concept of minimal risk serves two basic functions in regulation. First, it may be used as a "sorting mechanism," directing the attention of the IRB to studies posing greater risk. Second, it serves as a threshold, limiting the amount of non-therapeutic risk to which vulnerable research subjects may be exposed. The provision in the Common Rule allowing for expedited review is an example of the use of minimal risk as a sorting mechanism. If a study is found to pose only minimal risk, it may, with certain other caveats, receive approval by the IRB chair (or an IRB member chosen by the chair) without a full IRB review. The regulations state:

The Journal of Law, Medicine & Ethics

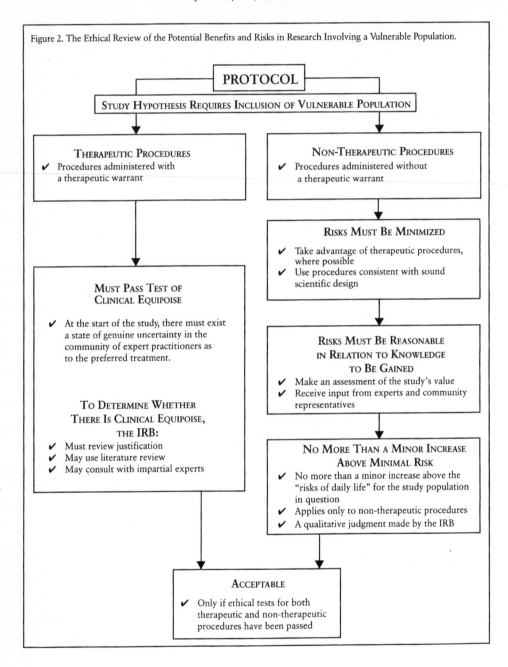

Figure 2. The Ethical Review of the Potential Benefits and Risks in Research Involving a Vulnerable Population.

Volume 28:4, Winter 2000

An IRB may use the expedited review procedure to review either or both of the following:

(1) some or all of the research appearing on the list and found by the reviewer(s) to involve no more than minimal risk,

(2) minor changes in previously approved research during the period (of one year or less) for which approval is authorized.

Under an expedited review procedure, the review may be carried out by the IRB chairperson or by one or more experienced reviewers designated by the chairperson from among members of the IRB. In reviewing the research, the reviewers may exercise all of the authorities of the IRB except that the reviewers may not disapprove the research. A research activity may be disapproved only after review in accordance with the non-expedited procedure set forth in § 46.108(b).[90]

Several problems are apparent with this provision. First, the requirement that non-therapeutic risks be both minimal risk and included in the list of "Research activities which may be reviewed through expedited review procedures" is curious. The list is obviously designed to include procedures that pose minimal risk to healthy adult subjects. For example, "moderate exercise by healthy volunteers" and "collection of blood samples by venipuncture ... from subjects 18 years of age or older" are permitted procedures. This eliminates from expedited review any study involving venipuncture in children or exercise by adults who are ill. This seems inconsistent with minimal risk, as defined, which does not limit the standard to healthy persons or adults.[91]

Second, the provision for expedited review offers an incomplete set of criteria. A given study might pose only minimal risk to subjects and yet raise serious ethical concerns that ought to make it ineligible for expedited review. One such case is a study that involves a vulnerable population. Studies involving vulnerable populations require special scrutiny by the IRB and should not be eligible for expedited review. Another such case is a study that has serious methodological flaws. Freedman observes that the ethical requirement that a study have a sound research design (validity) is absolute.[92] Thus, a study ought to be eligible for expedited review only if three conditions are fulfilled:

1. the study poses no more than minimal risk to participants;
2. it does not involve a vulnerable population; and
3. there are no serious methodological flaws.

Most important is the role of minimal risk as a threshold for allowable non-therapeutic risk in research involving vulnerable populations. Vulnerable populations in the Common Rule include children, prisoners, pregnant women, mentally disabled persons, or economically or educationally disadvantaged persons.[93] Given the heterogeneity of these populations, vulnerability itself must be a complex notion. Indeed, it encompasses groups who have one or more of the following characteristics: undue susceptibility to harm (e.g., pregnant women); incapability providing informed consent to study participation (e.g., children); or being so situated so as to render the voluntariness of consent suspect (e.g., prisoners).[94] In light of these characteristics, those qualifying as vulnerable are entitled to special protections in research (see Figure 2). Three protections are often invoked. First, a vulnerable group may only be included in research when their participation is essential to the hypothesis being tested. Second, if persons are incapable of providing informed consent, the consent of a proxy decision-maker is required. Third, the amount of non-therapeutic risk to which the vulnerable group may be exposed is limited to minimal or a minor increase over minimal.

The importance of the last protection can scarcely be overemphasized. Clinical equipoise ensures that therapeutic procedures in a study are comparable with each other and with alternatives in clinical practice in terms of their therapeutic indices. Thus, the incremental risk posed by study participation is that posed by non-therapeutic procedures. If vulnerable populations, such as children or incapable adults, are to be protected in any meaningful way, the risks of non-therapeutic procedures must be limited to a minor increase above minimal risk. This standard has the advantage of mirroring the custodial duty of parents to children and caretakers to incapable adults.

The NBAC proposes to eliminate this important protection. In its report *Research Involving Persons with Mental Disorders that May Affect Decisionmaking Capacity*, no limit is placed on the non-therapeutic risk to which an incapable adult may be exposed, provided certain consent provisions are obtained (Recommendation (12)).[95] This is shortsighted. When the limit of a minor increase above minimal risk is eliminated as a threshold for permissible non-therapeutic risk, no amount of risk is ruled out for research involving incapable persons. As long as the research question is important enough and informed-consent provisions are fulfilled, any amount of non-therapeutic risk is permissible. This change, if translated into regulation, will effectively undermine protections for incapable persons in research. Incapable persons will then be exposed to exploitation legitimated by the very regulations that were supposed to protect them.

IMPLICATIONS FOR U.S. REGULATIONS

It is clear that the Common Rule and the DHHS regulations were profoundly influenced by the works of the National Commission, as the different models of risk analysis that have been used by the National Commission are all reflected in the regulations. This incompatibility of ethical frameworks must be corrected if IRBs are to use the regulations to fulfill their mandate to adequately protect research subjects. What follows is a summary of the changes that I would recommend to the Common Rule and the DHHS regulations pertaining to risk analysis in order to achieve a single conceptual framework — namely, the "component analysis" approach. Specific recommendations for changes to Subparts B (pregnant women) and C (prisoners) of the DHHS regulations are not included.

To begin with, the concepts of therapeutic and non-therapeutic procedures ought to be specifically named and defined, as they are central to this approach to risk analysis. They should be defined as follows:

> § 46.102(k) *Therapeutic procedures* are study interventions administered with the intent of providing direct benefit to the research subject.
> § 46.102(l) *Non-therapeutic procedures* are study interventions that are not administered with therapeutic intent and are only intended to answer the scientific question of the study.

The general obligations of IRBs regarding the ethical analysis of the potential benefits and risks of research should be stated more clearly. I recommend the following:

> § 46.111(a) In order to approve research covered by this policy the IRB shall determine that both of the following requirements are satisfied:
> (1) Therapeutic procedures fulfill the requirements of clinical equipoise. That is, at the start of the study there must exist a state of genuine uncertainty in the community of expert practitioners as to the preferred treatment.
> (2) The risks associated with non-therapeutic procedures must be minimized (i) by using procedures which are consistent with sound research design and which do not unnecessarily expose subjects to risk, and (ii) whenever appropriate, by using procedures already being performed on the subjects for diagnostic or treatment purposes. Risks of non-therapeutic procedures must be reasonable in relation to the knowledge to be gained.

The definition of "minimal risk" has been a source of considerable controversy and confusion. The definition ought to be simplified and clarified as follows:

> § 46.102(i) *Minimal risk* means that the probability and magnitude of harm is no greater than that encountered in the daily lives of all (or the great majority) of persons in the population from which research subjects are to be recruited. It refers only to the risks associated with non-therapeutic procedures.

The role of the concept of minimal risk in expedited review needs to be clarified. The use of a list of procedures drawn up only for healthy adults is inconsistent with the concept's definition and use. Furthermore, minimal risk is not a sufficient condition for a research protocol to receive expedited review. Generally speaking, the study protocol must also be methodologically sound and not involve a vulnerable population. To this end, I would recommend that § 46.110(a) be deleted and that § 46.110(b) be changed as follows:

> § 46.110(b) An IRB may use the expedited review procedure to review either an entire protocol or a protocol amendment provided the review(s) determine:
> (1) the study methods are valid;
> (2) it does not involve a vulnerable population; and
> (3) it poses no more than minimal risk.

The ethical analysis of risk for research involving children can be simplified greatly with this conceptual approach. Simplifying these regulations will avoid confusion and help IRBs protect children who are research subjects. I would recommend deleting §§ 46.405, 46.406, and 46.407 and changing § 46.404 as follows:

> § 46.404 In order to approve research involving children covered by this policy, the IRB shall determine that all of the following requirements are satisfied:
> (a) the conditions of §§ 46.111(a)(1), 46.111(a)(2), and 46.111(a)(3) are satisfied;
> (b) answering the study's scientific hypothesis requires the inclusion of children as research subjects; and
> (c) risks associated with non-therapeutic procedures are no more than a minor increase over minimal risk.

A new section must be added to the DHHS regulations detailing protections for adults who are incapable of providing informed consent. The protections for incapable adults will, for the most part, be similar to those for children. I recommend the following:

§ 46.500 In order to approve research involving incapable adults covered by this policy, the IRB shall determine that all of the following requirements are satisfied:

(a) the conditions of §§ 46.111(a)(1), 46.111(a)(2), and 46.111(a)(3) are satisfied;

(b) answering the study's scientific hypothesis requires the inclusion of incapable adults as research subjects; and,

(c) risks associated with non-therapeutic procedures are no more than a minor increase over minimal risk.

ACKNOWLEDGMENTS

This article is dedicated to my three teachers, Benjamin Freedman z"l, Abraham Fuks, and Robert J. Levine. I am grateful for the helpful comments on earlier drafts of this paper by Drs. Chris MacDonald, Eric Meslin, Paul Miller, and Marjorie Speers. This work was commissioned by the U.S. National Bioethics Advisory Commission and funded by a Canadian Institutes of Health Research New Investigator Award and Operating Grant as well as a Dalhousie University Clinical Research Scholar Award.

REFERENCES

1. C. Weijer, "Thinking Clearly About Research Risk: Implications of the Work of Benjamin Freedman," *IRB*, 21, no. 6 (1999): 1–5.
2. B. Freedman and S. Shapiro, "Ethics and Statistics in Clinical Research: Towards a More Comprehensive Examination," *Journal of Statistical Planning and Inference*, 42 (1994): 223–40.
3. National Commission for the Protection of Human Subjects of Biomedical and Behavioral Research, *The Belmont Report: Ethical Principles for the Protection of Human Subjects of Biomedical and Behavioral Research*, DHEW Pub. No. (OS) 78-0012 (Washington, D.C.: U.S. Gov't Printing Office, 1978).
4. 45 C.F.R. § 46.111(a).
5. National Commission, *supra* note 3.
6. R.J. Levine, "The Boundaries Between Biomedical or Behavioral Research and the Accepted and Routine Practice of Medicine" and "The Role of Assessment of Risk Benefit Criteria in the Determination of the Appropriateness of Research Involving Human Subjects," in National Commission for the Protection of Human Subjects of Biomedical and Behavioral Research, *The Belmont Report: Ethical Principles and Guidelines for the Protection of Human Subjects of Research*, Appendix 1, DHEW Pub. No. (OS) 78-0013 (Washington, D.C.: U.S. Gov't Printing Office, 1978).
7. R.J. Levine, *Ethics and the Regulation of Clinical Research*, 2d ed. (New Haven: Yale University Press, 1988): at 37.
8. G. Chouinard, "A Placebo-Controlled Clinical Trial of Remoxipride and Chlorpromazine in Newly Admitted Schizophrenia Patients with Acute Exacerbation," *Acta Psychiatrica Scandinavica*, 358 (1990): 111–19.

9. C. Weijer, "Placebo-Controlled Trials in Schizophrenia: Are They Ethical? Are They Necessary?" *Schizophrenia Research*, 35 (1999): 211–18.
10. P. Zimbardo, "Inducing Hearing Deficit Generates Experimental Paranoia," *Science*, 212 (1981): 1529–31.
11. M. Lewis and P. Zimbardo, "The Ethics of Inducing Paranoia in an Experimental Setting," *IRB*, 3, no. 10 (1981): 9–11.
12. S. Phillips, "Asking the Sensitive Question: The Ethics of Survey Research and Teen Sex," *IRB*, 16, no. 6 (1994): 1–7.
13. *Id.*
14. J.P. Struewing et al., "The Risk of Cancer Associated with Specific Mutations of BRCA1 and BRCA2 Among Ashkenazi Jews," *N. Engl. J. Med.*, 336 (1997): 1401–08.
15. K.C. Glass et al., "Structuring the Review of Human Genetics Protocols Part II: Diagnostic and Screening Studies," *IRB*, 19, no. 3–4 (1997): 1–11, 13.
16. Levine, *supra* note 7, at 42–57.
17. Levine, "The Role of Assessment of Risk Benefit Criteria in the Determination of the Appropriateness of Research Involving Human Subjects," *supra* note 6, at 2.5–2.44.
18. B. Gray, "Bioethics Commissions: What Can We Learn from Past Successes and Failures?" in R. Bulger, E. Bobby, and H. Fineberg, eds., *Society's Choices: Social and Ethical Decision Making in Biomedicine* (Washington, D.C.: National Academy Press, 1995): 261–306.
19. National Commission for the Protection of Human Subjects of Biomedical and Behavioral Research, *Research on the Fetus: Report and Recommendations*, DHEW Pub. No. (OS) 76-127 (Washington, D.C.: U.S. Gov't Printing Office, 1975); National Commission for the Protection of Human Subjects of Biomedical and Behavioral Research, *Research Involving Prisoners: Report and Recommendations*, DHEW Pub. No. (OS) 76-131 (Washington, D.C.: U.S. Gov't Printing Office, 1976); National Commission for the Protection of Human Subjects of Biomedical and Behavioral Research, *Research Involving Children: Report and Recommendations*, DHEW Pub. No. (OS) 77-0004 (Washington, D.C.: U.S. Gov't Printing Office, 1977); National Commission for the Protection of Human Subjects of Biomedical and Behavioral Research, *Research Involving Those Institutionalized as Mentally Infirm: Report and Recommendations*, DHEW Pub. No. (OS) 78-0006 (Washington, D.C.: U.S. Gov't Printing Office, 1978); National Commission for the Protection of Human Subjects of Biomedical and Behavioral Research, *Institutional Review Boards: Report and Recommendations*, DHEW Pub. No. (OS) 78-0008 (Washington, D.C.: U.S. Gov't Printing Office, 1978); National Commission, *The Belmont Report*, *supra* note 3.
20. Levine, *supra* note 7, at 297–98.
21. National Commission, *Research on the Fetus*, *supra* note 19, at 6.
22. *Id.*
23. *Id.*
24. *Id.* at 73.
25. *Id.* at 74.
26. Levine, *supra* note 7, at 298.
27. 45 C.F.R. § 208(a).
28. National Commission, *Research Involving Prisoners*, *supra* note 19, at x.
29. *Id.* at xi.
30. *Id.*
31. *Id.* at 20.
32. *Id.* at 15.
33. National Commission, *Research Involving Prisoners*, *supra* note 19, at 20.

34. 45 C.F.R. § 46.306(a)(2)(A); 45 C.F.R. § 46.303(d).

35. National Commission, *Research Involving Children*, *supra* note 19.

36. Levine, *supra* note 7, at 239.

37. National Commission, *Research Involving Children*, *supra* note 19, at xx.

38. 45 C.F.R. § 46.120(i).

39. National Commission, *Research Involving Children*, *supra* note 19, at 20.

40. *Id*. at 2.

41. *Id*. at 5.

42. *Id*. at 5–6.

43. *Id*. at 7.

44. National Commission, *Research Involving Children*, *supra* note 19, at 7–8.

45. *Id*. at 139.

46. *Id*. at 148.

47. See discussion in the text under the subheading "Ethical Analysis of Entire Protocols" *supra*.

48. *Id*. at 7.

49. 45 C.F.R. § 46.102(i).

50. National Commission, *Research Involving Children*, *supra* note 19, at 2.

51. National Commission, *Research Involving Those Institutionalized as Mentally Infirm*, *supra* note 19.

52. *Id*. at 8.

53. National Commission, *Institutional Review Boards*, *supra* note 19, at xx.

54. *Id*. at 23.

55. *Id*. at 19–20.

56. National Commission, *The Belmont Report*, *supra* note 3.

57. *Id*.

58. Levine, "The Boundaries Between Biomedical or Behavioral Research and the Accepted and Routine Practice of Medicine," *supra* note 6, at 1.9–1.10.

59. Levine, *supra* note 7, at 250–51.

60. 45 C.F.R § 46.111(a).

61. *Id*.

62. 45 C.F.R. § 46.208(a).

63. 45 C.F.R. § 46.404–07.

64. 45 C.F.R. § 46.111(a)(1)–(2).

65. B. Freedman, A. Fuks, and C. Weijer, "Demarcating Research and Treatment: A Systematic Approach for the Analysis of the Ethics of Clinical Research," *Clinical Research*, 40 (1992): 653–60; Weijer, *supra* note 1.

66. B. Freedman, "Equipoise and the Ethics of Clinical Research," *N. Engl. J. Med.* 317 (1987): 141–45.

67. R. Peto et al., "Design and Analysis of Randomized Clinical Trials Requiring Prolonged Observation of Each Patient: I. Introduction and Design," *British Journal of Cancer*, 34 (1976): 585–612; R. Peto and C. Baigent, "Trials: The Next 50 Years," *British Medical Journal*, 317 (1998): 1170–71; C. Weijer, K.C. Glass, and S. Shapiro, "Why Clinical Equipoise, and not the Uncertainty Principle, is the Moral Underpinning of the RCT," *British Medical Journal*, 321 (2000): 756–57.

68. Freedman, *supra* note 66.

69. K.M. Taylor, R. Margolese, and C.L. Soskolne, "Physicians' Reasons for Not Entering Eligible Patients in a Randomized Clinical Trial of Surgery for Breast Cancer," *N. Eng. J. Med.*, 310 (1984): 1363–67.

70. Freedman, *supra* note 66.

71. B. Freedman, "Placebo-Controlled Trials and the Logic of Clinical Purpose," *IRB*, 12, no. 6 (1990): 1–6.

72. World Medical Association Declaration of Helsinki,

"Ethical Principles for Medical Research Involving Human Subjects" (October 2000) (visited Dec. 11, 2000) <www.wma.net/e/policy/17-c_e.html>.

73. J. Kane, "Schizophrenia," *N. Engl. J. Med.*, 334 (1996): 34–41.

74. B. Freedman, K.C. Glass, and C. Weijer, "Placebo Orthodoxy in Clinical Research. I: Empirical and Methodological Myths," *Journal of Law, Medicine & Ethics*, 24 (1996): 243–51; B. Freedman, K.C. Glass, and C. Weijer, "Placebo Orthodoxy in Clinical Research. II: Ethical, Legal, and Regulatory Myths," *Journal of Law, Medicine & Ethics*, 24 (1996): 252–59; Weijer, *supra* note 9.

75. 45 C.F.R. § 46.102(d).

76. 45 C.F.R. § 46.111(a)(1).

77. 45 C.F.R. § 46.111(a)(2).

78. B. Freedman, "Scientific Value and Validity as Ethical Requirements for Research: A Proposed Explication," *IRB*, 9, no. 6 (1987): 7–10.

79. C. Weijer, "Protecting Communities in Research: Philosophical and Pragmatic Challenges," *Cambridge Quarterly of Healthcare Ethics*, 8 (1999): 501–13.

80. C. Weijer, G. Goldsand, and E.J. Emanuel, "Protecting Communities in Research: Current Guidelines and Limits of Extrapolation," *Nature Genetics*, 23 (1999): 275–80.

81. C. Weijer and E.J. Emanuel, "Protecting Communities in Biomedical Research," *Science*, 289 (2000): 1142–44.

82. Australia National Health and Medical Research Council (NHMRC), *National Statement on Ethical Conduct in Research Involving Humans* (Canberra: NHMRC, 1999); Medical Research Council of Canada, Natural Sciences and Engineering Research Council of Canada, Social Sciences and Humanities Research Council of Canada, *Tri-Council Policy Statement: Ethical Conduct for Research Involving Humans* (Ottawa: Public Works and Government Services Canada, 1998); Council for International Organizations of Medical Sciences (CIOMS), *International Ethical Guidelines for Biomedical Research Involving Human Subjects* (Geneva: CIOMS, 1993); Council of Europe, *Convention for the Protection of Human Rights and Dignity of the Human Being with Regard to the Application of Biology and Medicine: Convention on Human Rights and Biomedicine* (Oviedo: European Treaty Series, 1997); Royal College of Physicians of London, *Guidelines on the Practice of Ethics Committees in Medical Research Involving Human Subjects* (London: Royal College of Physicians of London, 1996); 45 C.F.R. § 46.

83. 45 C.F.R. § 46.102(i).

84. B. Freedman, A. Fuks, and C. Weijer, "In Loco Parentis. Minimal Risk as an Ethical Threshold for Research upon Children," *Hastings Center Report*, 23, no. 2 (1993): 13–19.

85. 45 C.F.R. § 46.102(i).

86. *Id*.

87. L. Kopelman, "Estimating Risk in Human Research," *Clinical Research*, 29, (1981): 1–8.

88. Freedman, Fuks, and Weijer, *supra* note 84, at 16.

89. *Id*.

90. 45 C.F.R. § 46.110(b).

91. 45 C.F.R. § 46.102(i).

92. Freedman, *supra* note 78, at 9.

93. 45 C.F.R. § 46.111(b).

94. C. Weijer, "Research Involving the Vulnerable Sick," *Accountability in Research*, 7 (1999): 21–36.

95. National Bioethics Advisory Commission, *Research Involving Persons with Mental Disorders that May Affect Decisionmaking Capacity* (Rockville: National Bioethics Advisory Commission, 1998).

Defining and Describing Benefit Appropriately in Clinical Trials

Nancy M. P. King

Institutional review boards (IRBs) and investigators are used to talking about risks of harm. Both low risks of great harm and high risks of small harm must be disclosed to prospective subjects and should be explained and categorized in ways that help potential subjects to understand and weigh them appropriately. Everyone on an IRB has probably spent time at meetings arguing over whether a three-page bulleted list of risk description is helpful or overkill for prospective subjects. Yet only a small fraction of all the time and attention lavished on risk disclosure has been devoted to discussing whether and when potential benefit to subjects can reasonably be claimed and, if so, how it should be described in the consent form and process.

Traditionally, IRBs and regulators have worked to ensure that clear lines can be drawn between research that, by definition, carries no potential for direct benefit — because it uses healthy volunteers or because it is not foreseeably focused on the development of treatments — and research that does have the development of effective treatments as its goal.[1] Because of this, we have allowed ourselves to assume that all clinical research using patients as subjects and directed toward developing treatments offers a reasonable potential for direct benefit to subjects. This assumption is incorrect in many cases, resulting in what has been called the "therapeutic misconception."[2]

When the consent form and process go into great detail about the risks of harm and little is said about the potential for benefit, it is understandable that all those involved in clinical research — prospective subjects, investigators and other study personnel, referring physicians, regulators and policy makers, and the general public — generally assume that the intervention being studied is the best

Journal of Law, Medicine & Ethics, 28 (2000): 332–343.
© 2000 by the American Society of Law, Medicine & Ethics.

treatment option and that it would not be offered to prospective subjects if it was not going to work.

The therapeutic misconception has become more widespread because of recent technological optimism and public relations blitzes that preview even the most preliminary preclinical research results in the popular press.[3] This trend is far from new, but increasingly common. Indeed, the press conference has become a standard method of promoting research. For example, a recent cartoon depicts several white-coated researchers in front of a bank of microphones: "And while the drug hasn't been tested on humans, it works on mice and the stock market."

Unfortunately, this kind of discussion and promotion can result in confusion and betrayal of trust when patient-subjects realize that the optimistic assessment of their chances of benefit was really a misconception. Articles with headlines like "Patient or Guinea Pig? Dilemma of Clinical Trials"[4] and "When the Dying Enroll in Studies: A Debate Over False Hopes"[5] have become commonplace in the popular press over the last several years.

The Common Rule[6] actually doesn't say much about benefit. In order for research to be approved, it requires that "risks to subjects are reasonable in relation to anticipated benefits, if any, to subjects, and the importance of the knowledge that may reasonably be expected to result" (that is, the benefit to society from the results of the research).[7] And benefits to subjects or others "which may reasonably be expected from the research" should be described in the consent form and process.[8]

Thus, for all research using patients as subjects, IRBs and investigators must do more than distinguish between research that is and is not focused on the development of treatments. In addition, for all research focused on the development of treatments, it is essential, first, to determine whether participation in the research holds out a reason-

The Journal of Law, Medicine & Ethics

able prospect of direct benefit for subjects and, second, to describe and discuss the prospect of direct benefit sufficiently to permit informed decision-making by prospective patient-subjects. That is, there must be a *reasonable chance* of benefit in order for a prospective subject to make a *reasonable choice* about participation based on anticipated benefit.[9] Note that "reasonable" is not synonymous with "rational." Reasonableness requirements take into account circumstances and values, not just statistics, but can nonetheless be subjected to deliberation and discussion.

It is especially important to try to determine whether there is a reasonable chance of benefit to subjects because, under the current regulatory scheme, so much hinges on distinguishing between research that does offer subjects the potential for direct benefit and research that does not. Being able to claim that there is potential benefit for subjects is linked to:

- research bearing more than minimal risk and involving children,[10] pregnant women and fetuses,[11] persons with questionable decisional capacity,[12] and prisoners;[13]
- waiver of consent in emergency research;[14]
- emergency use of a "test article" without IRB approval, including without consent;[15]
- use of so-called "treatment 'investigational new drugs'" (INDs);[16] and
- insurance reimbursement for research costs.[17]

Thus, there is a natural tendency for investigators and IRBs to indulge in "benefit creep." That is, to ensure that research considered beneficial to *society* can go forward, investigators and IRBs may exaggerate or even invent benefit to subjects.

What IRBs Can Do

Even outside of these particular research categories and populations, it is important to correct what has become the pervasive and routine underdescription and overestimation of benefit in clinical research. There are four things IRBs should do, discussed below.

Keep the types of benefit separate

There are three distinguishable types of benefit possible from research:

- *direct* benefit to subjects, which is properly defined as benefit arising from receiving the intervention being studied;
- *collateral* benefit to subjects (the National Bioethics Advisory Commission calls this "indirect" benefit[18]), which is benefit arising from being a

subject, even if one does not receive the experimental intervention (for example, a free physical exam and testing, free medical care and other extras, or the personal gratification of altruism);
- *aspirational* benefit,[19] or benefit to society and to future patients, which arises from the results of the study.

Payment to subjects, though technically a collateral benefit, is classified and treated separately in research ethics and policy.[20]

In clinical research designed to develop future treatments, it is direct benefit that is of greatest interest to patient-subjects. And it is, unfortunately, quite common to combine and confuse direct benefit with aspirational benefit. One of the ways this happens is through the background and purpose sections of consent forms. These sections at the beginning of the consent form often contain extensive descriptions of what the research hopes to prove — that is, of the generalizable knowledge and societal benefit sought — in terms that are easy to confuse with what patient-subjects hope for themselves. This problem is compounded when the purpose section in an early-phase trial describes the aspirational benefit expected from the entire line of research, not just from the particular trial. This fosters confusion between what the investigators hope to show by the end of the clinical trials process and what individual subjects can anticipate in that trial.[21]

It is also common to combine and confuse direct and collateral benefit, as investigators do when they express their firm belief that "patients get the best treatment on-study" because they are at the best academic medical centers and getting more attention than they would off-study. Indeed, direct and collateral benefit are confused any time the discussion of benefit is limited to "benefit from participating in this research" rather than focusing on both "benefit from receiving the intervention being studied" *and* "other benefits from participating."[22]

To give a recent example, the 1998 study of IRBs by the National Institutes of Health's Office of Extramural Research, "Evaluation of NIH Implementation of Section 491 of the PHS Act, Mandating a Program of Protection for Research Subjects," contains only one paragraph about benefit:

> Investigators were also asked to identify the types, level, and likelihood of benefits to subjects that were anticipated when their protocols were submitted. Analysis revealed the majority of investigators expected for each type of benefit both a medium or high level of beneficial effect and a 50 percent or greater chance of the benefit occurring.[23]

This is pretty optimistic, but the optimism is made more understandable when you realize that the report's types of benefit — medical, social, psychological, educational — do not distinguish between direct and collateral benefit at all.

Examine any claim of potential benefit carefully

Some clinical trials with patients as subjects clearly do not offer the prospect of direct benefit. Some IRBs recognize this and require investigators to be candid in the consent form. For example, one of the first gene transfer research protocols for cystic fibrosis took place at the University of North Carolina. Corrected genetic material was combined with a modified virus "vector" designed to transport the material into the subject's cells, and was instilled into subjects' nasal passages. Since cystic fibrosis profoundly affects patients' lungs and other organs, this experiment could not make a difference in their disease even if it were completely successful in "transfecting" cells in the subjects' noses. The consent form appropriately said: "You will not benefit."[24]

Such clear statements are rare. Nonetheless, in many early-phase clinical trials, the prospect of direct benefit may be too small, too attenuated, too unlikely, too uncertain to hold out as reasonable to expect. Phase I trials like the nasal gene transfer study, which test the safety and toxicity of drugs, biologicals, or other interventions not yet tried in humans, generally fall into this category; yet consent forms for many Phase I oncology trials, for example, contain a great deal of optimistic, treatment-oriented language addressing potential benefit. When benefit cannot reasonably be expected, the consent form should say, "You will not benefit."

For early-stage research, investigators should be required to demonstrate to the IRB that "You will not benefit" is *not* what should be in the consent form. Currently, it is often presumed that benefit can be shown. The presumption should be reversed in order to elicit better and more complete evidence about the potential for benefit.

What is a reasonable chance of direct benefit? That is a critical and difficult question. IRBs and investigators haven't often looked at this question, and in my view, many guidance documents like *The Belmont Report*,[25] the IRB Guidebook[26] issued by the Office for Human Research Protections (formerly the Office for Protection from Research Risks), and the Food and Drug Administration's Information Sheets[27] are better at illustrating the problem than offering a solution. Yet other scholarly and guidance documents are clearer and require more. For example, the National Commission for the Protection of Human Subjects of Biomedical and Behavioral Research states that to be considered direct, the possibility of benefit must be "fairly immediate" and the expectation of success should be well-founded scientifically.

This definition provides a little more specificity, even though it still leaves some terms to be defined.[28] Significantly, it makes clear that any "reasonable chance" threshold requirement is *evidentiary* in nature — that is, within the province of the IRB and scientific knowledge. Only the reasonable *choice* requirement is personal because what counts as a reasonable choice, after appropriate disclosure and discussion, is left to the prospective subject.

Investigators and IRBs need better guidance in making and evaluating claims of potential benefit to subjects. But even without setting a reasonable chance threshold, IRBs can do much to improve disclosure and discussion and to enable reasonable choice about benefit.

Discuss the dimensions of benefit

There are three dimensions of potential benefit that should be described and discussed in the consent form and process, just as they are discussed with respect to risks of harm:

- the nature of the potential benefit;
- the magnitude (size and duration) of the potential benefit; and
- the likelihood of the potential benefit.

It is immediately evident that these dimensions overlap in some respects, as they do for risks. It is also clear that it is somewhat difficult to be specific about these dimensions as applied to the type of benefit of greatest interest — direct benefit — since this is exactly what is being studied. But this "uncertainty factor" is equally true for risks of harm, and we talk about risks in the same kind of detail all the time — indeed, it is strongly encouraged.[29]

Most importantly, though, as thoughtful IRB members will recognize, detailed statements about anticipated benefit must be very carefully articulated in order to avoid precisely the conflation that must be avoided: confusing societal benefit — that is, future effects of the research results — with direct benefit from receiving the experimental intervention.[30] Will more description inevitably produce more overselling? I don't think so, provided that the description is accurate in its depiction of the uncertainties and limitations of the evidence.

Nature

What kind of benefit is expected? In some early-phase research, the kind of benefit may be difficult to specify, as the research design will be focused on measuring toxicity and evaluating safety. Some protocols may measure surrogate endpoints — laboratory measures thought to serve as markers for long-term, harder-to-measure improvements in morbidity and mortality. Sometimes, it is not clear to IRBs or to potential subjects what clinical effects are anticipated to correspond with the measured endpoints. But a general description of the nature of the benefit, accompanied by a clear statement of the uncertainties, unknowns, and unproven status of the intervention being studied, is possible and necessary.

Magnitude

How great is the potential benefit expected to be, and how long is it expected to last? These two components of magnitude are rarely discussed in consent forms, leading to the natural assumption that the intervention being studied promises a complete and permanent cure, when often the most that could ever be expected is partial: a reduction in symptoms or an improvement in a condition. In research on most surgical procedures and some drugs and biologicals, the beneficial effects that could be realized are permanent; but more often, they are temporary, in ways that are obvious (e.g., effects of the study drug last only as long as you are taking it) or not so obvious (e.g., effects of the intervention are expected to wear off or fade over time). "We do not know how long any beneficial effects might last" is always a true statement about an unproven intervention being studied.

Likelihood

How likely is it that any given subject will experience a direct benefit? This is, of course, quite difficult to predict, but several things are surely true. First, the likelihood can at least be partially signaled by the results of preclinical (laboratory and animal) research. Although 100 percent effectiveness in a test tube does not portend the same success rate in human trials, a low incidence of effectiveness in preclinical trials does generally suggest a low likelihood in human trials.

Second, the likelihood of effectiveness will probably be quite low in the earliest phases of clinical trials and may change (along with specificity about the other dimensions of potential benefit) in later phases, as more information is gathered about effectiveness — either about how to maximize it or about its failure to materialize.

Third, the likelihood of effectiveness is affected by design elements, such as placebo or standard treatment arms, dose escalation designs, and the assignment of subjects to different dosing cohorts or regimens. Even when the likelihood of beneficial effect from the intervention is relatively high, it is lowered for individual subjects by the probability that they could be assigned to a placebo arm or to a cohort receiving a low dose. Likelihood need not be characterized by percentages, but all necessary information must be used in any characterization. Thus, if animal studies showed that two of twelve rabbits had a change in a surrogate measure at the highest dose level, but only one of those two rabbits had a change great enough to show clinical effect in hu-

mans and only the third dosing cohort (3–6 subjects) in a Phase I study is going to receive a dose comparable to that given to the twelve rabbits, the likelihood that any of the subjects in this Phase I trial is going to benefit directly from participation is, at best, very low — and should be so described.

For example, in mid-October 1999, the first human trials of endostatin for tumor suppression were started. Dr. Judah Folkman emphasized in an interview with the *Chicago Tribune* that despite the enormous optimism and publicity surrounding his research — three subjects were picked by lottery from thousands of "hopeful applicants" — success in mice does not necessarily portend even partial success in humans. After all, he noted, "Most drugs fail."[31]

Acknowledge uncertainty without ambiguity

Instead of detailed discussion designed to promote careful assessment and reasonable decision-making, prospective subjects are more likely to read "boilerplate" statements, such as the following, in the benefit section of the consent form:

- "It is not known whether your participation in this research study will have a beneficial effect."
- "You may not benefit from this research study."
- "Personal benefit cannot be guaranteed."
- Or the standard version used in much oncology research, "A potential benefit is control of your disease, if you should respond to these treatments. However, it is possible that your condition could worsen despite treatment."

Often, this is the only description of potential benefit in the entire document, aside from the aspirational benefit description in the purpose section. The vagueness of these statements is particularly troubling because they are so general that they could be applied to any standard treatment of proven effectiveness and, therefore, do nothing to distinguish research from treatment or to signal the uncertainty appropriate to most research settings. Surely we can do better than this.

Several examples of improved benefit boilerplate statements follow:

- "This medical research project is not expected to benefit you" (scholars from the University of Pennsylvania's Bioethics Center have recommended that this statement be prominently placed near the beginning of all consent forms for Phase I studies).[32]
- "What you need to know before entering a clinical trial: You are not a patient" (the headline on a sidebar in a *U.S. News Online* story about

Volume 28:4, Winter 2000

the brief suspension of Duke University's federal authorization to perform human subjects research in April 1999).[33]

Are these better? Yes. Are they good enough? No. The problem is that detail and evidence are required when direct benefit is being discussed. Boilerplate is simply inadequate; it is essential to particularize.

The following statement, compiled from three consent forms for early-stage research that had unusually detailed benefit sections, may serve as one example of particularization:

> This research project is primarily testing the safety of an experimental intervention with which we have little experience. It is not likely that participation will benefit you. Results of earlier research have shown that a few subjects experienced reduction in symptoms, but most did not benefit in any way. We hope that the tumor may become smaller for a period of time, but we do not know if this will occur or for how long any benefit will last.

It is obvious how much more this attention to detail requires of both investigators and IRBs — namely, to craft and review descriptions of potential benefit whenever it can be reasonably claimed and to be sure that claims of potential benefit are adequately supported and not overstated. But because so little attention has been given to describing and discussing benefit in research, improvements here could greatly improve decision-making.

A REASONABLE CHANCE OF DIRECT BENEFIT

Better disclosure of and discussion about the potential for direct benefit could also provide needed insight into whether a "reasonable chance of benefit" threshold can be established for clinical research. What should count as a reasonable chance of benefit? How should it be measured and by whom? Can a threshold be set?

A definition?

The easiest way to talk about direct benefit is by using lawyerly language, familiar from informed consent case law, using as a reference point the famed "reasonable person." One possible definition follows: *A reasonable chance of direct benefit exists when a reasonable person under all the circumstances would consider the nature, magnitude, and likelihood of direct benefit sufficient to reasonably choose to participate in research in anticipation of the benefit.*

"A reasonable person" really means *all* reasonable people. This is implicit, but not discussed, in the application of the reasonable-person standard to informed decision-making. It makes obvious sense because otherwise only one reasonable person would be needed to establish a standard for everyone. Yet all that is required is that the potential for direct benefit be generally considered sufficient to choose on that basis. It does *not* mean that all reasonable people would so choose, because, as we also know from the law, reasonable minds may differ.

The important thing about the reasonableness of the chance lies in the definition's implicit demand that *evidence* be presented with respect to all three dimensions of direct benefit and that, in combination, they be judged sufficient to support a decision to become a subject in order to gain the chance to benefit. It is essential that supporting evidence appropriate to the stage of research be presented to potential subjects[34] — including laboratory and animal evidence, and human data if available. A plausible, logical theory is not enough.

Remember that a reasonable chance of direct benefit and a reasonable choice about participation are not the same. The proposed definition of reasonable chance does not mean that all reasonable people would choose to participate. That would wrongly equate the evidentiary reasonable-chance standard with the only reasonable choice. Instead, a reasonable chance means that all reasonable people would consider the information sufficient to attempt to secure the benefit. The emphasis is on the presentation of evidence sufficient to support a benefit-seeking choice.

Skepticism about claims of direct benefit in clinical research is essential. Nonetheless, the evidence required to claim direct benefit from an investigational intervention should not be expected to be the same as what is required to prove that an intervention is beneficial as treatment. It stands to reason that, because of uncertainty and the need to gather evidence, benefit claims about an intervention that is unproven and being studied should necessarily require less evidence than benefit claims about standard treatment.

Finally, reasonable minds may differ. Saying no to research participation is always a reasonable choice, even when there is a reasonable chance of direct benefit. Deciding about research participation depends upon a variety of potential reasons, including, but certainly not limited to, differences in values and preferences as applied to the evidence about benefit and different valuations of the burdens of research participation.

Thus, (1) there must be a reasonable chance of direct benefit from an intervention being studied before the possibility of direct benefit may be offered to potential subjects; and (2) the possibility of direct benefit must be well-described to potential subjects in terms of all the dimensions of benefit.

Because the chance of direct benefit supports a decision to enroll in research in anticipation of that benefit, this is a *disclosure* issue, not a matter of *risk-benefit assessment*

The Journal of Law, Medicine & Ethics

in the first instance. The absence of a reasonable chance of direct benefit in early-phase research will not normally affect the ability of the research to satisfy conditions of value and validity[35] or the balance between risks of harm and aspirational benefit.[36] Nor will the absence of a reasonable chance of direct benefit preclude well-informed potential subjects from choosing to participate in research on other grounds, ranging from altruism to collateral benefit to the belief that trying for a very long shot at direct benefit is worth it under all the circumstances.

The last possibility is especially likely to be true in circumstances where available treatments are so imperfect and the burden of disease is so great that long-shot treatments would be considered worth trying by some reasonable patients. It would be paternalistic to consider this reason for research participation invalid, yet it is extremely difficult, in practice, to minimize the potential for the therapeutic misconception. One essential way of doing so is to explain that no direct benefit is expected for subjects and why. Only Jay Katz's formulation — "Remember, you will be a subject; you will not be my patient"[37] — can adequately frame the necessary disclosure and discussion here.

The circumstances and the alternatives

Assessment of whether there is a reasonable chance of benefit is, of course, always "under all the circumstances." That modifier covers a lot of ground. Indeed, the circumstances are likely to be so complex and variable that no single threshold standard can be set. It seems more plausible to consider context-specific threshold requirements — specific to the disease or condition, the subject population and the degree of disease burden, available treatments and their benefits and burdens, and other relevant contextual features. Reasonableness judgments are likely to be contingent and time-consuming for IRBs and may benefit from input from scientific and disease constituencies at a national level.

It is therefore tempting to take a shortcut — to assume that every investigational intervention offered to a patient-subject carries a reasonable chance of benefit, since every time an offer is accepted, it signals the reasonableness of the choice. This shortcut is wrong, though, because offers made in a last-chance mode might easily be supported by insufficient evidence and be grounded more in desperation than in expectation. This shortcut would simply routinize the therapeutic misconception.

A reasonable chance and clinical equipoise

Another tempting but wrong-headed shortcut would be to equate the existence of equipoise with a reasonable chance of benefit. It is tempting to do this because clinical equipoise[38] requires a difference of opinion among reasonable minds about whether the investigational intervention is likely

to be better than standard treatment or better than nothing. But ensuring that equipoise exists is not the same as establishing a reasonable chance of benefit.

Equipoise takes into consideration a range of factors, not solely nor primarily the potential for direct benefit. The ultimate focus of equipoise is the entire risk-of-harm/chance-of-benefit calculus, encompassing aspirational benefit in particular. That is, equipoise is a reasonable difference of opinion about what *will be* the better *treatment* for future patients — not about what *is* better for current subjects.[39] Importantly, the precise nature and focus of clinical equipoise may shift according to different stages in the clinical trials process, and in early-phase trials, the focus of equipoise may be limited. For example, in Phase I safety studies, equipoise is primarily or exclusively about safety. The question, "Is the investigational intervention at least as safe as standard treatment?" expresses the equipoise that must be disturbed, one way or another, by a completed Phase I trial; yet, the successful completion of that first trial is not yet determinative of safety. It is not until the successful end of the entire clinical trials process that equipoise can definitively be disturbed in favor of the investigational intervention, which thereby earns the title "new treatment."

The oncology example

Oncology research takes place in a very complex and particular context: Available treatments are unproven, unsatisfactory, and often toxic; potential subjects and investigators alike feel a sense of urgency and even desperation; and there exists a publicly acknowledged commitment to increasing cancer patients' participation in research. Most of the time, patients are expected to have exhausted all standard and otherwise available treatment options before enrolling in research, so that they will not be tempted to forgo imperfect but accepted treatments off-study in hopes of a very long shot on-study. As a result, early-phase clinical trials in oncology have been said to enroll not only the most desperate patients as subjects, but also those least likely to benefit from a new intervention — at least from a new variant of the same classes of interventions to which they have not responded previously. However, many physicians, investigators, and patients believe that the academic medical setting and close monitoring offered as collateral benefits in trials make research the best treatment option. And increasingly, patients who have not exhausted all conventional treatment options are choosing — and being encouraged to choose — research participation earlier.[40]

One consequence of these trends is increased blurring between research and treatment. The ideal of genetic tumor typing is the development of a regimen specifically tailored to the disease and the genetic makeup of each individual.[41] Since "tailored treatments" cannot be studied like conventional agents, this ideal views each patient as an experiment with an *n* of 1, seeking the development of generalizable knowledge before and during individual interventions rather than through the traditional "gold standard" clinical trial process.

Is it possible, then, to consider early-phase oncology research as offering a reasonable chance of direct benefit to subjects? In traditional oncology research — from which the best data about whether Phase I trials show any tumor effects are derived — the answer is clearly no. Even so, however, little information is provided that would inform potential subjects better. Well-known and often-quoted data show very low likelihoods of tumor response, generally placed at less than 5 percent for subjects in Phase I trials.[42] A higher percentage of tumor responses is seen in Phase II trials, as most doses in this phase are clustered near the maximum tolerated dose identified in Phase I.[43] But most of these data do not quantify tumor response beyond its standard definition of greater than 50 percent shrinkage, and none appear to provide any indication of response duration.

More importantly, tumor response is not usually defined in either the consent form or the consent process. Since patient-subjects generally hope for remission or cure, tumor response is at least somewhat likely to fall below the level of clinical benefit that potential subjects may consider "worth it" as part of a "reasonable chance" determination.

It seems clear that conventional oncology research suffers from very poor disclosure and that assessing the reasonableness of the chance of benefit in a given trial is not possible without better disclosure of existing data and better discussion of what is known and not known. At present, it appears that no Phase I trial can offer a reasonable chance of direct benefit — and that more information about the burdens of research participation and the alternatives of palliative and supportive care is imperative. Yet it is certainly also possible that a few classes of interventions may have a sufficiently different evidentiary basis to support the claim of a reasonable chance of benefit sooner in the trial process — still not in Phase I, because of uncertainties and unknowns, but perhaps in Phase II if stronger evidence of efficacy has been gathered in Phase I than usually appears.[44]

The gene transfer example

Whether gene transfer research holds out a reasonable chance of direct benefit is an especially complicated question to address. Gene transfer's direct benefit claims have received perhaps even less attention than most because of its presumed safety — "it can't hurt, so why not just try it?" — until the death of Jesse Gelsinger in a Phase I study in the fall of 1999.[45]

Most gene transfer research has turned out to be oncology research, raising similar or identical concerns about the low likelihood of direct benefit and the enrollment only of subjects with no remaining viable treatment options. But some gene transfer research is directed toward chronic but not life-threatening diseases and to circumstances in which patients with relatively stable disease are asked to serve as subjects.

The oncology model, applied to the very different intervention of gene transfer, can promote a "biggest bang for your buck" mentality, much as in oncology. When investigators look first to patients for whom all else has failed, it is easy to think that because these patients are the sickest and the most in need of a successful intervention, they are also the most likely to benefit from the intervention being studied. However, subjects' desperate circumstances cannot increase the likelihood of benefit. When there is only preclinical evidence to support efficacy in humans, that is enough evidence to maintain equipoise, but not enough to disturb it.

In contrast, currently stable patients with chronic disease are much more like so-called healthy volunteers. They may be less likely to think of themselves — or to be thought of by investigators — as likely to benefit, because they are less in need of something that works. People with genetic diseases like cystic fibrosis, hemophilia, and various enzyme deficiency disorders have all been enrolled in research with no reasonable chance of direct benefit, and fairly often they are told exactly that. The tricky part here is to address the argument that gene transfer is so unprecedented a field, with such irresistible therapeutic logic, that disclaiming direct benefit will understate reality and mislead potential subjects in a different way.

Claims of direct and substantial benefit to subjects enrolled in some Phase I gene transfer trials have been in the news lately.[46] If a Phase I trial does not collect efficacy data sufficient to make a claim about direct benefit meaningful, no such claim can be plausible: A claimed reasonable chance of benefit that is not adequately supported by evidence is not a reasonable chance. But the increasingly common combination of Phase I and Phase II trials, the unique way that gene transfer is thought to work, and the high disease burden of most genetic disorders may combine to make early claims of direct benefit plausible in some studies, if they are well-supported.

COLLATERAL BENEFIT, TREATMENT, AND JUSTICE

When investigators argue that "patients do better on-study," so that enrolling in research is their best treatment option, they are making a collateral benefit claim.[47] The provision of collateral benefit in a research project raises issues of justice in two ways. First, providing a potentially higher standard of care to those enrolled in research than those receiving standard treatment potentially discourages the improvement of standard treatment. Second, because collateral benefits are entirely under the control of research

The Journal of Law, Medicine & Ethics

investigators and sponsors, their provision poses the risk of manipulating or possibly even coercing participation from subjects who are disadvantaged or otherwise vulnerable. At the very least, questions are raised about the standard of care and about the best ways to provide and finance health care for those in need.

Yet the problem of collateral benefit may be more complicated still. Remember that what distinguishes collateral benefit from direct benefit is that direct benefit is linked to the intervention under study and collateral benefit is available to all subjects simply by virtue of being in the study. There are several new research design trends that seek to make it difficult to distinguish between these two types of benefit. Conflation of direct and collateral benefit serves the argument that research is the best treatment, which in turn makes it difficult to remember that patients may also be subjects.

Some thoughtful investigators and policy makers have begun to broaden their definitions of the intervention being studied as well as to design studies that include several stages in order to maximize the potential for direct benefit to subjects.[48] This is most readily seen in psychiatric research, especially drug trials and comparisons of drug and non-drug interventions, and is largely a response to public concern about placebo designs, challenge studies, and wash-out periods. Proponents of this viewpoint do not consider the potential benefit from the study drug in isolation from the rest of the study. They do not regard study design features that minimize risk or provide collateral benefit (e.g., monitoring and testing, rescue medications, non-study physician available to monitor subjects — all means of minimizing risks to subjects; crossover designs and post-study open label extensions — two means of ensuring that all subjects gain at least limited access to the drug being studied) in isolation, either. Instead, they take it all together, rolling risk-minimization features and collateral benefit features into one package, and view the whole study as providing direct benefit. According to this view, the whole study has been designed to maximize the potential for direct benefit to all subjects.[49]

Robert Levine has called this view, which takes all the components of the study as a whole, "the fallacy of the package deal."[50] He has condemned it when it is used to label an entire study "nontherapeutic," as has been done in the past, because it contains some unproven and/or purely research components. But its use as described here turns the "fallacy of the package deal" to the opposite effect — to label an entire study "therapeutic" despite the clearly experimental character and unproven benefit of its central component, i.e., the drug being studied.

This view rightly recognizes that a treatment program has many interconnected features and components and that maximizing potential benefit for patients requires a grasp of this dynamic complexity. Analogizing from the treatment setting, this view considers a research protocol to be a plan for cutting-edge treatment — but the analogy goes too far. A research protocol is not treatment, no matter how much all parties wish it so. Treatment requires genuine attention to the best interests of the patient as an individual, including individual attention and individual tailoring or complete changing of any regimen for maximal efficacy.[51] Even if the organization, scope, and duration of a clinical trial were compatible with these goals, the uncertainties and unknowns attendant upon use of an unproven intervention make individual tailoring almost meaningless, especially in early-phase trials. Moreover, the trialists' mandate to collect data systematically makes individual tailoring largely incompatible with the development of generalizable knowledge.[52]

Nonetheless, this view of trials as cutting-edge treatment supports the research systematization trend now gaining momentum in oncology and HIV/AIDS research in particular. Patients with some conditions have little access to interventions of any sort outside research. Pediatric oncology is the best example; most children with cancer are enrolled in research because the community of practice agreed to develop an all-encompassing research agenda in order to make progress against the disease.[53] Most patients with HIV disease are enrolled in research, but for a different reason: They cannot afford to pay for highly active anti-retroviral therapy regimens themselves. A great many HIV patients have lost their health insurance, have exceeded their lifetime policy limits, or have never been insured; thus, enrolling in research may be their only access to any drug treatment.[54]

In contrast, in some very unsettled areas of disease and treatment, investigators have found it difficult to enroll subjects in studies of unproven interventions because those interventions are available off-study; are believed by patients, physicians, and the general public to be better than standard treatments; and are often paid for by health insurance. The classic example is high-dose chemotherapy followed by bone marrow transplantation (or, more recently, stem cell transplantation) for solid tumors, especially for breast cancer. Despite a paucity of evidence showing that this type of highly risky, burdensome, and indeed dangerous regimen is effective, dying women initiated a flood of lawsuits during the 1980s and 1990s against their health insurers and managed care organizations to get this expensive intervention paid for.[55] Many patients lost these suits; more won. Many insurers paid up; more changed their policies to improve coverage for enrollment in research "likely to be beneficial," though the likelihood of benefit was rarely discussed since death was otherwise inevitable. Blue Cross announced early on in this long battle that it would subsidize clinical trials in order to gather some meaningful evidence about the efficacy of this extremely risky and burdensome intervention. At length, in late 1999, studies that had taken many more years to complete than had been originally hoped, because of slow enrollment, all showed that overall survival and quality of life were not meaningfully improved by this type of regimen.[56] But in the meantime, every community hospital was doing it.[57] And as a result, the cancer research community has announced its intention to ensure that every cancer patient will also be a research subject. The reasoning? It makes better data available faster and patient-subjects will be treated with a uniformly high, academic-medicine-based standard of care.

CONCLUSION

If increasing the enrollment of patients as subjects in research is a good thing, it is good for the following reasons: Medical research will expand, knowledge will increase, and perhaps future patients will benefit if the new knowledge produces better treatments.[58] Even if all these benefits materialize, it is still not necessarily true that patients will get better treatment if they enroll in research — nor that they will benefit from receiving the intervention being studied. If data are needed, if more needs to be learned, investigators can surely tell patients several important things:

- their help is needed to look for better treatments for future patients;
- in exchange for their help, they will receive either the best current treatment or something unproven in a study setting;
- investigators, study sponsors, and IRBs will do their utmost to protect them from harm;
- disclosure and discussion will be thorough and honest, telling them what benefit they can and cannot expect from receiving an unproven intervention and from being a research subject, as compared with receiving standard treatment.

Why does this disclosure and discussion seem so insufficient to many investigators and even to some IRBs? Some have argued that it is not enough because people do not want to be guinea pigs; instead, they want to be taken care of. It is possible to take good care of subjects in clinical trials; indeed, it is the investigator's duty to do so. Yet when no standard treatment works very well, no physician can fulfill a duty to take care of the patient if care means only cure — although, of course, it should mean more than that.

If patients who are subjects are properly cared for, only those who prefer to be deceived will want to be enrolled in research and told it will help them. Others may choose to enroll to advance science or to help future patients; still others will choose not to take part in research. And certainly there are investigators who may simply be unwilling or unable to have honest and respectful conversations with patients. Perhaps they fear that other investigators will continue to be deceptive and will thus enroll more subjects; or perhaps they fear that too few patients would enroll in research if they knew how unlikely direct benefit is for subjects.

If the only way to address these fears is to make sure that every patient is a research subject, then we have strayed very far from any morally reasonable goal in health care or in research. Improving disclosure about all dimensions of potential benefit to subjects has the capacity to promote more reasoned discussion about what can and cannot be expected in research. From there, improving public discourse about the goals of clinical research seems possible, necessary, and long overdue.

ACKNOWLEDGMENTS

I would like to thank my colleagues in a past and a current ELSI project for their contributions to my thinking on this subject. This work was supported in part by a Kenan Award from the University of North Carolina at Chapel Hill and is part of a book manuscript in preparation.

REFERENCES

1. This is the outdated but persistent distinction between "nontherapeutic" and "therapeutic" research. See, for example, World Medical Association Declaration of Helsinki, "Recommendations Guiding Medical Doctors in Biomedical Research Involving Human Subjects," revised 1996, reprinted in *JAMA*, 277 (1997): 925–26; see also A.M. Capron, "Ethical and Human-Rights Issues in Research on Mental Disorders That May Affect Decision-Making Capacity," *N. Engl. J. Med.*, 340 (1999): 1430–34; F. Rolleston and J.R. Miller, "Therapy or Research: A Need for Precision," *IRB*, 3, no. 7 (1981): 1–3; R. Levine, "The Need to Revise the Declaration of Helsinki," *N. Engl. J. Med.*, 341 (1999): 531–34.

2. P.S. Appelbaum, L.R. Roth, and C. Lidz, "The Therapeutic Misconception: Informed Consent in Psychiatric Research," *International Journal of Law & Psychiatry*, 5 (1982): 319–329; P.S. Appelbaum et al., "False Hopes and Best Data: Consent to Research and the Therapeutic Misconception," *Hastings Center Report*, 17, no. 2 (1987): 20–24; P.S. Appelbaum, "Commentary: Examining the Ethics of Human Subjects Research," *Kennedy Institute of Ethics Journal*, 6 (1996): 283–287. It has also been called the "therapeutic illusion." J. Katz, "Statement by Individual Committee Member," in Advisory Committee on Human Radiation Experiments, *Final Report* (Oxford University Press, 1996): 545.

3. L.R. Churchill et al., "Genetic Research as Therapy: Implications of 'Gene Therapy' for Informed Consent," *Journal of Law, Medicine & Ethics*, 26 (1998): 38–47. See also G. Kolata, "Separating Research From News," *New York Times*, July 18, 2000.

4. D. Grady, "Patient or Guinea Pig? Dilemma of Clinical Trials," *New York Times*, Jan. 5, 1999.

5. G. Kolata, "When the Dying Enroll in Studies: A Debate Over False Hopes," *New York Times*, Jan. 29, 1994.

6. The Common Rule is the shorthand name for the set of federal regulations that govern federally funded research with human subjects. The regulations, which implement Pub. L. 93–348 (the National Research Act of 1974), were harmonized into

The Journal of Law, Medicine & Ethics

the Common Rule in 1991 for 17 federal departments and agencies, and are codified separately for each. The Common Rule itself was published in the Federal Register, 56 Fed. Reg. 28,012 (June 18, 1991). The codifications most familiar to those involved in research oversight are the U.S. Department of Health and Human Services regulations, 45 C.F.R. pt. 46, and the Food and Drug Administration regulations, 21 C.F.R. pts. 50 and 56. The FDA has not adopted the Common Rule; its regulations are somewhat modified, though overall quite similar.

7. § ___.111(a)(2).

8. § ___.116(a)(3).

9. I am indebted to Alex Capron for the "reasonable chance/ reasonable choice" formulation.

10. 45 C.F.R. pt. 46, subpt. D, "an intervention or procedure that holds out the prospect of direct benefit for the individual subject."

11. 45 C.F.R. pt. 46, subpt. B, "the purpose of the activity is to meet the health needs of the mother" or "the particular fetus"; a revised subpart B, which has for some time been awaiting final signoff, would change this.

12. National Bioethics Advisory Commission, *Research Involving Persons with Mental Disorders That May Affect Decisionmaking Capacity, Report and Recommendations of the National Bioethics Advisory Commission* (December 1998) [hereinafter cited as NBAC Report] ("protocol that ... offers the prospect of direct medical benefit to the subject").

13. 45 C.F.R. pt. 46, subpt. C, research on innovative practices "which have the intent and reasonable probability of improving the health and well-being of the subject."

14. FDA, 21 C.F.R. § 50.24; DHHS, 61 Fed. Reg. 51,531 (preclinical studies and other evidence "support the potential for the intervention to provide a direct benefit to the individual subjects").

15. FDA, 21 C.F.R. § 56.102(d) ("life-threatening situation in which no standard acceptable treatment is available" — potential benefit implicit); 21 C.F.R. § 50.23(b) (informed consent also waived if "immediate use of the test article is, in the investigator's opinion, required to preserve the life of the subject").

16. FDA, 21 C.F.R. § 312.34-35 (data show that drug "may be effective"). A "treatment IND" is the use of an investigational new drug (IND) for treatment. The FDA issues "IND numbers" to unapproved drugs to authorize their testing for eventual approval.

17. See, for example, R. Pear, "Managed-Care Plans Agree to Help Pay the Costs of Their Members in Clinical Trials," *New York Times*, Feb. 9, 1999; "NIH, HMO Group Pact Will Enable Increased Member Access To Clinical Trials," *The Blue Sheet*, Feb. 17, 1999; G. Kolata and K. Eichenwald, "Group of Insurers Will Pay for Experimental Cancer Therapy," *New York Times*, Dec. 16, 1999; R. Pear, "Clinton to Order Medicare to Pay New Costs," *New York Times*, June 7, 2000. Both individual states and the federal government are moving toward mandating insurer coverage of late-phase clinical trials on a case-by-case basis according to their potential for direct benefit as well as coverage of routine medical expenditures in research if they would be covered outside the research setting.

18. NBAC Report, *supra* note 12, at 45, citing National Commission for the Protection of Human Subjects of Biomedical and Behavioral Research, *Research Involving Those Institutionalized as Mentally Infirm* (1978): at 31, and E.W. Keyserlingk et al., "Proposed Guidelines for the Participation of Persons with Dementia as Research Subjects," *Perspectives in Biology and Medicine*, 38 (1995): 319-62, at 327-28.

19. L.R. Churchill, "Toward a More Robust Autonomy: Re-

vising the *Belmont Report*," paper prepared for NBAC (presented April 17, 1999).

20. N. Dickert and C. Grady, "What's the Price of a Research Subject? Approaches to Payment for Research Participation," *N. Engl. J. Med.*, 341 (1999): at 198.

21. For example, a purpose statement that declares, "The purpose of this research is to develop a new kind of cancer treatment, which works by helping the body's immune system to attack cancer cells," could be misleading in a consent form for a Phase I study when the intervention has not yet been tried in humans. Potential subjects could easily take this to mean that in this Phase I study they will receive a "new treatment" that "works."

22. See NBAC Report, *supra* note 12; Keyserlingk et al., *supra* note 18.

23. *Final Report* (June 15, 1998): at 21 (visited Dec. 11, 2000) <http://ohrp.osophs.dhhs.gov/hsp_report/hsp_final_rpt.pdf>.

24. R.C. Boucher and M.R. Knowles, "Clinical Protocol: Gene Therapy for Cystic Fibrosis Using E1-Deleted Adenovirus: A Phase I Trial in the Nasal Cavity, The University of North Carolina at Chapel Hill," *Human Gene Therapy*, 5 (1994): 615-639. In the Purpose section, the consent form states: "I understand that this study is not designed for treatment, and that I will not get any medical benefit from this nose study of adenoviral gene transfer" (at 636). In the Benefits section, the form states: "I will not benefit directly from the nose study of adenoviral gene transfer" (at 638).

25. National Commission for the Protection of Human Subjects of Biomedical and Behavioral Research, *The Belmont Report: Ethical Principles and Guidelines for the Protection of Human Subjects of Research*, DHEW Pub. No. (OS) 78-0012, (Washington, D.C.: U.S. Gov't Printing Office, 1978). The *Belmont Report* was reprinted in the Federal Register in 1979 and is now available online at <http://ohrp.osophs.dhhs.gov/humansubjects/guidance/belmont.htm>.

26. The *IRB Guidebook* was published in hard copy in 1993, and is currently available at <http://ohrp.osophs.dhhs.gov/irb/irb_guidebook.htm>.

27. The *FDA Information Sheets* were last updated in 1998. They are available at <http://www.fda.gov/oc/oha/irb/toc.html> as well as in hard copy.

28. NBAC Report, *supra* note 12, at 44, citing National Commission for the Protection of Human Subjects of Biomedical and Behavioral Research, *Research Involving Those Institutionalized as Mentally Infirm* (1978): at 31. See also J.W. Berg, "Legal and Ethical Complexities of Consent with Cognitively Impaired Research Subjects: Proposed Guidelines," *Journal of Law, Medicine & Ethics*, 24 (1996): 18-35, at 24-25.

29. For example, the guidance document provided for investigators preparing gene transfer research protocols (Appendix M of the NIH Guidelines, "Points to Consider in the Design and Submission of Protocols for the Transfer of Recombinant DNA Molecules into One or More Human Subjects") requires "clear itemization" in the consent form of "types of adverse experiences, their relative severity, and their expected frequencies." It suggests that risks of harm be categorized as mild, moderate, and severe, and that any verbal descriptions of frequency, such as rare, uncommon, or frequent, be explained. It also mandates mention of the possibility of unforeseen harms (Appendix M-III-B-1-e). See N.M.P. King, "Rewriting the 'Points to Consider': The Ethical Impact of Guidance Document Language," *Human Gene Therapy*, 10 (1999): 133-39.

30. I am indebted to Dr. Jon Gordon for first calling my

Volume 28:4, Winter 2000

attention to this concern.

31. J. Crewsdon, "Human Trials of Cancer Treatment Set to Begin," *Chicago Tribune*, reprinted in *Herald-Sun*, Durham, N.C., Oct. 18, 1999; see also F. Russo, "The Clinical-Trials Bottleneck," *Atlantic Monthly*, May 1999, at 30–36 ("no more than 20 percent" of experimental interventions succeed in Phase III trials, where success is defined as extending median survival by 25 percent); Kolata, *supra* note 3.

32. J. Moreno et al., "Updating Protections for Human Subjects Involved in Research," *JAMA*, 280 (1998):1954.

33. "Human Guinea Pigs," *U.S. News Online*, May 24, 1999 (visited Dec. 12, 2000) <http://www.usnews.com/usnews/issue/990524/nycu/trials.b.htm>.

34. See N.M.P. King, "Experimental Treatment: Oxymoron or Aspiration?" *Hastings Center Report*, 25, no. 4 (1995): 6–15; L.R. Churchill et al., *supra* note 3; J. Goldner, "An Overview of Legal Controls on Human Experimentation and the Regulatory Implications of Taking Professor Katz Seriously," *Saint Louis University Law Journal*, 38 (1993): 63–134, at 125.

35. The essential goal of clinical research is to "develop or contribute to generalizable knowledge." Common Rule, §__.102(d). In order to achieve this goal, proposed research must demonstrate both *value* and *validity* — that is, the research must ask a question that is of scientific and societal importance (value) and the research design must have the capacity to answer that question, in either the affirmative or the negative (validity). E. Emanuel et al., "What Makes Clinical Research Ethical?" *JAMA*, 283 (2000): 2701–2711.

36. Of course, a continuing failure to produce data supporting direct benefit in later phases of research will affect the promise of the line of research and its aspirational benefit.

37. J. Katz, personal communication (November 1997).

38. B. Freedman, "Equipoise and the Ethics of Clinical Research," *N. Engl. J. Med.*, 317 (1987): 141–45.

39. The extensive debate about the ethics of randomization in Phase III clinical trials is largely about when enough evidence exists to assert that one treatment is superior. This complex literature is beyond the scope of the present discussion of early-phase trials.

40. See the NCI booklet "Taking Part in Clinical Trials: What Cancer Patients Need to Know," available online at <http://cancertrials.nci.nih.gov/understanding/bookshelf/treatment/index.html>. This change is based not only on the reasons stated but also on the growing use of diagnostic technologies to give information on tumor cell types and their probable responses to conventional treatments, as well as on the development of new classes of investigational interventions that may have effects on treatment-refractory disease.

41. See, for example, J. Groopman, "Dr. Fair's Tumor," *The New Yorker*, Oct. 26/Nov. 2, 1998, at 78–102.

42. See, for example, C. Daugherty, "Impact of Therapeutic Research on Informed Consent and the Ethics of Clinical Trials: A Medical Oncology Perspective," *Journal of Clinical Oncology*, 17 (1999): 1601–17.

43. C. Daugherty et al., "Perceptions of Cancer Patients and Their Physicians Involved in Phase I Trials," *Journal of Clinical Oncology*, 13 (1995): 1062–72.

44. Some have argued for redesigning Phase I trials, especially in oncology and other serious diseases, to cluster intervention dosing around the probable maximum tolerated dose (MTD) as predicted by lab and animal studies. See, for example, B. Brody, Chapter 8, in *The Ethics of Biomedical Research: An International Perspective* (Oxford: Oxford University Press, 1998); K. Kipnis, "Vulnerability in Research Subjects: An Ethical Taxonomy," paper prepared for NBAC (July 2000). However, it is not clear that this would substantially increase the likelihood of direct benefit in Phase I trials. That would be true only if the drug is actually effective, if the duration of the trial is sufficient to produce meaningful clinical effects, and if the projections about the MTD turn out to be reasonably accurate. With no previous human experience and probably rather sketchy preclinical data, that is a lot of ifs. See also M. Miller, "Phase I Cancer Trials: A Collusion of Misunderstanding," *Hastings Center Report*, 30, no. 4 (2000): 34–43, at 39–40.

45. See, for example, "The Biotech Death of Jesse Gelsinger," *New York Times Magazine*, Nov. 28, 1999. Gelsinger, who had just turned eighteen, was enrolled in a Phase I safety and toxicity study in which corrected genetic material, combined with a modified adenovirus vector, was injected into subjects with a genetic deficiency of an essential enzyme called ornithine transcarbamylase, which affects liver function. The injection apparently caused an overwhelming inflammatory response. At the time, safety concerns in the field of gene transfer research were directed primarily toward the risk of inadvertently altering subjects' germlines (a safety issue for the subjects' future offspring) and long-term risks of causing mutations in subjects (an issue similar to the possibility that successful cancer treatment could cause new malignancies decades from now). Little attention was directed toward risks of immediate and direct harm since the worst that had been publicly discussed was "flu-like symptoms" after an injection of genetic material in a modified viral carrier "vector," like adenovirus. The consent form for the study in which Gelsinger died promised no direct benefit to subjects, but Gelsinger's father testified before the U.S. Congress last February that he and his son were given somewhat different and misleading information during the consent process. Jesse Gelsinger's death has spurred significant new oversight activity in all human subjects research. See, for example, D. Shalala, "Protecting Research Subjects — What Must Be Done," *N. Engl. J. Med.*, 343 (2000): at 800.

46. See, for example, J. Stephenson, "Gene Therapy Trials Show Clinical Efficacy," *JAMA*, 283 (2000): 589–90.

47. All claims of benefit, including collateral benefit, should address all three dimensions of benefit. In some respects, collateral benefit claims may be questioned, but that discussion is beyond the scope of this paper.

48. See Daugherty, *supra* note 43.

49. See, for example, W.T. Carpenter and R.R. Conley, "Sense and Nonsense: An Essay on Schizophrenia Research Ethics," *Schizophrenia Research*, 35 (1999): 219–225, at 223. See also *supra* note 44.

50. R. Levine, "Uncertainty in Clinical Research," *Law, Medicine & Health Care*, 16 (1988): 174–82.

51. See *The Belmont Report*, *supra* note 25. The *Belmont Report* defines treatment (or "practice") as "interventions that are designed solely to enhance the well being of an individual patient … and that have a reasonable expectation of success."

52. J. Katz, "Human Experimentation and Human Rights," *Saint Louis University Law Journal*, 38 (1993): 7–54, at 25–26. But see G. Norquist et al., "Expanding the Frontier of Treatment Research," *Prevention & Treatment*, 2 (1999):1–5.

53. G. Kolata and K. Eichenwald, "In Pediatrics, A Lesson in Making Use of Experimental Procedures," *New York Times*, Oct. 3, 1999.

54. Patients who are uninsured, underinsured, or otherwise economically vulnerable are, in general, at some risk of exploitation when researchers, even with the best of intentions, offer them research participation as a treatment substitute. R. Levine, *Ethics and Regulation of Clinical Research*, 2d ed., (New Haven: Yale

The Journal of Law, Medicine & Ethics

University Press, 1988): 82–84; G. Kolata and K. Eichenwald, "For the Uninsured, Experiments May Provide the Only Treatment," *New York Times*, June 22, 1999.

55. See, for example, D. Light, "Life, Death, and the Insurance Companies," *N. Engl. J. Med.*, 330 (1994): 498–500; S. Boren, "I Had a Tough Day Today, Hillary," *N. Engl. J. Med.*, 330 (1994): 500–502.

56. P.A. Rowlings et al., "Factors Correlated With Progression-Free Survival After High-Dose Chemotherapy and Hematopoietic Stem Cell Transplantation for Metastatic Breast Cancer," *JAMA*, 282 (1999): 1335–43; W.J. Gradishar, "High-Dose Che-

motherapy and Breast Cancer," *JAMA*, 282 (1999): 1378–80.

57. G. Kolata and K. Eichenwald, "Health Business Thrives on Unproven Treatment, Leaving Science Behind," *New York Times*, Oct. 2, 1999.

58. Unfortunately, the ability to disseminate and apply the best current knowledge gleaned from clinical trials is compromised by publication bias in the reporting of study data. See, for example, D. Rennie, "Fair Conduct and Fair Reporting of Clinical Trials," *JAMA*, 282 (1999): 1766–68. This raises the problem of how the results of clinical research can and should influence practicing physicians.

[23]

WHAT RESEARCH WITH STORED SAMPLES TEACHES US ABOUT RESEARCH WITH HUMAN SUBJECTS

DAVID WENDLER

ABSTRACT

There is widespread discussion concerning the safeguards appropriate for human research subjects. Less discussed is the fact that the safeguards one deems appropriate depend, in large part, on the model of research participation that one assumes. Therefore, to determine what safeguards are appropriate, it is necessary first to clarify the competing models of research participation. The ostensibly obscure debate over informed consent for research on stored biological samples is of particular interest in this regard because such research can involve varying subsets of the three central elements of research involvement. As a result, analysis of this debate provides an opportunity to identify the competing models of research participation. Based on this analysis, this paper describes a new model of research participation that is emerging, and considers its implications for clinical research.

To implement human subjects protections, one must first identify which individuals are involved in research. Most analyses address this need by assuming some paradigm cases of research involvement, for instance, an individual with metastatic cancer receiving experimental treatment as part of a research protocol. Although this reliance on paradigm cases is sufficient in many cases, it obscures the fact that involvement in research includes three distinct elements: 1. *exposure* to risks; 2. *performance* of research mandated behaviors; 3. *contribution* to answering a research question. Without further analysis, then, it is unclear whether the need for human subjects protections is a function of all three elements, or some subset of them.

To consider a specific example, the standard drug trial involves individuals facing risks (risk element) as a result of taking an

34 DAVID WENDLER

experimental drug (performance element) in a way that helps investigators determine whether the drug might be clinically useful (contribution element). Because all three elements co-occur in the standard cases, it is unclear which one(s) ground the need for familiar human subjects protections: Do investigators need to obtain the informed consent of individuals who partici-pate in drug trials because they are being exposed to risks and/or because they are being asked to take certain medicines and/or because they are contributing to a specific research project?

Research on stored biological samples offers a surprising opportunity to answer this question because it can involve varying subsets of the three elements of research involvement. For instance, research on personally identified stored samples can pose risks to sources even though investigators never interact with the sources or ask them to do anything. The present paper attempts to identify the competing models of research involve-ment by assessing when research with stored samples is thought to require human subjects protections.

The present discussion, particularly as it concerns human subject regulations, focuses on the situation in the United States. In part, this is because much of the discussion concerning research on stored samples has been occurring in the United States. Moreover, limiting the discussion to the situation in a single country allows me to bracket any cross-national differences in policies regarding research with stored samples and focus on the relevant conceptual issues.

THE CURRENT DEBATE

When should investigators obtain sources' informed consent for research on stored biological samples? Most writers agree that investigators need not obtain sources' informed consent for research on completely anonymous samples. And many agree that investigators should obtain informed consent for research on samples that retain personal identifiers. This consensus has focused much of the debate on research using 'anonymizable' samples – samples that have personal identifiers which, for the purposes of the research, could be removed before the research is conducted.

The U.S. College of Medical Genetics argues that whether research on anonymizable samples requires sources' consent depends upon how burdensome it would be to obtain it.[1] Most

---

[1] American College of Medical Genetics. Statement on storage and use of genetic materials. *Am J. Hum. Genet.* 1995; 57: 1499–1500.

WHAT RESEARCH WITH STORED SAMPLES   35

accounts evaluate different levels of burden based on the research's risks. When research poses only minor risks, there is little reason to solicit sources' consent; hence, almost any level of burden required to contact them would be deemed excessive. However, as research poses increasing risks to sources, investigators should be required to accept increasing burdens to obtain their consent.

The primary risks of research on stored samples involve unwanted information flow. Such research may reveal facts about sources, and their futures, that they did not know, and did not want known.[2] Anonymizing samples eliminates these risks by eliminating the possibility of tracing results back to sources. Thus, on the view that the burden of contacting sources should be evaluated against the risks of the research, investigators need not solicit sources' consent for research on anonymizable samples. Instead, investigators can anonymize the samples and proceed with their research (provided anonymizing samples is consistent with the goals of the research). Reilly, Boshar and Holtzman: 'Truly anonymous studies circumvent the need to address ... issues such as fear of unauthorized release of genetic information ...'[3] In the supporting words of the American Society of Human Genetics (ASHG): anonymizing samples protects sources from the risks of genetic research and thus 'eliminates the need for recontact to obtain informed consent.'[4]

Critics respond that this view ignores much of the point of obtaining sources' informed consent. In addition to notifying sources of any risks, informed consent allows sources to control whether their samples are used for research purposes. On this

---

[2] Research on stored samples may also reveal unwanted facts about the *groups* to which sources belong. However, to simplify things, I shall focus on research that poses risks only to the individuals involved in the research. (I shall also assume that the research under consideration does not offer any potential for medical benefit to subjects.) Group risks are of theoretical interest because they present the possibility that individuals may be harmed by research they do not participate in. Adopting the terminology used below, this possibility reveals that protocols which require consent on the subject model are not, as one might initially suppose, a subset of the protocols which require consent on the experiential model. The U.S. NBAC considers this issue briefly in its report 'Research Involving Human Biological Materials: Ethical issues and Policy Guidance', *Report and Recommendations of the National Bioethics Advisory Commission.* Vol. I. Rockville, MD. August 1999: 73.

[3] P.R. Reilly, M.F. Boshar, S.H. Holtzman. Ethical Issues in Genetic Research: disclosure and informed consent. *Nat. Genet.* 1997; 15: 17.

[4] The American Society of Human Genetics. Statement on informed consent for genetic research. *Am. J. Hum. Genet.* 1996; 59: 473.

36   DAVID WENDLER

basis, an Ethical, Legal, and Social Implications of the human genome project (ELSI) working group argues that sources' consent should be obtained whenever possible: 'if the source can be identified, that source should be asked for his or her consent.'[5] Similarly, participants in a workshop on research with tissue samples concluded that anonymizing samples based on the absence of any risks to subjects is: 'problematic because researchers had an opportunity to seek consent but did not exercise it.'[6]

Importantly, these two approaches adopt the same view when samples lack personal identifiers and when removal of personal identifiers would be inconsistent with the scientific goals of the research. In the first case, those who understand informed consent as a mechanism for notifying sources of potential risks argue that the research can proceed without consent because anonymizing the samples eliminates any risks. Those who understand informed consent as a mechanism for allowing sources to control whether their samples are used for research purposes agree, in this case, because the anonymity of the samples eliminates the possibility of contact. When personal identifiers cannot be removed, the emphasis on risks implies that informed consent should be obtained in order to notify sources of the risks. Those who emphasize allowing sources to control the use of their samples agree because the personal identifiers provide investigators with the opportunity for contact.

Research on samples with personal identifiers that can be removed is of theoretical interest because it is here that the two dominant views on obtaining sources' consent diverge. Those who focus on risks recommend that investigators anonymize samples and conduct their research without sources' consent; those who emphasize allowing sources to control the use of their samples argue that the identifiers should be used to contact sources. The claim that informed consent may be waived for anonymizable research appears to trace to the earliest model for understanding clinical research. Early on research procedures tended to pose risks to subjects without much chance of medical benefit. Add to this the fact that the most egregious research abuses involved individuals being subjected to especially risky

[5] NIH-DOE Working Group on the Ethical, Legal, and Social Implications of Human Genome Research. February, 1995. ELSI Working Group Statement on Research on Previously Collected Tissue Samples: 1.

[6] E.W. Clayton, K.K. Steinberg, M.J. Khoury, et al. Informed consent for genetic research on stored tissue samples. *JAMA*. 1995; 274: 1788. I note that not everyone in the workshop agreed with this view.

WHAT RESEARCH WITH STORED SAMPLES   37

procedures, and one gets the view that individuals' involvement in clinical research is defined by the risks they face, by what they are being subjected to.[7]

A number of writers have pointed out that research can affect individuals, by having them do things or doing things to them, even when it poses no risks to them. Given that individuals have an interest in what happens to them, these writers conclude that investigators should obtain individuals' informed consent whenever research affects them personally. To take a notable example, Robert Veatch argues that the doctrine of informed consent is based, not on individuals' right to avoid risks, but on their right to control the course of their lives.[8] The U.S. National Commission agreed, defining a human subject as a 'person about whom an investigator conducting scientific research obtains data through intervention or interaction with the person.'[9] Current U.S. federal regulations on human subjects research are based on this 'experiential' model, rather than the earlier subject model.[10]

Although the experiential model offers the most prominent alternative to the subject model, it does not imply that investigators necessarily ought to obtain sources' informed consent for anonymizable research. For instance, when samples have been obtained, and will be anonymized, sources are unaffected by whether the research takes place or not. Hence, those who base the need for informed consent on individuals' right to control the course of their lives have no reason to require sources' consent in these cases. The fact that some writers argue for sources' consent, nonetheless, suggests that they are appealing to some third model of research involvement.

The alternative models of research involvement can be characterized in terms of alternative accounts of individuals'

[7] For instance, the earliest U.S. regulations for ethics review committees (IRBs) define a subject of research as an individual who 'may be at risk.' DHEW. 1971. The Institutional Guide to DHEW Policy on Protection of Human Subjects. Publication No. (NIH). Washington, D.C. U.S. Govt Printing Office: 72–102.

[8] R. Veatch. 1978. Theories of Informed Consent: Philosophical Foundations and Policy Implications. The Belmont Report. Appendix II DHEW Publication No. (Os) 78–0014. Washington, D.C. U.S. Govt Printing Office.

[9] The National Commission for the Protection of Human Subjects of Biomedical and Behavioral Research. 1978. Report and Recommendations: Institutional Review Boards. DHEW Publication No. (OS) 78: 0008. Washington, D.C. U.S. Govt Printing Office.

[10] United States Department of Health and Human Services. 1991. Protections of Human Subjects. Title 45 Code of Federal Regulations Part 46.102 f.

38   DAVID WENDLER

relevant interests. The subject model traces to the claim that
individuals' primary interests relevant to research are their
interests in avoiding harm. On this view, whether specific
individuals are involved in research in a way that should trigger
human subjects protections depends upon whether the research
poses risks to them. The experiential model recognizes a broader
range of interests as relevant to individuals' research involvement,
requiring that one consider whether the research might affect the
individuals in any way, not simply whether it might harm them.
The impetus for a possible third model for understanding
research involvement starts with the question of whether
individuals have interests relevant to clinical research independent
of the risks it poses, or how it affects them personally.

SOURCES' INTERESTS AND THE ARGUMENT FROM CONTRIBUTION

To start, what reason could there be to solicit sources' informed
consent for research that poses no risks to them and does not
affect them personally? What is left for sources to consent to?
Stripping away how the research affects sources personally leaves
the research itself: why it is being conducted, what its goals are,
who is supporting it, and so on. This suggests that any plausible
argument for obtaining informed consent for research on
anonymizable samples will have to show that sources should be
able to determine whether their samples are used for specific
research purposes independently of whether these projects affect
them personally. One way to defend such a position is by means
of the following 'Argument from Contribution':

1. Sources have an interest in whether their samples are used
   for specific research purposes independently of whether the
   research affects them personally.
2. Individuals should have a say in states of affairs in which they
   have an interest.
3. Therefore, sources should have a say in whether their samples
   are used for specific research purposes independently of
   whether the research affects them personally.
4. For sources to have a say in whether their samples are used
   for specific research purposes, investigators must obtain their
   informed consent.
5. Therefore, investigators should obtain sources' informed
   consent even when the research does not affect them
   personally.

WHAT RESEARCH WITH STORED SAMPLES   39

Starting with the second premise, one can think of an individual's interests as referring to the various aspects of a flourishing life for that individual: if X is part of a flourishing life for P, then P has an interest in (the obtaining of) X.[11] Conversely, if X conflicts with a flourishing life for P, then P has an interest in X's not obtaining. For the most part, the various aspects of a flourishing life are states of affairs. So, for instance, on the assumption that a flourishing life includes good health and close personal relationships, individuals have an interest in the obtaining of these states of affairs.[12]

In addition to the obtaining or not of specific states of affairs, the flourishing life also includes some degree of personal autonomy. It is not important simply that particular states of affairs come about, that one's life consists of a series of desirable states of affairs. A flourishing life also involves individuals actively shaping their own lives by determining what experiences they have and what projects they contribute to. Of course no one gets to control every aspect of one's life, and no sane person would want to. As will be important later on, individuals can cede control over certain aspects of their lives without them being any less human or any less flourishing.

It is important to distinguish two aspects of having a say over a particular state of affairs: the *weight* of one's claim to have a say and the *nature* of one's say. The weight of an individual's claim to a say is a function, roughly, of how central the state of affairs is to their life.[13] Individuals have a weighty claim to a say over those states of affairs that are central to their lives, such as the careers they follow, whether they marry, and what happens to their appendages, and a less weighty claim over states of affairs less central to their lives, such as who their neighbors are. The weight of one's claim to a say provides a rough measure of the burdens

[11] The states of affairs in which P has an interest should be contrasted with the states of affairs in which P is interested. For a (brief) account of the latter, see S. Kagan. 1989. *The Limits of Morality*. Oxford. Oxford University Press, especially p. 3.

[12] Roughly speaking, which states of affairs count as aspects of a flourishing life for P can be understood objectively or subjectively. On an objective account, it is simply a fact, independent of P's psychology, that certain things are part of a flourishing life for her. On a subjective account, whether X is part of a flourishing life for P depends in some way on P's psychology, for instance, on P's actual or idealized *preferences*.

[13] 'Weight' in the sense intended here is often understood in terms of the 'strength' of the relevant desire (for instance, see Griffin p. 15). I avoid this terminology because it invites confusion with strength understood as felt intensity or motivational force.

society must accept in respecting one's say. Since I have a very weighty claim to determine what happens to my body, only societal interests of the highest order can outweigh my say over what happens to my body.

The *nature* of the say that one has over a particular state of affairs is, roughly, a measure of the extent to which one gets to determine whether the state of affairs comes about. A plausible assumption is that the nature of one's say is determined by the weight of one's claim to having a say. If I have a very weighty claim, then I get the determinative voice, and if I have a much less weighty claim, I get, in effect, only a single vote. In fact, the nature of one's say also depends upon the extent to which others have a say. For instance, I have a weighty interest, and typically others do not have a weighty interest, in issues central to my life, such as what happens to my body. It follows that my weighty interest in what happens to my body often implies that I get to control this aspect of my life. But this is not always the case. Forced military service involves my weighty claim to having a say over what happens to my body being overridden by the competing weighty claims of others to national defense. At the opposite extreme, my very weak claim to having a say over a particular state of affairs, what happens to a particular sea shell, for example, can amount to de facto personal control because no one else has any claim over the state of affairs in question.

Granting that one often does not get personal control over the states of affairs in which one has an interest, it might seem that one nonetheless gets personal control over whether one contributes to the state of affairs in question. Others may be able to outweigh my vote for mayor, but they cannot force me to vote for a specific individual. In fact, control over one's own contribution is defeatable as well. The example of individuals being forced to serve in the military and, thereby, forced to contribute to the war effort, is one example. Similarly, individuals who strongly oppose urban sprawl do not get to decide whether their tax dollars are used to connect the newest executive suburb to the opera house.

To this point, the discussion has been concerned primarily with states of affairs that affect individuals personally – whether they marry, what happens to their bodies. In these cases, it is plausible to argue that individuals should have a say because it is plausible to say that they have an interest. It is less obvious, as premise 1 of the Argument from Contribution assumes, that individuals also have interests in states of affairs that do not affect them personally. Indeed, one might assume that without the

WHAT RESEARCH WITH STORED SAMPLES 41

possibility of a personal experience, there is no ground on which to base an interest, no way in which the state of affairs in question could be about one's life.

NON-EXPERIENTIAL INTERESTS

Certain states of affairs can be part of a flourishing life for us, hence, we can have an interest in whether these states of affairs obtain, even though they never affect us personally. To take a concrete example, individuals' future driving records can have implications for their driving instructors' lives. Whether the students were taught well, and go on to spotless records, or weren't and go on to many accidents, is relevant to the instructors' lives. It says something about how well the students were taught, hence, something about how good the instructors were. Notice that this implication remains even when the students' driving futures do not affect the instructors personally, for instance, even when the students never have an accident with their instructors. The fact that we can have interests in states of affairs that do not affect us personally raises the question of what, if not one's personal experiences, determines the scope of one's interests.

Consider Derek Parfit's example of meeting a stranger on a train, finding out that he may have a fatal disease, and developing a desire that things work out for the best.[14] Presumably, it would be a good thing if, six months later, the stranger is cured. However, as Parfit points out, the stranger's cure is not in Parfit's interests, despite the fact that Parfit may be very interested in whether the stranger is cured. The reason, Parfit argues, is that one has interests in only those states of affairs that are 'about one's own life.'

Although this sounds right, it presses the question of which states of affairs are *about* one's life. Why is the future fate of driving students relevant to their instructors' lives, but the future health of the stranger isn't relevant to Parfit's life? Notice that the answer does not depend upon the *strength* of the individual's desire. Parfit may desire the stranger's cure more than the instructor desires the future safety of his ex-students. Nonetheless, the stranger's cure does not seem to be about Parfit's life in the way that the students' driving futures are about their instructor's life. How might we explain this difference?

[14] D. Parfit. 1984. *Reasons and Persons*. Oxford. Oxford University Press: 494.

42   DAVID WENDLER

James Griffin suggests that, in addition to what we experience directly, our interests also include those states of affairs that 'I take into my life as an aim or goal.'[15] On Griffin's account, although Parfit desires the stranger's return to health, he does not, as the story goes, take this on as a personal goal: he does not commit himself to working to bring about the stranger's cure.

Griffin's crucial insight is that mere desiring is not sufficient to ground an interest because it is too passive. The fact that I take on a particular goal makes the state of affairs referred to a part of my life in the sense that this is now one of my goals. However, it does not seem to follow that the occurrence of the state of affairs in question necessarily has implications *for* my life. We would not say that I lived a better or worse life simply because this goal of mine is or is not realized; it depends upon *how* the goal is realized.

We assume, in the standard cases, that once an individual takes on a particular goal, she will actively work toward realizing that goal. The problem for Griffin's account is that such activity is not required by the mere fact of having the goal – one can have goals that one does nothing to bring about (although the fact that one does nothing may provide evidence that one does not really have the goal in question). Imagine that after worrying for several weeks, Parfit takes on the stranger's cure as a personal goal. If the stranger is cured, we would not say, now that this is one of Parfit's goals, that Parfit's life is necessarily better for it. In a similar way, we do not say that the students' future driving records say something about the instructor's life simply because she has the goal, assuming she does, of her students being accident free. We say this because the instructor actually did something to realize this goal: she taught her students how to drive. Indeed, in this case at least, the instructor's contribution seems to render irrelevant her having the relevant goal, or even the relevant desire. Even if the instructor develops the strong desire that her ex-students crash and burn, their future driving records would still say something about what kind of instructor she was.[16] Put generally, *working* toward a particular goal entails that its realization says something about one's life because it is

---

[15] J. Griffin. 1986. *Well Being*. Oxford. Oxford University Press: 22.

[16] The instructor could make more substantial changes which might entail that the students' driving futures is no longer in her interest. For instance, she might decide to commit herself to a life of helping as few people as possible. In some such cases (particularly if one accepts a subjective account of a flourishing life), we might want to say, given this change, that the students' future driving records are no longer in, and may even be contrary to the instructor's interests.

WHAT RESEARCH WITH STORED SAMPLES   43

now, in an important sense that it was not before, one's own project.[17]

The present line of reasoning suggests that we can have interests in states of affairs that do not affect us personally because we can contribute to whether they obtain.[18] And this suggests that the confirmation of the first premise in the Argument from Contribution – sources have an interest in whether their samples are used for specific research purposes independently of whether the research affects them personally – requires showing that sources contribute (in the relevant sense) to such research.

THE NATURE OF SOURCES' CONTRIBUTION

A number of pathologists have pointed out that non-genetic (e.g. epidemiological) research on stored samples has been going on for years without bioethicists, or anyone else, claiming that the researchers need to obtain sources' informed consent. Since genetic research with *anonymized* samples is no more risky, and has no more effect on individual sources, this argument suggests that investigators should be able to conduct genetic research on anonymized samples without sources' informed consent. Before considering whether this view is right, consider the following: why did the advent of widespread genetic research trigger demands that researchers obtain sources' informed consent in a way that earlier epidemiological research had not?

Part of the answer, I suspect, is that genetic research is newer and we have less sense of what it might lead to. As a result, we tend to judge it as being riskier. Granting this, epidemiological research also typically involves investigators analyzing fairly general properties of the tissue in question. For instance, epidemiologists consider whether individuals who received drug

---

[17] To press Griffin's account further, it seems that the stranger's cure being about my life requires that I actually make a contribution, not simply that I attempt to do so. If I send the stranger money for new treatments, but he is cured before it arrives, then his cure is not about my life. Even though I took on his cure as a personal goal and tried to do something to realize this end, I did not in fact make a contribution.

[18] A related question arises here. Do individuals have an interest in controlling information about them independent of their own experiences or the projects to which they contribute? On the present account it is not clear that they do. However, some have concerns about the availability of personal information per se and seem to regard it as relevant to their lives. In the end, this may not be a complete account of individuals' interests, but it does capture the interests that are relevant to the debate over anonymized research.

44   DAVID WENDLER

X developed abnormality Y at an increased rate relative to the general population. In contrast, genetic research often involves investigators analyzing individual properties of a given tissue sample. When searching for the genes implicated in breast cancer, investigators search extended regions of sources' genotypes to isolate the differences between those who develop the disease versus those who don't. In this case, the individual properties of the sources' DNA become central, the investigators are no longer analyzing various tissues, they are analyzing the tissue of specific persons. As a result, it seems more plausible to argue that the persons in question make an individual contribution to the research.

The sense that sources make a personal contribution to genetic research is reinforced by historical views on genes. Historically, many people have viewed the genetic code as central to, and even constitutive of, one's identity. Given this presumed strong connection between individuals and their DNA, it is not surprising that people would regard the use of tissue samples for genetic research as representing more of an individual contribution to that research than the use of tissue samples for epidemiological research.

The subject model defines individuals' involvement in clinical research in terms of their exposure to research risks, while the experiential model defines research involvement in terms of individuals interacting with investigators and being asked to do certain things. The present line of reasoning suggests a third model that understands individuals' involvement in clinical research in terms of their making a contribution to particular research projects. Although I cannot provide a complete account of the contribution model here, it will be important to understand the nature of individuals' possible contribution to research.

On the 'contribution' model, whether an individual is involved in clinical research, hence, whether human subjects protections apply to them, can be understood in terms of whether information about the individual is used to answer the scientific question being asked. Put simply, whether an individual is a contributor to a research project in this sense depends upon whether information about the individual will be included as data in the analysis of the study. If it will be, then the individual is a contributor to the research project. And since individuals have an interest in the projects to which they contribute, it follows that individuals who contribute in this way have a claim to a say over whether they make this contribution. Therefore, to the extent sources contribute to genetic research in this sense, they have an

WHAT RESEARCH WITH STORED SAMPLES   45

interest in how their samples are used whether or not the research affects them personally.[19]

Research on stored samples helps to distinguish the experiential model from the contribution model by clarifying at least one way in which an individual's contribution to a research project need not be active. In particular, it clarifies that one can contribute to a research project in the sense that one's DNA is included in the project's data analysis without one having to do anything for the project, indeed without one even having to know of the project's existence. In the standard cases, all that is required is that one provided a DNA sample, along with information about one's phenotype, and the investigators now include correlations between the two in their data.

Although the stored sample debate helps to distinguish the three models of research involvement, it is important to recognize that such research is unusual in this sense. In the standard cases, individual's involvement in research involves all three elements. That is, although the three models present alternative understandings of involvement in research, they do not present mutually exclusive understandings. Recognizing the contribution model as a distinct way of conceptualizing research involvement helps to clarify an otherwise anomalous feature of the debate in the U.S. over consent for research on stored samples.

THE IMPORTANCE OF WHEN SAMPLES ARE OBTAINED

The U.S. federal regulations do not apply to research on *existing* tissue samples provided: 'the information is recorded by the investigator in such a manner that subjects cannot be identified, directly or through identifiers.'[20] As a result, investigators who

---

[19] One could argue that the contribution model is simply an expansion on the experiential model (as opposed to a new model of research involvement) in the sense that the contribution model recognizes an additional aspect of individuals' experience, contributing to a research project, as relevant to their research involvement. In the end, it is not clear that any substantive issues hang on whether one considers the contribution model to be a new model versus a new expansion of an old model. With that said, there is an important question of why the three models of research involvement emerged in this particular order – subject, experiential, contribution? Briefly, I suspect the answer has to do with the research community's coming to recognize an increasingly broader range of subjects' interests relevant to their research participation.

[20] United States Department of Health and Human Services. 1991. Protections of Human Subjects. Title 45 Code of Federal Regulations Part 46: 1014.

46   DAVID WENDLER

plan to anonymize previously obtained samples prior to the initiation of their research are not required to obtain ethics review committee (IRB) approval, nor sources' informed consent. The 'preamble' to the regulations explains why not: 'In developing the HHS proposed regulations care was taken to provide protection for human subjects involved in those activities that present risk to subjects, while exempting from coverage by the regulations many forms of research that do not involve risks or involve only slight or remote risks.'[21]

The U.S. regulations' treatment of samples that will be obtained in the future is very different. Research on tissue samples that will be left over, and made anonymous, following future clinically indicated surgery does not pose any risks to the sources. Nonetheless, in this case, the lack of risks is not deemed sufficient to waive ethics review and sources' consent. Instead, research on samples yet to be obtained must undergo ethics review. In addition, such research must obtain sources' informed consent unless it 'could not practicably be carried out without the waiver [of informed consent].'[22] In other words, in moving from previously obtained to prospectively obtained samples, the U.S. federal regulations move from a default of waiving consent to one of requiring consent.

The ASHG also changes its proposed safeguards as it moves from research on existing samples to research on samples that will be obtained prospectively. In the former case, the ASHG endorses waiving informed consent; in the latter case, the ASHG recommends that investigators 'communicate with potential subjects in advance and involve them in the research by obtaining informed consent.' To take one more example, the U.S. National Bioethics Advisory Commission (NBAC) endorses waiving sources' consent for minimal risk research on existing samples on the grounds that doing so does not pose any risks to sources, and does not threaten their rights and welfare. Why then doesn't the NBAC recommend waiving informed consent for research on samples that will be obtained in the future provided the research poses minimal risks and the waiver of consent does not jeopardize sources' rights and welfare?

When samples are obtained does not necessarily affect a protocol's risks or potential benefits, nor what the protocol asks of sources. Nonetheless, it may affect how one conceptualizes the

---

[21] Federal Register. 1981. Final regulations amending basic HHS policy for the protection of human research subjects. 46: 8369.
[22] *Op. cit.* note 20, page 116.

WHAT RESEARCH WITH STORED SAMPLES 47

role of sources. When it comes to research on *existing* tissue samples, the interaction between sources and those obtaining the samples has already occurred, the sources fade from view and, in evaluating the research, one is left with the interaction between an investigator and a clump of cells. Given that this interaction does not include sources, one has less reason to consider whether they might have any interests in whether they contribute to the research in question. Instead, one assesses only whether they face any risks. In other words, one adopts the subject model of sources' role.

Changing the example to one in which the samples will be obtained tomorrow, rather than yesterday, does not necessarily change whether the research will affect sources. However, it does change the interaction that one focuses on in evaluating the research: one considers the removal of samples from people's bodies rather than laboratories' refrigerators and ends up with the contribution model. The tense is relevant to the need for informed consent, then, because it brings the sources into view, thus raising the expectation that investigators will consider their broader interests.

I should point out that although the prospect of obtaining tissue in the future leads many to adopt the contribution model, it does not affect everyone in this way. The College of American Pathologists (CAP) argues that the U.S. federal regulations' exemption for research on existing samples should be expanded to cover research on samples that will be obtained prospectively, provided the samples are obtained for clinical reasons and the tissue is left over after 'all work necessary for the patient's care has been completed.'[23] In effect, the CAP is asking that the U.S. federal regulations apply the subject model consistently. This makes sense. For the most part, pathologists deal with tissue, not sources. Even when the tissue is obtained tomorrow, pathologists will not be interacting with the sources. Thus, they are never in a position of taking tissue from sources while wondering whether the sources have any preferences on how the tissue will be used. Finally, identifying the contribution model as distinct from the subject and experiential models allows us to consider its practical implications.

---

[23] College of American Pathologists. Uses of Human Tissue. 1996: 7. (A consensus statement by the College of American Pathologists and 16 other organizations, available from the college at 325 Waukega Road, Northfield, IL, U.S.A 60093 or http://www.cap.org/)

48   DAVID WENDLER

PRACTICAL IMPLICATIONS

Imagine that an investigator is offered any tissue samples that are left over after clinically indicated surgery that will be performed in two months. If the investigator submits her proposal to conduct research on these samples to the ethics review committee *before* the samples are obtained, the ethics review committee would be reviewing a proposal to conduct research on prospectively obtained samples. Hence, under the U.S. regulations, the protocol would have to obtain ethics review, as well as sources' informed consent provided it can be obtained practicably.

With this in mind, a savvy investigator doing exactly the same research could avoid the requirement for informed consent simply by delaying submission of the protocol until after the samples have been obtained, at which point the ethics review committee would be reviewing a proposal to conduct research on existing samples. Assuming the now-existing samples are anonymized, the research would be exempt from ethics review, hence, the researcher would not be required to obtain sources' informed consent.

As the U.S. regulations turn to existing samples, they shift to the subject model. In the process, the requirement to obtain sources' consent when it is practicable to do so drops out. Using this loophole, unsavory investigators could obtain tissue samples under an innocuous research study and then propose a controversial study for which the investigator has reason to believe sources would not have consented. Since the research now involves existing stored samples, the investigator could avoid ethics review and the need for sources' consent by anonymizing the samples.

Next, the U.S. ELSI working group argues that: 'Any proposals for anonymous research on previously stored tissue samples should be reviewed by an IRB (ethics review committee).'[24] Along the same lines, Clayton et al. suggest that ethics review committees could 'usefully review research proposals to [ ] make currently identifiable tissue samples anonymous without the sources' consent.' The proposal continues: 'Some participants urged that consideration be given to amending the regulations to require such reviews.'[25] Even Knoppers and Laberge, who question these recommendations on several counts, agree with

[24] *Op. cit.* note 6, p. 1788.
[25] *Ibid.*

WHAT RESEARCH WITH STORED SAMPLES   49

this suggestion: 'Clayton et al. wisely suggest IRB review before removal of identifiers.'[26]

Presumably, this suggestion seems wise because the risks of genetic research are largely unknown. Therefore, rather than develop a general policy on when sources' informed consent should be required, and when samples can be anonymized without consent, it makes sense to allow an independent group to make this determination on a case by case basis. Unfortunately, given the current U.S. regulations, this recommendation is not as neutral as it might appear. The requirement that all research proposing to anonymize tissue samples first undergo ethics review would result in investigators having to obtain informed consent whenever doing so is 'practicable'. On the assumption that it is practicable to obtain sources' consent in many cases, this requirement would lead to an unintended increase in the number of times that investigators would be required to obtain sources' consent. To address these practical difficulties, consider the possibility of applying the contribution model consistently to all research using biological samples.

POLICY IMPLICATIONS FOR RESEARCH ON BIOLOGICAL SAMPLES

The weight of individuals' claim to a say over whether they contribute to a particular research project depends upon how central making this contribution is to their lives. In the majority of cases, it seems plausible to assume that it is important for individuals to determine whether their samples are used for research purposes since doing so allows sources to decide whether they contribute to the general project of increasing medical knowledge and helping others. This suggests that sources have a moderately weighty claim to determine whether their samples are used for research purposes at all. It seems less important, in most cases, for individuals to control whether their samples are used to study one disease or another. Whether I contribute to medical research at all says something important about my life; whether I contribute to research on arthritis as opposed to research on diabetes says less about my life. This suggests that, in general, sources have a less weighty claim to determine precisely for which research projects their samples are used. However, the specific nature of certain research projects

---

[26] B.M. Knoppers, C. Laberge. Research and Stored Tissues: persons as sources, samples as persons? *JAMA* 1995; 274: 1807.

50   DAVID WENDLER

can give sources a weighty interest in determining whether their samples are used. For instance, some oppose abortion and dedicate their lives to ending its provision. Such individuals have a weighty interest in controlling whether they contribute to research projects that involve abortion.

The weight of individuals' claims to having a say must be balanced against any interest they have in *not* having a say. To obtain individuals' informed consent, investigators must first provide them with information about the study. For instance, with respect to research on stored samples, sources might be told that, if they agree, their DNA will be tested for a particular mutation. In certain instances, sources may be better off without this information. Knowing that one's DNA is being tested for a particular mutation may put individuals in the position of having to decide whether to inform their employers that their DNA may have tested positive for this mutation. Given that employers may use this information to the individual's detriment, the process of informing sources could put them in the position of having to lie or disclose potentially harmful information.

To balance sources' interests in having a say against their occasional interest in not being given certain information requires an assessment of the risks of being informed in particular cases. Might being informed of the nature of a particular study jeopardize sources' jobs or insurance status? Is there evidence that the information in question poses risks to family members? The answers to these questions will depend upon the kind of study in question and, thus, must be assessed on a case by case basis.

Sources' moderately weighty interest in determining whether their samples are used for research purposes at all suggests that their consent should be required for research using samples for which consent for research purposes has never been obtained. Once consent for research purposes has been obtained, sources' less weighty interest in determining the specific projects to which they contribute suggests that investigators should obtain consent for additional research studies provided it is relatively easy to do so. This suggests that something like the practicability standard should be applied to all research, even research that involves previously obtained samples. When contacting sources is not feasible, consent can be waived provided consent for research purposes has been obtained previously, and there is no reason to think that the research in question is central to sources' interests in the way that research on abortion is for some.

The claim that individuals can make a contribution to research on stored samples that does not affect them personally is not

WHAT RESEARCH WITH STORED SAMPLES   51

limited to genetic research. To take an earlier example, sources contribute to epidemiological research in the sense that some of their tissue is used to conduct the research in question. Thus, on the contribution model, investigators have a reason to obtain sources' consent for epidemiological research even when the research will be done anonymously. However, for reasons discussed earlier, sources make less of a personal contribution to epidemiological research. As a result, they have less of an interest in controlling whether they contribute to such research and investigators have less of a reason to solicit their consent. Two conclusions are possible here.

First, one could conclude that epidemiologists ought to solicit sources' informed consent when it is relatively easy to do so. Alternatively, one might conclude that since sources' interest in epidemiological research is less weighty, the burden of obtaining consent outweighs sources' interests in having a say. In support of this approach, and pending empirical evidence to the contrary, it seems plausible to assume that epidemiological research represents an example of research for which sources are willing to allow investigators to decide whether their tissue is used. Assuming this is right, it seems reasonable to waive the requirement for informed consent for epidemiological research.

To take a second example, on the contribution model, individuals are involved in research that gathers data from their medical records. As a result, individuals have an interest in having a say in whether they contribute to such research. With that said, such research seems to represent less of a contribution on the part of sources in the sense that sources contribute information only, they don't contribute part of themselves.[27] This suggests individuals have a much less weighty interest in determining whether their medical records are used for research purposes, hence, investigators have little reason to obtain their informed consent in these cases. Therefore, it appears, on the contribution model, that consent can be waived for research on medical records provided there is no reason to think the research may be of special concern to sources. Of course, although individuals' status as contributors does not imply a need to obtain their consent in this case, their status as individuals with an interest in avoiding harms may. That is, consent should be obtained for research that poses serious risks even when individuals' contribution to the research is minimal.

---

[27] This example suggests that any complete account of the contribution model will have to admit of varying degrees of contribution.

52 DAVID WENDLER

IMPLICATIONS FOR OTHER ISSUES IN BIOETHICS

The contribution model recognizes that individuals may be involved in research, in the sense of contributing to the research in question, even when it does not pose any risks to them and does not ask them to do anything. To the extent this model applies to research participation in general, it may help illuminate other debates in the ethics of human subjects research. To take just one example, Robert Truog has argued that the requirement for informed consent should be waived for a trial of two antibiotics that have similar side effect profiles when it is unknown which medication is better.[28] Truog points out that, given the similar risk/potential benefit profiles, patients are unlikely to prefer one medication over the other. He concludes that the process of obtaining consent is unlikely to serve the patients in any meaningful way.

Truog bases his argument on the claim that the obligation to seek consent depends upon 'the risk-benefit ratios of the intervention and the alternatives, as well as the degree to which the patient would be expected to have preferences about the various options for diagnosis or treatment that are under investigation.'[29] Recognition of the contribution model makes clear that these are not the only factors relevant to whether consent should be obtained: the fact that individuals are being asked to contribute to the research project provides a prima facie claim that their consent should be obtained.

Whether this prima facie claim is overridden in the kinds of cases that Truog imagines depends upon the weight of individuals' claim to have a say and the nature of the say they should have. The present point is not to determine whether, in these cases, individuals' interests are sufficiently weighty to require their consent. Instead, the point is that the purpose of obtaining individuals' informed consent for research participation goes beyond giving them a choice between their various research options, and includes giving them a say in whether they contribute to the research project in question.[30] Hence, the fact that individuals are very likely indifferent

---

[28] R. Truog. Is informed consent always necessary for randomized, controlled trials. *New England J Med* 1999; 340: 804–806.

[29] *Ibid.*

[30] In addition, any psychological benefits of contributing to research require that individuals *know* they are making a contribution. This would be another reason to obtain their consent.

between their research options does not necessarily imply that there is no reason to obtain their informed consent.

CONCLUSION

The debate over when investigators should obtain consent for research on anonymizable biological samples suggests a new paradigm for understanding individuals' involvement in research. On the subject model, there is no reason to solicit sources' informed consent because research using anonymized samples poses no direct risks to sources. Similarly, on the experiential model, there is no reason to solicit sources' informed consent because, and this is particularly clear for samples that were obtained in the past, anonymized research may not affect sources personally. The fact that some writers argue for informed consent, nonetheless, points to a third model of sources' involvement in research.

The contribution model recognizes that individuals' interests extend beyond their own experiences. In particular, individuals have interests in the projects to which they contribute. By taking these interests into account, it becomes clear that many of the arguments for and against obtaining sources' informed consent have been overstated. Those who argue that investigators have no reason to obtain informed consent for anonymizable research implicitly assume an overly narrow understanding of sources' relevant interests, one that ignores their potential interests in determining whether they contribute to the research in question. Others recognize that investigators have a reason to obtain sources' informed consent for anonymizable research, but often conclude that consent should be obtained whenever possible. This view implicitly assumes that individuals' interests in having a say always outweighs any reasons not to obtain consent. There are two problems with this view.

First, individuals can have competing interests in not having a say. In addition, individuals often have less weighty interests in controlling precisely which research projects they contribute to. Thus, serious burdens in obtaining their consent can outweigh their interest in determining whether they contribute to a specific research project. Finally, individuals' autonomy interests do not imply that they should control every aspect of their lives, including determining every project to which they contribute. Individuals can cede control over particular projects. In the case of research with biological samples, individuals can ethically give consent for future research purposes in general without having

54 DAVID WENDLER

to know about and approve every individual use of their samples.

David Wendler
Department of Clinical Bioethics
National Institutes of Health
Building 10, Room 1C118
Bethesda, MD USA 20892
wendler@nih.gov

[24]

Uncertainty in Clinical Research

Robert J. Levine

"It is a fact of life that human beings find it difficult to maintain a consistent, self-conscious appreciation of the extent to which uncertainty accompanies them on their daily rounds and to integrate that uncertainty with whatever certainties inform their conduct. Physicians are not exempt from this human proclivity."

—Jay Katz[1]

Among Jay Katz's numerous distinguished contributions to the field of law and medicine is his clarification of the concept of uncertainty and its impact on the practice of medicine. He has explored and explained how and why physicians typically avoid dealing with the problematic existence of uncertainty except in the realm of theory. He has made it clear that physicians' avoidance or disregard of the problem of uncertainty is a major barrier to communications between doctors and patients.

The purpose of this essay is to reflect on some manifestations of uncertainty in the design and conduct of clinical research. The focus is on the randomized clinical trial (RCT), generally regarded as the gold standard for the evaluation of therapeutic agents. The purpose of the RCT is to resolve certain types of uncertainties. Is drug A effective in the treatment of disease D?, for example. Or, is drug A more or less effective than drug B in the treatment of disease D? What kinds of uncertainty justify beginning an RCT? How well do we communicate such uncertainties to prospective subjects? Does the RCT resolve uncertainty? These are the questions I shall address in this paper.

Justification to Begin

For the purpose of illustration, let us consider a simple RCT design—one that will compare therapy A with therapy B in the treatment of disease D. It is generally agreed that a necessary condition for ethical justification of such an RCT is that the investigators be able to state an honest null hypothesis—a formal statement of equivalence of the two therapies being compared.[2] The null hypothesis is articulated in this form: Therapy A is equal to therapy B in the treatment of disease D.[3]

The null hypothesis is considered "honest" if it has two characteristics. First, it must take into account all previous studies designed to evaluate the efficacy of either therapy A or therapy B as well as those designed to compare the efficacy of A and B. It is not permissible to disregard data derived from any such studies; rather, some explanation is required as to why data that appear to contradict the null hypothesis are not to be considered convincing. Second, the statement of equivalence must take into account all the important consequences —both harmful and beneficial—of the two therapies. For example, in an RCT comparing radical mastectomy with wide excision in the treatment of early breast cancer, many critics considered a statement that the same number of women were expected to be alive after five years inadequate. It disregarded, they felt, the expected mutilation and disability in those randomized to undergo radical surgery.[4]

The RCT is designed to test the null hypothesis. Mathematically, it is impossible to prove the null hypothesis unless one can demonstrate the equivalence of therapies A and B in the entire universe of patients having disease D. What one can do is to reject this hypothesis. This is accomplished by finding a superior result with one of the two therapies. For example, if a superior result is found in patients receiving therapy A and if this occurs sufficiently often to be considered statistically significant, one may reject the null hypothesis, A = B. We may state, instead, with appropriate reservations, that A is superior to B. Statistical significance refers to the likelihood that the observed difference in results might have occurred by chance. Typically, we agree that if the observed difference would occur by chance less than five times in 100 (or 0.05), the observed difference is statistically significant. The probability (p) of chance occurrence of less than 0.05 is expressed conventionally, "$p < 0.05$."

Charles Fried introduced the term "equipoise" to refer to the state of therapeutic equivalence necessary to justify the conduct of an RCT.[5] The concept of equipoise refers to a state of perfect balance of therapies A and B. It presupposes that there is no important information suggesting the superiority of either A or B and further that, considering the balance of risks and benefits for each therapy, there are no rational grounds for choosing one or the other. Such conditions of equipoise virtually never exist. As we consider the justification of any particular RCT, we almost always find that one or both of the two presuppositions either does not obtain or if they do they probably will soon cease to obtain. I shall return to this point.

But first let us consider why this condition of equipoise is considered so vital in the ethical justification of RCTs. To a large extent this reflects the patient-centered ethic of medicine. Put simply, the doctor is required to recommend what he or she believes is the best therapy for the patient. As Shaw and Chalmers put it:[6]

"If the clinician knows, or has good reason to believe, that a new therapy (A) is better than another therapy (B), he cannot participate in a comparative trial of therapy A versus therapy B. Ethically, the clinician is obligated to give therapy A to each new patient with a need for one of these therapies.

"If the physician (or his peers) has genuine doubt as to which therapy is better, he should give each patient an equal chance to receive one or the other therapy. The physician must fully recognize that the new therapy might be worse than the old. Each new patient must have a fair chance of receiving either the new and, hopefully, better therapy or the limited benefits of the old therapy."

Shaw and Chalmers recognize the possibility that reasonable doctors may differ on whether an honest statement of a null hypothesis can be made. According to their formulation, those who believe that the null hypothesis could be true should participate in the RCT. Others who are already convinced of the superiority of

therapy A or therapy B should abstain from participation in the RCT; instead they should recommend to their patients that they accept treatment with the therapy they consider superior.

As Shaw and Chalmers observe, early usage of new therapies commonly is performed in an uncontrolled fashion. This often leads to false impressions about their safety and efficacy. Poorly controlled pilot studies often generate inadequate information that tends to inhibit the subsequent conduct of adequate RCTs. For example, the results of an early pilot study may show that a new therapy A seems far superior to the standard therapy B; thus, the statement of therapeutic equivalence necessary to justify a comparison between A and B will tend to be challenged, perhaps inappropriately. To avoid such problems, Shaw and Chalmers encourage the use of RCTs as early as possible in the course of testing a new therapy. In fact, in a subsequent publication, Chalmers, et al. urge randomization with the very first use of a new therapy; i.e., the first patient eligible to receive a new drug should have a 50–50 chance of receiving either it or the standard alternative drug.[7]

For several good reasons it is not customary to introduce new therapies by random allocation with the very first patient.[8] Clinical investigators generally demand some preliminary evidence that the new therapy will have at least some beneficial effect. RCTs are expensive and those who finance such trials do not, in general, wish to make major investments in studying agents that are not likely to prove effective. Moreover, in the period before beginning an RCT, studies are done that are designed not only to establish preliminary evidence of efficacy but also to determine the optimum dose to be studied during the RCT.[9] All things considered, it would be quite irresponsible to begin an RCT without quite a bit of preliminary information about the safety and efficacy of a new drug.

Thus, when RCTs are begun, there is generally available sufficient information about the drugs to be studied to indicate that they are effective and to provide a basis for selection of the proper doses to be administered to patient-subjects—doses most likely to secure the intended benefits without producing unacceptable adverse effects. The availability of such preliminary data makes justification of placebo-controlled RCTs particularly problematic. In such studies, one is generally comparing a drug "known" to have a therapeutic effect with a placebo which is selected because it is believed not to have such an effect.[10] Thus, many physicians will challenge the legitimacy of the null hypothesis in a placebo-controlled trial, particularly those in which the purpose of the active agent is to mitigate that component of a disease process that leads to lethal or disabling complications. Similar controversies over the legitimacy of the

Volume 16: 3–4, Winter 1988

null hypothesis are commonly seen when new drugs are to be compared with relatively ineffective standard therapies in the treatment of lethal diseases—e.g., chemotherapy resistant cancers.[11]

During the conduct of an RCT, data are accumulated relevant to the relative merits of the therapies that are being compared. In an RCT that will eventually reject the null hypothesis, therapy A = therapy B, with the passage of time the accumulated data will be increasingly suggestive of the superiority of either drug A or drug B. Thus, even when the initial statement of therapeutic equivalence made to justify the beginning of the RCT is noncontroversial, during the course of the study there usually is increasingly strong reason to dispute any claim that the two therapies being compared are equivalent.

Shaw and Chalmers describe vividly the threats to the integrity of the RCT if the investigators are allowed to be aware of emerging trends during the course of the RCT.[12] They recommend keeping "the results confidential from the participating physician until a peer review group says that the study is over. When appropriate, an understanding of the need for confidence until a conclusion is reached, fortified by an explanation of the built-in safety mechanisms, should be a part of the information imparted in obtaining informed consent." It is customary in large scale RCTs to have Data Monitoring Committees.[13] These groups monitor data developed in the course of the RCT for purposes of determining whether the RCT should be discontinued or whether the RCT or the consent procedures should be modified; their deliberations are kept secret from both investigators and subjects unless and until they determine that the RCT should be either interrupted or modified.

Confidentiality of preliminary findings is recognized as so vital to the integrity of RCTs that in 1980 the Health, Education, and Welfare Ethics Advisory Board (EAB) recommended a limited exemption for such data from the Freedom of Information Act.[14]

At this point, I hope it is clear to the reader that there is a problem with the traditional approach to justification of RCTs. All too often, before the RCT is begun there are data available to support challenges to the claims of therapeutic equivalence or equipoise required for such justification. Physician-investigators are asked to try to disregard these data—to suspend disbelief—so that they may participate in these studies without violating their patient-centered ethic. During the course of the RCT, data are developed that make the initial claims of equipoise seem increasingly indefensible. We shield these data from physician-investigators and patient-subjects alike so that they will not behave in ways that would undermine the validity of the RCT.

Benjamin Freedman has argued persuasively that these problems with equipoise derive from a particular understanding of that concept which he calls "theoretical equipoise."[15] "Theoretical equipoise exists when, overall, the evidence on behalf of two alternative treatment regimens is exactly balanced. This evidence may be derived from a variety of sources, including data from the literature, uncontrolled experience, considerations of basic science and fundamental physiologic processes, and perhaps a 'gut feeling' or 'instinct' resulting from (or superimposed on) other considerations. . . ."

Freedman characterizes theoretical equipoise as "overwhelmingly fragile," "conceptually odd and ethically irrelevant." He recommends a different understanding of equipoise as more satisfactory in all respects—viz., "clinical equipoise." "To understand the alternative, preferable interpretation of equipoise, we need to recall the basic reason for conducting clinical trials: there is a current or imminent conflict in the clinical community over what treatment is preferred for patients in a defined population P. The standard is A, but some evidence suggests that B will be superior (because of its effectiveness or its reduction of undesirable side effects, or for some other reasons). . . . Or there is a split in the clinical community, with some clinicians favoring A and others favoring B. Each side recognizes that the opposing side has evidence to support its position, yet each still thinks that overall its view is correct. . . . A clinical trial is instituted with the aim of resolving this dispute. . . .

"We may state the formal conditions under which a trial would be ethical as follows: At the start of the trial, there must be a state of clinical equipoise regarding the merits of the regimens to be tested, and the trial must be designed in such a way as to make it reasonable to expect that, if it is successfully concluded, clinical equipoise would be disturbed. In other words, the results of the successful trial should be convincing enough to resolve the dispute among clinicians.

"A state of clinical equipoise is consistent with a decided treatment preference on the part of the investigators. They must simply recognize that their less-favored treatment is preferred by colleagues whom they consider to be responsible and competent."

I agree with Freedman that the concept of clinical equipoise is decidedly more relevant than theoretical equipoise to the ethical justification of RCTs. Clinical equipoise better describes the state of knowledge about comparative efficacy at times when most RCTs are begun as well as during their conduct. Those responsible for determining that RCTs are justified ethically often persuade themselves that the state of knowledge more closely approximates theoretical equipoise than it actually does. Consequently, as we shall see, they create barriers to effective communications with patient-subjects.

Law, Medicine & Health Care

Communications with Patient-Subjects

"The importance that physicians have attributed throughout medical history to faith, hope and reassurance seems to demand that doctors be bearers of certainty and good news. Therefore, the idea of acknowledging to patients the limitations of medical knowledge and of doctors' capacities to relieve suffering is opposed by an ancient tradition."

—Jay Katz[16]

Such beliefs about what patients expect and need from their doctors have been reflected in controversies over whether prospective subjects of RCTs ought to be informed that therapy will be decided by chance. Thomas Chalmers reflected tersely the beliefs of many of his colleagues when he said in 1967: "If they (patients) were in their right senses, they would find a doctor who thought he knew which was the best treatment, or they would conclude that if the differences were so slight. . . , they would prefer to take their chances on no operation."[17] Since 1967 there has developed near consensus that prospective subjects of RCTs should be informed that their therapy will be chosen by chance.[18] Among those who have joined in this consensus is Chalmers; all prospective subjects of RCTs at his institution are informed that their therapy will be decided by chance, apparently without inhibiting the recruitment of prospective subjects.[19]

This consensus notwithstanding, we still see occasional expressions of concern by physicians and scientists on this point. For example, in 1984, Taylor, et al. surveyed the surgeons participating in a cooperative protocol designed to compare two forms of primary therapy for breast cancer;[20] they wanted to learn why there was a disappointingly low rate of patient accrual for this RCT. They found that only 27 percent of surgeons enrolled "all eligible patients." The others offered the following explanations: " 1) Concern that the doctor-patient relationship would be affected by an RCT (73 percent), 2) Difficulty with informed consent (38 percent), 3) Dislike of open discussion involving uncertainty (22 percent), 4) Perceived conflict between the roles of scientist and clinician (18 percent), 5) Practical difficulties in following procedures (9 percent), and 6) Feelings of personal responsibility if the treatments were found to be unequal (8 percent)."

Another manifestation of the belief that patients need their doctors to be "bearers of certainty and good news," is the proposal by Marvin Zelen of various prerandomization designs for RCTs. In these designs, randomization is accomplished before informed consent during which subjects are told what therapy has been selected for them. Almost all commentators on the ethical justification of such prerandomization designs have decided that they are not responsive to the ethical

grounding for the requirement of informed consent.[21] Moreover, in most of the small number of RCTs in which these designs have been employed, they did not achieve the expected increase in efficiency.[22]

Implicit in reaching the consensus that prospective subjects of RCTs should be informed that their therapy will be chosen by chance was an understanding that there must also be a disclosure of uncertainty regarding the relative merits of the therapies to be compared. There was no need for a separate determination in this regard; it was simply self-evident that one could not disclose the fact that therapy would be chosen by chance without also disclosing uncertainty. If uncertainty about the relative merits of the therapies to be compared were not revealed, it would make no sense whatever to prospective subjects that their therapies were to be decided by chance.

Let us now consider how we communicate this uncertainty to prospective patient-subjects of RCTs. Here is a typical statement from a consent form for a multi-center RCT in the field of oncology: "It is not yet known which drug is better although both have been shown to be active." What meaning is conveyed by such a statement?

"It is not known," suggests that there is simply no information available that would lead anyone to a judgment that either therapy A or therapy B is more likely to be the better treatment for patients in general or for any patient in particular. In short, it suggests that knowledge on this point is in a state of theoretical equipoise. As already discussed, in many cases this is not an accurate representation of the state of knowledge as patients are recruited to participate in RCTs. In many, but not all, RCTs designed to compare two or more active therapies, the state of knowledge at the outset may be sufficiently close to theoretical equipoise to justify stating, "It is not known." But even in such cases, shortly after the RCT is begun, data become known (at least to members of Data Monitoring Committees) which are contradictory to such statements.

Statements reflecting theoretical equipoise made to prospective subjects of placebo-controlled RCTs are even more problematic. In such cases, patients are asked to believe that "it is not known" whether the active drug will prove to be better or worse than placebo (generally

Volume 16: 3–4, Winter 1988

explained in consent forms as "an inert substance").[23] One must wonder why any rational person would agree to participate in an RCT in which there are only two possibilities—viz., to receive "an inert substance" or a drug which is "not known" to be either better or worse than the inert substance.

I have argued elsewhere that in placebo-controlled RCTs in which the active drug is designed to mitigate that component of a disease process that leads to lethal or disabling complications, there ought to be full disclosure of preliminary data indicating that the active drug is likely to prove effective.[24] In such RCTs, placebo administration ought to be considered a nontherapeutic procedure which presents more than minimal risk. The risk is that of withholding effective therapy—i.e., the risk of the lethal or disabling complications that the active therapy is designed to prevent. Ethically and legally it is not permissible to withhold information about risks which surpass the threshold of "minimal risk."

In such placebo-controlled RCTs, when therapies known to be effective for the same condition are available, their availability as alternatives to participating in the RCT must also be disclosed to the prospective subject. Let us consider some of the implications and ramifications of disclosure to prospective subjects of the hazards of placebo administration, the results of preliminary studies and the availability of alternatives.

Let us imagine that we have just finished presenting to a man with moderately severe hypertension information on which will be based his informed consent to participate in a placebo-controlled RCT of a new antihypertensive drug. He responds: "Do you mean to say you are asking me to spend six months taking either an inert substance or one that you have no cause to suspect is either better or worse than that inert substance when the risk of taking a placebo entails approximately a 28 percent chance per year of having a severe complication such as stroke, malignant hypertension, heart failure, or death?[25] You offer me an invitation to participate in such an RCT when I could instead take any of the many antihypertensive drugs which are already approved by the FDA and which would reduce my risk of a major complication to 1.6 percent per year? Why would any rational person do that?" Why, indeed!

It is not the purpose of this paper to assess the ethical justification of placebo-controlled RCTs.[26] Rather, I want to point out that in our communications with prospective subjects of such RCTs, we may encounter formidable problems.

Several commentators have recognized that if we present full information to prospective subjects of RCTs, the rate of refusal to participate would likely be so great as to jeopardize any possibility of completing the RCT. In general, they point out that physicians following a patient-centered ethic will be unwilling to enroll patients in such RCTs and patients who are pursuing primarily or exclusively their personal health-related interests will refuse to cooperate.

Here are some of the solutions they have asked their readers to consider. Arthur Schafer suggests that we must consider shifting "from a patient centered to a social-welfare centered ethic."[27] Don Marquis suggests, "perhaps what is needed is an ethics that will justify the conscription of subjects for medical research."[28] Paul Meier suggests that we should rely on the altruism of the patient: ". . . Most of us would be quite willing to forgo a modest expected gain in the general interest of learning something of value."[29] I mention these proposals only to illustrate the gravity of the problems that may be encountered in communications with patient-subjects; in appreciation of these problems several commentators have found it necessary to propose radical revisions of our traditional understandings of medical ethics in the interests of conducting certain types of RCTs. The merits of these and other related proposals have been discussed by Freedman[30] and Levine.[31]

I suggest that informed consent to RCTs should require conveying to prospective subjects the concept of clinical equipoise. As compared with theoretical equipoise, it is, as discussed earlier, a more accurate reflection of the true state of affairs regarding knowledge about the merits of the therapies to be compared. As such, it is more responsive to the ethical purposes of informed consent than is the current tendency to rely on theoretical equipoise.

Will revising our approach to informed consent to reflect clinical equipoise help us with any of the practical problems I have mentioned? I believe it will help with recruitment of subjects for two types of RCTs: First, it should be helpful in recruiting patient-subjects for placebo-controlled RCTs when there is no alternative "standard therapy." A good case in point was the placebo-controlled RCT of azidothymidine (AZT) in the treatment of AIDS conducted in 1986.[32] In this clinical trial many subjects did not believe that it was "not known" whether AZT was more effective than placebo in reducing the morbidity and mortality from AIDS. Indeed, many physicians and scientists had expressed their doubts regarding the statements of therapeutic equivalence. Consequently, many subjects doubted the integrity of the RCT and those who conducted it. They engaged in various behaviors which were detrimental to the validity of the study—e.g., falsification of inclusion criteria and surreptitious sharing of their pills.[33]

It would have been more conducive to confidence in this RCT if subjects had been informed that "some but not all doctors believe that AZT is effective in the treatment of AIDS. The purpose of this RCT is to resolve this controversy. If this controversy can be resolved, there will be reason for manufacturing a sufficient quantity of AZT to treat all eligible patients."

In RCTs comparing two active therapies, I believe it would be similarly helpful to inform prospective subjects in a fashion that reflects the concept of clinical equipoise, If such an approach had been used, for example, in the RCTs comparing radical mastectomy with less mutilating procedures, I believe that the harsh criticisms of these studies would have been blunted.

On the other hand, I rather doubt that changing the approach to informed consent in placebo-controlled trials in which there are available as alternatives safe and effective standard therapies will resolve any of the problems that I have mentioned. In such clinical trials, planning informed consent so as to reflect the concept of clinical equipoise could have heuristic value. In some, but not all, cases one might decide that no rational patient would be likely to accept enrollment in the RCT. In such cases the planners might decide to substitute for the placebo-controlled RCT one having either historical or active controls.

As noted earlier, during the course of an RCT that will eventually reject the null hypothesis, therapy A = therapy B, with the passage of time the accumulated data will be increasingly suggestive of the superiority of either drug A or drug B. Knowing this, patients may express desires to be informed of interim results. One might say, for example, "I do not want to wait for statistical significance. It is sufficient for my purposes to know that drug A seems to be superior even though the probability that this result could have occurred by chance is 10 percent." Here again the concept of clinical equipoise should prove useful to guide communications with subjects. They may (and should) be informed that the purpose of the RCT is to resolve controversy among clinicians and that such resolution ordinarily requires a finding of superiority that is significant at the 5 percent level.[34] They should further be informed that it is only at that point that the RCT will be considered completed and that for good reasons, no preliminary findings will be revealed earlier to either patients or investigators.

There is one more point I wish to make about the typical approach to disclosure of alternatives in RCTs designed to compare two (or more) active therapies. All too often statements in consent forms fail to reflect adequately alternatives to participation in the RCT which some, perhaps most, patients might consider preferable to any of the therapies to be administered in the RCT. Problems are particularly likely to arise in the field of oncology when the cancer is rapidly progressive and resistant to therapy and the therapies to be compared are highly toxic.

Consider this statement from a consent form de-signed by a cooperative oncology group for such an RCT: "Alternatives which could be considered in your case include different drugs or drug combinations, or radiation therapy. Another alternative is no further therapy, which would probably result in continued growth of the tumor. At this time it is felt that no other therapy is more beneficial than the treatments now proposed."

It is true that "no further therapy" would probably —indeed, almost certainly—be associated with "continued growth of the tumor." Not revealed, however, is the fact that either of the two therapies being compared most likely would similarly be associated with such continued tumor growth. Moreover, each of the two therapies is likely to cause severe nausea, vomiting, bone marrow depression, life-threatening infections and other serious and uncomfortable complications. While some patients in the RCT might have satisfactory remissions, most will experience some reduction in the number of days they have to live and in their quality of life during those few remaining days. On balance, the average patient in the RCT will die sooner and will be less comfortable during his or her remaining days than those who choose "no further therapy."

Without chemotherapy, patients eligible for enrollment in this RCT will experience "continued growth of the tumor" which, in turn, will be associated with relentless progression of disability and, eventually, death. In the ancient tradition to which Jay Katz refers, it is essential to offer such patients "good news," some grounds for hope, some reassurance. The "good news" is that they may elect to participate in an RCT in which they will receive one of two new therapies each of which "have been shown to be active." But is it fair to say that "no other therapy is more beneficial than the treatments now proposed"?

When patients have diseases that are likely to be lethal within a relatively short period of time, it is vitally important that the doctor and patient have careful discussions designed to reach agreements about therapeutic objectives; they may choose to 1) pursue a cure or remission, 2) maintain biologic function, or 3) maximize comfort.[35] Such choices are essential because pursuit of any of these objectives entails interventions likely to undermine the accomplishment of either of the others.[36] For example, in the RCT from which the statement of alternatives now being discussed was derived, a choice to enroll presupposes as the therapeutic objective the pursuit of a cure or remission. This entails acceptance of detriments to biologic function (e.g., bone marrow depression) and discomfort (e.g., nausea and vomiting).

The problem with the disclosure of alternatives as presented in the consent form is that it is preemptive. It is suitable only for those who have chosen to pursue remission with full awareness of the adverse conse-

Volume 16: 3–4, Winter 1988

quences they may expect. Only in such cases is it appropriate to say "it is felt that no other therapy is more beneficial than the treatments now proposed."

In situations of the sort I am now describing, many patients are likely to choose as their therapeutic objective the maximization of comfort (or palliative treatment). For this reason, the Institutional Review Board at Yale-New Haven Medical Center commonly requests the addition to consent forms of language to the following effect:

"Before you agree to participate in this protocol, you should consult with your personal physician. Please show your physician a copy of this protocol and consent form and ask for his or her advice as to whether you should agree to participate in this protocol."

Do RCTs Resolve Uncertainty?

"Only during the last 150 years, thanks to the unprecedented advances in medical science, have physicians begun to acquire the intellectual sophistication and experimental tools to distinguish more systematically between knowledge and ignorance, between what they know, do not know, and what remains conjectural. . . . Without the emergence of medical science, the legal doctrine of informed consent probably could not have been promulgated."

—Jay Katz [37]

Is Jay Katz's confidence in medical science justified? Are RCTs so successful in resolving uncertainty about the merits of medical therapies? There are some grounds for concern.

In recent years, the RCT as it is typically designed, conducted and analyzed has been subjected to a variety of criticisms. A full discussion of these criticisms is beyond the scope of this paper.[38] I shall mention just two of them here.

Alvan Feinstein identifies as a major problem the fact that there are conflicting schools of thought about how RCTs ought to be conducted:[39] the "pragmatic" school which includes most clinical practitioners and the "fastidious" school which includes most biostatisticians. The former "usually want the trial to answer pragmatic questions in clinical management. For this purpose, the plans would incorporate the heterogeneity, occasional or frequent ambiguity, and other 'messy' aspects of ordinary clinical practice. The advocates of the opposing viewpoint fear that this strategy will yield a 'messy' answer. They prefer a 'clean' arrangement, using homogeneous groups, reducing or eliminating ambiguity, and avoiding the spectre of biased results."

Currently, the fastidious viewpoint seems dominant in the conduct of RCTs. Consequently, according to Feinstein, RCTs are not good predictors of what will occur in the practice of medicine. Among other reasons, the RCT, being a carefully contrived laboratory model in which the patient-subjects are carefully selected and the conditions of therapy rigidly controlled, does not simulate very well the practice of medicine. For example, the majority of the patients encountered by the practicing physician would have been excluded from the RCT designed to validate the therapy owing to such "exclusion criteria" as coexisting disease.

In addition, there is tendency to overlook the acquisition and analysis of what Feinstein calls "soft data." Soft data are concerned with symptoms caused and relieved by the new therapies; often these are most important in determining whether patients will accept a new therapy or consider it superior to an alternative.[40]

Another major controversy concerns the approach that should be used to the statistical analysis of data yielded by an RCT. More precisely, there have been formidable challenges to the use of standard statistical methods suggesting that Bayesian analysis would be likely to yield different and perhaps more valid results. Using Bayesian methods of statistical analysis, Diamond and Forrester examined the results of several major published RCTs and concluded that they were probably invalid.[41] For example, they concluded that the University Group Diabetes Program probably did not establish that tolbutamide increases cardiac mortality, and that the Aspirin and Myocardial Infarction Study probably did not establish a protective effect of aspirin.[42]

As a result of these and other considerations, some clinicians (and some statisticians) are not accepting the results of RCTs as decisive in resolving disputes about the efficacy of therapies, at least in some cases. These are problems that must be taken seriously. To Jay Katz I now respond with a qualified agreement. Yes, "physicians have begun to acquire the . . . tools to distinguish . . . between what they know, do not know, and what remains conjectural." But we are not systematically re-

Law, Medicine & Health Care

placing uncertainties with certainties. We must continue to be skeptical about our "certainties" and persistent in our pursuit of better intellectual tools to distinguish between knowledge and ignorance. In the foreseeable future it will be necessary for us to continue to grapple with the problem of uncertainty, to learn how best to deal with it and to communicate about it with subjects and prospective subjects of research.

References

Acknowledgment: I thank Susan L. Katz for her helpful criticisms of an early draft of this paper.

1. J. Katz, *The Silent World of Doctor and Patient* (New York: Free Press, 1984), 165–66.

2. R.J. Levine, *Ethics and Regulation of Clinical Research,* 2d ed. (Baltimore: Urban & Schwarzenberg, 1986), 187ff.

3. Although this is the typical form of expression of the null hypothesis, it would be more accurate to say "therapy A = therapy B in the accomplishment of objective O in population P," where objective O is the endpoint under examination (e.g., lowering of blood pressure) and population P is a subset of those patients with disease D (e.g., essential hypertension) who have the necessary attributes (inclusion criteria and lack of exclusion criteria) to be eligible for participation in the RCT.

4. R.J. Levine, supra note 2, at 188–89.

5. C. Fried, *Medical Experimentation: Personal Integrity and Social Policy* (New York: American Elsevier Company, 1974), 51 ff.

6. L.W. Shaw and T.C. Chalmers, "Ethics in Cooperative Trials," *Annals of the New York Academy of Sciences,* 169 (1970): 487–95.

7. T.C. Chalmers, J.B. Block, and S. Lee, "Controlled Studies in Clinical Cancer Research," *New England Journal of Medicine,* 287 (1972): 75–78.

8. R.J. Levine, supra note 2, at 187–88.

9. A.E. Cato and L. Cook, "Clinical Research," in G.M. Matoren, ed., *The Clinical Research Process in the Pharmaceutical Industry* (New York: Marcel Dekker, Inc., 1984), 217–38.

10. R.J. Levine, supra note 2, at 202–07.

11. D. Marquis and R. Stephens, E.S. Siris and M.M. Kemeny, and R.J. Levine, "The Doctor's Unproven Beliefs and the Subject's Informed Choice," *IRB: A Review of Human Subjects Research* 10, 2 (May/June 1988): 3–5; H.Y. Vanderpool and G.B. Weiss, "False Data and Last Hopes: Enrolling Ineligible Patients in Clinical Trials," *Hastings Center Report,* 17, 2, (April 1987): 16–19.

12. L.W. Shaw and T.C. Chalmers, supra note 6.

13. L. Friedman and D. Demets, "The Data Monitoring Committee: How It Operates and Why," *IRB: A Review of Human Subjects Research* 3, 4, (April 1981): 6–8.

14. Ethics Advisory Board, Department of Health and Human Services, "The Request of the National Institutes of Health for a Limited Exemption from the Freedom of Information Act," Report Submitted to the Secretary, DHHS, May 21, 1980.

15. B. Freedman, "Equipoise and the Ethics of Clinical Research," *New England Journal of Medicine,* 317 (1987): 141–145.

16. J. Katz, supra note 1, at 189.

17. T.C. Chalmers, "The Ethics of Randomization as a Decision Making Technique and the Problem of Informed Consent," in USDHEW Report of the 14th Annual Conference of Cardiovascular Training Grant Program Directors (Bethesda, MD: National Heart Institute, 1967). As cited by C. Fried, supra note 5.

18. R.J. Levine, supra note 2, at 194 ff.

19. T.C. Chalmers, "The Clinical Trial," *Milbank Memorial Fund Quarterly,* 59 (1981): 324–339.

20. K.M. Taylor, R.G. Margolese, and C.L. Soskolne, "Physicians' Reasons for Not Entering Eligible Patients in a Randomized Clinical Trial of Surgery for Breast Cancer," *New England Journal of Medicine,* 310 (1984): 1363–67.

21. A full discussion of prerandomization designs is beside the point of this article; such a discussion may be found in R.J. Levine, supra note 2, at 194–97.

22. S.S. Ellenberg, "Randomization Designs in Comparative Clinical Trials," *New England Journal of Medicine* 310 (1984): 1404–08.

23. Actually, most consent forms for placebo-controlled RCTs which I have seen do not use the expression, "it is not known." Many of them provide information based upon which prospective subjects could make either of two seemingly inconsistent inferences: 1) The consent form usually refers to preliminary evidence that the active drug is effective and labels the placebo as "an inert substance." In presenting the risks of placebo, it may also refer to the perils of withholding active therapy. From such information the prospective subject could reasonably infer that the investigator already believes that the active drug is more likely than not to prove superior to placebo. 2) Institutional Review Boards (IRBs) generally constrain investigators from making clear statements that the investigational drug is likely to be effective, reasoning that if this were already known, it would invalidate the null hypothesis used to justify the RCT. Following this reasoning, grounded in the concept of theoretical equipoise, it is considered unethical to tell subjects that a new drug is likely to be effective until the RCT demonstrates that it is. IRBs generally require that subjects be informed that "the purpose of this study is to determine whether the drug is effective." Since in order to do this it will be compared with placebo, the subject could infer that "it is not known whether the new drug is better or worse than placebo."

24. R.J. Levine, "The Use of Placebos in Randomized Clinical Trials," *IRB: A Review of Human Subjects Research,* 7, 2 (March/April 1985): 1–4.

25. Id.

26. For further discussion of such justification, see R.J. Levine, supra note 2, at 202–06.

27. A. Schafer, "The Ethics of the Randomized Clinical Trial," *New England Journal of Medicine,* 307 (1982): 719–24.

28. D. Marquis, "Leaving Therapy to Chance," *Hastings Center Report,* 13, 4 (August 1983): 40–47.

29. P. Meier, "Terminating a Trial—the Ethical Problem," *Clinical Pharmacology & Therapeutics,* 25 (1979): 633–40.

30. B. Freedman, supra note 15.

31. R.J. Levine, supra note 2, at 202ff.

32. M. Fischl, et al., "The Efficacy of Azidothymidine (AZT) in the Treatment of Patients with AIDS and AIDS-

Volume 16: 3–4, Winter 1988

Related Complex," *New England Journal of Medicine,* 317 (1987): 185–91.

33. G.B. Melton, et al., "Community Consultation in Socially Sensitive Research: Lessons from the Clinical Trials of Treatments for AIDS," *American Psychologist* (in press).

34. For further elaboration of this point including the specifics of what ought to be disclosed and explained, see R.J. Levine, supra note 2, at 200–01.

35. Committee on Policy for DNR Decisions, Yale-New Haven Hospital, "Report on Do Not Resuscitate Decisions," *Connecticut Medicine* 47 (1983): 477–83.

36. Id.; R.J. Levine, and K.A. Nolan, "Do Not Resuscitate Decisions: A Policy," *Connecticut Medicine,* 47 (1983): 511–12.

37. J. Katz, supra note 1, at xvi.

38. I have discussed the leading criticisms of RCTs in R.J. Levine, supra note 2, at 207–210.

39. A.R. Feinstein, "An Additional Basic Science for Clinical Medicine: II. The Limitations of Randomized Trials," *Annals of Internal Medicine,* 99 (1983): 544–50.

40. A.R. Feinstein, "An Additional Basic Science for Clinical Medicine: IV. The Development of Clinimetrics," *Annals of Internal Medicine,* 99 (1983): 843–48.

41. G.A. Diamond and J.S. Forrester, "Clinical Trials and Statistical Verdicts: Probable Grounds for Appeal," *Annals of Internal Medicine,* 98 (1983): 385–94.

42. A full discussion of why some statisticians prefer Bayesian methods is beyond the scope of this discussion. For a very lucid exposition of the problem in which the relevant concepts are made accessible to the relatively unsophisticated reader, see J.O. Berger and D.A. Berry, "Statistical Analysis and the Illusion of Objectivity," *American Scientist,* 76 (1988): 159–65.

[25]

EQUIPOISE AND THE ETHICS OF CLINICAL RESEARCH

BENJAMIN FREEDMAN, PH.D.

Abstract The ethics of clinical research requires equipoise — a state of genuine uncertainty on the part of the clinical investigator regarding the comparative therapeutic merits of each arm in a trial. Should the investigator discover that one treatment is of superior therapeutic merit, he or she is ethically obliged to offer that treatment. The current understanding of this requirement, which entails that the investigator have no "treatment preference" throughout the course of the trial, presents nearly insuperable obstacles to the ethical commencement or completion of a controlled trial and may also contribute to the termination of trials because of the failure to enroll enough patients.

I suggest an alternative concept of equipoise, which would be based on present or imminent controversy in the clinical community over the preferred treatment. According to this concept of "clinical equipoise," the requirement is satisfied if there is genuine uncertainty within the expert medical community — not necessarily on the part of the individual investigator — about the preferred treatment. (N Engl J Med 1987; 317: 141-5.)

THERE is widespread agreement that ethics requires that each clinical trial begin with an honest null hypothesis.[1,2] In the simplest model, testing a new treatment B on a defined patient population P for which the current accepted treatment is A, it is necessary that the clinical investigator be in a state of genuine uncertainty regarding the comparative merits of treatments A and B for population P. If a physician knows that these treatments are not equivalent, ethics requires that the superior treatment be recommended. Following Fried, I call this state of uncertainty about the relative merits of A and B "equipoise."[3]

Equipoise is an ethically necessary condition in all cases of clinical research. In trials with several arms, equipoise must exist between all arms of the trial; otherwise the trial design should be modified to exclude the inferior treatment. If equipoise is disturbed during the course of a trial, the trial may need to be terminated and all subjects previously enrolled (as well as other patients within the relevant population) may have to be offered the superior treatment. It has been rigorously argued that a trial with a placebo is ethical only in investigating conditions for which there is no known treatment[2]; this argument reflects a special application of the requirement for equipoise. Although equipoise has commonly been discussed in the special context of the ethics of randomized clinical trials,[4,5] it is important to recognize it as an ethical condition of all controlled clinical trials, whether or not they are randomized, placebo-controlled, or blinded.

The recent increase in attention to the ethics of research with human subjects has highlighted problems associated with equipoise. Yet, as I shall attempt to show, contemporary literature, if anything, minimizes those difficulties. Moreover, there is evidence that concern on the part of investigators about failure to satisfy the requirements for equipoise can doom a trial

From the McGill Centre for Medicine, Ethics and Law, McGill University, Lady Meredith Bldg., 1110 Pine Ave. W., Montreal, PQ H3A 1A3, Canada, where reprint requests should be addressed to Dr. Freedman.

Supported in part by a research grant from the Social Sciences and Humanities Research Council of Canada.

as a result of the consequent failure to enroll a sufficient number of subjects.

The solutions that have been offered to date fail to resolve these problems in a way that would permit clinical trials to proceed. This paper argues that these problems are predicated on a faulty concept of equipoise itself. An alternative understanding of equipoise as an ethical requirement of clinical trials is proposed, and its implications are explored.

Many of the problems raised by the requirement for equipoise are familiar. Shaw and Chalmers have written that a clinician who "knows, or has good reason to believe," that one arm of the trial is superior may not ethically participate.[6] But the reasoning or preliminary results that prompt the trial (and that may themselves be ethically mandatory)[7] may jolt the investigator (if not his or her colleagues) out of equipoise before the trial begins. Even if the investigator is undecided between A and B in terms of gross measures such as mortality and morbidity, equipoise may be disturbed because evident differences in the quality of life (as in the case of two surgical approaches).[3-5,8] In either case, in saying "we do not know" whether A or B is better, the investigator may create a false impression in prospective subjects, who hear him or her as saying "no evidence leans either way," when the investigator means "no controlled study has yet had results that reach statistical significance."

Late in the study — when P values are between 0.05 and 0.06 — the moral issue of equipoise is most readily apparent,[9,10] but the same problem arises when the earliest comparative results are analyzed.[11] Within the closed statistical universe of the clinical trial, each result that demonstrates a difference between the arms of the trial contributes exactly as much to the statistical conclusion that a difference exists as does any other. The contribution of the last pair of cases in the trial is no greater than that of the first. If, therefore, equipoise is a condition that reflects equivalent evidence for alternative hypotheses, it is jeopardized by the first pair of cases as much as by the last. The investigator who is concerned about the ethics of recruitment after

142   THE NEW ENGLAND JOURNAL OF MEDICINE   July 16, 1987

the penultimate pair must logically be concerned after the first pair as well.

Finally, these issues are more than a philosopher's nightmare. Considerable interest has been generated by a paper in which Taylor et al.[12] describe the termination of a trial of alternative treatments for breast cancer. The trial foundered on the problem of patient recruitment, and the investigators trace much of the difficulty in enrolling patients to the fact that the investigators were not in a state of equipoise regarding the arms of the trial. With the increase in concern about the ethics of research and with the increasing presence of this topic in the curricula of medical and graduate schools, instances of the type that Taylor and her colleagues describe are likely to become more common. The requirement for equipoise thus poses a practical threat to clinical research.

Responses to the Problems of Equipoise

The problems described above apply to a broad class of clinical trials, at all stages of their development. Their resolution will need to be similarly comprehensive. However, the solutions that have so far been proposed address a portion of the difficulties, at best, and cannot be considered fully satisfactory.

Chalmers' approach to problems at the onset of a trial is to recommend that randomization begin with the very first subject.[11] If there are no preliminary, uncontrolled data in support of the experimental treatment B, equipoise regarding treatments A and B for the patient population P is not disturbed. There are several difficulties with this approach. Practically speaking, it is often necessary to establish details of administration, dosage, and so on, before a controlled trial begins, by means of uncontrolled trials in human subjects. In addition, as I have argued above, equipoise from the investigator's point of view is likely to be disturbed when the hypothesis is being formulated and a protocol is being prepared. It is then, before any subjects have been enrolled, that the information that the investigator has assembled makes the experimental treatment appear to be a reasonable gamble. Apart from these problems, initial randomization will not, as Chalmers recognizes, address disturbances of equipoise that occur in the course of a trial.

Data-monitoring committees have been proposed as a solution to problems arising in the course of the trial.[13] Such committees, operating independently of the investigators, are the only bodies with information concerning the trial's ongoing results. Since this knowledge is not available to the investigators, their equipoise is not disturbed. Although committees are useful in keeping the conduct of a trial free of bias, they cannot resolve the investigators' ethical difficulties. A clinician is not merely obliged to treat a patient on the basis of the information that he or she currently has, but is also required to discover information that would be relevant to treatment decisions. If interim results would disturb equipoise, the investigators are obliged to gather and use that information. Their

agreement to remain in ignorance of preliminary results would, by definition, be an unethical agreement, just as a failure to call up the laboratory to find out a patient's test results is unethical. Moreover, the use of a monitoring committee does not solve problems of equipoise that arise before and at the beginning of a trial.

Recognizing the broad problems with equipoise, three authors have proposed radical solutions. All three think that there is an irresolvable conflict between the requirement that a patient be offered the best treatment known (the principle underlying the requirement for equipoise) and the conduct of clinical trials; they therefore suggest that the "best treatment" requirement be weakened.

Schafer has argued that the concept of equipoise, and the associated notion of the best medical treatment, depends on the judgment of patients rather than of clinical investigators.[14] Although the equipoise of an investigator may be disturbed if he or she favors B over A, the ultimate choice of treatment is the patient's. Because the patient's values may restore equipoise, Schafer argues, it is ethical for the investigator to proceed with a trial when the patient consents. Schafer's strategy is directed toward trials that test treatments with known and divergent side effects and will probably not be useful in trials conducted to test efficacy or unknown side effects. This approach, moreover, confuses the ethics of competent medical practice with those of consent. If we assume that the investigator is a competent clinician, by saying that the investigator is out of equipoise, we have by Schafer's account said that in the investigator's professional judgment one treatment is therapeutically inferior — for that patient, in that condition, given the quality of life that can be achieved. Even if a patient would consent to an inferior treatment, it seems to me a violation of competent medical practice, and hence of ethics, to make the offer. Of course, complex issues may arise when a patient refuses what the physician considers the best treatment and demands instead an inferior treatment. Without settling that problem, however, we can reject Schafer's position. For Schafer claims that in order to continue to conduct clinical trials, it is ethical for the physician to offer (not merely accede to) inferior treatment.

Meier suggests that "most of us would be quite willing to forego a modest expected gain in the general interest of learning something of value."[15] He argues that we accept risks in everyday life to achieve a variety of benefits, including convenience and economy. In the same way, Meier states, it is acceptable to enroll subjects in clinical trials even though they may not receive the best treatment throughout the course of the trial. Schafer suggests an essentially similar approach.[5,14] According to this view, continued progress in medical knowledge through clinical trials requires an explicit abandonment of the doctor's fully patient-centered ethic.

These proposals seem to be frank counsels of desperation. They resolve the ethical problems of equipoise by abandoning the need for equipoise. In any event, would their approach allow clinical trials to be conducted? I think this may fairly be doubted. Although many people are presumably altruistic enough to forgo the best medical treatment in the interest of the progress of science, many are not. The numbers and proportions required to sustain the statistical validity of trial results suggest that in the absence of overwhelming altruism, the enrollment of satisfactory numbers of patients will not be possible. In particular, very ill patients, toward whom many of the most important clinical trials are directed, may be disinclined to be altruistic. Finally, as the study by Taylor et al.[12] reminds us, the problems of equipoise trouble investigators as well as patients. Even if patients are prepared to dispense with the best treatment, their physicians, for reasons of ethics and professionalism, may well not be willing to do so.

Marquis has suggested a third approach. "Perhaps what is needed is an ethics that will justify the conscription of subjects for medical research," he has written. "Nothing less seems to justify present practice."[4] Yet, although conscription might enable us to continue present practice, it would scarcely justify it. Moreover, the conscription of physician investigators, as well as subjects, would be necessary, because, as has been repeatedly argued, the problems of equipoise are as disturbing to clinicians as they are to subjects. Is any less radical and more plausible approach possible?

THEORETICAL EQUIPOISE VERSUS CLINICAL EQUIPOISE

The problems of equipoise examined above arise from a particular understanding of that concept, which I will term "theoretical equipoise." It is an understanding that is both conceptually odd and ethically irrelevant. Theoretical equipoise exists when, overall, the evidence on behalf of two alternative treatment regimens is exactly balanced. This evidence may be derived from a variety of sources, including data from the literature, uncontrolled experience, considerations of basic science and fundamental physiologic processes, and perhaps a "gut feeling" or "instinct" resulting from (or superimposed on) other considerations. The problems examined above arise from the principle that if theoretical equipoise is disturbed, the physician has, in Schafer's words, a "treatment preference" — let us say, favoring experimental treatment B. A trial testing A against B requires that some patients be enrolled in violation of this treatment preference.

Theoretical equipoise is overwhelmingly fragile; that is, it is disturbed by a slight accretion of evidence favoring one arm of the trial. In Chalmers' view, equipoise is disturbed when the odds that A will be more successful than B are anything other than 50 percent. It is therefore necessary to randomize treatment assignments beginning with the very first patient, lest equipoise be disturbed. We may say that theoretical equipoise is balanced on a knife's edge.

Theoretical equipoise is most appropriate to one-dimensional hypotheses and causes us to think in those terms. The null hypothesis must be sufficiently simple and "clean" to be finely balanced: Will A or B be superior in reducing mortality or shrinking tumors or lowering fevers in population P? Clinical choice is commonly more complex. The choice of A or B depends on some combination of effectiveness, consistency, minimal or relievable side effects, and other factors. On close examination, for example, it sometimes appears that even trials that purport to test a single hypothesis in fact involve a more complicated, portmanteau measure — e.g., the "therapeutic index" of A versus B. The formulation of the conditions of theoretical equipoise for such complex, multidimensional clinical hypotheses is tantamount to the formulation of a rigorous calculus of apples and oranges.

Theoretical equipoise is also highly sensitive to the vagaries of the investigator's attention and perception. Because of its fragility, theoretical equipoise is disturbed as soon as the investigator perceives a difference between the alternatives — whether or not any genuine difference exists. Prescott writes, for example, "It will be common at some stage in most trials for the survival curves to show visually different survivals," short of significance but "sufficient to raise ethical difficulties for the participants."[16] A visual difference, however, is purely an artifact of the research methods employed: when and by what means data are assembled and analyzed and what scale is adopted for the graphic presentation of data. Similarly, it is common for researchers to employ interval scales for phenomena that are recognized to be continuous by nature — e.g., five-point scales of pain or stages of tumor progression. These interval scales, which represent an arbitrary distortion of the available evidence to simplify research, may magnify the differences actually found, with a resulting disturbance of theoretical equipoise.

Finally, as described by several authors, theoretical equipoise is personal and idiosyncratic. It is disturbed when the clinician has, in Schafer's words, what "might even be labeled a bias or a hunch," a preference of a "merely intuitive nature."[14] The investigator who ignores such a hunch, by failing to advise the patient that because of it the investigator prefers B to A or by recommending A (or a chance of random assignment to A) to the patient, has violated the requirement for equipoise and its companion requirement to recommend the best medical treatment.

The problems with this concept of equipoise should be evident. To understand the alternative, preferable interpretation of equipoise, we need to recall the basic reason for conducting clinical trials: there is a current or imminent conflict in the clinical community over what treatment is preferred for patients in a defined population P. The standard treatment is A, but some evidence suggests that B will be superior (because of its effectiveness or its reduction of undesirable side effects, or for some other reason). (In the rare case when the first evidence of a novel therapy's superiority would be entirely convincing to the clinical community, equipoise is already disturbed.) Or there is a split in the clinical community, with some clinicians favoring A and others favoring B. Each side recognizes that the opposing side has evidence to support its position, yet each still thinks that overall its own view is correct. There exists (or, in the case of a novel therapy, there may soon exist) an honest, professional disagreement among expert clinicians about the preferred treatment. A clinical trial is instituted with the aim of resolving this dispute.

At this point, a state of "clinical equipoise" exists. There is no consensus within the expert clinical community about the comparative merits of the alternatives to be tested. We may state the formal conditions under which such a trial would be ethical as follows: at the start of the trial, there must be a state of clinical equipoise regarding the merits of the regimens to be tested, and the trial must be designed in such a way as to make it reasonable to expect that, if it is successfully concluded, clinical equipoise will be disturbed. In other words, the results of a successful clinical trial should be convincing enough to resolve the dispute among clinicians.

A state of clinical equipoise is consistent with a decided treatment preference on the part of the investigators. They must simply recognize that their less-favored treatment is preferred by colleagues whom they consider to be responsible and competent. Even if the interim results favor the preference of the investigators, treatment B, clinical equipoise persists as long as those results are too weak to influence the judgment of the community of clinicians, because of limited sample size, unresolved possibilities of side effects, or other factors. (This judgment can necessarily be made only by those who know the interim results — whether a data-monitoring committee or the investigators.)

At the point when the accumulated evidence in favor of B is so strong that the committee or investigators believe no open-minded clinician informed of the results would still favor A, clinical equipoise has been disturbed. This may occur well short of the original schedule for the termination of the trial, for unexpected reasons. (Therapeutic effects or side effects may be much stronger than anticipated, for example, or a definable subgroup within population P may be recognized for which the results demonstrably disturb clinical equipoise.) Because of the arbitrary character of human judgment and persuasion, some ethical problems regarding the termination of a trial will remain. Clinical equipoise will confine these problems to unusual or extreme cases, however, and will allow us to cast persistent problems in the proper terms. For example, in the face of a strong established trend, must we continue the trial because of others' blind fealty to an arbitrary statistical bench mark?

Clearly, clinical equipoise is a far weaker — and more common — condition than theoretical equipoise. Is it ethical to conduct a trial on the basis of clinical equipoise, when theoretical equipoise is disturbed?

Or, as Schafer and others have argued, is doing so a violation of the physician's obligation to provide patients with the best medical treatment?[4,5,14] Let us assume that the investigators have a decided preference for B but wish to conduct a trial on the grounds that clinical (not theoretical) equipoise exists. The ethics committee asks the investigators whether, if they or members of their families were within population P, they would not want to be treated with their preference, B? An affirmative answer is often thought to be fatal to the prospects for such a trial, yet the investigators answer in the affirmative. Would a trial satisfying this weaker form of equipoise be ethical?

I believe that it clearly is ethical. As Fried has emphasized,[3] competent (hence, ethical) medicine is social rather than individual in nature. Progress in medicine relies on progressive consensus within the medical and research communities. The ethics of medical practice grants no ethical or normative meaning to a treatment preference, however powerful, that is based on a hunch or on anything less than evidence publicly presented and convincing to the clinical community. Persons are licensed as physicians after they demonstrate the acquisition of this professionally validated knowledge, not after they reveal a superior capacity for guessing. Normative judgments of their behavior — e.g., malpractice actions — rely on a comparison with what is done by the community of medical practitioners. Failure to follow a "treatment preference" not shared by this community and not based on information that would convince it could not be the basis for an allegation of legal or ethical malpractice. As Fried states: "[T]he conception of what is good medicine is the product of a professional consensus." By definition, in a state of clinical equipoise, "good medicine" finds the choice between A and B indifferent.

In contrast to theoretical equipoise, clinical equipoise is robust. The ethical difficulties at the beginning and end of a trial are therefore largely alleviated. There remain difficulties about consent, but these too may be diminished. Instead of emphasizing the lack of evidence favoring one arm over another that is required by theoretical equipoise, clinical equipoise places the emphasis in informing the patient on the honest disagreement among expert clinicians. The fact that the investigator has a "treatment preference," if he or she does, could be disclosed; indeed, if the preference is a decided one, and based on something more than a hunch, it could be ethically mandatory to disclose it. At the same time, it would be emphasized that this preference is not shared by others. It is likely to be a matter of chance that the patient is being seen by a clinician with a preference for B over A, rather than by an equally competent clinician with the opposite preference.

Clinical equipoise does not depend on concealing relevant information from researchers and subjects, as does the use of independent data-monitoring committees. Rather, it allows investigators, in informing subjects, to distinguish appropriately among validated knowledge accepted by the clinical community, data on treatments that are promising but are not (or, for novel therapies, would not be) generally convincing, and mere hunches. Should informed patients decline to participate because they have chosen a specific clinician and trust his or her judgment — over and above the consensus in the professional community — that is no more than the patients' right. We do not conscript patients to serve as subjects in clinical trials.

THE IMPLICATIONS OF CLINICAL EQUIPOISE

The theory of clinical equipoise has been formulated as an alternative to some current views on the ethics of human research. At the same time, it corresponds closely to a preanalytic concept held by many in the research and regulatory communities. Clinical equipoise serves, then, as a rational formulation of the approach of many toward research ethics; it does not so much change things as explain why they are the way they are.

Nevertheless, the precision afforded by the theory of clinical equipoise does help to clarify or reformulate some aspects of research ethics; I will mention only two.

First, there is a recurrent debate about the ethical propriety of conducting clinical trials of discredited treatments, such as Laetrile.[17] Often, substantial political pressure to conduct such tests is brought to bear by adherents of quack therapies. The theory of clinical equipoise suggests that when there is no support for a treatment regimen within the expert clinical community, the first ethical requirement of a trial — clinical equipoise — is lacking; it would therefore be unethical to conduct such a trial.

Second, Feinstein has criticized the tendency of clinical investigators to narrow excessively the conditions and hypotheses of a trial in order to ensure the validity of its results.[18] This "fastidious" approach purchases scientific manageability at the expense of an inability to apply the results to the "messy" conditions of clinical practice. The theory of clinical equipoise adds some strength to this criticism. Overly "fastidious" trials, designed to resolve some theoretical question, fail to satisfy the second ethical requirement of clinical research, since the special conditions of the trial will render it useless for influencing clinical decisions, even if it is successfully completed.

The most important result of the concept of clinical equipoise, however, might be to relieve the current crisis of confidence in the ethics of clinical trials. Equipoise, properly understood, remains an ethical condition for clinical trials. It is consistent with much current practice. Clinicians and philosophers alike have been premature in calling for desperate measures to resolve problems of equipoise.

I am indebted to Robert J. Levine, M.D., and to Harold Merskey, D.M., for their valuable suggestions.

REFERENCES

1. Levine RJ. Ethics and regulation of clinical research. 2nd ed. Baltimore: Urban & Schwarzenberg, 1986.
2. *Idem.* The use of placebos in randomized clinical trials. IRB: Rev Hum Subj Res 1985; 7(2):1-4.
3. Fried C. Medical experimentation: personal integrity and social policy. Amsterdam: North-Holland Publishing, 1974.
4. Marquis D. Leaving therapy to chance. Hastings Cent Rep 1983; 13(4):40-7.
5. Schafer A. The ethics of the randomized clinical trial. N Engl J Med 1982; 307:719-24.
6. Shaw LW, Chalmers TC. Ethics in cooperative clinical trials. Ann NY Acad Sci 1970; 169:487-95.
7. Hollenberg NK, Dzau VJ, Williams GH. Are uncontrolled clinical studies ever justified? N Engl J Med 1980; 303:1067.
8. Levine RJ, Lebacqz K. Some ethical considerations in clinical trials. Clin Pharmacol Ther 1979; 25:728-41.
9. Klimt CR, Canner PL. Terminating a long-term clinical trial. Clin Pharmacol Ther 1979; 25:641-6.
10. Veatch RM. Longitudinal studies, sequential designs and grant renewals: what to do with preliminary data. IRB: Rev Hum Subj Res 1979; 1(4):1-3.
11. Chalmers T. The ethics of randomization as a decision-making technique and the problem of informed consent. In: Beauchamp TL, Walters L, eds. Contemporary issues in bioethics. Encino, Calif.: Dickenson, 1978:426-9.
12. Taylor KM, Margolese RL, Soskolne CL. Physicians' reasons for not entering eligible patients in a randomized clinical trial of surgery for breast cancer. N Engl J Med 1984; 310:1363-7.
13. Chalmers TC. Invited remarks. Clin Pharmacol Ther 1979; 25:649-50.
14. Schafer A. The randomized clinical trial: for whose benefit? IRB: Rev Hum Subj Res 1985; 7(2):4-6.
15. Meier P. Terminating a trial — the ethical problem. Clin Pharmacol Ther 1979; 25:633-40.
16. Prescott RJ. Feedback of data to participants during clinical trials. In: Tagnon HJ, Staquet MJ, eds. Controversies in cancer: design of trials and treatment. New York: Masson Publishing, 1979:55-61.
17. Cowan DH. The ethics of clinical trials of ineffective therapy. IRB: Rev Hum Subj Res 1981; 3(5):10-1.
18. Feinstein AR. An additional basic science for clinical medicine. II. The limitations of randomized trials. Ann Intern Med 1983; 99:544-50.

[26]

EQUIPOISE, KNOWLEDGE AND ETHICS IN CLINICAL RESEARCH AND PRACTICE

RICHARD ASHCROFT

ABSTRACT

It is widely maintained that a clinical trial is ethical only if some form of equipoise between the treatments being compared obtains. To be in equipoise between two treatments A and B is to be cognitively indifferent between the statement 'A is strictly more effective than B' and its negation. It is natural to claim that equipoise regarding A and B is necessary for randomised assignment to treatments A and B to be beneficent and non-maleficent and is sufficient for such an assignment to be fair. Cashing this out precisely is difficult, and various forms of equipoise have been discussed which consider whose equipoise is relevant to the decision. This is to make judgement of equipoise something to be managed socially, while its prima facie significance is supposedly cognitive. Recent reconstructions of equipoise-like concepts in epistemology give clues about how to understand equipoise cognitively. In this paper I examine some of this work and discuss how successful it has been. I suggest that while this work is promising, it still has far to go, and that while equipoise remains the best theory we have of the cognitive justification for clinical trials, it is nonetheless incoherent.

INTRODUCTION

Clinical equipoise is the standard rationale for enrolling patients into clinical trials.[1] We can define it as follows. Suppose we have two treatments, and a patient in a certain condition, and a

---

[1] Edwards J.L., Lilford R.J., Braunholtz D.A., Jackson J.C., Hewison J., Thornton J., 'Ethics of randomised trials' in *Health Services Research Methods: A Guide to Best Practice* edited by Black N., Brazier J., Fitzpatrick R., Reeves B., London: BMA Books, 1998 ch.9; Freedman B. 'Equipoise and the Ethics of Clinical Research' *New England Journal of Medicine* 1987; 317: 141–5

physician (or other healthcare worker) trying to decide what to prescribe. The physician has a decision problem, which is to choose the better treatment for this patient. He or she is ignorant as to which of the two treatments is superior. In this situation we can say that he or she is in *equipoise* regarding the two options.

In such a situation, it is reasonable to suppose that the assignment of treatments could be done by a random device. Consequently, enrolling a patient into a randomised controlled trial which compares the effectiveness of the treatments is reasonable. Conversely, it is generally thought that if equipoise does not obtain, assignment of treatment by randomisation is not acceptable. For, if the physician is not in equipoise, that is to say, is not indifferent between the treatments, then he or she is obliged to give the patient the preferred treatment. This is what benificence and non-maleficence require. Note here that the argument from equipoise to random assignment is intended to show that random assignment is morally and therapeutically reasonable. The scientific case for randomisation (to eliminate various biases) is different, and itself controversial.[2]

The standard worry about clinical trials is that doctors are not in equipoise regarding every patient, nor can they be said to be in equipoise regarding the intrinsic merits of the treatments once trial data begins to come in. It is sometimes claimed that most trials are unethical in this way, if not at the outset, then certainly once some data is in. Various ingenious designs have been proposed to overcome this problem, although their statistical reliability and equivalence to the simple RCT are questionable.[3]

In this paper I will discuss some of the epistemological problems of equipoise. It is clear from the foregoing, I think, that getting the ethics of clinical trials right depends absolutely on getting the epistemology right. The bad news is that the epistemological situation is no less murky; the good news is that there are resources 'out there' to make an attack on the problem possible. My main conclusion is that we have no viable conception of equipoise, and that while it certainly theorises the justification of the clinical trial along the right lines, we need

[2] Lilford R.J., Jackson J., 'Equipoise and the Ethics of Randomization' *Journal of the Royal Society of Medicine* 1995; 88: 552–559; Ashcroft R.E., Chadwick D.W., Clark S.R.L., Edwards R.H.T., Frith L., Hutton J.L., 'Implications of Socio-Cultural Contexts for Ethics of Clinical Trials' *Health Technology Assessment* 1997; 1 no. 9 esp. ch. 2.
[3] Zelen M., 'Randomized Consent Designs for Clinical Trials: An Update' *Statistics in Medicine* 1990; 9: 645–656; Kadane J.B. (ed.) *Bayesian Methods and Ethics in a Clinical Trail Design* New York: John Wiley, 1996.

316   RICHARD ASHCROFT

to do a lot more work before we can regard the ethical problems of the clinical trial as solved.

EQUIPOISE: KNOWLEDGE, IGNORANCE AND BELIEF

Equipoise is not simply preference neutrality. The physician may not prefer treatment A to treatment B, or vice versa. But what is important is not whether this is his or her preference, but whether he or she has *reason* to prefer one treatment to the other. Preferences for treatment should be rationally corrigible. That is, they should be such that if a set of 'final ends', life purposes or fundamental values is chosen, then preferences for means and instrumental goods should be adjustable in the light of knowledge and rational reflection so as best to achieve those final ends. For example, treatment is normally considered an instrumental good. Some authors argue that final ends can be chosen rationally, but most authors take final ends as fixed by non-rational sources.[4]

It may be that the patient prefers one treatment to the other, however. Let us set aside cases where the preferred treatment is only available through the trial, so that the patient can actually choose which treatment he or she receives. Are patient preferences subject to the same constraint of rational corrigibility? Perhaps not. At least, autonomy theories lead us to think that it is none of the physician's business to inquire into (competent) patients' rationales. But most people would regard it as desirable to have the treatment which is actually superior (even if we don't know which). Patients' preferences here are referred to a wider set of values than the physician's. For instance in a trial of surgical against chemical interventions, it may be that effectiveness is not the only relevant value for the patient.[5] But here, following Susan Hurley, the thought should be that underlying preferences are judgements of value which are reasons.[6] Herein lies part of the significance of consent: patient preferences need bear no relation to the preferences of their

[4] Richardson H.S., *Practical Reasoning About Final Ends* Cambridge: Cambridge University Press, 1994; Broome J., 'Can A Humean be moderate?' in Broome J. *Ethics Out of Economics* Cambridge: Cambridge University Press, 1999 pp. 68–87.

[5] Ashcroft J.J., Leinster S.J., Slade P.D., 'Breast Cancer — Patient Choice of Treatment: Preliminary Communication' *Journal of the Royal Society of Medicine* 1985; 78: 43–6.

[6] Hurley S.L., *Natural Reasons: Personality and Polity* Oxford University Press, 1989, part I 'Relations Between Mind and Value'.

physicians. If we rephrase equipoise as the state in which the physician has no reason to choose one treatment over the other and vice versa, then we should inquire what sort of reasons are required here. Naturally the most important kind are epistemic reasons. Others are, of course, important. The decision regarding treatment is always a practical judgement, involving belief and desire components, and the desires furnish important contributory reasons too. What doctors want, or ought to want, and what connection this should have to what patients want, is too big a subject for me here, and in any case are distinct problems from the narrowly epistemic one I am considering here.

The epistemic equipoise argument is this: patients should be enrolled into clinical trials if there is no reliable epistemic reason (evidence) to favour one treatment over the other. 'Favouring' here relates to effectiveness and safety. Sometimes the argument is raised that equipoise makes no sense as a justification for trials simply because the only reason to test a new treatment is that it is believed to be superior to existing treatments. In many cases this is not the rationale at all, for instance in equivalence trials, but consider those cases where the new treatment does hold out the prospect of decisive superiority. The whole debate turns on the role of belief. Pro-triallists argue that such belief does not amount to sufficient reason to bypass comparative trials, and anti-triallists argue that it does. By 'pro-triallist' I mean someone who thinks that (a) we need sound randomised trial evidence to reduce uncertainty to 'moral certainty' and (b) we should seek such reductions where we can get them and (c) such reductions are the only reliable ones available. By anti-triallist I mean someone who denies one of (a), (b) or (c), and, in particular, someone who denies (c) i.e., someone who asserts that we can have reliable knowledge of effectiveness without necessarily applying the statistical standard of reliability implied by (a). No one, I think, dissents from (b) as a matter of general policy. The anti-triallist and the pro-triallist simply disagree about how often (b) makes a claim on us, and what the requirements for fulfilling that claim are. For example, AIDS activists and sufferers from terminal illnesses sometimes take our level of ignorance regarding an experimental treatment to be much less or alternatively are prepared to take more risks (live with more uncertainty) than the population at large, just because their condition lacks effective remedies.[7]

---

[7] Schüklenk U., *Access to Experimental Drugs in Terminal Illness: Ethical Issues* New York: Pharmaceutical Products Press, 1998.

Book review

Tomossy GF and Weisstub DN, editors
Human Experimentation and Research
2003
Aldershot, UK: Ashgate
Hardback
652 pages
£115.00
ISBN: 0 7546 2226 6

Received: 8.3.04

318   RICHARD ASHCROFT

Figuring out what to say about belief vis-à-vis the two treatments here is a surprisingly difficult problem. For instance, what is the content of the belief? Surely some sort of proposition regarding the effectiveness of the new treatment or perhaps a proposition regarding the relative effectiveness of the two treatments. But what are the semantics of such a proposition? Is 'effectiveness' a property? For instance, if we assert that 'Aspirin is effective for the prevention of secondary stroke' are we claiming that aspirin has some property of 'being effective for the prevention of the secondary stroke'? (Compare the way we understand 'snow is white' to be true if and only if the stuff snow has the property of being white). 'Effectiveness' would be rather a peculiar property; and I suggest that it is not obvious what sort of predicate it is. In any case, I know of no successful analysis of this sort of belief.

Notice that the pro-triallist is claiming that we do not *know* which treatment is superior, or anything of specifically therapeutic importance about the novel treatment. But the anti-triallist may be arguing one of two things. Either the argument is that in fact we do know enough to proceed with unrandomised prescription to all. Or the argument is that the pharmacological, animal model and early-phase, uncontrolled trial evidence is itself sufficient warrant for belief in the new treatment to be sufficient reason to proceed with non-trial use. More strictly, such evidence is sufficient not only for belief (as a practical premise in a practical syllogism) but actually for knowledge. The argument for early-stopping of controlled trials is logically similar, although there are some technical sophistications that provide a clearer model of justification than the qualitative arguments used by anti-triallists. That the sophistications are clearer or more explicit does not necessarily make them better (or worse).[8]

The argument from knowledge is, clearly, stronger, since requirements for knowledge are strict conditions on beliefs. The issue which the anti-triallists rightly pick up is one of equivocation. To say that we do not know something covers a whole range of credal states, from frank ignorance through degrees of doubt to the states philosophers identify when discussing whether to know p requires also knowledge that one knows that p. From the point of view of the ethics of belief, all this range of

[8] Baum M., Houghton J., Abrams K., 'Early Stopping Rules — Clinical Perspectives and Ethical Considerations' *Statistics in Medicine* 1994; 13: 1459–1469.

ignorance or lack of knowledge is profoundly unhelpful. What, the anti-triallists ask, is the standard of knowledge which the triallist is using in order to say that without a trial we do not know? That is, is the triallist saying that only claims vindicated by a suitable clinical trial are known to be true? Clearly not. For there is a range of types propositional knowledge that are acceptable without trial evidence, even in medicine. Also, a criterion of knowledge which invokes trials as the standard by which to justify trials would be obviously circular.

If trials generate knowledge in some paradigmatic sense, it is because they can be referred to some external standard of reliability. Qualitatively, this can be shown easily enough — trials have a number of design features which warrant reliability judgements, including randomisation, controlled comparison, specific inclusion and exclusion criteria and so on.[9] But while this shows that trial evidence is reliable if anything is, it does not show that anything else is not reliable. One traditional source of knowledge is the experience of the educated, skilled and experienced practitioner, who possesses the intellectual virtue of practical wisdom and good judgement (phronesis).[10] And while this claim is not currently fashionable, recent work on testimony and on practical skills makes it clear that such sources of belief can be sources of knowledge.[11] Furthermore, this skill is universally agreed to be required in the application of trial evidence to treatments of individual patients. So if non-trial evidence of effectiveness is problematic, it cannot be so only because it is not trial evidence.

To get further into this would be to take me too far into epistemology proper. But it is important to note the dependence of the ethics of trials on something like equipoise, and the dependence of equipoise on judgements of cognitive indifference, or ignorance, and the relation ignorance has to the standards of knowledge one has in the background. Even the keenest proponent of trials accepts that in some cases trials are not necessary because the non-trial evidence has been so overwhelming — e.g. penicillin as an antibiotic or aspirin as an analgesic.

What then does the equipoise principle say, in the light of these arguments about knowledge and trials? Let p be the

---

[9] Op.cit. n.3.

[10] Shapin S., *A Social History of Truth: Civility and Science in Seventeenth Century England* University of Chicago Press, 1994.

[11] Coady C.A.J., *Testimony: A Philosophical Inquiry* Oxford University Press, 1992; Galison P., *How Experiments End* University of Chicago Press, 1987.

320   RICHARD ASHCROFT

proposition 'The new treatment A is strictly more effective in treating this condition in this class of patients than the old treatment B'. Equipoise is saying, 'I do not know that p', which is to say that even if we believe that p we don't have sufficient justification, or perhaps simply that p is false. We can disregard the latter alternative which is a book-keeping point only — we cannot be said to know false propositions. Someone who believes p to be false will normally say not, 'I do not know that p', but 'I know that not-p'. The alternative is to say that we should suspend judgement about p, since we believe p but believe also that this is not a justified belief, or simply that we neither believe or disbelieve that p.

In other words, equipoise is a situation involving beliefs, rather than knowledge. Knowledge that p has the property that if we believe p, are justified in believing p, and p is true, then p is an item of common knowledge, rather than the justified, true belief of a particular subject. Equipoise is about beliefs, and beliefs that are held or not held, or held to be false, by given subjects. Equipoise, in other words, is a propositional attitude.

So, whose equipoise? And what if I am in equipoise and you are not? And how can equipoise be removed and replaced by knowledge?

The varieties of equipoise

In the classical equipoise formulation proposed by Benjamin Freedman the important form of equipoise was *clinical* equipoise, that is, equipoise in the mind of the intending physician regarding treatment options.[12] In many ways this remains the best formulation. For clinical equipoise is a necessary condition on entering a patient into a trial, and if any clinician is not in clinical equipoise regarding a patient or a trial, then this (or any other of his patients) should not be entered by him or her into the trial. The ethical duty of the physician here is clear enough.

But, say the pro-triallists, if the clinician is not in equipoise, perhaps he or she ought to be.[13] In practice, pro-triallists are

---

[12] Op.cit. n.1.

[13] Chalmers I., Chalmers T.C., 'Randomisation and Patient Choice' *Lancet* 1994; 344:892–3; Chalmers I., 'What do I want from health research and researchers when I am a patient?' *BMJ* 1995; 310:1315–1318; Harrison J. 'Clinical trials: A Patient's view' *MRC News* 1998; 79:22-23; Lees R., 'If I had a stroke...' *Lancet* 1998; 352: (suppl. III) 28–30; Chalmers I., 'What is the prior probability of a proposed new treatment being superior to established treatments?' *BMJ* 1997; 314: 74–75.

unwilling to press this point, because there is a politics of 'clinical freedom'. But many will press the argument in general that absence of RCT evidence (or other high-quality data) is the same thing for medical practice as absence of justification for belief. Or at least absence of justification for 'public' beliefs. Clinicians, like other sorts of expert, disagree. Disagreement about the merits of treatments implies, in itself, reason to doubt, and perhaps a requirement to settle doubts in the situation where both parties cannot be right — it seems clear that where this obtains, two groups of patients are receiving different treatments, and unless these treatments are genuinely equivalent (which we do not know) or these patients are genuinely different (likewise), one group is ipso facto not receiving the better treatment. This argument is what gives us another notion of equipoise, which some think superior to clinical equipoise. This is *collective* or *professional* equipoise.[14]

But we can go further than this. Perhaps all this talk of professionals' knowledge is too paternalistic, in that it overlooks patient preferences. Pragmatic trials, where two treatments of known efficacy are compared, either to show superiority or equivalence in terms of narrow technical effectiveness, are often charged with being unethical because while the professionals may be indifferent between them, patients are certainly not. For example, trials of radical and conservative surgery in breast cancer have certainly been challenged on this ground.[15] And here it is sometimes thought that the relevant equipoise ought to be further extended to cover patient indifference. Narrow patient equipoise (usually just *patient* equipoise) holds that no patient should be enrolled in the trial unless he or she is themselves in equipoise (more correctly, *full indifference*, since the patient is entitled to non-cognitive preferences which the doctor is not, on the autonomy theory). Wide patient equipoise, or *community equipoise*, requires patients (and their carers, families etc.) to be in equipoise.[16] This is perhaps relevant in only a few cases — cases where there is an identifiable and politically self-conscious and cohesive patient population such as gay men and lesbians with HIV or community

[14] Johnson N., Lilford R.J., Brazier W., 'At What Level of Collective Equipoise Does a Clinical Trial Become Ethical?' *Journal of Medical Ethics* 1991; 17: 30–4.

[15] Op.cit. n.5.

[16] Alderson P., 'Equipoise as a Means of Managing Uncertainty: Personal, Communal and Proxy' *Journal of Medical Ethics* 1996; 22: 135–9; Gifford F., 'Community-Equipoise and the Ethics of Randomized Clinical Trials' *Bioethics* 1995; 9: 127–148.

322   RICHARD ASHCROFT

and cultural groups like the Maori or Inuit.[17] One could go on and on constructing equipoises. Perhaps we should require *industry equipoise* as an ethical norm for pharmaceutical companies, to restrict the production of 'me-too' drugs.

For equipoise to be a justification of a clinical trial in practice, some social control over the judgement of equipoise must exist. Who gets to decide? Who gets to decide when equipoise is replaced by knowledge? The latter question may be simpler than the former, in that we could all accept the trial methodology as reliable and secure, but even the 'we' here is normally some identifiable group — some (probably not all) patients who consent (rather than those who do not); Research Ethics Committees; funders; purchasers; and the trial management team. Remember also that in the USA insurers will usually not pay for experimental treatments, so even outside the trial one key group gets to decide when equipoise applies and when it does not, by deciding what counts as 'experimental'.[18]

Socialists and Bayesians

If we take the claim that equipoise is regulated socially, we may take a position I will call 'socialist'. The socialists are those who take the line roughly described just now, about social control of epistemic ignorance and its experimental consequences. The socialist claim takes weaker and stronger forms. The strongest form, essentially social-constructivist, is that cognitive claims are through-and-through social, and I believe this is a possible line to take, although I will say nothing about it here. Suffice it to say that even if it is correct, we still need to understand the social grammar of the language of equipoise, and how the justification-discourse functions.[19] Initial work has been done on these lines by Steven Epstein and Marc Berg, although they do not discuss equipoise directly.[20] The weaker view is that there

---

[17] Garfield S., *The End of Innocence: Britain in the Time of AIDS* London: Faber, 1994 ch.7; Campbell A.V., 'Ethics in a Bicultural Context' *Bioethics* 1995; 9: 149–154.

[18] Freeman H.P., 'The Impact of Clinical Trial Protocols on Patient Care Systems in a Large City Hospital: Access for the Socially Disadvantaged' *Cancer* 1993; 72:2834–8.

[19] Mulkay M.J., Gilbert G.N., *Opening Pandora's Box: A Sociological Analysis of Scientists' Discourse* Cambridge University Press, 1994.

[20] Epstein S., 'Democratic Science? AIDS Activism and the Contested Construction of Knowledge' *Socialist Review* 1991; 21:35–64; Berg M., *Rationalizing Medical Work: Decision Support Techniques and Medical Practices* Cambridge, Mass.: MIT Press, 1997.

EQUIPOISE, KNOWLEDGE AND ETHICS   323

may be a clear concept of equipoise, but either we do not yet have it, or we do, but this is not generally reflected in practice. Under this view, the usage of the conceptions of equipoise is not tied to the concept itself, and so in effect the discourse is controlled, if at all, by social means. I am sympathetic to this view, in that it seems to fit the facts. Under the weak socialist account, if we are to hold off the strong socialist programme, the pro-triallist must supply an account of rational acceptance or belief (and consequently an account of when we should rationally suspend judgement — that is, take up equipoise). It is my view that this socialist challenge can apparently be met by borrowing 'Bayesian' ideas from that school of epistemology. But I will argue the problem is likely to reappear in another, epistemic form.

Bayesian epistemology concerns rational inductive inference.[21] It is concerned not so much with knowledge, which it conceives as propositional knowledge taken to be true with probability 1, as with acceptance. A proposition is accepted, subject to certain constraints, when it is believed with at least a certain minimum degree of belief — e.g, with degree of belief 0.95. Degrees of belief are represented by subjective probabilities, that is they have a measure on a scale 0 to 1, which, subject to certain technical criteria, obey Bayes's theorem in conditional probability. The importance of Bayesian epistemology is that application of Bayes's theorem is supposed to give us a mechanism to update all our beliefs conditional on new evidence. In other words, it gives us a rational mechanism for rational correction and expansion (or contraction) in beliefs.[22]

The beauty of the Bayesian approach is that it is explicitly probabilistic. And wedded to a decision theory, where the outcomes are assigned utilities, we have a powerful tool for expressing the language of clinical trials. Clinical trials can be of two basic kinds, from a statistical point of view. Either they are hypothesis tests, where we take as null hypothesis the proposition that the two treatments are equivalent; or they are estimation techniques, for estimating the size of the treatments effects (in placebo controlled trials). Estimations are usually accepted with margins of error selected such that the 'true' value will lie within the estimation band with probability 0.95 — sometimes with higher probability. In either case, a decision is taken regarding

---

[21] Kaplan M., *Decision Theory as Philosophy* Cambridge University Press, 1996.
[22] Levi I., *The Enterprise of Knowledge: An Essay on Knowledge, Credal Probability and Chance* Cambridge, Mass.: MIT Press, 1980.

324   RICHARD ASHCROFT

the relative acceptability of false positive and false negative results, and in part this is decided with respect to the magnitude of difference between treatments that is decided to make changing treatment policy worthwhile.[23]

The first point to note is that this is a model of belief wherein the cash value of belief is how one applies it in decisions and actions. This does seem to be a step forward. Equipoise is meaningless unless thought of in the context of decision-making about actual treatment. Perhaps this gives us some insight into the difficulty of analysing the propositions about which indifference is expressed. It might be that indifference between proposals to act is a better account of equipoise than indifference between accepting statements of fact. The propositional attitude we call equipoise turns out to be essentially practical.

This possibility, that scientific belief is essentially evaluative, in that knowledge is always referred to some actual or potential decision situation, has been discussed, and accepted in modified form, by Isaac Levi.[24] Unlike most Bayesians, who are personalists (i.e. probabilities are subjective in that they measure personal degrees of belief), Levi is an objectivist about these probabilities. He takes the view that probabilities are to be interpreted in terms of an inductive logic, following Carnap (although for important technical reasons he departs from the standard view of inductive logic in allowing that agents need not have numerically precise degrees of belief, while maintaining that there are objective constraints in how to acquire and respond to evidence). In this context he argues that scientific cognition is practical in this sense, but that the values to which it is referred are not just any values, but specifically scientific, truth-seeking, values. On the basis of this account he has constructed a sophisticated decision theoretic epistemology, with persuasive analyses of belief, acceptance, knowledge, ignorance and epistemic utility. On this account, we know something when we accept it as true with sufficiently low probability of false positives. 'Sufficiently low' is analysed in terms of the seriousness of error. What is at stake if we reject this hypothesis when it is true?

Levi's account is designed to reflect statisticians' and scientists' actual practice in seeking to extend our stock of knowledge, and also to avoid some of the main challenges to the dominant,

[23] Mayo D.G., *Error and the Growth of Experimental Knowledge* University of Chicago Press, 1996.
[24] Levi I., *Decisions and Revisions: Philosophical Essays on Knowledge and Value* Cambridge University Press, 1984 chs. 1, 2.

personalist Bayesian theory of rational belief.[25] Personalist Bayesian theories present problems for understanding equipoise as a rational state and rational justification for clinical trials. To survey these briefly, as in the qualitative analysis of equipoise, personalist accounts are hamstrung by being essentially accounts of states of individual belief. As such, even if I start in equipoise, it is not transparent why this should oblige you to do so; and even if post-trial I am no longer in equipoise (once I reconditionalise my personal probability distribution) there is no determining reason for you to move out of equipoise too. Your personal probability distribution need not be even qualitatively equivalent to mine. Moreover, the utilities you assign to the various decision-outcomes clearly need not be the same as mine even under the strictest rationalising conditions. In the end, we need to invoke further constraints on belief warranted by authority — albeit scientific rather than political authority.

Arguably Levi's theory overcomes or avoids most of these problems, although I have no wondrous proof of this, and it would certainly take more than the margin of this article![26] However, the use of 'seriousness of error' in the medical context, as the hinge on which decisions regarding acceptance are to turn, is to open up once again the same problems of 'whose equipoise' and fixing rules about when it can be considered to have been replaced by acceptance of one treatment or the other as superior remains political, in the broadest sense, rather than rational. The service Levi does us is to show that medical knowledge has a practical, and not a theoretical, character; and in particular that the value we put on seriousness of error is an inescapable part of the judgement of acceptance, and hence of equipoise. Levi's account of probabilities goes a long way, I think, to describing what is rational in the equipoise theory, but it also shows what the social content of the equipoise decision is, to whit, in decisions about the seriousness of error.

The open question is whether this decision is something other than individual consent to participate, or whether there is some further collective decision to be made. As it stands, the answer appears to be yes: consider the risk prone subject whose standards for acceptance of the superiority of the new therapy are low (say because he regards the seriousness of a false negative rejection of

[25] For a clear account of personalist Bayesianism see Howson C, Urbach P., *Scientific Reasoning: The Bayesian Approach* La Salle, IL: Open Court, 1992 (second edition).

[26] Op.cit. n.25, chs. 9, 11, 13.

326   RICHARD ASHCROFT

this therapy as very high). What makes it acceptable to insist that this subject can only have the treatment through randomisation? On a genuine equipoise theory, this should be answered by saying that this subject has no good reason to believe that the new treatment is superior, no matter how serious the consequence of a false negative. The 'no good reason' here must be grounded in objective evidential relations to the proposition in question. Levi's theory gives no better answer to this than any other available theory of equipoise, no matter that his theory has at least many advantages over its rivals, and I conclude that we have no watertight theory of equipoise which licenses holding both that we are right to be in equipoise and that the risk-taker is wrong to insist. Unless we can cash out an objective content to seriousness of error which does not reduce to private preference, I suggest that we are better to pursue an explicitly socialist line. We should do so because the socialist account appears at least *descriptively* adequate regarding the dynamics of collective belief. It will not do for the socialist to celebrate too soon, however, as the socialist will still need to give an account of how to be reasonable in collective decision-making, and this will need to incorporate judgements about scientific evidence. The demands of epistemology in doing ethics are stringent, and not easily to be set aside.

CONCLUSION

I have shown that to make sense of equipoise as currently understood we have to supplement it with a theory of acceptance and ignorance. On the best available account, however, the attempt to replace political judgement with inductive logic is unsuccessful. If the argument for clinical trials rather than personal judgement in treatment evaluation, and consequently the argument that trials are ethical because of rational indifference, rests on this foundation, then I claim that this argument is not proven. We have two complementary lines of inquiry, therefore: the first is to consider the Evidence Based Medicine movement frankly as an attempt to redraw the lines of medical cognitive authority. The second is to follow Levi's and Susan Hurley's lines of inquiry and try to show that medical inquiry, while value-laden, is laden with rationally corrigible and objective values which warrant equipoise. But decision-theoretic and other Bayesian theories on their own do not help us.

Centre for Ethics in Medicine
University of Bristol

[27]

Ethical considerations concerning treatment allocation in drug development trials

S Senn Department of Epidemiology and Public Health, Department of Statistical Science, University College London, UK

It is claimed that much of the opposition to placebos is based on the misunderstanding that their use implies the withholding of effective treatments. It is also argued that the ethical feasibility of a trial must be judged by comparing the likely prognosis of patients in the trial to their expectations outside the trial. Furthermore, a longer-term perspective of the patients needs is necessary; the ethical dilemmas involved cannot be resolved at the point of sickness. Some device such as the 'original position' of the philosopher John Rawls is needed. Finally, it is argued that placebo run-ins involve a violation of consent and should be eliminated from clinical trials.

Introduction

There is a general suspicion that the randomized clinical trial (RCT) can only proceed by sacrificing some requirements of individual to collective ethics.[1] We would like to have good reasons for prescribing one treatment rather than another. Given enough patients, the RCT appears to deliver it. However, life involves decision-making under uncertainty and, by necessity, we sometimes have to back our hunches. Except very rarely, when balanced on that rare cusp of indifference known as *equipoise*,[2] any prescribing physician is likely to prefer, however slightly, one treatment to another. Thus, in entering patients in a clinical trial, physicians will be condemning some patients to receive treatments they suspect are inferior.[2] This, it is claimed, is unethical. For serious and in particular acute diseases, this would seem to preclude the possibility of carrying out controlled trials. (For various chronic conditions it is often argued that some temporary loss on the patient's part is acceptable.[3] This debate will not be entered into here and it will be implicitly assumed in what follows that trials in serious, acute and possibly life-threatening diseases are being considered.)

Moral space for experimentation has usually been sought by trying to extend the region of exact equipoise to one of broader rough comparability. This is because, for example, on a Bayesian analysis, if a physician starts out in equipoise, say with a flat prior centred on zero difference in effect between treatments, then at some stage before reasonably strong belief in the superiority of one treatment or another is reached, weak belief in its superiority must be obtained and such belief violates equipoise. Spiegelhalter *et al.* have tried to deal with this by proposing a 'range of equivalence' within which experimentation can continue.[4] Kadane *et al.* have used an alternative approach.[5] They

404   *S Senn*

consider a community of priors corresponding to a range of opinions held by participating physicians. A treatment is admissible provided that at least one physician prefers it to all others. Experimental use of a treatment within a trial can continue as long as at least one participating physician still believes it is the best. (This begs the question as to how such physicians are to be chosen in the first place.) Peto and Baigent take a frequentist view in which *knowledge* rather than *belief* is stressed and make appeal to an *uncertainty principle*, whereby, 'a patient can be entered if, and only if, the responsible clinician is substantially uncertain which of the trial treatments would be most appropriate for that particular patient'.[6] Peto and Baigent do not define 'substantially uncertain'.

In this paper, an alternative ethic is proposed that does not require trialists to be the medical equivalent of Buridan's ass: that allows them to randomize patients both in the patients' and society's interest. This revised view regards justice and autonomy as twin poles of medical ethics and, it will be claimed, also satisfies the demands of beneficence and non-maleficence. It supports the previously stated view that clinical trialists have to consider both individual and collective ethics[7] and justifies the latter in terms of the former.

The three party system

Many discussions of medical ethics centre on the doctor–patient relationship. However, from one point of view this is incomplete. There are no millionaires on a desert island and a common justification of taxation, in opposition to libertarian views, is that society is entitled to undertake (some) re-distribution because wealth is only possible in society. Similarly, there are no medicines unless we look beyond the physician and his or her patient. Physicians do not produce their own simples. A just society also represents the interests of patients, not excluding those being treated but also including those yet to fall ill, a category to which most patients once belonged. It is thus necessary to include a third party in the medical ethic, society as a whole.

In all modern democracies, one role that society has taken upon itself is the licensing of drugs. Pharmaceutical industry sponsors are required to prove quality, safety and efficacy of medicines before being permitted to sell them to physicians, patients and reimbursers. Efficacy and, to some extent, safety are examined through the medium of the clinical trial. The registered pharmacopoeia thus provides an armoury to which all physicians (in principle) have access. This armoury defines, or at least delimits, standard best possible care. We can thus regard society as defining through the regulatory process the standard of care (potentially) available.

This role of society removes an ethical conflict from the doctor provided that s(he) observes the following principle. The *expected* value to the patient of any treatment offered in a clinical trial to which the patient is recruited should be at least as good as that available outside the trial. This means that the fact that society has prohibited certain treatments from general use and only permits their use within the clinical trial, perhaps using a clinical trial exemption (CTX), in the UK, or investigational new drug (IND) in the USA, renders equipoise irrelevant. A physician who says that (s)he cannot enter patients in a clinical trial, because although neither treatment is inferior to

Treatment allocation in drug development trials 405

standard care, one (the experimental treatment) is superior to the other, condemns all patients to receiving an inferior treatment.

Thus, one view of the ethics of patient participation in drug development programmes is that physicians are entitled to recommend to their patients that they should enter a clinical trial as long as the physicians believe that no treatment being compared is inferior to standard care. Experimentation continues until either society is convinced that a treatment being examined, must now be added to those generally available and should no longer be restricted to clinical trials, or the physician becomes convinced that the treatment is, after all, inferior. Equipoise is not then the necessary condition for starting the trial. On the contrary, equipoise is the point which either a sceptical regulator or an optimistic sponsor must reach (and exceed) in order to stop the trial.

This requires no conflict on the physician's part between doing the best for the patient and doing the best for society by doing good science. It raises the question, however, as to whether a just society is entitled to organize itself in such a way. It might be argued that society is simply resolving the physician's ethical conflict by usurping a responsibility to which it is not entitled: that of deciding which drugs are permitted. An answer to this charge can be found by using John Rawls's approach to justice.[8]

Justice and the point of sickness

As Rawls recognized,[8] many ethical dilemmas of a just society cannot be resolved by referring only to 'now'. Medical dilemmas are no exception. They cannot be resolved by considering them at the point of sickness. Consider, for example, two facts of modern life in Britain: first, the apparent chronic long-standing shortage of cash within the National Health Service (NHS); second, that many young people spend their spare cash and time on summer holidays in Ibiza and other holiday destinations where they indulge in binge-drinking and casual sexual relations in a way that shocks older generations. It seems that this money could be better spent on the NHS, which in any case may have extra burdens of care placed upon it due to the unwise excesses of British youth. Do we not stand condemned as a society by not organizing taxation to make sure that this money is better spent?

One answer is the Rawlsian one that if placed in the so-called 'original position' (where we do not know what place we shall have in society) we would not necessarily choose to have more money spent on health and less on holidays. Even using the more modest perspective of insurance, many young people would not choose to forgo their holidays in exchange for the guarantee that they could have hip replacements and a host of other operations and treatments in old age if and when needed. Similarly, although the comparison of different generations is difficult, those currently infirm would not necessarily have chosen to forego pleasure in youth for a promise of health care in old age. From this perspective, Alan Maynard's concept of 'a fair innings' can be seen as just.[9]

An application of the Rawlsian theory of justice to the problem of drug regulation and clinical trials might be as follows. We are to consider in the *original position* whether we wish to join one of two societies. In the first there is no regulation of medicines. A physician is simply placed under the obligation of providing the patient with that treatment (s)he believes most efficacious. No controlled clinical trials are possible. As a consequence the study of treatment is less efficient, medical progress is slower and less certain and lives are lost.[10] In the second sort of society, treatments are not registered until there is a reasonable consensus that they are efficacious. This consensus is achieved through clinical trials. A side effect of this is that physicians are not always free to give what they consider best treatment. The only opportunity to receive such treatment may be to enter a clinical trial in which its allocation will not be certain. On the other hand, in the second society, standard care is almost certain to be better than in the first. Which society would we choose?

It is plausible that we would, in fact, prefer the second society when placed in the original position. This is not to say that we will prefer it at the point of sickness. From the prospective patient's point of view, the best position is to be guaranteed that society will be run along the second model unless and until that individual falls ill, when the first will apply. Such behaviour is, of course, manifestly unfair: the patient seeks an advantage that only others can provide and that (s)he is unwilling to repay.

If this view is accepted, for example, it could then be argued that the behaviour of certain members of the auto-immune deficiency syndrome (AIDS) lobby some years ago, in attempting to 'bounce' the Food and Drug Administration (FDA) into lower standards for registering therapies for this disease, was immoral.[11] This is because such lower standards, although clearly in the interest of patients then current, were neither in the interests of future patients nor would they have been in the interest of current patients in the original position. Even if potential patients had been told they would eventually contract the disease, they would not have known whether they would be amongst early or late cohorts. As such, they might have preferred the FDA to maintain the usual standards.

Thus, although the details of how a rational drug regulation system should be implemented are a matter for a careful decision analysis that has yet to be made, the Rawlsian perspective suggests that such a system need not be unfair. The regulatory system is to be used as a means of separating permitted from experimental treatments. The population of patients in clinical trials, therefore, are those who, with the help of their physicians, have taken the decision that their expectations are better served by having a chance of being allocated an experimental therapy believed or hoped to be superior.

The role of placebos

It might be thought that the requirement that patients should have no expected loss when compared with standard care by entering a clinical trial, excludes the use of placebos. This is not true. Both critics[12] and defenders[13] of the placebo have misunderstood their nature. Before examining exactly what that is, however, one red-herring will be disposed of, namely that placebos may be justified because they are often an effective treatment.

Treatment allocation in drug development trials 407

This argument is unacceptable for various reasons, not least because there is considerable doubt as to whether placebos are effective.[14-16] If the justification for the use of placebos is that they continue to be necessary in clinical trials because only through *concurrent* control can the effect of treatment be established, then the corollary is that to claim that placebos are effective we should also have established *their* efficacy in a controlled manner. This requires three-armed trials in which an active and placebo group are compared to a no-treatment group. Very few such trials have been run. It is plausible that much of the so-called placebo effect is often regression to the mean.[17-19] This makes little difference to the utility of placebos as comparators but it does suggest that they may not be useful therapies in their own right. Whether or not this argument is accepted, however, there is a second and more serious objection. If effective therapies are to be determined through controlled clinical trials, then it follows that any effective therapy must be one that is more effective than placebo. Hence, whether or not a placebo is partially effective, where a treatment has been established to be partially effective, it must, by definition, be more effective than placebo. Thus, if this treatment is part of the standard armoury, the use of a placebo involves an expected loss compared to that available outside the trial and is thus unacceptable.

The reason that placebos are, after all, acceptable is that the use of placebo does not, contrary to what is often maintained, necessarily imply that therapy is being withheld. In fact, a placebo is always specific to a therapy. It is nearly always necessary in order to blind a trial to use placebo, even where two active treatments are being compared. If, in order to use a placebo, all effective therapy had to be withdrawn, then it would indeed be quite impossible to run placebo-controlled trials. Food, drink and air are all effective treatments, as becomes obvious if we consider what will happen to the patient if they are denied. Yet no one thinks that the use of placebo necessarily involves starving or smothering the patient. In other words, the question as to which therapies are to be given is logically independent as to whether placebo is being used or not: a placebo can be given instead or as well as an existing therapy.

The existence of standard care defines a 'baseline' by which experimental strategies should be judged. All clinical trials involve the use of one or more of the following compared to this 'baseline': maintenance (M); elimination (E), which is never more than partial; augmentation (A); and substitution (S), this last being a combination of E and A. Consider, as a case in point, the introduction of new treatments for AIDS in the era since the development of zidovudine . Such trials have consisted of an M group receiving standard therapy (often, nowadays consisting of several treatments) and an M + A group receiving an experimental treatment in addition. In order to blind the experimental treatment, a placebo will need to be used. These are then placebo-controlled trials, the 'placebo group' being the M group. Senn lists several papers reporting such trials, many of which are described as placebo-controlled by their authors.[20]

We can thus see that the common opinion of critics of the placebo, that the existence of an effective remedy makes the use of placebo control unethical, is false. Where the Declaration of Helsinki states, 'The benefits, risks, burdens and effectiveness of a new method should be tested against those of the best current prophylactic, diagnostic, and therapeutic methods. This does not exclude the use of placebo, or no treatment, in

408   *S Senn*

studies where no proven prophylactic, diagnostic or therapeutic method exists',[21] it actually opens the door to a type of trial, an active control trial, which would be unethical. This is because an effective remedy (the control) would be being withheld from the experimental group, who would be entitled to this treatment if not entered onto the trial and would be given instead a treatment of unproven efficacy. Similarly the claim by Rothman that, 'As medical knowledge accumulates, the number of placebo trials should fall' is misguided for the same reason.[12]

If the new treatment proves particularly effective, a situation may then arise, where: (1) the combined therapy now becomes standard; and (2) it is suspected that the contribution that the original standard therapy makes to the combined efficacy may not justify its toxicity. This may then lead to a further trial in which there is an M group (combined therapy maintained) and an E group (original standard therapy eliminated). Again this will involve the use of a placebo. The E group will need to be provided with a placebo to the original standard therapy.

This is not merely a quibble. The real ethical issue is: what treatment is the physician justified in giving his or her patients? This decision has to be made in the light of: (1) society's legitimate control of available treatments; (2) the physician's beliefs about efficacy of treatments; and (3) society's interest in the scientific investigation of new therapies.

A practical problem

It can thus be seen that regulation and the conduct of clinical trials can be organized on a principle of justice that does not harm requirements of beneficence and non-maleficence. These have to be judged not at the point of sickness but with respect to the patient's legitimate interests in the original position. In the original position there is no necessary conflict between the interest of society and those of the individual: society is to be organized to benefit all individuals. It is simply necessary to take at least a lifetime view of the interest of individuals. There is, however, a potential practical conflict. The persons administering the systems of clinical research and drug regulation are not in the original position nor are they (in the main) patients. There may thus be a temptation to press the present to serve the future beyond what is justified. The practical principle of justice outlined above requires that treatments should not just be studied but also implemented and this requires a trade-off between current and future demands.

Such trade-offs have been studied by a number of Bayesian statisticians, most noticeably by Don Berry and co-workers.[22] The basic idea is that we wish to treat a potentially large number of future patients by establishing the best treatment using current patients. However, we do not draw a rigid distinction between current and future patients and wish to optimize the treatment of patients overall. This leads to a dynamic allocation of treatments in which results to date guide choices for further experimentation.[22] Such designs are known as *bandit designs*. How much experimentation is allowed is determined by the discount rate applied to future patients. If the discount rate is infinite, experimentation, in the sense of a scientific choice between possible treatments, becomes impossible, since only what is currently believed best for the next patient is relevant. (This is, in fact, the perspective adopted in the continuous reassessment method of O'Quigley and co-workers.[23,24]) Given a large number of future patients and a low discount rate, however, even randomized designs may be (nearly) acceptable from this perspective.[22] A useful review is given by Palmer and Rosenberger.[25]

The requirements of autonomy: an unethical use of placebos

One might be tempted to take the Rawlsian analysis further and say that not only is experimentation justified by consideration of our interests in the original position but it also justifies coercion: that patients should be entered into clinical trials without their consent. In my view, this takes the matter too far. Patients do not have the right to demand therapies from society, except on terms that society has agreed. But by the same token, society does not have the right to demand co-operation from the patient. Matters are to be organized so that it is rational to want to enter clinical trials, not so that patients need to be forced into them.

Thus, there is a separate principle of autonomy that applies which suggests, amongst other matters for example, that the patient should be free to seek an alternative physician if (s)he does not like the advice given by his or her current one.

Curiously, although much ink has been wasted on the ethics of placebos as controls in clinical trials, remarkably little has been said about the use of placebo run-in periods. These are periods in which all patients are given placebo in a single-blind fashion. Such run-ins always involve a violation of informed consent, although this problem is usually fudged in some way.[20,26] The only true standard of informed consent must be willingness to show the trial protocol to the patient if the patient so desires and refusal to rely on a presumption of ignorance on the patient's part. Such presumption is 'the argument from the stupidity of others'[26,27] and has no part in serious approaches to medical research.

Conclusion

If the argument that has been presented here is accepted, then the ethical problem in using placebos in clinical trials may be resolved by the following steps.

1. Recognizing that the use of placebo in a clinical trial carries with it no necessary implication that effective treatment should be withheld. Such treatment can form background care for all patients in both arms. Whether or not standard treatment is to be withheld is a separate issue.
2. Recognizing that society has a right, acting in the interests of all patients in the 'original position', to restrict the availability of certain medicines to clinical trials.
3. Ensuring that patients are not entered into clinical trials unless it is expected that they will suffer no loss in doing so.
4. Practising informed consent.

410   *S Senn*

The last of these four points is extremely important. The ethical perspective of clinical trials being offered here is that it has to be a co-operative exercise: one organized by society on mutual principles for the potential need of any member. Such a society must view knowledge on the part of patients as being beneficial rather than harmful. Patients need to learn why clinical trials benefit us all. Trust is of the essence. Deliberate deception of patients, as in the use of placebo run-ins,[26] has no part in such a society.

Acknowledgements

I am grateful to Professor Mike Baum and Professor John Bunker for helpful discussions. This paper is a written version of a public lecture given in acceptance of the George C Challis Award of the University of Florida, December 2001, and I am grateful to the Statistics Department of the University of Florida for this designation and to the George C Challis foundation for the award.

References

1   Lilford RJ, Jackson J. Equipoise and the ethics of randomization. *Journal of the Royal Society of Medicine* 1995; **88**: 552–9.
2   Freedman B. Equipoise and the ethics of clinical research. *New England Journal of Medicine* 1987; **317**: 141–5.
3   Stein CM, Pincus T. Placebo-controlled studies in rheumatoid arthritis: ethical issues. *Lancet* 1999; **353**: 400–3.
4   Spiegelhalter DJ, Freedman LS, Parmar MKB. Bayesian approaches to randomized trials. *Journal of the Royal Statistical Society, Series A* 1994; **157**: 357–87.
5   Kadane J. *Bayesian method and ethics in clinical trials design.* New York: Wiley, 1996.
6   Peto R, Baigent C. Trials: the next 50 years. Large scale randomised evidence of moderate benefits. *British Medical Journal* 1998; **317**: 1170–1.
7   Lellouch J, Schwartz D. L'essai therapeutique: ethique individuelle ou ethique collective. *Revue de l'Institute International de Statistique* 1971; **39**: 127–36.
8   Rawls J. *A theory of justice.* Oxford: Oxford University Press, 1972.
9   Maynard A. Evidence-based medicine: an incomplete method for informing treatment choices [see comments]. *Lancet* 1997; **349**: 126–8.
10 Baum M, Vaidya JS. The price of autonomy. *Health Expectations* 1999; **2**: 78–81.
11 Thornton H, Baum M. Ethics of clinical trials: the 'forbidden fruit' phenomena. *Breast* 1996; **5**: 1–4.
12 Rothman KJ. Placebo mania. *British Medical Journal* 1996; **313**: 3–4.
13 Levine RJ. The need to revise the Declaration of Helsinki. *New England Journal of Medicine* 1999; **341**: 531–4.
14 Kienle GS, Kiene H. The powerful placebo effect: fact or fiction? *Journal of Clinical Epidemiology* 1997; **50**: 1311–8.
15 Kaptchuk TJ. Concerns about run-in periods in randomized trials. *JAMA* 1998; **279**: 1526–7.
16 Hrobjartsson A, Gotzsche PC. Is the placebo powerless? An analysis of clinical trials comparing placebo with no treatment. *New England Journal of Medicine* 2001; **344**: 1594–602.
17 Kaptchuk TJ. Powerful placebo: the dark side of the randomised controlled trial. *Lancet* 1998; **351**: 1722–5.
18 McDonald CJ, Mazzuca SA, McCabe GP, Jr. How much of the placebo 'effect' is really statistical regression? *Statistics in Medicine* 1983; **2**: 417–27.
19 Senn SJ. How much of the placebo 'effect' is really statistical regression? [letter]. *Statistics in Medicine* 1988; **7**: 1203.
20 Senn SJ. The misunderstood placebo. *Applied Clinical Trials* 2001; **10**: 40–6.
21 World Medical Association 52nd Assembly. World Medical Association Declaration of Helsinki Ethical Principles for Medical Research Involving Human Subjects. Edinburgh: World Medical Association, 2000, 5.

Treatment allocation in drug development trials   411

22 Berry DA, Eick SG. Adaptive assignment versus balanced randomization in clinical trials—a decision-analysis. *Statistics in Medicine* 1995; **14**: 231–46.

23 O'Quigley J, Pepe M, Fisher L. Continual reassessment method—a practical design for phase-1 clinical-trials in cancer. *Biometrics* 1990; **46**: 33–48.

24 O'Quigley JO, Shen LZ. Continual reassessment method: a likelihood approach. *Biometrics* 1996; **52**: 673–84.

25 Palmer CR, Rosenberger WF. Ethics and practice: alternative designs for phase III randomized clinical trials. *Controlled Clinical Trials* 1999; **20**: 172–86.

26 Senn SJ. Are placebo run ins justified? *British Medical Journal* 1997; **314**: 1191–3.

27 Senn SJ. *Statistical issues in drug development.* Chichester: John Wiley, 1997.

[28]

When Are Placebo-Controlled Trials No Longer Appropriate?

Baruch A. Brody, PhD

Center for Medical Ethics and Health Policy, Baylor College of Medicine, Houston, Texas

ABSTRACT: This paper presents a standard for assessing the validity of placebo-controlled trials in circumstances in which such trials might be unjustly denying appropriate therapies to members of the control group. This standard categorizes the types of risks that can or cannot be imposed upon consenting research subjects in such control groups. The paper also shows how needed research can be conducted while respecting the proposed ethical standard. Both the problem and the proposed standard are illustrated by reference to the major trials of the thrombolytic agents. *Controlled Clin Trials 1997; 18:602–612*   © Elsevier Science Inc. 1997

KEY WORDS: *Placebo control groups, research ethics, thrombolytic agents, equipoise, informed consent*

PART I: INTRODUCING THE PROBLEM

Since Sir Bradford Hill's trial of streptomycin in 1948 to treat pulmonary tuberculosis, the well-designed clinical trial has quite properly emerged as the gold standard for clinical research. Such trials (1) are prospective, (2) involve carefully defined populations, interventions, and endpoints, (3) contain a control group as well as an intervention group, (4) randomly assign subjects to the control group or the intervention group, (5) blind both the subjects and the treating professionals to that assignment, (6) are adequately sized, and (7) are approved in advance by an IRB and are monitored during the trial by a Data Safety and Monitor Board (DSMB).

The absence of any one of these features weakens the scientific validity of the clinical trial, with different features having different degrees of importance. Sir Bradford Hill's trial did not blind the subjects/patients and the investigators because of the burden of maintaining the blind, but that did not significantly weaken the scientific validity of that trial. On the other hand, no feature is more important for the scientific validity of the trial than feature three, the existence of a control group as well as an intervention group. Without a comparison of outcomes between these two groups, we learn nothing about the efficacy of the intervention being tested. While such control groups can be historical or concurrent, the use of historical control groups is usually less satisfactory scientifically, in part because that use precludes randomization (feature four) and in part because there is a concern that other changes besides the intervention might be responsible for the differences between the control group and the intervention group. These considerations mean that scientific validity is usually greatly strengthened by the use of concurrent control groups, either placebo control groups, active control groups, or dosage control groups. There are, of course, further scientific advantages to the use of placebo control groups over the two other forms of concurrent control groups. As Dr. Temple [1] has pointed out, these include the ability to run smaller trials, the lessening of the incentives to sloppiness, and the need to make fewer assumptions of an implicitly historical nature. But these are scientific advantages rather than absolute needs for scientific validity, and that means that they might be outweighed in at least some cases by other concerns such as ethical concerns.

What are these ethical concerns? The crucial concern is that the subjects in the control group are being unfairly denied certain beneficial medical interventions. Which interventions? In the drug setting, which is the setting with which I am concerned in this paper, two possibilities suggest themselves. The first occurs when there already is an available drug approved for a given indication and the clinical trial is testing a new drug for that same indication. If the trial involves a placebo control group, then it might be suggested that the members of that group are being unfairly denied the available, already approved drug whose favorable risk-benefit ratio for the indication in question has presumably been established before approval. The second occurs when no drug has yet been approved for a given indication, the clinical trial is testing a drug for that indication, the drug is available and already approved for other indications so that clinicians are entitled to prescribe it for this new indication, and there already is substantial evidence (although not enough evidence to secure approval) of a favorable risk-benefit ratio for the new indication. If the trial involves a placebo control group, then it might be suggested that the members of that group are being unfairly denied the already available drug whose favorable risk-benefit ratio for the new indication is supported by substantial evidence.

This ethical concern does not arise for clinical trials in which there is no available already approved drug for the indication in question and either (1) the drug being tested for that indication in the clinical trial is not available outside the setting of the trial because it is not yet approved for use for any indication or (2) there is not yet substantial evidence supporting the use of the drug being tested for the indication in question. In such cases, there is no available beneficial intervention being unfairly denied to members of the placebo control group. Different ethical issues arise when interim data from the trial substantially support the use of the drug being tested for the indication in question, but they are not our concern in this paper.

With these considerations in mind, the question of this paper can now be stated relatively precisely: under what conditions do the scientific advantages of using a placebo control group justify its employment in a clinical trial even if that means denying to members of the placebo group a different available drug already approved for the indication in question because it has a favorable risk-benefit ratio or denying to members of the placebo group the drug being tested which is otherwise available and whose use for the indication in question is supported by substantial evidence of a favorable risk-benefit ratio?

This question can be illustrated by the history [2] of the clinical trials of the intravenous administration of APSAC, tPA, and streptokinase. The major placebo-controlled trials of the intravenous administration of these drugs to patients with a myocardial infarction (AIMS [3], ASSET [4], GISSI [5], ISIS-2 [6]) occurred after the intracoronary administration of streptokinase had been approved by the FDA in 1982 for patients with a myocardial infarction because it saved a substantial number of lives. The patients in the placebo control groups were being denied a very beneficial medical intervention. Was that just? Moreover, many of these trials continued after the publication in 1986 of the GISSI data which certainly offered substantial support for the lifesaving benefits for patients with myocardial infarctions of the intravenous administration of streptokinase. Since intravenously administered streptokinase was already approved for other indications, the patients in the placebo control groups in the continuing trials were being denied an available medical intervention whose benefit for this indication was supported by substantial evidence. Was that just?

A number of points should be noted about this example. To begin with, the interventions being denied to the placebo control group in these trials were either demonstrated to be lifesaving (intracoronary streptokinase) or were substantially supported as lifesaving (intravenous streptokinase). Even those who generally advocate the use of placebo control groups recognize this type of case as different because of the lifesaving nature of the intervention. Secondly, certain techniques often used to mitigate the unfairness to the placebo group were not available in this example. For example, a program of salvage therapy for patients in the control group doing poorly that switched them to the treatment group was unlikely to be helpful because of the limited time frame in which thrombolytic therapy must be administered if it is to be helpful. So there were powerful ethical reasons for not using placebo control groups in these trials. At the same time—and this is the third point to be noted about this example—the use of placebo control groups in these trials enabled the benefits of intravenously administered thrombolytic therapy to be clearly demonstrated relatively quickly. This led to the approval and widespread use of these thrombolytic agents, saving many thousands of lives annually. Were there any alternatives that could have accomplished the same thing? If not, does that justify the use of the placebo control groups in these trials?

In the remaining sections of this paper, I will (1) consider six suggestions that might help resolve these issues and argue that they do not; (2) put forward a new standard for the use of placebo-controlled trials in the circumstances we are considering; and (3) apply that standard to the example of the trials of the thrombolytic agents, suggesting alternatives to the trials that were actually run.

PART II: SIX SUGGESTIONS

Our problem is not new, and many suggestions have been made that can be of some use in dealing with various aspects of it. In this section, I will consider six suggestions. While each will turn out to have some merit, none will be adequate for a full resolution of the problem.

The first suggestion is that we need to begin clinical trials earlier. If the very first patient to receive a new intervention, or an old intervention for a new indication, did so in the context of a randomized controlled trial, we would not confront the problem of denying to the placebo control group an intervention about which there was substantial evidence that it had a favorable risk-benefit ratio.

There are many questions that can be raised about the practicality of this first suggestion, even though it is an attractive suggestion. It is easiest to implement for new drugs, since they first become available, after the issuance of an investigational new drug (IND) approval, for use in clinical trials. The use of other interventions such as already approved drugs for new indications is less controllable, so the suggestion would be harder to implement for them. But the crucial point is that even if fully implemented, this suggestion would offer only a partial solution to our problem. Its implementation would insure that no placebo control group was denied a new drug, or an already approved drug being tested for a new indication, in a clinical trial after there was already substantial evidence of its favorable risk-benefit ratio for that indication. But none of this would help with the case in which the placebo control group was being denied another drug already approved for the same indication, so this suggestion, even if fully implemented, would only partially solve our problem. In this second type of case, many scientifically desirable placebo-controlled trials could still not be run.

To return to our example, the full implementation of this suggestion would have meant that the first subject to receive an intravenously administered thrombolytic agent for a myocardial infarction would have received it in the context of a placebo-controlled clinical trial. In that trial, the placebo control group would have not received any thrombolytic agent intravenously, but that might have been acceptable since there would not have been any evidence from clinical trials about the effectiveness of intravenously administered thrombolytic agents. But the placebo control group in that trial would also not have received any thrombolytic agent administered intracoronary, and that would have been problematic since the intracoronary use of streptokinase for myocardial infarctions had already been approved because of its demonstrated benefits for that indication. How then could one have ethically conducted a placebo-controlled clinical trial of any intravenously administered thrombolytic agent? In fact, Anderson [7] in 1985 concluded for these reasons that one could not, and he ran a series of trials on APSAC as concurrent active controlled trials.

The second suggestion is that our problem can be solved by blinding treating clinicians to ongoing results that might favor the intervention over the placebo; these results should be available only to an independent DSMB. This suggestion is very useful in dealing with the problem for which it was developed [8], the conflict of interest faced by an investigator/clinician who is aware of interim data favoring one arm in a clinical trial. How could that clinician keep his or her patients in the trial if they were in the less-favored arm? By being blinded to interim data, he or she cannot face this conflict of interest. But our problem is not the conflict of interest posed by knowledge of interim data. Our problem is about the design of the trial itself, and it arises even before the trial begins. Blinding those involved to interim data is, then, irrelevant to our problem.

A third suggestion is that our problem is solved by the informed-consent process in which the subjects/patients consent to randomization. So long as they are informed about the existence of the placebo control group and about the potential risks (as well as the potential benefits) of receiving only a placebo, and as long as they consent to being randomized, those in the placebo control group cannot have been unjustly denied anything. Their valid consent insures that the denial of an active treatment is not unjust.

It is important to note that this suggestion makes several presuppositions about the informed-consent process. To begin with, the process must make sure that the patients/subjects understand the potential risks of being in the placebo control group as well as the potential risks of receiving the intervention being tested. This understanding requires their knowledge of the evidence supporting the use of the drug being tested for the intervention in question, if there is any, and their knowledge of the available, already approved drugs for the indication in question that are being withheld from the placebo control group, if there are any. Secondly, the process must fulfill the requirements for the consent's being valid. The consenting subject must be competent to make the choice about participating and must have sufficient time to consider the issue.

Our example of the trials of the thrombolytic agents illustrate the theoretical difficulties in satisfying the second presupposition. They are good examples of emergency research. It is now well understood that the conditions under which emergency research is performed (the questionable competency of the patient/subject in light of his/her medical problems and in light of the effects of the initial treatments and the questionable amount of time for careful consideration of the risks and benefits of participating in the research) may make obtaining valid informed consent impossible. For that reason, new standards for doing emergency research without consent have emerged [9]. So it is unclear that consent, even when obtained (GISSI, for the reasons just mentioned, did not require obtaining consent), could justify denying treatment to the placebo control group. Moreover, a look at the consent forms actually used in these trials illustrates what I believe is a common failure to inform the patients adequately about already approved treatments which they will not receive in the trial. For example, even the long consent form used by ISIS-2 investigators in the United States [10], while mentioning the possibility of not participating in the trial and getting intracoronary streptokinase instead, did not mention that intracoronary streptokinase was already approved for use for myocardial infarctions because of its demonstrated efficacy in substantially reducing mortality.

Let us, for the moment, disregard these issues and suppose that the above-listed presuppositions were fully met. Let us suppose that the patients/subjects had validly consented to being randomized into a placebo-controlled trial because they had received all the relevant information, were competent to consent, and voluntarily consented after sufficient time to consider whether or not to participate. Does this mean, as the third suggestion says, that the members of the placebo control group were not being unjustly denied an active treatment? I think not. I think that the third suggestion has failed to keep in mind that obtaining valid consent from the subjects/patients is a necessary, but not a sufficient, condition for the moral legitimacy of a clinical trial. Obtaining that consent satisfies only the requirements of the principle of autonomy. Other universally recognized requirements, grounded in the principle of nonmaleficence, are that the risks to the subjects/patients be minimized and that the risk-benefit ratio be favorable. It is questionable that these other requirements can be satisfied if there is another available drug already approved for the indication in question being denied to members of the placebo control group. It is also questionable that they can be satisfied if there already is substantial evidence that the available drug being tested, and therefore being denied to the placebo control group, has a favorable risk-benefit ratio for the indication in question. In the cases about which we are concerned, especially when dealing with lifesaving interventions such as thrombolytic agents, it seems, therefore, that even obtaining valid consent may not be sufficient to justify withholding active interventions from the placebo control group.

The fourth and fifth suggestions refer to a state of equipoise, a state of uncertainty as to whether being in the treatment arm or the placebo arm of a placebo-controlled trial is preferable. According to the fourth suggestion [11], running a placebo-controlled trial is acceptable so long as the individual researchers are in this state of equipoise. According to the fifth suggestion [12], running a placebo-controlled trial is acceptable so long as the relevant community of experts is in this state of equipoise to the extent that at least some members are not yet convinced as to the benefits of being in one arm rather than the other. According to both suggestions, equipoise of the relevant sort means that patients/subjects in the placebo control group are not being unjustly denied interventions.

I am dissatisfied with this approach because it seems to be excessively descriptive rather than normative. It allows placebo-controlled trials to be run as long as some appropriate individual or group is not sufficiently convinced by the evidence of the benefit of the withheld intervention. One of the things we know from the history of science is that people are often not convinced by scientific evidence long after they should have been convinced. If the state of equipoise should have been ended by the accumulated evidence for the benefit of the intervention, but it was not because of personal or sociological factors, why should that justify the continued use of a placebo-controlled trial?

This concern is troubling enough when we are dealing with the withholding from the members of the placebo control group of the drug being tested after there already is substantial evidence of a favorable risk-benefit ratio for its use for the indication in question but before the drug is approved for that indication. This is, of course, the context for which this approach was developed. For example, once the data from GISSI showed a substantial improvement in survival rates after receiving intravenous streptokinase rather than a placebo, why should the mere fact that some individual or group of individuals remained uncertain about the benefits of intravenously administered thrombolytic agents be sufficient to justify the withholding of these agents in further placebo-controlled trials? Shouldn't their uncertainty have to be justified for these trials to be justified? That, it should be noted, seems to have been why the TIMI investigators [13] canceled their plans for a placebo-controlled trial of intravenously administered tPA even while other placebo-controlled trials continued.

These equipoise suggestions are even more troubling when what is being withheld from the placebo control group is some other drug already approved for the indication in question. To apply these suggestions in that setting, one would have to say that as long as some appropriate individual or individuals are not yet convinced that it is better to receive the already approved drug than to receive a placebo, it is permissible for investigators to run placebo-controlled trials of the new drug. But in this type of case, a normative judgment has been made by the national drug regulatory agency that the already approved drug has a favorable risk-benefit ratio for that indication. Why should the mere fact that there is some remaining uncertainty on the part of some individual investigator or some group of investigators, whatever the merits of their uncertainty, justify withholding the other already approved drug from the members of the placebo control group? Shouldn't their uncertainty have to be justified? For example, once intracoronary streptokinase was approved by the FDA for use in myocardial infarctions because it was demonstrated to save lives, why should the mere remaining uncertainty of some individual or group of individuals about whether it was beneficial be sufficient to justify withholding it from the members of a placebo control group so that intravenously administered thrombolytic agents could be tested in a placebo-controlled trial? Shouldn't that defense of a placebo-controlled trial have to be based on a normative justification of their uncertainty?

Unlike the first five suggestions, the sixth and final suggestion [14], accepts the possibility that those randomized to placebo control groups may in some cases be unjustly denied the benefits of either the drug being tested or some other already approved drug. It nevertheless feels that this may be justified because of the resulting social gains from the information gathered from these trials. Perhaps, it suggests, our whole problem grows out of an understandable, but excessive, emphasis on an individualistic rather than a social perspective.

This last suggestion is certainly correct in reminding us that social gains may sometimes be sufficient to justify individual injustices; concerns about justice do not always have lexical priority over concerns about social benefits. But in deciding which should take priority, many questions need to be considered. Among them are the following:

1. Do we really have to choose between justice to the individual subjects/patients and promoting social gains through research, or can we design trials controlled in other ways so that we can realize both goals?
2. What is the permissible extent of the injustices to the individuals in the placebo control group if a placebo-controlled trial is run?
3. What is the needed extent of the incremental social gain from the placebo-controlled trial as opposed to some other type of trial?
4. Who should make the decision as to which value should take priority and what should be told to the subjects about the choice that has been made?

A standard dealing with all of these questions must be developed before the last suggestion is adopted as a basis for resolving our problem, and until now it has not been developed.

While none of the suggestions are satisfactory as they stand, several important themes have emerged from our critical analysis that should be incorporated into any solution to our problem. In the design of controlled clinical trials, we need to consider allowing sufficiently important social benefits from some trial designs to take precedence over sufficiently modest injustices to individuals from those same designs. In doing so, the informed consent of those suffering the injustices will be an important necessary condition for the justification of those designs, even if it is not a sufficient condition for their justification. This type of justification requires a normative theory of the priority of values. In the next section, I will present a solution incorporating all of these themes.

PART III: A NEW STANDARD

The new standard I wish to propose is directed to the cases we are considering: (1) those cases in which there already is an available drug approved for the indication in question and the trial is testing a new drug for that same indication or (2) those cases in which there is no drug approved for the indication in question, the trial is testing an available drug already approved for other indications, and there is substantial evidence of a favorable risk-benefit ratio for this new use of the drug. In such cases, the standard says that a randomized placebo-controlled trial is justified only if (1) the subjects have validly consented to being randomized, unless we are dealing with research that does not require valid consent and (2) a reasonable person of an average degree of altruism and risk-aversiveness might consent to being randomized.

This standard does recognize that social benefits sometimes, but not always, justify imposing injustices on subjects/patients by withholding from them treatments for which there is substantial support. Valid consent is a necessary, but not sufficient, condition for doing so. There is an additional normative standard, viz., that the injustice be sufficiently small that reasonable people who are self-interested but also have an average degree of altruism might find the social gain sufficient to justify their personal loss. This normative judgment, made by the IRB approving the research, supplements the personal judgment made by the individual subject/patient agreeing to participate. In this way, the standard in question incorporates all of the themes that emerged in our analysis.

The basic theme behind this new standard is that we are entitled to take into account the altruism as well as the self-interest of research subjects. This theme is not new. Paul Meier invoked it in 1979 [15] when he wrote, "As a matter of normal social behavior, most of us would be quite willing to forgo a modest expected gain in the general interest of learning something of value. However, we should want to be assured that what we agree to give up is indeed modest and not a truly large amount."

I am suggesting that we turn this theme into a standard. Valid consent of subjects would still be required in most cases (a possible exception is the case of emergency research), so there normally is no element of conscripting subjects into the war against disease, a theme that has sometimes been employed by those trying to justify such placebo-controlled research. At the same time, there is an appropriate balance between what is given up and what is learned. The balance is that what the subjects/patients give up is modest, and this is operationalized in the idea that it must be a loss that a person with an average degree of altruism and risk-aversiveness would be willing to accept. If the loss to the subjects/patients is greater than that, then the research is illicit even if there are great gains to be obtained from learning the results of the placebo-controlled trial.

It is useful to compare this standard with some of the standards found in the statements of various regulatory and professional groups. The Declaration of Helsinki [16] incorporates the least permissive standard. It requires that "In any medical study, every patient—including those of a control group, if any—should be assured of the best proven diagnostic and therapeutic method." That would certainly rule out placebo-controlled trials in the first of our cases, where there already is an approved drug for the indication in question. It might also rule them out in the second of our cases, where there already is substantial evidence supporting the new use of the drug being investigated; that would depend upon how much evidence there is and upon what Helsinki means by "best proven." The trouble with the standard in the Declaration of Helsinki is that it makes no allowance for subjects/patients validly consenting to assuming even modest risks to aid the search for medical knowledge. The Royal College of Physicians [17] is more helpful in this respect, as it allows "withholding effective treatment for a short time, whether or not it is substituted by a placebo," while requiring that the subject/patient validly consent to this withholding. But its standard does not define the extent of the risks that can be imposed on these subjects/patients, and that is a shortcoming that needs to be corrected. The FDA, in a discussion of placebo controlled trials [18], has partially corrected that defect by making it clear that "placebo-controlled trials, whatever their advantages in interpretability, are obviously not ethically acceptable where existing treatment is life-prolonging." But I would urge that the losses resulting from receiving existing treatment can be sufficiently great in terms of diminution of quality of life or of functioning to rule out a placebo-controlled trial even when there is no issue of life prolongation. For that reason, I find the FDA's correction insufficient. The standard I have proposed adds, I believe, the needed additional correction.

With these standards in mind, we return to the trials of the thrombolytic agents. The results of applying these standards are quite troubling. Once the intracoronary administration of streptokinase had been approved for the treatment of myocardial infarctions because of its demonstrated improvement in survival, what was the justification for denying it to those in the placebo arm of the trials of intravenously administered thrombolytic agents? It was certainly not justified according to the Declaration of Helsinki. But neither was it justified according to the FDA's observation that placebo-controlled trials cannot be employed when existing treatment is life-prolonging. And it certainly is not justified by our standard. Would a reasonable person of average altruism agree to participate in these trials if that meant risking giving up a substantial improvement in survival rate if one were assigned to the placebo arm? Such a person might, if he or she had a sufficiently better chance of survival by receiving the newer intervention than by receiving intracoronary streptokinase. One might risk getting nothing in the hope of getting something much better. But there was certainly no reason to suppose that intravenously administered thrombolytic agents would sufficiently improve the likelihood of survival over intracoronary thrombolytic agents to sustain that choice.

I conclude, therefore, that Anderson was right when he argued from the beginning that placebo-controlled trials of intravenous thrombolytic agents were not justified. The TIMI investigators were even more justified, then, when they canceled their planned placebo-controlled trial of intravenous tPA after the results of GISSI were announced.

What were the alternatives to those placebo-controlled trials? Several come to mind: (1) There were many institutions in the United States and elsewhere in which the intracoronary administration of a thrombolytic agent could not have been provided in the mid 1980s and in which it would not have been feasible to transfer patients in a reasonable time to other institutions that could have provided an intracoronary thrombolytic agent. Our standard would not apply to patients/subjects in such institutions. In those institutions, a placebo-controlled trial of intravenous thrombolytic agents would not have deprived members of the placebo control group of anything that was both available and of proven value, at least until the results of GISSI were available. So the initial trials to validate intravenously administered thrombolytic agents could have been run as placebo-controlled trials in those institutions. (2) After such trials had established the benefits of intravenous administration, active controlled trials to prove the equivalence of intravenously administered thrombolytic agents with thrombolytic agents administered intracoronary could still have been run in any institution, and those would have been valuable trials to run since they would have validated this easier and more widely available mode of administration. Similarly, actively controlled trials of other thrombolytic agents to prove their equivalence to streptokinase could have been run. (3) Those who believed that some of the other thrombolytic agents (tPA, APSAC) were better than streptokinase could have run active controlled trials designed to prove that superiority, with those randomized to receive streptokinase serving as the control group. As is well known, such trials to prove superiority are less subject to the concerns about active controlled trials than trials to prove equivalence.

I recognize that such a program of trials would have raised many technical issues of interpretation and coordination. At the same time, I believe that everyone has to recognize that the placebo-controlled trials that were run, whatever their advantages, were, in the words of the FDA, "obviously not acceptable where existing treatment is life-prolonging." The above-sketched program is just one attempt to show how the scientific/medical needs for data from controlled trials could have been better reconciled with the moral imperative to properly protect the subjects/patients in clinical trials.

To conclude: I have presented a standard for assessing the validity of placebo-controlled trials in circumstances in which such trials might be unjustly denying appropriate therapies to members of the control group. It builds upon ideas expressed by Paul Meier and Stuart Pocock, and it modifies other ideas expressed by the FDA, to categorize the types of risks that can or cannot be imposed upon research subjects/patients in such placebo-controlled trials, even when they consent to participate. I have also tried to show how, even in difficult cases, the needed scientific/medical information could be obtained while respecting this ethical standard.

REFERENCES

1. Temple R. Government viewpoint of clinical trials. *Drug Info J* 1982;10–17.

2. Brody, BA. *Ethical Issues in Drug Testing, Approval, and Pricing.* New York: Oxford University Press; 1994.

3. AIMS Trial Study Group. Effect of intravenous APSAC on mortality reduction in acute myocardial infarction. *Lancet* March 12, 1988;545–549.

4. ASSET Study Group. Trial of tissue plasminogen activator for mortality reduction in acute myocardial infarction. *Lancet* Sept. 3, 1988;525–530.

5. GISSI, Effectiveness of intravenous thrombolytic treatment in acute myocardial infarction. *Lancet* Feb. 22, 1986;397–401.

6. ISIS Steering Committee. Intravenous streptokinase given within 0–4 hours of onset of myocardial infarction reduced mortality in ISIS-2. *Lancet* Feb. 28, 1987;502.

7. Anderson J et al. Multicenter reperfusion trial of intravenous anisoylated plasminogen streptokinase activator complex (APSAC) in acute myocardial infarction. *J Am Coll Cardiol* 1988;11:1153–1163.

8. Chalmers, TC. The ethics of randomization as a decision-making technique and the problem of informed consent. In: Abrams N and Buckner M, eds. *Medical Ethics*. Cambridge: MIT Press;1983:514–518.

9. Consensus Statement. Informed consent in emergency research. *JAMA* 1995;273: 1283–1287.

10. ISIS-II Protocol; Appendix B.

11. Fried C. *Medical Experimentation*. Amsterdam: North Holland; 1974.

12. Freedman B. Equipoise and the ethics of clinical research. *N Engl J Med* 1987;317: 141–145.

13. Stipp D. A clot-dissolving drug is more effective in federal test of heart-attack patients. *Wall Street Journal* 11 February, 1986.

14. Pocock S. When to stop a clinical trial. *Brit Med J* 1992;305:235–239.

15. Meier P. Terminating a trial—the ethical problem. *Clin Pharm and Ther* 1979;25:637.

16. Levine R. *Ethics and Regulation of Clinical Research*. New Haven: Yale University Press; 1988:287–289.

17. Royal College of Physicians. *Guidelines on the Practice of Ethics Committees in Medical Research Involving Human Subjects*. London: Royal College; 1990:section 7.100.

18. FDA. Placebo-controlled and active-controlled drug study design. In: *Clinical Investigator Information Sheets*. Washington: FDA;1989.

Part IV
Globalization and Corporation – Trust and Participation

[29]

International Research: Ethical Imperialism or Ethical Pluralism?[1]

Ruth Macklin*

Albert Einstein College of Medicine, Department of Epidemiology and Social Medicine

Conflicts have arisen in international research when countries in which research is being carried out lack the ethical rules or mechanisms for review employed in the United States and Europe. It is objected that a requirement to adhere to regulations promulgated by the US government constitutes "ethical imperialism." But if researchers in some countries need not be bound by ethical standards widely accepted in the conduct of research, it could open the door to an ethical relativism allowing virtually any standard a country desires to accept. One example is the variations in informed consent, especially in countries that accord lesser importance to the individual than do the US and Europe. A recent controversy centered on a series of placebo-controlled, HIV/AIDS trials sponsored by the United States and conducted in several developing countries. These trials could not ethically be carried out in the United States because a proven effective treatment exists. Attempts to avoid similar controversies in forthcoming HIV/AIDS vaccine trials have been initiated by the joint United Nations AIDS program, with a process of regional consultations in the countries where the research will be conducted.

Keywords: international research; ethical imperialism; informed consent; HIV/AIDS; Declaration of Helsinki

A prominent view holds that research involving human subjects must embody ethical universals rather than be tailored to the norms

---

[1]Portions of this paper are adapted from my forthcoming book *Against Relativism*. New York: Oxford University Press.

and practices of particular cultures. One expression of the universal view states: "If it is unethical to carry out a type of research in a developed country, it is unethical to do that same research in a developing country." This requirement for uniformity seeks to ensure that justice prevails in the conduct of research that crosses national boundaries. It is also designed to protect vulnerable populations from exploitation. An underlying assumption of this "protectionist" stance is that people in developing countries are somehow vulnerable to exploitation in a way that people in developed countries are not. That assumption bears examination, and has, in fact, been challenged by developing country researchers and health advocates in a series of meetings on HIV/AIDS vaccine research to be described later in this article.

A different view—we may call it "ethical pluralism"—holds that rules governing research practices may vary according to the cultural norms accepted in the country where the research is carried out. "Respect for diversity" underlies the approach of ethical pluralism, which rejects the notion that a single set of ethical standards for research should prevail in our culturally diverse world.

The United States has elaborate and detailed federal regulations governing biomedical and behavioral research, whereas many countries in the world have no such laws, regulations, or procedures for protecting human subjects, and others have the only barest minimum. Conflicts are bound to arise in international collaborative research where a country in which research is being carried out lacks the norms or mechanisms that have become accepted standards by the sponsoring agency. If researchers in those countries must adhere to regulations promulgated by the US government, the objection is raised that it constitutes "ethical imperialism." But if researchers in some countries need not be bound by ethical standards widely accepted in the conduct of research, it would open the door to an ethical relativism allowing virtually any standard a country desires to accept.

Differences among cultures—especially with regard to the primacy of the individual—have led some people to argue that informed consent is a concept understandable and applicable in the West but is irrelevant to social and cultural norms in Africa and Asia. For example, at a conference sponsored by the World Health Organization in December 1980, the WHO's Proposed International Ethical Guidelines for Human Experimentation were first presented. One conference participant from the United States (Miller, 1981) described the guidelines as "essentially based on American standards of ethical review as well as on the international codes"—the Nuremberg Code and the Declaration of Helsinki. This concern was also voiced by some participants from developing countries at the conference (Miller), who objected to elements of the proposed guidelines on grounds of ethical imperialism: "How far, they wondered, can Western countries impose a certain concept of human rights? In countries where the common law heritage of individuality, freedom of choice, and human rights do not exist, the . . . guidelines may seem entirely inappropriate."

Interestingly, just the opposite worry has been voiced by individuals from developing countries. In recent decades and even today, some research has been carried out in developing countries that could not be conducted in North America and Western Europe. Critics of a "double standard" from both the West and from developing countries argue that if a research project is deemed ethically questionable or unethical in a developed country it ought not to be conducted in a developing country, especially one that lacks a process for research review. Even where there does exist a mechanism for ethical review of research in a developing country, the norms of that country might not recognize as wide an array of individual rights as is common in the West, so ethical review committees could find it perfectly acceptable to proceed with a research design that would not be approved in North America or Europe. It is at least an apparent contradiction to seek to have it both ways, arguing on the one hand that research considered unethical in the US should not be conducted in Africa or Asia, and at the same time contending that ethical values vary from one place to another so it is ethical imperialism to impose Western values on non-Western cultures.

Variations in Informed Consent

Nevertheless, when required by international sponsors to employ rigorous procedures to obtain voluntary, informed consent from subjects, some researchers in non-Western countries have complained that it is "ethical imperialism" to impose North American procedures requiring strict adherence to informed consent on cultures in which patients normally do not have to give consent to treatment or research maneuvers.

Several years ago I was a member of a group assembled by the Centers for Disease Control (CDC) to discuss a number of ethical issues that arose in a proposed collaborative study between the CDC and medical researchers in China. The study was to take place in a rural area where there was a high incidence of birth defects. The study design involved the use of a placebo for some participants, while others would receive a substance that researchers thought might reduce the likelihood of birth defects. The Chinese collaborator was resisting the ethical requirement of obtaining individual informed consent from prospective subjects. Some CDC officials thought that the Chinese researcher's objections were valid, given the differences in biomedical research and practice in the US and the People's Republic of China. Our standards of informed consent to treatment seem rarely to apply in the PRC, and up to that time there had been relatively few clinical trials similar to those common in the US and Europe.

The Chinese physician stated his opposition to the informed consent requirement on two separate grounds. First, obtaining consent from patients is an altogether alien notion in medical practice, so to introduce it into the research context would be unfamiliar to many Chinese participants and likely to arouse suspicion. A population unacquainted with biomedical research would have difficulty understanding why physicians would seek their permission to do something, since doctors normally do what they believe is best for patients without the need to ask. Second, the Chinese physician argued, if potential subjects were told that half would get placebo, no one would enroll because the concept of a placebo (or, at least, a placebo-controlled study) is unheard of in China. If people knew there was a possibility that they would get a dummy pill instead of an active substance no one would agree to participate and so, he argued, whatever information they are given should not include mention of the placebo control. In addition to the two main reasons the researcher stated, an additional complication is the Chinese cultural tradition of involving the family and even the larger community in individual health-related matters. In sum, the researcher said that if the CDC required the informed consent of Chinese participants, it would be impossible for him to carry out the study.

Some CDC officials questioned whether it would constitute ethical imperialism to impose on China, researchers requirements drawn from US regulations. Several of us at the meeting argued that it was not specific US government regulations that were being imposed, but rather, world-wide principles articulated in documents such as the Declaration of Helsinki, an international statement first adopted in 1964 by the World Medical Association and amended several times since then at periodic meetings of the World Medical Assembly (most recently in 1996).

After much discussion, the group reached a consensus that the use of placebos in research would be unethical if subjects are not informed that they will either receive active medication or placebo. The discussion was complicated by the literal translation of "placebo" offered by the Chinese researcher. He gave a Chinese translation of the phrase "makes people comfortable," which accurately conveys the meaning of "placebo" in the treatment setting but is misleading in the context of research. The group insisted that he use different Chinese words that would convey the true meaning of "placebo" in the research setting.

Several years after that meeting at the Centers for Disease Control, I learned what the Chinese researcher had actually done. The physician who was the principal investigator attended a conference in the US and described the cultural compromise he and his collaborators had reached.[2] He reiterated his belief that no one would agree to join the study if the researchers sought consent only from the individual women who were potential subjects. In Chinese culture women have to involve their husbands, their family, their community leaders. The researchers developed a process of "community consent," which involved different levels of the community, at the county, township, and village levels. All had to agree for subjects to be enrolled. Researchers spoke with government leaders at every level. Next, they talked to the health authorities at each level. Professional people from all these levels also had to understand and approve the research. Then, finally, there was the family. The entire family then had to approve, but the actual role of the family depended on who was the head. The physician would tell the woman "it is good for health reasons" for her to take the pill. After this whole process was completed, the woman came to the physician/researcher, who explained everything to her. The physician, not the woman, signed the consent form. It took about three months for all these steps to be accomplished.

---

[2]The researcher was present at a conference devoted to ethics and research held at the University of North Carolina, Chapel Hill, North Carolina, in November 1995.

Although the procedures differed considerably from those typically employed in Western countries, the solution the researchers arrived at sought to adapt the Western requirement of obtaining informed consent from the individual to the family-and community-oriented situation in China. While the women participants in the study appeared to be reasonably well informed, they alone did not consent to participate in the study. One aspect of the procedure that would not be acceptable to most research ethics committees in the US is the physician's statement that "for health reasons, it is good for the woman to take the pill." That could not truthfully be claimed (at least, not in advance) for those women who received a placebo instead of the study medication, nor could positive health benefits be guaranteed for the experimental drug. The researcher maintained that in the absence of some such statement, no one would consent to participate and the study could not be carried out.

It is critically important to distinguish between the specific procedures embodied in US regulations and the fundamental principle demanding that we respect as individuals the persons who are enlisted as subjects of research. Respect for persons is properly understood as the ethical principle designed to protect the rights of human subjects of biomedical and behavioral research, in particular, the right to self-determination. The reason why informed consent is an ethical requirement even when the proposed research carries a very low or virtually nonexistent risk of harm, as in some social or behavioral investigations, is that people can be wronged even when they are not harmed. To carry out perfectly benign studies on human beings without their knowledge or consent would wrong them because their right to self-determination is violated. In the absence of their granting voluntary, informed consent, research subjects would be treated as a mere means to the ends of others, as objects or instruments rather than as persons worthy of respect.

But what about cultures in which individuals are not granted the right of self-determination in other areas of life? It is just this focus on the individual that is criticized as uniquely American or at least, Western. Lisa Newton (1990), a philosopher from the United States, argued that "[i]t is 'ethical imperialism' at its worst to assume that the informed consent requirement, which does indeed serve one (only one) moral principle in the Western setting, is in itself such a universal ethical standard" (p.11). Newton contends that there is today a growing doubt surrounding the value of individualism and individual rights, so "the investigator might better stick to the research and accept the local assessment as to adequate protection of individual rights."

Exactly the opposite position is stated by another American bioethicist, Ruth Faden, and co-author Carel B. Ijsselmuiden (1992), a physician from South Africa, who writes: "Appeals to cultural sensitivity ...are no substitute for careful moral analysis. We see no convincing arguments for a general policy of dispensing with, or substantially modifying, the researcher's obligation to obtain first-person consent in biomedical research conducted in Africa" (p. 833). Interestingly, Ijsselmuiden and Faden add that defenders of such a policy "have relied on limited and often dated anthropologic literature that does not reflect the rapid cultural changes brought about by colonialism and independence, warfare, and urbanization" (p. 833).

The danger of a reliance solely on local assessment is that in societies where there is no tradition whatsoever of individual rights, the local assessment may reject the very concept that individual research subjects have rights and therefore, they may be enrolled simply with the permission of the village chief. Even if it is the custom for a village chief to decide what everyone in that village is permitted or required to do in the ordinary activities of the village, it does not follow that the chief should be granted the same authority to submit members of his village to research maneuvers at the hands of biomedical or social scientists. Lisa Newton's observation that there is today a growing doubt surrounding the value of individualism and individual rights may well be accurate, but that doubt exists mainly in the minds of academics who live comfortable lives in a nation whose Bill of Rights stands as a bedrock of constitutional democracy. No corresponding doubts are to be found among advocates of democratic reform in China or in the many Latin American countries in which dictators reigned until very recently. In countries whose members struggle against dictators or oppression at the hands of autocratic rulers, reformers strive for recognition of individual rights.

The conduct of international collaborative research requires ongoing attention to these concerns. In one instance, a research proposal from an African country designed to study fertility awareness and pregnancy avoidance stated that "village chiefs will also assure the women of the need to cooperate...." The program officer from the international agency to which the proposal was submitted wrote back to the principal investigator: "This implies pressure from the village chiefs, and also implies that the women who participate in the study will be known to them." The program officer's letter added: "... you state 'the consent that we anticipate is almost taken for granted in our own part of the country'. Again, as you well understand, consent should be informed and entirely voluntary." In his reply, the principal investigator expressed his knowledge of and willingness to comply with these ethical requirements. The researcher's letter said:

> ... In Nigeria, there is no ethical problem in dealing with human subjects relating to information gathering. The intensity of research activities in various parts of Nigeria also reveals that Nigerian women are more than willing to answer questions relating to their sexuality....[E]merging new experiences corrected the earlier insinuations that Nigerian rural women might be unwilling to discuss what might be regarded as private affairs.
>
> In the present circumstance, the village chiefs are routinely informed of any project to be executed in their villages as part of courtesy to them as the head of the village and for him to be in the know of things going on around him. He, in any case, does not know the individual women to be interviewed. In our case, we do not anticipate any ethical problem on this: indeed the consent of the village chief is taken for granted because it is freely and willingly given. The responses to questions from women are to be held confidential. Those unwilling to be interviewed are normally not coerced to respond. Therefore the issue of pressure does not arise at all.[3]

It is evident that the Nigerian researcher was well aware of the ethical requirements of the sponsoring agency and sought to assure the sponsor that the ethical precepts of voluntariness of participation and preserving confidentiality would be adhered to. What happened in the actual conduct of the research is, of course, impossible to know.

One journal article (Loue, S., Okello, D. and Kawuma, M., 1996) described a workshop on research ethics in Uganda that addressed the problem of acquiescence by another family member in order for an individual to participate in research. The Ugandan setting appears to be similar to the research in China described above, where not only the husband but also other groups had to be consulted before individual subjects could be enrolled. In Uganda, however, the situation was further complicated by the simultaneous existence of customary or traditional practices and modern, civil law. The latter states that an eighteen-year-old male living at home has the legal

---

[3] These details and the correspondence were provided to me by the program officer, in connection with my role as a temporary adviser to the program. Names and institutions are omitted here to protect confidentiality.

right to make his own decision. But customary law dictates that the son must first obtain his father's permission. Ugandan women are even further restricted by the need to obtain the permission of their partner before they may agree to serve as a research subject.

Participants in the Ugandan workshop arrived at a compromise solution between the conflicting demands of customary law and the principle of respect for autonomy as it applies to research. The group recommended a 48-hour waiting period between the time researchers solicit subjects' participation and the time they sign a consent form. During that period, subjects may confer with family members, if they wish, before deciding finally whether to participate. A family member could ask the researcher questions about the research that might arise in the course of a family discussion. The workshop group agreed, however, that another family member could not offer an individual as a research subject if that person was unwilling. The Ugandan group did not view the concept of autonomy as entirely alien to their culture when applied to the research context. Instead, they arrived at a compromise not unlike the one fashioned by the Chinese researcher who collaborated with the CDC. It thus seems possible to respect the autonomy of the individual and at the same time respect the cultural practice of involving the family.

The requirement in US research regulations that informed consent be documented in a written, signed form points to another example of cross-cultural differences. Especially in social science research, but in some biomedical research as well, researchers in other countries often balk at this requirement. Obtaining written, signed consent forms is sometimes described as an ethical "standard" that is acceptable in the United States but not in other cultures. If researchers in countries where people are reluctant to put their signature on "official" documents use oral consent only, are they adhering to a lower standard, one that is ethically questionable, if not unethical?

In some situations, strict adherence to the requirement that written consent be obtained would throw up a barrier to carrying out the research. At meetings I attended and in numerous individual interviews, researchers in Latin America stated that people in their country believe they are signing away their rights; or they may view signing a consent form as a "waiver" of some sort. Especially in countries that have until recently had authoritarian or military governments, people are wary of signing papers. According to social scientists I met with in more than one country, written consent is virtually never obtained for social and behavioral studies.

The procedure of written, signed consent forms is just that—a procedural requirement and not an ethical "standard." It is not a substitute for the consent process, and there may be ethically sound reasons for waiving this procedural requirement. One obvious reason is that the presence of a signed consent form places the subjects at risk. Social scientists conducting abortion research in the Philippines said that one reason written consent is not obtained is the need to preserve confidentiality. In places where abortion is illegal, the existence of a signed consent form in abortion research reveals the likelihood that the woman had an abortion. The same point was made in Chile by a group carrying out epidemiological research on AIDS. If the very existence of signed consent forms places subjects at risk of psychological, social, or legal harm, then it is not only ethically permissible, but ethically desirable to forgo signed consent forms. This is true in the United States as well as in those countries less accustomed to obtaining written consent for participation in research.

Another obvious reason for waiving the requirement for written consent is that some studies involve illiterate subjects. The fact that people are illiterate may not be grounds for disqualifying them, and it is certainly not grounds for abandoning an oral explanation and gaining their permission to serve as subjects. It is, however, sufficient reason to abandon the need for a written document describing what they have been told and requiring that they make an X on a signature line.

The key distinction here is between the *process* of informing and obtaining voluntary consent from prospective subjects, and the piece of paper they are asked to sign. The latter is a consent document, it is not informed consent. It is amazing but true that even today, many sophisticated professionals from Western countries continue to fail to distinguish between the process of obtaining people's permission to invade their bodies or ask intrusive questions, on the one hand, and the consent form that is intended to document that process, on the other. They also frequently misconstrue the purpose of an informed consent document. Many physicians believe that the purpose of informed consent is to protect the researcher or clinician from legal liability, and they cynically observe that "you can be sued anyway, so informed consent is not worth the paper it's written on." But this is radically to mistake the purpose. The informed consent document is meant to attest to the research subject's having been told what the researcher plans to do and having granted permission for the research maneuver.

A Controversy: Placebo-controlled HIV/AIDS Trials

In exploring the topic of accountability in international collaborative research, it would be useful to focus first, on one recent episode, and second, on an innovative process designed to anticipate future ethical problems. The recent episode was the furious controversy that surrounded a set of maternal-to-child transmission studies of HIV carried out in several developing countries, in which some research subjects were given placebos. An extended public debate, some of which took place in the pages of the *New England Journal of Medicine*, involved the sponsors of the research—the National Institutes of Health (NIH), the Centers for Disease Control (CDC), and UNAIDS (the United Nations Joint Program on HIV/AIDS), and their opponents who criticized the studies.[4]

The furor was prompted by an open letter (Public Citizen, 1997) addressed to US officials by the Public Citizen's Health Research Group, which compared the CDC and NIH-sponsored trials to the infamous Tuskegee experiments, and newspaper stories that followed. The Public Citizen advocacy group argued that a proven treatment regimen can reduce the rate of vertical transmission, so it is unethical to withhold that treatment from women in the trial. The proven regimen (known as "076" from the clinical trial in the United States that demonstrated its effectiveness) uses a high dose of AZT, begun midway through pregnancy and administered intravenously during childbirth to the woman. The international collaborative studies were carried out in developing countries that cannot afford the expensive "076" AZT regimen routinely used in the US and European countries. These clinical trials were testing a lower dose of AZT, which was much cheaper and therefore presumed to be affordable to the poorer countries that would make it available to pregnant women. The developing country studies also began AZT treatment much later in pregnancy, since women in those parts of the world do not routinely receive early prenatal care, and the AZT was administered orally rather than intravenously, in line with the availability of medical facilities. These departures from the proven 076 treatment regimen were made in order to adapt AZT for pregnant

---

[4]In addition to the sources cited, some of the positions and arguments described in this section are taken from discussions, meetings and conferences in which I participated while the debate was going on.

70   R. Macklin

women to the medical realities in the developing countries where the treatment would be introduced.

For ethical reasons, placebo-controlled trials testing this experimental treatment regimen could not be conducted in the United States. Once its efficacy had been established, the 076 AZT regimen became the standard treatment for HIV-positive pregnant women in the US and other developed countries. It would surely be unethical to withhold from women in a research study an effective treatment they could obtain as part of their routine medical care. It is evident that these studies did violate the somewhat simple rule: "If it is unethical to carry out a research study in a developed country, it is unethical to do that same research in a developing country." But is not nearly as clear that these studies were unethical, despite the violation of that rule.

The Public Citizen group contended that "at least 1002 newborn babies will die as a result of HIV infections they will contract from their mothers in unethical experiments funded by the NIH or the CDC. An additional 502 infants can be expected to die in six other experiments funded by foreign governments including Belgium, Denmark, France, the UNAIDS program, and South Africa." The group argued that these deaths are unnecessary because women in trials on vertical transmission should be given the treatment regimen proven to reduce the incidence of HIV infection acquired through vertical transmission. Sponsors of the trials replied by noting that more than 350,000 children get infected from perinatal transmission every year in developing countries. It is expected that a shorter regimen would decrease the transmission rate by 40–50%. Therefore, every year delay in getting the results of these studies implies that 140–170,000 children are going to be infected without having access to any intervention.

The reply to their critics by the sponsoring agencies had four parts: (1) the "standard of care" for HIV-positive women in these developing countries is no treatment at all, so they are not being made worse off by being in the study; (2) a placebo-controlled trial can be carried out with many fewer subjects and completed in a much shorter time than could an AZT-controlled study, so useful information pertinent to this population will be available much sooner; (3) the AZT treatment regimen that has become standard in the West is not now and will never be available to this population because of its prohibitive costs, so its use in a research study cannot be justified; (4) if it is proven to be effective, the much cheaper and more appropriate experimental regimen will be made available by governments to all pregnant women in these countries. The conclusion defenders of these trials reached (Brown, 1997) is that thousands more children's lives will be saved by conducting the shorter, placebo-controlled trial than by the longer, AZT-controlled study, so it is ethical to do the placebo-controlled study in those countries.

Public Citizen's Health Research Group sought to rebut the argument (Public Citizen, 1997), claiming that the research violates at least four of the ten principles of the Nuremberg Code, and in addition, Guideline 15 of the *International Ethical Guidelines for Biomedical Research Involving Human Subjects* (CIOMS-WHO, 1993) is violated. That Guideline states that the ethical standards of the sponsoring agency's country should prevail when research is conducted in another country, and that the ethical standards should be no less exacting than those in the sponsoring agency's country. The Public Citizen group claimed that because these trials could not be conducted in developed countries today, the researchers "have chosen to ignore these standards of ethical conduct accepted the world over and have sunk to standards below those acceptable in their home countries." A different, and lower standard was being applied to poor, developing countries than that employed in wealthier countries, and that constituted an unacceptable ethical relativism, they argued.

The opponents in this dispute began by adopting quite different initial premises. The Public Citizen Group began with the premise that the same study could not ethically be carried out in developed countries and concluded that therefore, it would be unethical to conduct it in developing countries. The sponsoring agencies began with the premise that risk-benefit ratios are radically different in developing countries and in the sponsoring agencies' countries. In the developed countries, all women potentially had access to the effective treatment regimen but in the developing countries none did. In the developing countries, subjects were not being placed at greater risk than if they were not in the study at all, and many more people could potentially benefit much sooner from the shorter, placebo-controlled trial. The two cases were therefore not similar, but different in relevant respects.

Defenders of the placebo-controlled trials included representatives from the developing countries in which the trials were conducted. Some argued that the studies were ethically acceptable because they satisfied the relevant procedural requirements for approving and conducting research. They pointed out that the

72   R. Macklin

placebo-controlled perinatal transmission studies were approved by ethical review committees in the developed countries that sponsored the trials and also in the developing countries where they were being conducted. Furthermore, they argued, researchers from the developing countries were carrying out the studies in their own countries and women enrolled in the studies granted their voluntary, informed consent to participate. Therefore, they concluded, since the placebo-controlled trials adhered to ethically adequate procedures, they are ethically acceptable. Based on the approval of health officials in his country, as well as local ethical review and approval, one African researcher remarked that the Public Citizen critique of these AIDS trials "reeks of ethical imperialism."

This controversy has all the earmarks of a genuine ethical dilemma. The research in question does appear to violate a condition stated in the international Declaration of Helsinki (1996): "In any medical study, every patient—including those of a control group, if any—should be assured of the best proven diagnostic and therapeutic method." In the placebo-controlled studies, no group is provided with the best proven therapeutic method. However, Robert J. Levine (1998), an expert in the ethics of human subjects research questioned the interpretation of the phrase, "the best proven treatment: "When Helsinki calls for the 'best proven therapeutic method' does it mean the 'best therapy available anywhere in the world'? Or does it mean the standard that prevails in the country in which the trial is conducted?" (p. 6). Levine's answer is that "the best proven therapy standard must necessarily mean the standard that prevails in the country in which the clinical trial is carried out" (p. 6).

Others argue that to adopt that standard is to exploit nations and people who are economically disadvantaged. One physician (Kim, 1998) writes:

Exploitation by industrialized countries of the human and natural resources of the developing world has a long and tragic history. It has never been difficult for economically wealthy countries to justify their acts by citing, for example, the supposed genetic or moral inferiority of those exploited. Substituting economic inferiority in these old arguments makes the enterprise no less offensive. (p. 838)

The placebo arm of these studies was suspended in Thailand and Ivory Coast in February 1998, when results demonstrated the unquestioned superiority of the short course of AZT over placebo. But the early completion of the trials did not end the debate between medical scientists and ethicists who had staked out positions on either side. The controversy had little to do with different norms or values in different countries and everything to do with the economic disparity between developed and developing countries. Resulting from that economic disparity is a different standard of medical care in wealthier countries from that which exists in poorer nations. As one observer (Piot, 1998) noted, "the real double standard lies not in the way the trials are being conducted, but in the inequity in access to medicines in different countries"(p. 839). Although combatants in this controversy hurled charges and countercharges of "ethical exploitation" and "ethical imperialism," the debate had nothing to do with whether ethical standards should be relativized to culture or should be universal.

Three questions remained unresolved in this episode of international collaborative research. The first is a question of procedural ethics. The Ugandan researcher who claimed that the stance of the Public Citizen group "reeked of ethical imperialism" argued that researchers from Uganda and representatives from the Ugandan Ministry of Health were full participants in the decision to initiate the trials. People from a given culture or country are in the best position to decide what is best for their country, and not some outsiders who are unrelated to the research and unfamiliar with the health needs of the region. Furthermore, local ethical committees reviewed and approved the research. Because these trials were preceded by the proper procedures, involving local and regional committees and officials, they must therefore be ethically acceptable. A reply to this procedural justification (Ijsselmuiden, 1998) addressed its weakness: "Since the Tuskegee study was conducted by Americans on Americans, this argument obviously does not stand. . . . Unethical research will not benefit developing countries in the long run, since it undermines human rights, which are the very foundation on which sustainable development needs to be built"(p. 838).

The second unresolved question that emerges from the placebo-controlled perinatal transmission controversy is whether existing international guidelines are adequate to address the present and future conduct of international collaborative research. Specific items in the current version of the Declaration of Helsinki and the CIOMS International Guidelines are open to different interpretations, the guidelines themselves may well be internally inconsistent, and careful consideration reveals that some statements or guidelines may be in need of revision. These two documents are significant, as they are used for guidance and often as a definitive source of authority by the World Health Organization, by investigators in both developed and developing countries, and by national and local committees that review ethical aspects of research. Guidelines and principles from these documents were cited both in support and in criticisms of the trials in the controversy over the placebo-controlled AZT trials.

We have already noted the problem of interpreting the phrase, "the best proven treatment," in the Declaration of Helsinki. Other phrases in that same document are equally problematic, for example: "Concern for the interests of the subject must always prevail over the interests of science and society." Critics charged that in the placebo-controlled trials, the interests of society prevailed over the interests of the subjects enrolled in the study. However, supporters of the study could cite a different Helsinki principle: "Biomedical research involving human subjects cannot legitimately be carried out unless the importance of the objective is in proportion to the inherent risk to the subject" (World Medical Association, 1996). According to this defense, although there did exist a risk to the subjects who received placebo, the importance of obtaining an affordable and practical regimen for reducing maternal-to-child HIV transmission for large numbers of people in poor countries is so overwhelming that it justifies the risk of not taking steps to prevent HIV transmission in the relatively small group of study participants.

Similar difficulties arise in the CIOMS international guidelines. One paragraph (CIOMS-WHO, 1993) states:

[In a randomized clinical trial] the therapies (or other interventions) to be compared must be regarded as equally advantageous to the prospective subjects: there should be no scientific evidence to establish the superiority of one over another. Moreover, no other intervention must be known to be superior to those being compared in the clinical trial, unless eligibility to participate is limited to persons who have been unsuccessfully treated with the other superior intervention or to persons who are aware of the other intervention and its superiority and have chosen not to accept it. (pp. 39–40)

Critics charged that the placebo-controlled trials of perinatal transmission fail to comply with these conditions.

These examples should suffice to illustrate the problem. Which ethical guidelines should be followed? What should be done when ethical guidelines or elements in those guidelines come into conflict? The Declaration of Helsinki is undergoing extensive revisions at the present time, but whatever improvements may come about, a need will still exist to interpret vague or ambiguous statements or concepts. Although the current CIOMS guidelines are only five years old, they too are going to be revisited in the wake of the perinatal transmission controversy and in light of anticipated controversy that could accompany HIV/AIDS vaccine trials scheduled to begin soon.

HIV/AIDS Vaccine Trials

A controversy could very well arise in a series of international HIV vaccine trials scheduled to begin in late 1998 in Thailand, and in 1999 in Brazil and Uganda. These will be the first phase III trials of vaccines and will require a very large study population in order to demonstrate efficacy. One of the thorniest questions surrounds the type and level of care and treatment to be made available to trial participants who become infected (despite high-level counseling on risk reduction) in the course of the trial. Some people contend that the treatment should be that which is routinely offered to HIV-infected individuals in the sponsoring country. Others argue that it is ethically necessary only to provide treatments at the level of what is routinely available in the host country. This is one of the key issues in seeking to promote justice and avoid exploitation in international collaborative research.

Thus the third question that arises out of the placebo-controlled perinatal transmission controversy is whether such disputes might be identified and addressed in advance of initiating the research. This is the path that UNAIDS has begun to embark on. The vaccine development program at UNAIDS sought to resolve the dilemma by adopting a procedural solution to this and other ethical concerns likely to arise once the vaccine efficacy trials commence. Program officers at UNAIDS, in consultation with prominent vaccinologists and ethicists, decided to hold a series of consultations to gather the views of relevant groups who live in the regions where the vaccine trials will take place. The first step was a planning meeting held in Geneva in September 1997, the purpose of which was to begin to identify the array of ethical issues and to plan for a larger meeting in June of 1998 in which leading stakeholders in the conduct of vaccine trials would be invited to participate.

The next step was preparation for the three-day regional workshops. A rather lengthy, multi-part scenario was created with the

aim of raising all the ethical concerns that could likely (or even conceivably) arise in the design, implementation, and follow-up of vaccine efficacy trials. The three workshops were conducted in April
1998 in Brazil, Thailand, and Uganda, and involved representatives
from local and national nongovernmental organizations, grass-roots
health advocates, vaccine researchers, ethicists, lawyers, and social
scientists. These workshops were followed in May by a meeting in
Washington, DC with participants from the NIH, the CDC, vaccine
experts, ethicists, individuals who had chaired the three regional
workshops, as well as others from the regions where the vaccine trials are to take place.[5] Also present were Dr. Sidney Wolfe and Dr.
Peter Lurie from the Public Citizen's Health Research Group, who
were two of the major critics of the placebo-controlled perinatal
studies. The final event in this consultation process was a larger
conference held in June 1998 in Geneva, just prior to the annual
World AIDS conference. At the Geneva meeting, the conclusions
reached at the regional workshops were reviewed and participants
discussed elements of a proposed "ethical guidance document" for
UNAIDS and collaborating researchers in the design and implementation of HIV vaccine efficacy trials.

One way of describing the ethical concerns related to international collaboration in vaccine efficacy trials is to divide them into
three broad categories: 1) *procedural* issues of decisionmaking; 2)
substantive issues regarding features of trial design, treatment and
care of trial participants; and 3) issues of justice. The description of
these concerns below draws on the above-noted series of meetings
sponsored by UNAIDS.

Procedural issues

These issues pertain mainly to the process by which sponsors of the
trials and researchers and communities in the host country should
make decisions before and during the trial. This is the classic "who
should decide?" question, which involves not only the "*who*", but
also *how* the decision-making should take place, and when. The subject

---

[5]In my role as the chair of the Ethical Review Committee at UNAIDS, I participated
in the organization and planning of the above-noted meetings and workshops and
attended all but the regional workshop in Thailand.

matter of the decisions includes aspects of the trial design, treatment and care of participants who become infected during the course of the trial, who should receive vaccines of some proven efficacy once the trial is completed, what sort of compensation or remedy will be provided for harm to participants, (including harm to interests from breach of confidentiality), and other substantive matters.

Participants in the regional workshops and at the final meeting in Geneva strongly agreed that communities in the host countries should be involved in developing and conducting vaccine trials in a fully collaborative partnership. Despite the difficulty of defining the "community" that should be involved, all agreed it should not be limited to researchers, government officials, or other "experts" in the host countries. Virtually all participants concurred that it is time to abandon the "protectionism" of the past, which viewed developing countries as vulnerable to exploitation simply on grounds of their less-developed economic status. Instead, specific features that might render research subjects vulnerable need to be identified, such as inadequate protections of human rights or authoritarian governments lacking democratic processes for decisionmaking.

The adequacy of mechanisms for conducting scientific and ethical review is another significant procedural issue. Scientific and ethical review is by now well established in the countries and agencies that sponsor international collaborative research, but these procedures are at different stages of development in the countries where the vaccine trials will take place. Participants in the series of meetings sponsored by UNAIDS agreed that adequate mechanisms for review must be in place in the host countries prior to the initiation of vaccine efficacy trials. In some situations, another layer of review at the international level may be desirable. As the capacity for scientific and ethical review becomes established in developing countries, it provides further grounds for rejecting the paternalistic notion that developing countries are vulnerable and stand in need of protection from developed-country researchers.

To refer to these ethical issues as "procedural" is not to diminish their importance, but rather to identify the specific type of ethical concerns they raise. Proper procedures can still yield ethically questionable or unethical results. For example, an ethical review committee, even when properly constituted, could reach a conclusion that would be considered unethical according to ethical principles.

Substantive issues

Substantive ethical questions go to the heart of the design of vaccine trials and the care and treatment of participants. For example, even if it is agreed that a placebo control arm is methodologically necessary and ethically acceptable at the outset of vaccine trials, at what stage of development of candidate vaccines does it become ethically unacceptable to use a placebo control—even if it remains methodologically superior to other designs?

A key substantive question is what sorts of care and treatment should be available to vaccine trial participants. An undeniable ethical requirement is provision of the best available counseling for risk reduction for all trial participants. All three regional groups held this requirement to be unquestioned. To demonstrate how the substantive ethical requirements are intertwined with the procedural ones: participants in the Uganda workshop strongly agreed that risk-reduction counseling should be carried out by trained personnel independent of the research, to eliminate any potential for conflict of interest on the part of the researchers seeking answers to the scientific question of efficacy of the candidate vaccine. Investigators cannot obtain answers to the main research question if risk-reduction counseling is so effective that no one enrolled in the trial engages in risk behavior that results in HIV infection.

One of the thorniest questions surrounds the type and level of medical treatment to be made available to trial participants who become infected in the course of the trial despite high-level counseling on risk reduction. Some people contend that the treatment to be made available should be that which is routinely offered to HIV-infected individuals in the sponsoring country. Others argue that it is ethically necessary only to provide treatments at the level of what is routinely available in the host country. This controversy has been cast in the unfortunate language of "the standard of care"—unfortunate because that terminology was not devised for these purposes and can be misleading, if not pernicious as a basis for deciding what is ethically necessary or desirable. "Standard of care" is a legal term denoting the level of conduct a physician or health provider must meet in treating a patient in order not to be guilty of negligence. It generally (Annas, 1993) means: "what a reasonably prudent physician (or specialist) would do in the same or similar circumstances" (p. 4). Defined in this way, the concept of "standard of care" is not readily applicable to what types or level of treatments should be provided to participants in research during a trial. If a country or a region routinely provides no care, there is no standard and no care. It is an *absence* of care.

The best treatment for HIV infection uses antiretroviral drugs and is commonly known as "triple therapy." It has been shown to be effective in lowering the viral load of HIV-infected individuals and, if strictly adhered to, it delays or prevents progression to an active disease state. Triple therapy is offered early to people in the US after the discovery that they are HIV-positive. But that treatment is complex, burdensome to adhere to, and very expensive. It is not routinely available to the vast majority of HIV-infected individuals in developing countries.

The chief ethical problem arises out of the need to measure different endpoints in vaccine trials. The primary endpoint of an efficacy trial is to determine whether the vaccine prevents infection from taking hold in individuals exposed to the virus. Many leading vaccine researchers believe that a vaccine is unlikely to have that effect, but it may have the important secondary effect of keeping the viral load low, thereby preventing progression to disease. Herein lies the problem: because triple therapy, as currently provided on a routine basis in the United States, effectively lowers the viral load, it would interfere with the ability to measure the secondary endpoint—the efficacy of an HIV vaccine in preventing disease.

Since triple therapy is routinely available outside a research study, it could not ethically be withheld from vaccine trial participants in the US who become infected. That would make them worse off than they would be if they were not participants in the trial. However, in countries such as Thailand and Uganda, antiretroviral therapy is unavailable to all but a very small minority of people who can afford to pay, and is not provided to the vast majority of those who become infected. Hence the analogy with the perinatal trials: a research design that would not be ethically acceptable in the United States would have to be used in conducting the trial in a developing country. Critics could charge that once again, this is a double standard that constitutes exploitation of the population in the developing country.

In what ways can this dilemma be addressed? One attempt might be to distinguish between that which is, strictly speaking, part of the research design and that which is treatment lying outside the conduct of the research. According to this view, the provision of antiretroviral treatment for individuals who become HIV-infected is a matter of clinical care, not an integral part of the research design of vaccine trials that measure secondary endpoints. Accordingly, while the research design must adhere to international ethical standards of research, the provision of clinical care of HIV-positive individuals who seroconvert during the trial may be a function of what is practically available in each country. Although some people might be persuaded by this line of reasoning, it is unlikely to convince others who maintain that this distinction between conducting research and providing treatment is artificially drawn in order to circumvent the ethical problem.

What, then, is the "right" level of care: the lowest that is generally available? The "best available care" in the country or community where the trial is to take place?

The three regional workshops reached different conclusions on this point. The Brazil group arrived at the following strong consensus: "It would not be ethical to deny...antiretroviral...treatment to participants solely for the purpose of making a vaccine trial more valid or statistically powerful." Moreover, the Brazil group (Guenter, unpublished) agreed that "treatment for those who become infected should be provided at the level of that offered in the sponsoring country. It should continue at least for the duration of the trial, and further provision should be negotiated" (pp. 11–12).

The workshop in Thailand (Guenter, unpublished) reached the following consensus:

For those who contract HIV infection during the course of the trial... treatment should be provided at a level consistent with that available in the host country. There is no imperative to provide a level of care consistent with that in the sponsoring country, or with the highest available in the world. (pp. 11–12).

The consensus of the Uganda workshop participants (Guenter) was as follows:

The appropriate type and level of treatment should be decided upon by the host country. It is not necessary that the type and level of treatment coincide with . . . that available to the population of the sponsor country, nor the highest attainable world-wide. However, it must be made reasonably available for the lifetime of the participants. (pp. 11–12).

The Uganda group agreed that it is not ethical to conduct a trial in a given population solely for the purpose of avoiding populations where early treatment is routinely provided.

At the concluding meeting of the series in Geneva, participants (many of whom had attended the regional workshops and the Washington meeting) could not reach consensus on a substantive standard for the level of treatment to be provided. The group did, however, agree to a procedural solution. The level of treatment for people who become infected during an HIV-vaccine trial should be determined in advance by the host country in negotiations with the sponsor, but the standard should in any case be no lower than the highest practically attainable level of treatment.

Justice issues

Issues relating to justice are possibly the most difficult for reaching consensus because there exist different conceptions of justice that are incompatible with one another. A very general formulation of the requirement known as distributive justice related to research is stated in terms of fairness or equity: "The benefits and burdens of research should be distributed equitably." Few people would quarrel with that, but disagreements begin when we seek to identify the specific benefits and burdens and to determine just what equity requires. One conception of justice focuses on relative needs: those in greatest need deserve the most benefits. A market conception of justice (if that conception deserves to be called "justice" at all) is: "To each according to an ability to pay." The problem in international collaborative research, in a world of unequal distribution of wealth, is to decide whether justice requires rectifying the existing inequities of wealth regarding what should be made available during and after a trial. How to act justly in a world fraught with injustice is a general question addressed by philosophers but virtually ignored by political leaders and policy makers driven by national interests and market forces. But those involved in vaccine research and development, including governmental sponsors like the NIH, must provide answers to the following key questions:

What should be available to whom after the trial is completed? Should trial participants who received a placebo be entitled to the vaccine, if proven effective? Should individuals or groups deemed to be at high risk for infection in the country where the vaccine is tested receive the product? Should all with a perceived need in the country receive the vaccine? Should the vaccine be supplied to other developing countries with a high incidence and prevalence of HIV

infection? The CIOMS international guidelines include the following statements:

Externally sponsored research designed to develop a therapeutic, diagnostic or preventive product must be responsive to the health needs of the
host country. It should be conducted only in host countries in which the disease or other condition for which the product is indicated is an important
problem. As a general rule, the sponsoring agency should agree in advance
of the research that any product developed through such research will be
made reasonably available to the inhabitants of the host community or
country at the completion of successful testing. (pp. 44–45).

Participants in the series of workshops conducted by UNAIDS were
not able to come up with a precise account of what it means for a
product to be made "reasonably available." Attendees at the meeting in Washington, DC sharply disagreed both about the meaning
of the phrase and also to whom a product should be made reasonably available. Some argued that the obligation is owed only to vaccine trial participants who were in the control arm of the study, but
others claimed that is inadequate. Some made the proposal that the
vaccine should be made available in the country in which the trial
takes place, since that is the relevant moral unit. According to this
view, the other alternatives are ethically indefensible or impractical:
for example, all of East Africa is too large an area, whereas only the
trial participants or the community in which the trial takes place is
too small.

   Despite the lack of agreement on the meaning and scope of "reasonable availability", participants in all of the workshops agreed on
the need to develop and require a mechanism to determine an ethically appropriate solution. Agreements should be forged in advance
of initiating a trial regarding what will be made reasonably available,
by whom and to whom. Attendees at the workshops from developed
and developing countries all concurred that full collaboration is
required between sponsoring and host countries in planning and
conducting vaccine trials. This should be a true partnership, not a
hierarchical or paternalistic approach. If industrialized country sponsors and pharmaceutical companies adhere to the guidance document
for HIV vaccine efficacy trials issued under the auspices of UNAIDS,
it will usher in a new era in international collaborative research.
Both the process of regional consultations and the outcome of this
process should serve as a model for such collaborations for pharmaceutical products and diseases beyond vaccines for HIV/AIDS.

REFERENCES

Annas, G. (1993). *Standard of Care*. New York: Oxford University Press.

Brown, D. (1997, April 23). Medical Group Condemns US AIDS Drug Tests in Africa for Using Placebo. *Washington Post* p. A14.

Council for International Organizations of Medical Sciences and World Health Organization (1993). *International Ethical Guidelines for Biomedical Research Involving Human Subjects*. Geneva: Author.

Guenter, D. (Undated). *Final Report: UNAIDS-Sponsored Regional Workshops to Discuss HIV Vaccine Trials*. Unpublished.

Ijsselmuiden, C. (1998). Letter to the Editor. *New England Journal of Medicine* 338(12): 838.

Ijsselmuiden, C. and Faden, R. (1992). Images in Clinical Medicine. *New England Journal of Medicine* 326: 833.

Kim, R. (1998). Letter to the Editor. *New England Journal of Medicine* 338(12): 838.

Levine, R. (1998). The "Best Proven Therapeutic Method" Standard in Clinical Trials Technologically Developing Countries. *IRB: A Review of Human Subjects Research* 20(1): 6.

Loue, S., Okello, D. and Kawuma, M. (1996). Research Bioethics in the Ugandan Context: A Program Summary. *Journal of Law, Medicine & Ethics* 24(1): 47–53.

Miller, E. (1981). International Trends in Ethical Review of Medical Research. *IRB: A Review of Human Subjects Research* 3: 9.

Newton, L. (1990). Ethical Imperialism and Informed Consent. *IRB: A Review of Human Subjects Research* 12(3): 11.

Piot, Peter. (1998). Letter to the Editor. *New England Journal of Medicine* 338(12): 839.

Public Citizen. (1997, April 22). *Media Advisory*.

World Medical Association, Inc. (1996). *Declaration of Helsinki. Recommendations Guiding Physicians in Biomedical Research Involving Human Subjects*. France: Author.

[30]

Is Academic Medicine for Sale?

Marcia Angell, M.D.

IN 1984 the *Journal* became the first of the major medical journals to require authors of original research articles to disclose any financial ties with companies that make products discussed in papers submitted to us.[1] We were aware that such ties were becoming fairly common, and we thought it reasonable to disclose them to readers. Although we came to this issue early, no one could have foreseen at the time just how ubiquitous and manifold such financial associations would become. The article by Keller et al.[2] in this issue of the *Journal* provides a striking example. The authors' ties with companies that make antidepressant drugs were so extensive that it would have used too much space to disclose them fully in the *Journal*. We decided merely to summarize them and to provide the details on our Web site.

Finding an editorialist to write about the article presented another problem. Our conflict-of-interest policy for editorialists, established in 1990,[3] is stricter than that for authors of original research papers. Since editorialists do not provide data, but instead selectively review the literature and offer their judgments, we require that they have no important financial ties to companies that make products related to the issues they discuss. We do not believe disclosure is enough to deal with the problem of possible bias. This policy is analogous to the requirement that judges recuse themselves from hearing cases if they have financial ties to a litigant. Just as a judge's disclosure would not be sufficiently reassuring to the other side in a court case, so we believe that a policy of caveat emptor is not enough for readers who depend on the opinion of editorialists.

But as we spoke with research psychiatrists about writing an editorial on the treatment of depression, we found very few who did not have financial ties to drug companies that make antidepressants. (Fortunately, Dr. Jan Scott, who is eminently qualified to write the editorial,[4] met our standards with respect to conflicts of interest.) The problem is by no means unique to psychiatry. We routinely encounter similar difficulties in finding editorialists in other specialties, particularly those that involve the heavy use of expensive drugs and devices.

In this editorial, I wish to discuss the extent to which academic medicine has become intertwined with the pharmaceutical and biotechnology industries, and the benefits and risks of this state of affairs. Bodenheimer, in his Health Policy Report elsewhere in this issue of the *Journal*,[5] provides a detailed view of an overlapping issue — the relations between clinical investigators and the pharmaceutical industry.

The ties between clinical researchers and industry include not only grant support, but also a host of other financial arrangements. Researchers serve as consultants to companies whose products they are studying, join advisory boards and speakers' bureaus, enter into patent and royalty arrangements, agree to be the listed authors of articles ghostwritten by interested companies, promote drugs and devices at company-sponsored symposiums, and allow themselves to be plied with expensive gifts and trips to luxurious settings. Many also have equity interest in the companies.

Although most medical schools have guidelines to regulate financial ties between their faculty members and industry, the rules are generally quite relaxed and are likely to become even more so. For some years, Harvard Medical School prided itself on having unusually strict guidelines. For example, Harvard has prohibited researchers from having more than $20,000 worth of stock in companies whose products they are studying.[6] But now the medical school is in the process of softening its guidelines. Those reviewing the Harvard policy claim that the guidelines need to be modified to prevent the loss of star faculty members to other schools. The executive dean for academic programs was reported to say, "I'm not sure what will come of the proposal. But the impetus is to make sure our faculty has reasonable opportunities."[7]

Academic medical institutions are themselves growing increasingly beholden to industry. How can they justify rigorous conflict-of-interest policies for individual researchers when their own ties are so extensive? Some academic institutions have entered into partnerships with drug companies to set up research centers and teaching programs in which students and faculty members essentially carry out industry research. Both sides see great benefit in this arrangement. For financially struggling medical centers, it means cash. For the companies that make the drugs and devices, it means access to research talent, as well as affiliation with a prestigious "brand." The time-honored custom of drug companies' gaining entry into teaching hospitals by bestowing small gifts on house officers has reached new levels of munificence. Trainees now receive free meals and other substantial favors from drug companies virtually daily, and they are often invited to opulent dinners and other quasi-social events to hear lectures on various medical topics. All of this is done with the acquiescence of the teaching hospitals.

What is the justification for this large-scale breaching of the boundaries between academic medicine and for-profit industry? Two reasons are usually offered, one emphasized more than the other. The first is that ties to industry are necessary to facilitate technology transfer — that is, the movement of new drugs and devices from the laboratory to the marketplace. The term "technology transfer" entered the lexicon in 1980, with the passage of federal legislation, called the Bayh–Dole Act,[8] that encouraged academic in-

EDITORIALS

stitutions supported by federal grants to patent and license new products developed by their faculty members and to share royalties with the researchers. The Bayh–Dole Act is now frequently invoked to justify the ubiquitous ties between academia and industry. It is argued that the more contacts there are between academia and industry, the better it is for clinical medicine; the fact that money changes hands is considered merely the way of the world.

A second rationale, less often invoked explicitly, is simply that academic medical centers need the money. Many of the most prestigious institutions in the country are bleeding red ink as a result of the reductions in Medicare reimbursements contained in the 1997 Balanced Budget Act and the hard bargaining of other third-party payers to keep hospital costs down. Deals with drug companies can help make up for the shortfall, so that academic medical centers can continue to carry out their crucial missions of education, research, and the provision of clinical care for the sickest and neediest. Under the circumstances, it is not surprising that institutions feel justified in accepting help from any source.

I believe the claim that extensive ties between academic researchers and industry are necessary for technology transfer is greatly exaggerated, particularly with regard to clinical research. There may be some merit to the claim for basic research, but in most clinical research, including clinical trials, the "technology" is essentially already developed. Researchers are simply testing it. Furthermore, whether financial arrangements facilitate technology transfer depends crucially on what those arrangements are. Certainly grant support is constructive, if administered properly. But it is highly doubtful whether many of the other financial arrangements facilitate technology transfer or confer any other social benefit. For example, there is no conceivable social benefit in researchers' having equity interest in companies whose products they are studying. Traveling around the world to appear at industry-sponsored symposiums has much more to do with marketing than with technology transfer. Consulting arrangements may be more likely to further the development of useful products, but even this is arguable. Industry may ask clinical researchers to become consultants more to obtain their goodwill than to benefit from their expertise. The goodwill of academic researchers is a very valuable commodity for drug and device manufacturers. Finally, it is by no means necessary for technology transfer that researchers be personally rewarded. One could imagine a different system for accomplishing the same purpose. For example, income from consulting might go to a pool earmarked to support research or any other mission of the medical center.

What is wrong with the current situation? Why shouldn't clinical researchers have close ties to industry? One obvious concern is that these ties will bias research, both the kind of work that is done and the way it is reported. Researchers might undertake studies on the basis of whether they can get industry funding, not whether the studies are scientifically important. That would mean more research on drugs and devices and less designed to gain insights into the causes and mechanisms of disease. It would also skew research toward finding trivial differences between drugs, because those differences can be exploited for marketing. Of even greater concern is the possibility that financial ties may influence the outcome of research studies.

As summarized by Bodenheimer,[5] there is now considerable evidence that researchers with ties to drug companies are indeed more likely to report results that are favorable to the products of those companies than researchers without such ties. That does not conclusively prove that researchers are influenced by their financial ties to industry. Conceivably, drug companies seek out researchers who happen to be getting positive results. But I believe bias is the most likely explanation, and in either case, it is clear that the more enthusiastic researchers are, the more assured they can be of industry funding.

Many researchers profess that they are outraged by the very notion that their financial ties to industry could affect their work. They insist that, as scientists, they can remain objective, no matter what the blandishments. In short, they cannot be bought. What is at issue is not whether researchers can be "bought," in the sense of a quid pro quo. It is that close and remunerative collaboration with a company naturally creates goodwill on the part of researchers and the hope that the largesse will continue. This attitude can subtly influence scientific judgment in ways that may be difficult to discern. Can we really believe that clinical researchers are more immune to self-interest than other people?

When the boundaries between industry and academic medicine become as blurred as they now are, the business goals of industry influence the mission of the medical schools in multiple ways. In terms of education, medical students and house officers, under the constant tutelage of industry representatives, learn to rely on drugs and devices more than they probably should. As the critics of medicine so often charge, young physicians learn that for every problem, there is a pill (and a drug company representative to explain it). They also become accustomed to receiving gifts and favors from an industry that uses these courtesies to influence their continuing education. The academic medical centers, in allowing themselves to become research outposts for industry, contribute to the overemphasis on drugs and devices. Finally, there is the issue of conflicts of commitment. Faculty members who do extensive work for industry may be distracted from their commitment to the school's educational mission.

The New England Journal of Medicine

All of this is not to gainsay the importance of the spectacular advances in therapy and diagnosis made possible by new drugs and devices. Nor is it to deny the value of cooperation between academia and industry. But that cooperation should be at arm's length, with both sides maintaining their own standards and ethical norms. The incentives of the marketplace should not become woven into the fabric of academic medicine. We need to remember that for-profit businesses are pledged to increase the value of their investors' stock. That is a very different goal from the mission of medical schools.

What needs to be done — or undone? Softening its conflict-of-interest guidelines is exactly the wrong thing for Harvard Medical School to do. Instead, it should seek to encourage other institutions to adopt stronger ones. If there were general agreement among the major medical schools on uniform and rigorous rules, the concern about losing faculty to more lax schools — and the consequent race to the bottom — would end. Certain financial ties should be prohibited altogether, including equity interest and many of the writing and speaking arrangements. Rules regarding conflicts of commitment should also be enforced. It is difficult to believe that full-time faculty members can generate outside income greater than their salaries without shortchanging their institutions and students.

As Rothman urges, teaching hospitals should forbid drug-company representatives from coming into the hospital to promote their wares and offer gifts to students and house officers.[9] House officers should buy their own pizza, and hospitals should pay them enough to do so. To the argument that these gifts are too inconsequential to constitute bribes, the answer is that the drug companies are not engaging in charity. These gifts are intended to buy the goodwill of young physicians with long prescribing lives ahead of them. Similarly, academic medical centers should be wary of partnerships in which they make available their precious resources of talent and prestige to carry out research that serves primarily the interests of the companies. That is ultimately a Faustian bargain.

It is well to remember that the costs of the industry-sponsored trips, meals, gifts, conferences, and symposiums and the honorariums, consulting fees, and research grants are simply added to the prices of drugs and devices. The Clinton administration and Congress are now grappling with the serious problem of escalating drug prices in this country. In these difficult times, academic medicine depends more than ever on the public's trust and goodwill. If the public begins to perceive academic medical institutions and clinical researchers as gaining inappropriately from cozy relations with industry — relations that create conflicts of interest and contribute to rising drug prices — there will be little sympathy for their difficulties. Academic institutions and their clinical faculty members must take care not to be open to the charge that they are for sale.

MARCIA ANGELL, M.D.

REFERENCES

1. Relman AS. Dealing with conflicts of interest. N Engl J Med 1984;310:1182-3.
2. Keller MB, McCullough JP, Klein DN, et al. A comparison of nefazodone, the cognitive behavioral-analysis system of psychotherapy, and their combination for the treatment of chronic depression. N Engl J Med 2000;342:1462-70.
3. Relman AS. New "Information for Authors" — and readers. N Engl J Med 1990;323:56.
4. Scott J. Treatment of chronic depression. N Engl J Med 2000;342:1518-20.
5. Bodenheimer T. Uneasy alliance — clinical investigators and the pharmaceutical industry. N Engl J Med 2000;342:1539-44.
6. Faculty policies on integrity in science. Cambridge, Mass.: Harvard University, February 1996.
7. Abel D. Harvard mulls easing rules on research. Boston Globe. February 10, 2000:A1.
8. University and Small Business Patent Procedures Act of 1980.
9. Rothman DJ. Medical professionalism — focusing on the real issues. N Engl J Med 2000;342:1284-6.

[31]

Ethical Issues in Research Relationships Between Universities and Industry[1]

James T. Rule[a] and Adil E. Shamoo[b]

[a]*Center for Biomedical Ethics, University of Maryland at Baltimore. Department of Pediatric Dentistry, University of Maryland Dental School. 666 W. Baltimore Street, Baltimore, Maryland 21201-1503*
[b]*Department of Biochemistry and Molecular Biology, University of Maryland School of Medicine. 108 N. Greene Street, Baltimore, Maryland 21201-1503*

In the last twenty years, biotechnology and pharmaceutical corporations have invested large sums of biomedical research dollars with universities. In 1994, for

---

[1]This a report of a symposium that was held November 3,4 1995 in Baltimore Maryland. It was sponsored by the University of Maryland at Baltimore Center for Biomedical Ethics and supported by Friends, Research Institute Inc., Towson, MD. The Planning Committee included: James T. Rule, DDS, Acting Director, Center for Biomedical Ethics at UMAB and Professor, UMAB Dental School, Program Chairman; J. Leslie Glick, PhD, Graduate School of Management and Technology, UM University College; Thomas E. Hanlon, PhD, UMAB School of Medicine; Madison Powers, JD, PhD, Kennedy Institute of Ethics and Georgetown U.; M. Virginia Ruth, Dr PH, RN, UMAB School of Nursing; Mark Sargent JD, UMAB School of Law; Adil E. Shamoo, PhD, UMAB School of Medicine. Speakers and Panelists included: Lawrence K. Altman, MD, Medical Correspondent, *The New York Times*; Frederick Betz, PhD, Program Officer, NSF; David Blumenthal, MD, MPP, Chief, Health Policy, Massachusetts General Hospital; Joann A. Boughman, PhD, Vice President, Academic Affairs, UMAB; Robert P. Charrow, JD, Crowell & Moring, Washington, DC; Cynthia Crossen, Marketplace Editor, *Wall Street Journal*; Edward E. David Jr., PhD, President of EED Inc, Former Science Advisor of the President of the United States, Former President of Exxon Research, Former Executive Director of Bell Laboratories; Michael Davis, PhD, Senior Research Associate, Center for Study of Ethics in the Professions, Illinois Institute of Technology; V.M. Esposito, PhD, Chairman and CEO, MicroCarb Inc.; Mark S. Frankel, PhD, Director, Scientific Freedom, Responsibility and Law Program, AAAS; George J. Galasso, PhD, Associate Director, NIH; J. Leslie Glick, PhD, Editor-in-Chief, *Technology Management*; Allan L. Goldstein, PhD, Professor and Chair, Department of Biochemistry and Molecular Biology, George Washington University Medical Center; A. Arthur Gottlieb, MD, Professor and Chair, Department of Microbiology and Immunology, Tulane University School of Medicine; Ruth L. Greenstein, JD, Vice President for Administration and Finance, Institute for Defense Analyses, Alexandria, VA.; Sheldon Krimsky PhD, Professor, Department of Urban and Environmental Policy, Tufts University; Roland W. Schmitt, PhD, President Emeritus, Rensselaer Polytechnic Institute, Senior Vice President (Ret.), Science & Technology, General Electric, Chairman, Board of Governors, American Institute of Physics; Adil E. Shamoo, PhD, Editor-in-Chief, *Accountability in Research*; Edmund C. Tramont, MD, Professor and Director, Medical Biotechnology Center, University of Maryland Biotechnology Center; Steven S. Wasserman, PhD, Senior Research Coordinator, Center for Vaccine Development, UMAB.

example, the amount invested for research and development was approximately $1.5 billion.[1] The influx of money from industry and the recent decrease of federal research dollars, has presented ethical challenges both to the traditional roles of scientists and to the attitudes of universities receiving these funds.

Universities serve society by generating new knowledge through research, educating the future work force, and, more recently, contributing service to their community. On the other hand, industry contributes by providing society with the needed products and services. Ideally, in a capitalist system such as ours, the profit motive stimulates innovations, and competition fosters lower prices for consumers. When universities and industry work together in a democratic society, their competing interests are justly facilitated by government.

This idealistic relationship can be thrown into turmoil by a sudden surge in a new area such as biomedical technology, or by instances of overzealous abuses of public trust. In such cases, government has the duty to protect the public interest by issuing laws, rules, and guidelines. It is these conflicting concerns of private gain and public interest that brings forth ethical conflicts.

There can be significant uncertainty in both industry and academia about appropriate conditions under which industry funds are offered, accepted, and utilized by universities for biomedical research. This symposium brought together representatives from industry, universities, the federal government, and the press to discuss ethical issues of mutual interest and importance. Its objectives were to: (1) foster understanding in both groups of the mutually important ethical issues related to research sponsored by industry but performed at universities; (2) provide opportunities for extensive dialogue in the discussion of difficult issues; and (3) suggest approaches to resolve the problems and appropriate policy approaches to manage them.

WHAT IS HAPPENING NOW?

Unquestionably, university–industry research relationships are not only common, they are on the increase. A 1994 survey showed that 59% of life science companies supported research in universities, a 12% rise since 1984. Furthermore, 68% of the companies surveyed planned to increase their finding over the next three to five years, while only seven percent expected cuts in funding.[2]

Why is industry expanding its business with universities? Traditionally, their roles have been different. Universities have done the science, and industry has financed its application. Industry has also provided and used the technology. From the perspective of industry, in recent years the traditional roles have been reinforced by external influences.[3] Increases in world-wide competition have driven companies to shorten their research and development cycles. The old law of research and development has kicked in: "development drives out research." Industry today does less basic and pioneering research than it has in decades.[4] It, therefore, depends increasingly on research performed in academia.[5]

From the university perspective, the timing of these changes is crucial. Federal dollars for research have declined. Universities have increasingly turned to industry for basic research support. The traditional roles of academia and industry have, therefore, become even more entrenched. A new factor has emerged, however, that has caused uncertainty within universities and problems with university–industry relationships: technology transfer is an increasingly important new source of income for the university.[5] In 1993 universities received $350,000,000 from royalties and fees based on licensing and patenting agreements, and the number is rising.[2, 5]

As important as this income is for universities, its contribution is limited. Only 12% of all university research in the life sciences—7% in all fields—is funded by industry.[2] This compares with almost five times as much funding (58%) from federal sources and twice as much (24%) from the universities themselves, including funding from the state.[5] Additionally, although the $350,000,000 received by universities in 1993 for technology transfer sounds impressive, it still is only 0.25% of the total expenditures on higher education.[5]

BONANZA OR SLIPPERY SLOPE?

If one accepts the caveat that, *"the three most important factors in research are integrity, integrity, and integrity,"*[4] then how is integrity affected by academia–industry partnerships? Two distinctly different opinions emerge. One view holds that the interactions are essential, beneficial, and inevitable. They need only be managed intelligently and reasonably. The opposing view expresses caution for the integrity of the university. It holds that money clouds judgement, that interactions are risky, and that careful management and regulation are needed.

The Positive View

The expanding interaction between academia and industry reflects the reality of recent history. Industry has always been a source of research ideas for scientists.[5] Science and technology have always progressed together, never independently.[3] By working together, universities and industry create new opportunities that help all concerned. Universities get new ideas for research, the integrity of science is strengthened, and the education of students is enhanced.[5]

Another benefit is that individual academic researchers who are supported by industry publish more than faculty without much support from industry.[2] Additionally, these researchers report that their relationship with industry is intellectually stimulating, their students have better opportunities, and that the money from industry creates new jobs for the community.[2]

Despite common assumptions to the contrary, there is no reason to think that scientific integrity is at risk when universities and industry work together in basic research. Arguably, it is in everyone's interest to seek the truth, because ultimately there can be no practical applications to false discoveries. Furthermore, the public use of applied science and the public sharing of basic science are both exacting if informal tests of integrity.[5] Adding to the argument, if support from industry represented a challenge to integrity, it should be reflected in the reporting of scientific misconduct. In fact, reported cases of scientific misconduct are remarkably absent in university-based research supported by industry, unlike that of research supported from other sources.[2, 6, 7] This may be due, in part, to inherent incentives for integrity provided by the monitoring process of industry supported research and by its review by the FDA.[6]

One can reasonably conclude that too much attention has been paid to the nature and management of conflict between industry and academia. Arguably, it is now time to work towards the more effective translation of science into technology, in order to create the useful ends that represent the material benefits of science.[5] The future of the university is in partnerships with industry that are aided and abetted by government.[3, 5]

The Negative View

There is ample evidence that university–industry research relationships tend to create an environment that fosters ethical conflicts.[8] For example, when life science companies support PhD students, the great majority of them require the students to project the results.[2] Universities with financial interests in inventions may themselves become as secretive as industry in the protection of their technology.[9] When industry money is involved, there is a tendency for university scientists to voluntarily suppress opinions that are contrary to their personal benefits.[10] Individual investigators with support from industry tend to withhold important data in their publications, including information about methods, results, production know-how, and future avenues for research.[2] Investigators tend to voluntarily suppress data that is contrary to the interests of their sponsors. To illustrate, in a review of more that 100 publications of new drug clinical trials that were supported by industry, in no instances was the sponsor's drug found to be less effective than another company's product.[8] Investigators who have significant support from industry may no longer seek support from federal sources.[9] Investigators with industrial support tend to be influenced by prospects for commercialization when they make decisions about research proposals.[2] When scientists view themselves as trying to help industry, their research tends to be oriented towards the concerns of industry.[2] This can be understood if one realizes that there is always another renewal date in the offing. In legal conflicts involving industry, university professors are regularly hired to challenge other university professors.[10]

What is at stake is the objectivity and credibility of the university in the conduct of science.[2] *"In partnerships between academia and industry, the biggest danger is not trade secrets, not research bias, not the skewing of data. The biggest danger is the loss of soul of the university as a reservoir of independent minds, who can freely and securely offer a critical perspective on the conditions and directions of society, including its technological, political, economic, and social organization. The university is composed of tenured prima donnas who speak their mind and don't speak on behalf of their institution. This is a national resource for society."*[11]

Society needs such independent sources of judgement not only in science, but in everything from social engineering to national defence. The university— not government or the corporate world—is therefore the place where new ideas are best test-marketed. For the benefit of society, university–industry research relationships must be approached with caution. The potential financial benefits to individual investigators and to the university at large provides alluring but dangerous opportunities that must be approached with the overall progress and well being of our society in mind.

THE CENTRAL ISSUE: CONFLICT OF INTEREST

The increasing interdependence between universities and industry has dramatized existing ethical issues and created a few new ones. In one way or another, most of the issues revolve around conflicts of interest. These issues and some approaches to their resolution are presented in this section.

Except for emerging companies, industry tends to have well-developed policies for most conflict of interest situations.[12] The range of effectiveness in universities is much broader. Some universities have sound and well entrenched policies that could be used as models for other institutions. Others have not dealt adequately with the problems that confront them. Admittedly, many aspects of conflict of interest are difficult for universities to resolve due to the huge diversity of circumstances, resources, and attitudes about research within the various institutions.

Definitions and Examples

Conflict of interest can be defined as a set of conditions in which professional judgement about a primary interest tends to be unduly influenced by a secondary interest.[13] The primary interest is determined by one's obligations. Depending on the type of research involved, primary interests may center around issues of integrity, education, or health—possibly all three. In research involving patient care, primary interests include both the health of the subjects and the integrity of the research.

Secondary interests might include the financial interests of the company and the researcher. In health related research, these secondary interests should never outweigh the primary interests.[2] Conflicts of interest vary considerably in the nature of their secondary interests, in the likelihood that professional judgement would be influenced, and in the seriousness of harm that can result.[13] Sometimes secondary interests may be of such small consequence that their regulation is not worth it.[2]

The best way to understand the concept of conflict of interest is to imagine a gauge that has a little dirt trapped inside it. The gauge becomes stuck. You tap on the gauge, and the needle moves to give a reading. Is the reading accurate, or is the position of the needle still affected by some dirt in the works? It is the same with conflict of interest. When conflict of interest is present, it raises questions about whether there is dirt in the works.[14]

There are several types of conflicts of interest. The classical type is one in which a person has two conflicting *duties*. An example is seen with a university scientist who is a consultant for Company A. The job is to develop a drug for a certain disease. Later the same university scientist becomes a consultant for Company B to do the same thing. The scientist has clearly defined obligations to both companies because of his or her position, and they are in classical conflict.[6]

Not all conflicts of interest are of the classical type. Most conflicts of interest involve conflicts of values rather than conflicts of mandated duties.[14] These are widely seen in university–industry relationships. The values of companies tend to be oriented towards the making of profit and the manufacture of good products, while those of universities tend to focus on the education of students and the acquisition of new knowledge. An individual simultaneously employed by both institutions or a university official who negotiates contracts with companies may sometimes be influenced by competing interests that relate to the different values.[14]

Other examples of this type of conflict of interest include: (1) the scientist who sits on a FDA panel that is reviewing a new drug while she is simultaneously developing a similar drug of her own;[15] and (2) the scientist who owns stock in a biotech company that is developing a drug for a certain disease and who submits a grant to NIH that explores basic research on that disease.[6] In these cases the values become more personal, since personal gain (or the perception of personal gain) is at stake. Although it is possible that university scientists with income from industry could be both knowledgeable and disinterested, the reality is that the public tends to be suspicious of such situations.[6]

One of the most insidious and at times invisible conflicts of interest involving values occurs when a researcher avoids a certain line of inquiry due to a variety of personal concerns. The areas of research that can cause serious problems to the investigator could involve issues of health, environment, economics, social, and/or political topics. The concerns may vary from fear of retribution, fear of isolation from the scientific community, loss of status or income, and outright political pressure. This kind of conflict of interest may have a profoundly detrimental, chilling, and corrosive effect on the academic freedom of inquiry.

Another problem is the conflict of commitment. Conflicts of commitment occur when an individual has two things to do and cannot do both. When the tasks themselves are not be in conflict, there may only be a conflict of time or of timing. Such situations are not really conflicts of interest. However, when an academic scientist assumes time consuming consulting responsibilities for private concerns, this commitment may conflict with his or her university in ways that are truly a conflict of interests.[14]

The final type of conflicts are conflicting interests. People might enter science in part either for the joy of discovering "truth" or for the "glory" of success. These are conflicting interests but, in ordinary circumstances, do not become conflicts of interest. These conflicts are normal to science and are unavoidable.[14]

Is Conflict of Interest Unique to Industry Funded Research?

Arguments about the importance of conflict of interest in research revolve around the truth of the dictum that "money taints." The prevailing view seems to be that *of course* money taints. As soon as money is received, a loyalty is created, or at least a chance there is a loyalty. There is no such thing as pure research or truth, because it always has to be paid for.[8]

The conflicts that exist in research supported by the university and by government are arguably as important as those in research supported by industry.[17]

Furthermore, the more important the information, the more disputes there will be about its value.[3] No matter where the money comes from, there will always be issues of tenure, promotion, raises, mortgages to be paid, and other challenges to personal objectivity.[17] Research of any type puts career pressure on investigators to generate interesting data. There is always financial interest in the work of one's students, regardless of whether industry is supporting them. Publicly supported—as well as industry supported—clinical trials have financial interests, indirect though they may seem. Entrepreneurial investigators commonly leverage PHS grants for their own purposes.[17] Additionally, one's judgement can be tainted as much by the quest for fame as the quest for money.[5]

The preceding paragraphs acknowledge the pervasiveness of situations that foster conflict of interest, no matter what the funding source. Nonetheless, it is also true that the stakes can be much higher when money from industry is in the picture. Universities and their scientists are playing key roles in working with industry to move science from the laboratory to the market place. And they are getting rewarded for it. Money from technology transfer is becoming increasingly important to the university. And for individual university scientists, opportunities are unparalleled. For the first time, some university researchers are becoming millionaires.

If it is true that money taints, then perhaps larger amounts of money may taint more. In order to manage the conflict of interest issues related to dealing with industry, universities must develop effective and clear-cut policies. Often this has not yet happened. Such conflicts of interest as exist lie more within the university community than in industry. Up till now, universities in general have been influenced by, but not created effective policies to deal with, the new version of the golden rule: "He who has the gold, rules."[12]

Part of the problem may be that, since universities stand to gain financially from the activities of their most productive scientists, they are reluctant to regulate and restrict the behavior of those scientists. Universities should follow the lead of industry and effectively address the issues.[12]

How to Approach the Problem

There are several approaches to dealing with this problem, some of them worse than others. From the investigator's standpoint, there are three things that could be done.[14] First, the scientist can choose to avoid the situation altogether—an unlikely solution considering the growing interdependence between academia and industry. Second, he or she can eliminate the conflict within the situation by, for example, selling the stock or resigning the position—an equally onerous solution for most people. Third the conflict of interest can be disclosed, in which case there may still seem to be dirt in the gauge. The potential conflict of interest behavior of individual faculty scientists is being dealt with by conflict of interest policies. Such policies constitute a major approach to the management of these problems. Generally speaking, they give guidance to the approaches of conflict elimination and conflict disclosure. Despite the limitations of disclosure, it remains as the primary assurance of integrity, both for institutions and for their members.[4, 5] Furthermore, there is no evidence that disclosure impedes the development of academia–industry relationships.[2] Even so, the university community may not easily accept the concept of disclosure. Current data suggests that university scientists have almost no inclination to voluntarily disclose any information whatsoever about their financial interests in industry.[11]

The federal government has had longstanding concerns about conflict of interest that originated in apprehension about the public's perception of the integrity of federally supported research. These concerns triggered a lengthy process that culminated in a new set of conflict of interest guidelines jointly issued by the NIH and the NSF in 1995.[18]

This policy was designed both to promote objectivity in researchers and to restore and to promote confidence in the public sector. It covers all grants submitted for federal funding, sets permissible levels of investment equity in related industries, and affects everyone in a meaningful decision-making capacity, from the principal investigator to the nurse who decides which arm to inject.[18] Despite general acceptance of the need for such a policy, critics think it should be invoked only if a discernible problem arises.[6] Otherwise, it may force the individual researcher to disclose things which may not be related to the research being proposed. Also, the policy does not take into consideration the circumstances of individual investigators. A $10,000 equity in a company may be the life savings of one investigator, but be relatively meaningless for another.[6]

Another approach is for universities to formulate educational programs designed to sensitize scientists in training and their support staff to the ethical problems involved in the responsible conduct of research.[10, 14] Arguably, the educational approach should be a primary one. Many universities have already developed such programs, but in most cases the scope of such efforts is limited. Some institutions around the country have created formal courses on research ethics. Although the number of such courses is increasing, only a very small percentage of graduate students are currently participating. The further development of such courses should be advocated, and established scientists should encourage their students and post docs to take part.[4, 10, 14]

A final approach involves a significant effort among universities, industry, and government in a problem solving attempt to establish effective and ethical working arrangements among the players.[3, 4, 5, 12, 15, 19] During the conference there were many comments that either helped establish or endorse the need for such an effort. Because of the widespread interest in this approach, it will be dealt with as an independent section and presented below.

PROPOSAL: A CONFERENCE TO ESTABLISH ACADEMIA–INDUSTRY RESEARCH RELATIONSHIPS

The Problems

There are a host of problems that confront universities and industry when they want to conduct research together. Though often phrased in legal terminology, the issues are either questions of fairness between institutions or conflicts of academic values in scientific research.

Often the problems exist because universities tend to be inexperienced, naive, open, free, and undisciplined.[9] University scientists sometimes view themselves as being immune to university regulations, while their administrators fume at their attitudes.[20] Both administrators and scientists may fail to see that work in academic settings resembles work in industrial settings, in the sense that a hierarchy exists with people in charge. Consequently, university people may not be trained to be effective managers, nor are they trained in business ethics, in effective team management, in the evaluation of peers and subordinates, in the fundamentals of contract, and, sometimes, in good research practices. Under these conditions, management dilemmas tend to turn into ethical dilemmas.[12] Universities are badly in need of well thought out standards.[12]

Another problem is that several important issues require careful negotiation between the university and its industrial research sponsor. One of the issues is the ownership of intellectual property, essentially patents and copyrights. At present there is significant variation within universities with respect to patent arrangements.[20] In some universities patent issues are under dispute.[9] Controversy still exists over who owns the notebooks: the scientist, the university, or industry.[15] And no matter who owns the lab book, there is still the question of who owns the intellectual property.[20] Ownership issues have become a greater problem for universities due to more sources of income becoming available to them.[4] These issues need clarification because universities often do not fully realize the scope of their ownership potential with respect to research conducted in their facilities. Conversely, faculty inventors may be unaware that they are unjustly enriching themselves.[20]

Related to the ownership of intellectual property are some important financial issues. When opportunities arise for the commercialization of inventions, how are decisions made about which ones to select?[4] When both industry and academia stand to benefit, how is the division of spoils determined? What is the proper involvement for academic researchers in ownership of stock options, stock equity, and other financial rewards?[4, 9] When industry licenses a product, who should profit from the licensing agreements, in what form should the profit be (for example, front fees, milestone payments, and royalties), and how much?[4, 12, 15] More and more faculty are forming biotech companies or are officers in companies.[9] In these instances, what are the appropriate arrangements between the university and the scientist when the scientist is an officer in a company? Should the university receive gifts from the company?[15]

Issues related to secrecy, publication rights, and authorship may also become problems in negotiation. Although secrecy in universities has not yet been adequately studied,[2] concerns about the protection of information about university based technology, and the effect of enforced secrecy on students has previously been mentioned. What are appropriate guidelines for the withholding of technical information? What are appropriate guidelines for publication by universities and authorship by industries?[4] Should raw data from previously published reports be made available to scholars after an appropriate period of time?[10]

Issues pertaining to students require carefully thought out agreements. Under what circumstances is it acceptable for companies to pay for student stipends?[4]

There may be conflict of interest between the welfare of the student and the financial interest of the investigator.[2] Under what circumstances should graduate students or post docs be allowed to work on research of potential commercial value to faculty?[5] How can a balance be established that protects the right of students to publish (thus becoming more competitive in the job market), while meeting the requirements of industry for restriction of information.[2]

Finally, though not of least importance, when money from industry is present, what is the proper level of influence by a funding industry on research performers in universities? What are the mechanisms for determining research agendas and goals?[4]

A Proposal

In order to establish effective ethical and business guidelines for universities and industry to work together in research relationships, a concerted effort is required to further identify and address the problems.[12, 19] To insure its effectiveness, it would be essential for all significant interests to be represented. The format would be a national conference preceded by adequate advance deliberation by working groups.

Potentially the American Association for the Advancement of Science could play a leadership role in the development of these guidelines.[4] Alternatively, the process for establishing the guidelines could come from direct meetings between universities and industry.[15] In either case, a sound approach would be to find examples of university models that work and use those as the basis for discussion.[21] Prior to the initiation of the conference, a non-governmental board should be established to collect information on the state of research ethics. This has not yet been done.[4]

The process should involve scientists who are actively involved in research as well as administrators, technology transfer people, and representatives from the ethics community. Conditions should be established to maximize the development of trust. To this end, the legal viewpoint should be kept out of the process for as long as possible.[4]

One model that could serve as a reference for the development of guidelines is the concept of university based research centers, such as those advocated by the National Science Foundation for many years. These centers, which involve a consortium of funds from various industrial sources, stimulate the movement of research basic investigations. Fundamental to the creation of these centers has been the negotiation of a workable set of operating guidelines by all concerned.[3]

The collective experience of the NSF university based research centers is that they: establish a balance of interests among the participants; produce graduate theses that are better reconciled; facilitate the appropriate involvement of industrial sponsors in the setting of research agendas; produce PhDs for industry; and broaden the experience of students.[3]

REFERENCES

1 Haber, E. (1996) Industry and the university. *Nature Biotechnology* 14: 1501–1502.
2 Blumenthal, D. (1995) Academic–industry relationships in the 1990s: Continuity and Change. Oral presentation at symposium, *Ethical issues in research relationships between universities and industry*, Baltimore, MD.
3 Betz, F. (1995) Panel discussion at symposium, *Ethical issues in research relationships between universities and industry*, Baltimore, MD.
4 David, E.E., Jr. (1995) No-brainers and nonstarters: an outside perspective. Oral presentation at symposium, *Ethical issues in research relationships between universities and industry*, Baltimore, MD.
5 Schmitt, R.W. (1995) Conflict or synergy: university, industry, research relations. Oral presentation at symposium, *Ethical issues in research relationships between universities and industry*, Baltimore, MD., 1995.
6 Charrow, R.P. (1995) Grappling with conflicts: how to keep off the front page of the *Post* and the back page of a congressional subpoena. Oral presentation at symposium, *Ethical issues in research relationships between universities and industry*, Baltimore, MD.
7 Seashore-Louis, K., Swayze, J.D., Anderson, M.S., (1993) Ethical problems in academic research. *Academic Scientist* 81: 542–543.
8 Crossen, C.M. (1995) Drugs and money, Oral presentation at symposium, *Ethical issues in research relationships between universities and industry*, Baltimore, MD.
9 Goldstein, A.L. (1995) Academic Scientist as industrialist: experience at the interface-Part I. Oral presentation at symposium, *Ethical issues in research relationships between universities and industry*, Baltimore, MD.
10 Shamoo, A.E. (1995) Summary: what have we learned? Oral presentation at symposium, *Ethical issues in research relationships between universities and industry*, Baltimore, MD.
11 Krimsky, S. (1995) An evaluation of disclosure of financial interests in scientific publications. oral presentation at symposium, *Ethical issues in research relationships between universities and industry*, Baltimore, MD.
12 Esposito, V.M. (1995) Panel discussion at symposium, *Ethical issues in research relationships between universities and industry*, Baltimore, MD.
13 Thompson, D. (1993) Understanding financial conflicts of interests. *New England Journal of Medicine*, 329: 573–576.
14 Davis, M. (1995) Panel discussion at symposium, *Ethical issues in research relationships between universities and industry*, Baltimore, MD.
15 Gottlieb, A.A. (1995) Academic Scientist as industrialist: experience at the interface-Part II. Oral presentation at symposium, *Ethical issues in research relationships between universities and industry*, Baltimore, MD.
16 Greenberg, D.S. (1996) An unprecedented research kick, The Washington Post, Dec. 27, A23.
17 Glick, J.L. (1995) Panel discussion at symposium, *Ethical issues in research relationships between universities and industry*, Baltimore, MD.
18 Galasso, G.J. (1995) Federal conflict of interest policies. Oral presentation at symposium, *Ethical issues in research relationships between universities and industry*, Baltimore, MD.
19 Tramont, E.C. (1995) Panel discussion at symposium, *Ethical issues in research relationships between universities and industry*, Baltimore, MD.
20 Wasserman, S.S. (1995) Panel discussion at symposium, *Ethical issues in research relationships between universities and industry*, Baltimore, MD.
21 Frankel, M.S. (1995) Panel discussion at symposium, *Ethical issues in research relationships between universities and industry*, Baltimore, MD.

[32]

UNEASY ALLIANCE

Clinical Investigators and the Pharmaceutical Industry

THOMAS BODENHEIMER, M.D.

CLINICAL practice is changing rapidly. New cardiovascular drugs, antiinflammatory drugs, cancer chemotherapy, and other pharmacologic weapons are being added to physicians' therapeutic armamentarium virtually daily. Most clinical studies that bring new drugs from bench to bedside are financed by pharmaceutical companies. Many of these drug trials are rigorously designed, employing the skills of outstanding clinical researchers at leading academic institutions.

But academic medical centers are no longer the sole citadels of clinical research. The past 10 years have seen the spectacular growth of a new research model. Commercially oriented networks of contract-research organizations (CROs) and site-management organizations (SMOs) have altered the drug-trial landscape, forcing academic medical centers to rethink their participation in industry-funded drug research.

The infusion of industry dollars into an industry–investigator partnership has clearly improved clinical practice. Yet the medical literature contains many articles expressing concern about industrial funding of clinical research. Stelfox et al. found that authors whose work supported the safety of calcium-channel antagonists had a higher frequency of financial relationships with the drugs' manufacturers than authors whose work did not support the safety of these medications.[1] Davidson reported that results favoring a new therapy over a traditional one were more likely if the study was funded by the new therapy's manufacturer.[2] Cho and Bero demonstrated that articles from symposiums sponsored by a single drug company were more likely than articles without company support to have outcomes favorable to the sponsor's drugs.[3] Friedberg et al. reported that 5 percent of industry-sponsored pharmacoeconomic studies of cancer drugs reached unfavorable conclusions about the company's products, as compared with 38 percent of studies with nonprofit funding that reached similar conclusions.[4]

How much influence does industry have over the work and products of the research community? Can practicing physicians trust the information they receive about the medications they are prescribing? Does the shift from the academic to the commercial research sector give industry too much control over clinical drug trials?

In this report, I discuss some of the problems raised by pharmaceutical-industry funding of drug trials, problems that may deepen as trials are increasingly conducted by commercial organizations. I interviewed 39 participants in the process: 6 pharmaceutical executives, 12 clinical investigators, 9 people from university research offices, 2 physicians with CROs, 8 people who have studied the process of clinical drug trials, and 2 professional medical writers. Each interview consisted of standard questions plus an opportunity for the interviewees to discuss the industry–investigator relationship in a general way. Several interviewees preferred not to allow the use of their names in the article.

THE CLINICAL-DRUG-TRIAL SYSTEM

The Food and Drug Administration (FDA) requires manufacturers to show that their products pass tests of efficacy and safety.[5,6] For such drugs as antibiotics for acute infections, large populations and long time lines are seldom needed to establish efficacy and safety. With the new emphasis on prevention and treatment of chronic diseases, however, clinical drug research has changed. Many people must take antihypertensive drugs and lipid-lowering drugs for many years in order to prevent relatively few undesired clinical end points.[7] To establish the efficacy and safety of preventive products and products designed to treat chronic disease, clinical trials must be large, lengthy, and conducted at multiple centers, because a single site cannot recruit enough patients to ensure statistical validity.

The average cost of developing one new drug is estimated to be $300 million to $600 million.[8] Of the $6 billion in industry-generated money for clinical trials worldwide yearly, about $3.3 billion goes to investigators in the United States.[9] Seventy percent of the money for clinical drug trials in the United States comes from industry rather than from the National Institutes of Health (NIH).

THE SHIFT TO COMMERCIAL DRUG NETWORKS

Until recently, the pharmaceutical industry needed academic physicians to perform drug trials for three reasons: companies did not have the in-house expertise to design trials themselves, academic medical centers provided patients as subjects for trials, and companies needed the prestige of academic publications to market their products. Lately, industry's dependence on academia has weakened: industry employs top-level research physicians to design and interpret drug trials, and community physicians have become a reliable source of patients.

The New England Journal of Medicine

Moreover, pharmaceutical firms are frustrated with academic medical centers. Most medical schools and teaching hospitals require that industry–investigator agreements be approved by an office of sponsored research. Slow review of industry proposals by academic research offices and institutional review boards (which must review all trials to protect patients' safety[10]) delays the starting dates of trials. Since academic physicians have multiple responsibilities in teaching, research, and patient care, trials may proceed more slowly than the pharmaceutical firms desire. For each day's delay in gaining FDA approval of a drug, the manufacturer loses, on average, $1.3 million. Speed is paramount for pharmaceutical firms.

To expedite trials, industry is turning from academic medical centers to a growing for-profit marketplace whose key players are CROs and SMOs.[11-13] In 1991, 80 percent of industry money for clinical trials went to academic medical centers; by 1998, the figure had dropped precipitously to 40 percent.[14] Evidence suggests that the commercial sector completes trials more rapidly and more cheaply than academic medical centers.[11]

Because multicenter trials may involve hundreds of sites and investigators, few pharmaceutical manufacturers choose to manage the trials themselves. CROs, which employ physician-scientists, pharmacists, biostatisticians, and managers, offer manufacturers a menu of services. Large drug companies often create their own study designs and contract with CROs to develop a network of sites, implement the trial protocol at those sites, and send report forms to the sponsoring company, which performs the data analysis. Smaller pharmaceutical firms may hire a CRO to manage the entire trial, including study design, data analysis, and preparation of FDA applications and journal articles. Several hundred CROs compete for the drug-trial business; the largest are Quintiles Transnational and Covance.

CROs may use both academic medical centers and community physicians to recruit patients for a trial. In the community arm of drug trials, yet another intermediary has entered the picture, the SMO. CROs may subcontract with for-profit SMOs to organize networks of community physicians, ensure rapid enrollment of patients, and deliver case-report forms to the CRO. Some trials have four layers (manufacturer, CRO, SMO, and physician–investigator), a situation reminiscent of the multitiered managed-care model (employer, health maintenance organization, independent practice association, and physician). Three of the largest SMOs are Clinical Studies Limited, Hill Top Research, and Affiliated Research Centers. SMOs provide community-physician investigators with administrative support and help market investigators' services to pharmaceutical companies.[15] They have been criticized for producing data of poor quality, inadequately training investigators, and costing more than a system of independent sites unassociated with an SMO.[13,15]

Competition for drug-trial money has stiffened as hundreds of CROs, SMOs, academic medical centers, and independent nonacademic sites scramble for a larger piece of the pie. According to Gregg Fromell of Covance, a leading CRO, "academic medical centers have a bad reputation in the industry because many overpromise and underdeliver." In contrast, critics, including Dr. Sidney Wolfe of Public Citizen, view CROs and the commercial drug-trial network as handmaidens of pharmaceutical companies, concerned with the approval and marketing of drugs rather than with true science. Whereas the academic and commercial drug-trial sectors can be seen as distinct networks with conflicting cultures, they also interlock, since CROs often act as intermediaries between drug companies and academic investigators.

Several academic medical centers are fighting to regain lost market share, transforming themselves into research networks to compete with the commercial drug-trial sector.[14,16] Columbia University, Cornell University, and New York Presbyterian Hospital have created a Clinical Trials Network as a joint venture. With funding from both industry and NIH sources, the network brings together academic researchers and community-based physicians in cardiology, hepatology, neurology, and oncology. The network has instituted required training for all participants and has centralized contracting, budgeting, and reimbursement systems. The network plans to be financially self-sufficient in a few years. Director Michael Leahey says, "Our goal is to take clinical research back from for-profit companies and place it where it rightfully belongs — in networks that are partnerships between academic medicine and community practice. We are trying to formulate a real alternative to the for-profit drug-trial entrepreneurs."

In 1997 the University of Pittsburgh Medical Center Health System chartered the Pittsburgh Clinical Research Network (PCRN), a single point of contact between industry and clinical researchers in academic and community sites. PCRN provides the administrative procedures associated with clinical trials in such areas as contracting, institutional-review-board approval, and project management. Academic research expertise and a large hospital and community-practice network give PCRN resources unavailable to most commercial SMOs. PCRN's medical director, David Watkins, feels that "academic medical centers are sleeping giants that are beginning to awaken and respond to industry's needs."

Duke University and the University of Rochester are also leaders in developing academic clinical-research networks. Some academic medical centers will probably succeed in revamping their drug-trial business; others will fail.

HEALTH POLICY REPORT

INDUSTRY–INVESTIGATOR RELATIONSHIPS

Trial Design

A company seeking FDA approval for a product often designs a clinical trial in its research division and circulates the proposed design to recognized investigators in that field. If the company has no in-house expertise, outside investigators are asked to design the trial. In some cases, company and academic investigators form a steering committee to discuss a trial protocol. In an interview, Dr. Thierry LeJemtel, of the Albert Einstein College of Medicine Division of Cardiology, said that 20 years ago outside investigators designed the studies, but that now companies write the protocols and bring in outside investigators pro forma, with little intention of changing the study design. In-house control is more likely in the commercial sector than in the academic sector, because of the limited expertise of many community-physician investigators.

Sometimes an investigator will propose a drug trial to the drug's manufacturer. Two investigators interviewed, including Steven Cummings, professor of medicine and epidemiology at the University of California at San Francisco, found that companies' marketing departments, which often rule on studies to be conducted after a drug has received FDA approval, declined to fund clinically important studies at least partly because the results might reduce sales of the drug.

Companies may design studies likely to favor their products. Bero and Rennie, in an article worth study by all physicians, catalogue the methods companies can use to produce desired results.[17]

If a drug is tested in a healthier population (younger, with fewer coexisting conditions and with milder disease) than the population that will actually receive the drug, a trial may find that the drug relieves symptoms and creates fewer adverse effects than will actually be the case.[17] Rochon et al. found that only 2.1 percent of subjects in trials of nonsteroidal antiinflammatory drugs were 65 years of age or older, even though these drugs are more commonly used and have a higher incidence of side effects in the elderly.[18]

If a new drug is compared with an insufficient dose of a competing product, the new drug will appear more efficacious.[17] Rochon et al. concluded that trials of nonsteroidal antiinflammatory drugs always found the sponsoring company's product superior or equal to the comparison product; in 48 percent of the trials, the dose of the sponsoring company's drug was higher than that of the comparison drug.[19] According to Johansen and Gotzsche, most trials comparing fluconazole with amphotericin B used oral, not intravenous, amphotericin B, thereby favoring fluconazole, because oral amphotericin B is poorly absorbed.[20]

Clinical trials often use surrogate end points that may not correlate with more important clinical end points. Companies may study many surrogate end points and publish results only for those that favor their product.[7,17,21]

Data Analysis

A study's raw data are generally stored centrally at the company or CRO. Investigators may receive only portions of the data. Some principal investigators have the capacity to analyze all the data from a large trial, but companies prefer to retain control over this process.

A physician-executive at one company explained, "We are reluctant to provide the data tape because some investigators want to take the data beyond where the data should go." Several investigators, including Dr. LeJemtel, countered that industry control over data allows companies to "provide the spin on the data that favors them." In the commercial sector, where most investigators are more concerned with reimbursement than with authorship, industry can easily control clinical-trial data.

Publishing the Results

For academic investigators, publication in peer-reviewed journals is the coin of the realm. For pharmaceutical firms, in contrast, the essential product is the new-drug application to the FDA. In the absence of FDA approval, no journal article is worth a cent to a drug company. Yet publication in prestigious journals is important, to persuade physicians to prescribe the company's products.

Some multicenter trials have publication committees, which may be dominated by in-house or outside investigators, that write up the results for publication. In other cases, the company or CRO writes the reports for publication, circulating draft manuscripts to the investigators who will be listed as authors. Authorship may be determined by such criteria as who participated in designing the study, who enrolled the most patients, and who has a prominent name in the field.

Control over Publication

Many academic medical centers review contracts between industry and investigators, insisting on the investigator's right to publish the trial's results and allowing the company prepublication review, with a time limit of 60 to 90 days. Nikki Zapol, head of the sponsored-research office of Massachusetts General Hospital, estimates that 30 to 50 percent of contracts submitted by companies have unacceptable publication clauses that must be renegotiated.

In a survey of life-science faculty members, 27 percent of those with industry funding experienced delays of more than six months in the publication of their study results.[22] Chalmers argues that the results of substantial numbers of clinical trials are never published at all.[23]

In 1996, Canadian investigator Nancy Olivieri and colleagues found that deferiprone, used to treat thal-

The New England Journal of Medicine

assemia major, could worsen hepatic fibrosis. Apotex, the sponsoring company, threatened legal action if Olivieri published the findings. The contract between Apotex and Olivieri forbade disclosure of results for three years after the study without the company's consent. An article was eventually published.[24,25]

In 1987, the manufacturer of Synthroid (levothyroxine) contracted with University of California researcher Betty Dong to study whether Synthroid was more effective than competing thyroid preparations. In 1990, Dong found Synthroid to be no more effective than other preparations, including generic preparations. The sponsoring company refused to allow the findings to be published; the contract with Dong stipulated that no information could be released without the consent of the manufacturer. An article was finally published in 1997.[26]

Six investigators interviewed for this report cited cases of articles whose publication was stopped or whose content was altered by the funding company. In one case, according to Dr. Cummings, the company held up the prepublication review process for over half a year, then requested pages of detailed revisions that would have made the manuscript more favorable to the company's official marketing position. During the delay, the company secretly wrote a competing article on the same topic, which was favorable to the company's viewpoint.

In another case, the drug being investigated did not work. The investigator argued that scientific integrity required publishing the findings. The company never refused to publish, but it stalled until the investigator lost interest.

Another investigator, most of whose relations with industry have been without problems, related the case of two trials of the same drug, one more favorable to the company. Despite a protest from the investigator, the results of the less favorable trial were never published.

A fourth investigator found that a drug he was studying caused adverse reactions. He sent his manuscript to the sponsoring company for review. The company vowed never to fund his work again and published a competing article with scant mention of the adverse effects.

Dr. Curt Furberg, professor of public health sciences at Wake Forest University School of Medicine and principal investigator in a study whose results were unfavorable to the sponsoring company, refused to place his name on the published results of the study, because the sponsor was "attempting to wield undue influence on the nature of the final paper. This effort was so oppressive that we felt it inhibited academic freedom."[27]

A sixth investigator recounted two examples of suppressed manuscripts regarding negative studies whose results were sufficiently important to publish.

In scenarios such as these, the frequency of which

is unknown, companies repeatedly delay publication, eventually exhausting investigators who are busy with other projects. One industry executive explained that such cases result from priority setting within the company; with limited personnel to produce publications, certain trials take precedence over others. However, as one investigator described it, "when results favor the company, everything is great. But when results are disappointing, there is commonly an effort to spin, downplay, or change findings." A CRO executive added that "industry obstruction to publishing is a big problem. They are nervous if bad data comes out and gets into the mass media." Investigators in the commercial sector may be less concerned than those in academia with contract clauses guaranteeing their right to publish, thereby giving industry greater control over publications.

Authorship

In the past, publications were written by a study's principal investigator. More recently, a practice that one might call the nonwriting author–nonauthor writer syndrome has developed. Many interviews conducted for this report confirmed the wide prevalence of this syndrome in publications of drug-trial reports, editorials, and review articles. The syndrome has two features: a professional medical writer ("ghostwriter") employed by a drug company, CRO, or medical communications company, who is paid to write an article but is not named as an author; and a clinical investigator ("guest author"), who appears as an author but does not analyze the data or write the manuscript.[28-30] Ghostwriters typically receive a packet of materials from which they write the article; they may be instructed to insert a key paragraph favorable to the company's product.

The nonwriting author, who may be uninvolved in the research and have been requested to author the article to enhance its prestige, has final control over the manuscript. But many of these authors are busy and may not perform a thorough review. This guest-ghost syndrome[31,32] is a growing phenomenon, particularly in the commercial sector, where community-physician investigators have little interest in authorship.

In one study, 19 percent of the articles surveyed had named authors who did not contribute sufficiently to the articles to meet the criteria for authorship of the International Committee of Medical Journal Editors. Eleven percent had ghostwriters who contributed to the work but were not named as authors.[33,34] In justifying the nonwriting author–nonauthor writer syndrome, one industry executive explained that professional medical (ghost) writers are well trained, that investigators may be too busy to write, and that "nonwriting authors" are at fault if they do not carefully review ghostwritten manuscripts. An alternative view, articulated by Eric Campbell, of the Institute for Health Policy at Massachusetts General Hospital and Harvard Medical School, holds that "a manuscript represents the accumulation of the intellectual and physical processes conducted under the aegis of a study and should be produced by the people who have actually been involved in the design, conduct, and supervision of the research." Tim Franson, Vice President for Clinical Research and Regulatory Affairs at Eli Lilly, believes that "any parties, be they industry staff, investigators, or others who contribute to the content of articles should have their names listed on the article."

CONCLUSIONS

Without industry funding, important advances in disease prevention and treatment would not have occurred. In the words of Lee Goldman, chairman of the Department of Medicine, University of California at San Francisco, "companies translate biologic advances into useable products for patients. They do it for a profit motive, but they do it, and it needs to be done." Investigators interviewed for this report confirmed that many collaborations with pharmaceutical companies were conducted on a high professional level.

But when results are disappointing for a company, conflicts may develop. Dr. Furberg, with years of experience in industry-funded drug trials, stated: "Companies can play hardball, and many investigators can't play hardball back. You send the paper to the company for comments, and that's the danger. Can you handle the changes the company wants? Will you give in a little, a little more, then capitulate? It's tricky for those who need money for more studies."

Although academic–industry drug trials have been tainted by the profit incentive, they do contain the potential for balance between the commercial interests of industry and the scientific goals of investigators. In contrast, trials conducted in the commercial sector are heavily tipped toward industry interests, since for-profit CROs and SMOs, contracting with industry in a competitive market, will fail if they offend their funding sources. The pharmaceutical industry must appreciate the risks inherent in its partnership with the commercial drug-trial sector: potential public and physician skepticism about the results of clinical drug trials and a devaluation of the insights provided through close relationships with academic scientists.

A number of authors have recommended changes to resolve the problems of clinical drug trials.[11,35-37] An essential ingredient of any solution is increasing the independence of investigators to conduct and publish their research. Some investigators interviewed for this article felt that drug trials should be funded by industry but that design, implementation, data analysis, and publication should be controlled entirely by academic medical centers and investigators. The rise of the commercial sector — which reduces

rather than enhances the independence of investigators — appears to be moving drug trials in the opposite direction.

I am indebted to Janice Kohn for research assistance.

REFERENCES

1. Stelfox HT, Chua G, O'Rourke K, Detsky AS. Conflict of interest in the debate over calcium-channel antagonists. N Engl J Med 1998;338: 101-6.
2. Davidson RA. Source of funding and outcome of clinical trials. J Gen Intern Med 1986;1:155-8.
3. Cho MK, Bero LA. The quality of drug studies published in symposium proceedings. Ann Intern Med 1996;124:485-9.
4. Friedberg M, Saffran B, Stinson TJ, Nelson W, Bennett CL. Evaluation of conflict of interest in economic analyses of new drugs used in oncology. JAMA 1999;282:1453-7.
5. Chow S-C, Liu J-P. Design and analysis of clinical trials. New York: John Wiley, 1998.
6. Spilker BA. The drug development and approval process. (See: http://www.phrma.org.)
7. Psaty BM, Weiss NS, Furberg CD, et al. Surrogate end points, health outcomes, and the drug-approval process for the treatment of risk factors for cardiovascular disease. JAMA 1999;282:786-90.
8. Mathieu MP, ed. Parexel's pharmaceutical R & D statistical sourcebook 1998. Waltham, Mass.: Parexel International Corporation, 1999.
9. An industry in evolution. Boston: Centerwatch, 1999.
10. Woodward B. Challenges to human subject protections in US medical research. JAMA 1999;282:1947-52.
11. From bench to bedside: preserving the research mission of academic health centers. New York: Commonwealth Fund, 1999.
12. CRO mergers bring mixed results. Centerwatch 1997;4(6):1, 9-16.
13. Henderson L. The ups and downs of SMO usage. Centerwatch 1999; 6(5):1, 4-8.
14. Getz KA. AMCs rekindling clinical research partnerships with industry. Boston: Centerwatch, 1999.
15. Vogel JR. Maximizing the benefits of SMOs. Appl Clin Trials 1999; 8(11):56-62.
16. Academic medical centers: slowly turning the tide. Centerwatch 1997; 4(6):1-8.
17. Bero LA, Rennie D. Influences on the quality of published drug studies. Int J Technol Assess Health Care 1996;12(2):209-37.
18. Rochon PA, Berger PB, Gordon M. The evolution of clinical trials: inclusion and representation. CMAJ 1998;159:1373-4.
19. Rochon PA, Gurwitz JH, Simms RW, et al. A study of manufacturer-supported trials of nonsteroidal anti-inflammatory drugs in the treatment of arthritis. Arch Intern Med 1994;154:157-63.
20. Johansen HK, Gotzsche PC. Problems in the design and reporting of trials of antifungal agents encountered during meta-analysis. JAMA 1999; 282:1752-9.
21. Temple R. Are surrogate markers adequate to assess cardiovascular disease drugs? JAMA 1999;282:790-5.
22. Blumenthal D, Campbell EG, Anderson MS, Causino N, Louis KS. Withholding research results in academic life science: evidence from a national survey of faculty. JAMA 1997;277:1224-8.
23. Chalmers I. Underreporting research is scientific misconduct. JAMA 1990;263:1405-8.
24. Olivieri NF, Brittenham GM, McLaren CE, et al. Long-term safety and effectiveness of iron-chelation therapy with deferiprone for thalassemia major. N Engl J Med 1998;339:417-23.
25. Phillips RA, Hoey J. Constraints of interest: lessons at the Hospital for Sick Children. CMAJ 1998;159:955-7. [Erratum, CMAJ 1998;159: 1244.]
26. Rennie D. Thyroid storm. JAMA 1997;277:1238-43.
27. Applegate WB, Furberg CD, Byington RP, Grimm R Jr. The Multicenter Isradipine Diuretic Atherosclerosis Study. JAMA 1997;277:297.
28. Levy D. Ghostwriters a hidden resource for drug makers. USA Today. September 25, 1996.
29. Larkin M. Whose article is it anyway? Lancet 1999;354:136.
30. Ghost with a chance in publishing undergrowth. Lancet 1993;342: 1498-9.
31. Rennie D, Flanagin A. Authorship! Authorship! Guests, ghosts, grafters, and the two-sided coin. JAMA 1994;271:469-71.
32. Brennan TA. Buying editorials. N Engl J Med 1994;331:673-5.
33. Flanagin A, Carey LA, Fontanarosa PB, et al. Prevalence of articles

The New England Journal of Medicine

with honorary authors and ghost authors in peer-reviewed medical journals. JAMA 1998;280:222-4.

34. International Committee of Medical Journal Editors. Uniform requirements for manuscripts submitted to biomedical journals. JAMA 1997; 277:927-34. [Erratum, JAMA 1998;279:510.]

35. Wood AJJ, Stein CM, Woosley R. Making medicines safer — the need for an independent drug safety board. N Engl J Med 1998;339:1851-4.

36. Kunin CM. Clinical investigators and the pharmaceutical industry. Ann Intern Med 1978;89:Suppl:842-5.

37. Shine KI. Some imperatives for clinical research. JAMA 1997;278: 245-6.

[33]

Ethics Review for Sale? Conflict of Interest and Commercial Research Review Boards

TRUDO LEMMENS and
BENJAMIN FREEDMAN

University of Toronto; McGill University

AT A 1997 CONGRESSIONAL HEARING ON RESEARCH
involving human subjects, Representative Christopher Shays
(R-Conn.) was startled to hear of the existence of institutional
review boards (IRBs) set up as profit-making ventures (Stolberg 1997).
The congressional hearing marked one of the first public discussions
of the issue of private, commercial review of research involving human
subjects. Only recently has the phenomenon of commercial review attracted limited scholarly attention (Tendy 1996; Wadman 1997; Heath
1998; Kefalides 2000). More surprisingly, no governmental agency has
systematic data on commercial IRBs. This comes as a surprise, considering the fact that many commercial IRBs have been inspected for years by
the Food and Drug Administration (FDA) or received formal assurances
from the Office for the Protection from Research Risks (OPRR) (Office
of Inspector General 1998d).

The growth of the market for commercial research review is the latest
development in the history of IRBs. Since the 1960s, federal funding
agencies and the FDA have gradually introduced approval by an IRB as a
precondition for research involving human subjects. Originally required
only for research undertaken within specific research centers, granting
agencies soon expanded the requirement of IRB review to all federally
funded institutions. In 1981, the FDA also clarified that any medical

research used to support an application for approval of new drugs or medical devices, whether the research is performed within institutions or by private physicians, has to obtain approval from a duly constituted IRB. Many states have integrated the system of research review into their regulations and require IRBs to review all research protocols within an institution, regardless of the source of funding (Office of Inspector General 1998d).

Internationally, research review has also more clearly become a crucial element in the protection of research subjects over the last two decades. In 1975, for instance, the World Medical Association revised its Declaration of Helsinki to include a requirement that experimental procedures involving human subjects be reviewed by an independent committee (World Medical Association 1964; 1975). Furthermore, international guidelines for research requiring ethics approval were promulgated in 1991 and 1993 by the Council for International Organizations of Medical Sciences (Council for International Organizations of Medical Science 1991, 1993), and in 1995 by the World Health Organization (World Health Organization 1995). This international trend is reflected in the recent adoption of the International Conference on Harmonisation's Good Clinical Practice Guideline (hereafter ICH GCP Guideline) (International Conference on Harmonisation 1996) by several national regulatory agencies. The ICH GCP Guideline represents an effort on the part of several national regulatory agencies (in particular from the United States, Europe, and Japan) to develop a common standard for the conduct of clinical trials and the regulation of medical research (Hirtle, Lemmens, and Sprumont, 2000). The Guideline will likely set the international standard for clinical research involving human subjects, and it clearly identifies review by an independent committee as a precondition for medical research involving human subjects.

In this context of increasing need for efficient IRB review and significant growth in industry funded research, commercial IRBs found their niche. They have become very visible participants at the commercial exhibits of drug or therapeutics conferences, where fast research ethics review has become a marketable item, promoted in the well-designed brochures of contract research organizations (CROs) or commercial IRBs. Commercial research review is gaining importance as research and development of new drugs, particularly phase I studies, increasingly take place in research centers of pharmaceutical companies, in CROs, or through physicians independent from academic research centers (Office of Inspector General 1998c; Bodenheimer 2000). Researchers do not have access to IRBs established in academic centers. Thus, commercial IRBs have become crucial players in the rapidly expanding national and international drug and research industry.

Commercial IRBs can be divided in two categories: (1) freestanding commercial committees without institutional affiliation, established for the purpose of reviewing protocols for compliance with ethical and regulatory standards, often referred to as non-institutional review boards (NIRBs) or independent review boards, and (2) research review boards set up by CROs or pharmaceutical companies to review research for products developed or tested by the company itself, which we call proprietary IRBs. Often, the work of proprietary IRBs is an integral part of a wide array of services offered by the CRO. While NIRBs, by definition, review research undertaken elsewhere, proprietary IRBs typically review in-house studies. The division is far from absolute; some of the IRBs connected to CROs function as proprietary IRBs when reviewing protocols for research undertaken by the CROs themselves but also offer research review as a separate marketable product. For the sake of clarity, we will discuss proprietary and NIRBs as separate entities.

The purpose of this paper is to discuss one particular aspect of commercial research review that has been mentioned in the literature (Francis 1996; Office of Inspector General 1998a; Cho and Billings 1997) but has yet to be fully analyzed: the risk that fundamental conflicts of interest undermine the structure of commercial research review. Focusing on commercial IRBs, we point out why conflict-of-interest rules should be better developed and why they should prescribe more clearly what types of relationships are appropriate between IRBs or IRB members and research sponsors. In doing so, we recognize that the issue of the impact of financial interests on the independence of IRBs is not exclusive to commercial IRBs.

Nevertheless, we want to focus here on financial conflicts of interest that inhere in the structure and context of commercial IRBs. Two reasons justify our restricted focus. First, conflict of interest in academic research review has been discussed more extensively in the literature (Glass and Lemmens 1999; Cho and Billings 1997; Francis 1996; Jones 1995). As we will point out further, some of these conflicts are specific to research review in academic settings, and thus differ from the ones discussed here. The inherent financial conflict of interest underlying commercial IRB review has received less attention. Second, the conflicts of interest we analyze in commercial IRBs can be seen as a paradigm that has relevance for dealing with some forms of conflicts of interest affecting research review in the academic setting. We aim to clarify which conflicts are created by the commercialization of research review, and which are currently endemic to research in general. We argue that regulations do not adequately address the special nature of financial conflicts of interest affecting commercial and, increasingly, academic IRBs.

Commercial Review: A Thriving Business Escaping Public Scrutiny

The difference between commercial and academic IRBs lies primarily in the context in which they operate and, to some extent, in the goals of the medical research that these IRBs are reviewing. Traditional IRBs are generally established by nonprofit educational and research organizations, such as universities, nonprofit hospitals, granting agencies, or professional associations. Commercial IRBs, by contrast, mostly review studies on behalf of for-profit companies, such as CROs (Office of Inspector General 1998d). While this distinction is beginning to fade as a result of the significant increase in the proportion of industry-sponsored research in academic centers (Grob 1998; Maatz 1992; Kefalides 2000), it remains fair to distinguish private from academic IRBs in light of the former's focus on commercial studies. Even when private IRBs are involved in the review of research undertaken at academic health care centers, which is increasingly the case, they are primarily involved in the review of commercially sponsored research for these institutions (Office of Inspector General 1998d). Moreover, by focusing strictly on commercial IRBs, lessons can be learned about the potential need to restructure academic IRBs in the context of increasing academic entrepreneurialism. Several academic institutions have formed partnerships with CROs and set up academic IRBs to review in-house research, for example. These academic IRBs share many of the characteristics of proprietary IRBs, and our discussion of commercial IRBs is clearly relevant for determining what conflicts can arise from this situation.

The keys to the success of NIRBs seem to be the increasing demand for review of research protocols from CROs and independent physician-researchers, the speed of the review, the quality and variety of services offered, and the ability to review multisite projects (Office of Inspector

General 1998d; Heath 1998; Kefalides 2000). As Erica Heath, president of one of the largest American NIRBs, puts it: "We certainly cannot market approvals. But we can market in terms of speed, efficiency, expertise, customer relations, and complete information on readable forms" (Heath, personal communication, 1997). Unlike most academic IRBs, many NIRBs can guarantee a very short review time. The average review time of the NIRBs contacted by the Office of Inspector General was 11 days (Office of Inspector General 1998c). One survey found that some NIRBs guarantee review in as little as 5 days (Lemmens and Thompson 2000). Because of the high volume of protocols they review and the concomitant expertise of their members, many NIRBs are likely capable of giving coherent and clear instructions to improve protocols. Their reviews might be more predictable than those of some academic IRBs with more fluctuating and often less experienced membership. The latter have come under increasing criticism for their members' lack of training, administrative understaffing, and disregard of regulatory requirements (Office of Inspector General 1998a; 1998c; Kefalides 2000). Some NIRBs take a very active role in educational programs for IRB members. They sometimes have much stricter educational requirements for their members than many academic IRBs, which often hesitate to impose education on their volunteer members, who are frequently hard to recruit. Finally, many multisite trials can be efficiently reviewed by one NIRB, thus avoiding the lengthy process of going through multiple reviews, which often lead to contradictory instructions (Office of Inspector General 1998d; Heath 1998).

Proprietary IRBs offer a number of other advantages. They are directly accessible and may be under the authority of the CRO, so that research protocols can be reviewed even faster and upon special request. Setting up a proprietary IRB may be cheaper than paying an outside IRB, particularly if the CRO has a high volume of studies. Finally, a CRO may feel more comfortable in granting access to confidential information to an IRB that has a formal link with the company and adheres to its policies.

Surprisingly, notwithstanding their importance, official information on the number of NIRBs or proprietary IRBs functioning in the United States or Canada is lacking. Even the Department of Health and Human Services mentions in its official report only that there are "at least 15, and perhaps quite a few more" NIRBs and takes this guesstimate from a consortium of NIRBs (Office of Inspector General 1998d). Similarly, the Canadian Health Protection Branch has no official information on

NIRBs, although several of them are active in Canada and are recognized as playing an important role within the drug approval system.

The Health Industry Manufacturers Association's website recently listed 21 U.S. and one Canadian CROs or commercial IRBs (Health Industry Manufacturers Organization 2000). While preparing a survey on NIRBs, we found that there are at least two other Canadian NIRBs (Lemmens and Thompson 2000). Moreover, several European NIRBs and proprietary IRBs advertise their services at American conferences. These services include access to the booming European CRO industry, which benefits from the easy recruitment of human subjects in eastern European countries. While the Office of Inspector General's reports provide some information on NIRBs, there is no public information on proprietary IRBs set up within private commercial companies. The lack of clear, official information on NIRBs and the absence of any information on proprietary IRBs raise concerns in light of the public role these IRBs fulfill.

Since the congressional hearing, there have been signs in Canada, the United States, and Europe that governmental agencies are paying more attention to the phenomena of for-profit and proprietary review. In 1998, the three major federal funding agencies in Canada introduced a uniform Tri-Council Policy Statement on Ethical Conduct for Research Involving Humans (Medical Research Council, Social Sciences and Humanities Research Council, and Natural Sciences and Engineering Research Council 1998). The policy statement includes, among other things, more detailed instructions on how IRBs have to be set up. In discussing what constitutes a conflict of interest, there is a prudent reference to commercial IRBs. The statement gives, as an example of conflict of interest, a member's acceptance of "undue or excessive honoraria for their participation in the REB (e.g., *on commercial REBs*)" [the Research Ethics Board (REB) is the Canadian equivalent of the IRB] (Medical Research Council, Social Sciences and Humanities Research Council, and Natural Sciences and Engineering Research Council 1998). Unfortunately, the document offers no further discussion of commercial IRBs, nor does it clarify why commercial IRBs are singled out. As we will discuss further, undue payment may be a concern, but it is not clear why that would be an issue only for commercial IRBs.

In the United States, federal agencies involved in human subjects research took several initiatives following the congressional hearings on the protection of research subjects. The Department of Health and Human Services (Office of Inspector General 1998a; 1998b; 1998c; 1998d) and

the National Institutes of Health (Bell Associates 1998) published detailed reports that critically assess the adequacy of the current research
review system. One report of the Office of Inspector General focuses
exclusively on the emergence of "independent boards," another common term for NIRBs (Office of Inspector General 1998d). The first
official report on the subject, it indicates very clearly that commercial
NIRBs have become crucial players within the current review system
and identifies the advantages of NIRBs as well as their potential problems, with conflict of interest among the latter. The National Bioethics
Advisory Council is also looking into the adequacy of the current system of human subjects protection (Moreno 1998), and it is hoped that
they will deal with the phenomenon of private commercial review and
problems associated with it in their final recommendations. Recent suspensions of research institutions by OPRR have increased the calls for a
major reform of the system, and it remains to be seen what the role of
commercial IRBs in any new structure will be and whether the concerns
raised in this paper will be addressed.

In Europe, a recent scandal involving the alleged "importation" of
research subjects from eastern European countries (Estonia, Poland, and
perhaps even the war-torn former Yugoslavia) by a research company
located in Switzerland has raised awareness among regulatory agencies
of the loopholes in the regulation of medical research. It provoked an
official investigation into the activities of the CRO and the private IRB
responsible for reviewing the importation scheme (Hirtle, Lemmens,
and Sprumont 2000; Schaad 1999a; 1999b; 1999c). This case serves
to highlight some of the potential consequences arising from a lack of
clear conflict-of-interest guidelines. Sometime after the importation of
research subjects was exposed and became the subject of an investigation,
it was discovered that the director of the CRO had, for a long time, also
been the main administrator of the private ethics committee. While
this one incident does not represent a standard practice among CROs or
NIRBs, it does highlight the need for analysis and regulation of conflicts
of interest affecting such boards.

What Constitutes a Conflict of Interest?

While the concept of conflict of interest is clearly in vogue in discussions
around health policy and the term is used in many different contexts, it is

hard to find a clear definition of it. *Conflict of Interest in Academic Health Centers*, a 1990 report of the Association of Academic Health Centers (AHC), mentions the importance of professional norms for determining what conflicts of interest are. It states that a conflict exists "when legal obligations or widely recognized professional norms are likely to be compromised by a person's other interests" (Shipp 1992). James P. Orlowski and Leon Wateska define conflict of interest more narrowly as "a discrepancy between the personal interests and the professional responsibilities of a person in a position of trust" (Orlowski and Wateska 1992). Dennis Thompson defines a conflict of interest as "a set of conditions in which professional judgment concerning a primary interest (such as patient's welfare or the validity of research) tends to be unduly influenced by a secondary interest (such as financial gain)" (Thompson 1993). Other authors also stress that conflicts of interest arise when professional obligations clash with other interests (Shipp 1992; Erde 1996).

Secondary interests are not in themselves improper, but they should be subservient to primary interests. Secondary interests are often financial, but they can also be intangible ones, such as gaining professional advantage, prestige, or power. Following this definition, the central questions arise: what are the primary obligations of IRBs, what is the role of IRB members *qua* members, and how seriously can these obligations be affected by other interests? The impact of conflicts of interest can only be understood when the primary obligations of IRBs and IRB members are clarified.

IRBs have a protective public role. "The primary purpose [of IRB review]" according to the FDA Rules and Regulations, "is to assure the protection of the rights and welfare of the human subjects" (21 CFR 56). The ICH GCP Guideline refers to "the protection of the rights, safety and well-being of subjects" in its definitions of "independent ethics committee" and "institutional review board" (International Conference on Harmonisation 1996). As thus defined, an IRB's primary duty is to protect human subjects of research (Levine 1988).

In light of their public policy role, we argue that rules of administrative law ought to inspire us in refining the rules by which IRBs are organized. Rules of administrative law apply to a variety of judicial bodies and governmental agencies and may vary accordingly. It is not easy to determine which of these bodies resembles the IRBs most closely. In many respects, the role of IRBs can be situated somewhere between, for example, the roles of public curators and administrative licensing boards.

Licensing boards are similar to IRBs in that they often have an important public policy goal, they are given much discretion in the implementation of their policies, and their decisions often have a major impact on the activities they regulate. Moreover, administrative licensing boards are often specialized bodies, dealing with issues that require particular expertise from board members. The same is true for IRBs, which function within highly specialized areas of medical research. On the other hand, the IRB's role is clearly more intimately related to individual people's rights and welfare than, say, a land development, transportation, or liquor licensing board. Because of their protective role and their responsibility with respect to the rights, integrity, and well-being of individual research participants, IRBs have some of the characteristics of public curators. They are first and foremost obliged to look after the welfare and rights of research subjects. In addition, the IRB's mandate also resembles that of human rights commissions, when these are involved in policy rather than litigation. Finally, while specialized knowledge on the part of some IRB members is required, representation by the community and by members of different disciplines are core requirements for IRB review. Thus, IRBs differ from highly specialized administrative or professional bodies in that there is clearly public involvement and public responsibility directed toward the physical and emotional well-being of individual research participants.

Bias and Conflict of Interest in Administrative Law

Because of this resemblance to administrative bodies, administrative law on conflict of interest (discussed under the heading "bias") can inspire this debate. The independence and impartiality of judges and administrators are major principles of judicial and administrative review (Flick 1984). In common law, an essential principle of natural law is expressed in the adage *nemo judex in causa propria sua debet esse* ("no one ought to be judge in his or her own case"). In American law, conflict of interest falls under the due process clause, enshrined in the 14th Amendment to the Constitution, which guarantees the right to a fair hearing before an *impartial* tribunal.

This is not to say that IRBs ought to be treated entirely as tribunals. The rules on bias and conflict of interest in administrative law are a

556   *T. Lemmens and B. Freedman*

reflection of the general concern for independence and neutrality as essential ingredients for a good administration, particularly when administrators are given a specific public duty (Dickens 1995). They apply to a wide variety of administrative and judicial bodies.

As we have pointed out, IRBs are situated on a continuum somewhere in between administrative tribunals and administrative licensing boards. Where they are placed on this continuum between administrative and judicial bodies is important, if we want to apply rules of administrative law with respect to conflicts of interest in research review. While administrative adjudicators are held to the same requirement of impartiality as judges (*Tennessee Cable Television Association* v. *Tennessee Public Service Commission* 1992), the interpretation of what constitutes a conflict of interest may differ depending on the type of administrative board involved. Conflict-of-interest rules are context-specific; the assessment of conflict of interest can differ according to the type of administrative board or judicial body. The closer an entity approaches judicial decision-making, the stricter the rules of conflict of interest are. Clearly, judges presiding in a criminal procedure ought to have the highest level of detachment from financial or personal interest in a case. The same level of detachment is not necessary, possible, or always desirable when we are dealing with highly specialized administrative bodies. When dealing with a motion for preliminary injunction against an IRB's rejection of a research protocol, the Minnesota District Court recognized explicitly that there are due process standards in the IRB process, but that they are different from the ones in criminal procedures. "An IRB proceeding is, simply, not a federal criminal prosecution," the Court stated. "Such a proceeding is governed by contracts and federal regulations which do not require, or provide, the full panoply of criminal procedural rights" (*Halikas* v. *University of Minnesota* 1994).

IRBs need some specialists who, for example, may be very strongly committed to a certain area of research and may have strong personal bias toward seeing this research being undertaken. At the same time, membership of boards is precisely balanced, or is at least intended to be so, to ensure that these interests of individual members do not dominate the review process. For the same reason, a quorum of the IRB has to be weighed and, if majority rule rather than consensus is used, should not lead to a systematic outvoting of community members.

While IRBs are specialized entities, they do have general protective obligations toward the public. IRBs and their members have this protective role in a particular circumstance: research participants are often in a vulnerable position. They may suffer from disease; their financial and social situation may push them to participate in trials; in some cases, they may participate in research to try to obtain access to quality care. This situation warrants careful consideration because of the risk of undue influence or manipulation.

Writing about professional advisory relationships, Bernard Dickens (1995) points out that "dependent parties at disadvantage enter [these] relationships for their own protection against their ignorance and vulnerability to exploitation and abuse. These relationships impose special duties on those whose protection is sought and who undertake to afford that protection." The diligent exercise of responsible review by the boards should compensate partially for the vulnerable position of research subjects. In these circumstances, higher duties of protection are imposed on the party with more power. While IRB members have no direct relationship with research subjects, IRBs have special duties as organizations and their members have a professional obligation to fulfill their work in accordance with the mission of the IRB. Patients who participate as research subjects should be able to trust the health care institution in which they are treated to look after their well-being and respect their rights. The fiduciary nature of the doctor-patient relationship remains a cornerstone of medicine and should not be abandoned when physicians and patients are involved in research. Likewise, this fiduciary relationship should extend to the institutional bodies that are set up to protect patients and others who participate in medical research.

The need to create trust in IRBs as institutions can also be given a very practical justification. When IRBs function in a transparent way, they inspire public confidence. Public trust in the ethical conduct of trials is essential to the success of medical research, which relies on volunteer participation. Creating public trust in research and research review is therefore essential, not only to respect the subjects of research but also to ensure long-term research participation. Paul Finn's argument about the importance of conflict-of-interest rules for professionals rings very true in this context. He argues that "there can be a public interest in reassuring the community that even the appearance of improper behaviour will not be tolerated. The emphasis here seems to be the maintenance of the public's acceptance of, and the credibility of, important institutions in society which render 'fiduciary services'" (Finn 1987).

558   *T. Lemmens and B. Freedman*

The idea that public trust is an important aspect of conflict-of-interest rules seems to be confirmed by the standards used in American and common law to determine whether the impartiality of the administrative decision maker is affected by bias. In both systems of law, the test is whether it is reasonable to consider that secondary interests may have an influence on the decision-making process. The Canadian Supreme Court describes the "reasonable apprehension of bias" test as determining whether a "reasonably well-informed person" would consider the secondary interest to be so significant that it is likely to undermine the independence of the decision maker (*Pearlman* v. *Manitoba Law Society Judicial Committee* 1991). American law seems more lenient toward conflict of interest, by requiring that a party seeking to demonstrate bias must overcome the presumption of honesty and integrity on the part of decision makers and the presumption that decisions affecting the public are done in the public interest (McDonald 1999). Nevertheless, this can be done by using a "realistic appraisal of psychological tendencies and human weaknesses" (*Valley* v. *Rapides Parish School Board* 1997) to show a serious risk of actual bias or prejudgment. Other cases also refer to the test as simply requiring that an adjudicator's "impartiality might reasonably be questioned" (*Tennessee Cable Television Association* v. *Tennessee Public Service Commission* 1992), bringing the burden of proof closer to the common law standard.

In our view, recent controversies and research analyzing the impact of financial interests on the conduct and outcome of medical research show that financial interests can and do influence the behavior of those involved (Eichenwald and Kolata 1999a; 1999b; Reed and Camargo 1999; Stelfox, Chua, O'Rourke, et al. 1998; Lemmens and Singer 1998). These controversies understandably erode public trust. IRBs are supposed to counterbalance the concerns raised by these controversies and scandals by offering a system of independent, qualified, hands-off review. NIRBs and proprietary IRBs are financially dependent on the commercial actors they are supposed to control. It seems odd to hold as reasonable the presumption that financial interests can have a conscious or unconscious impact on these actors while ignoring that there is a serious risk of such impact on those who control them.

We hold that problems of conflict of interest in commercial IRBs are not adequately addressed through simple reliance upon the integrity of IRB members, or upon the fact that most IRB members are likely to adhere to high ethical standards. In a case concerning judicial bias one century ago, Justice Lush pointed out: "The law, in laying down this strict rule [against bias] has regard, not so much perhaps to the motives which might . . . bias the judge as to the susceptibilities of the litigant parties" (*Serjeant* v. *Dale* 1877). Although, as stressed earlier, IRBs perhaps need not submit to the stringent conflict rules that courts ought to observe, the significant public interest in protecting trust and maintaining confidence in the system calls for the development of adequate conflict-of-interest rules. As we will discuss further, this is even more important in light of the nature of research ethics review.

Interestingly, the importance of establishing public trust in IRBs is recognized explicitly by the ICH GCP Guideline. In its definition of "independent ethics committee," the Guideline states that such committees not only have to ensure protection, but also have to *provide public assurance of that protection* (International Conference on Harmonisation 1996) (our emphasis).

What, then, are the conflicts that should be avoided? The law differentiates among bias as a result of (1) pecuniary interests, (2) personal involvement of the decision maker, and (3) alleged prejudgment of the merits of a particular case (Schwartz 1995; Flick 1984; Hewitt 1972). In general, the law regards financial interests much more severely than it does other interests or biases. There is a reason for that; as John Stuart Mill points out, "the love of money is one of the strongest moving forces of human life" (Mill 1988). In the context of the highly profitable pharmaceutical industry, is it unreasonable to anticipate that decisions can be influenced by the promise of financial gains? Moreover, as Thompson recognizes, the existence of other motives or conflicting interests does not mean that we should not address financial ones; financial interests are more tangible. Many factors that are qualified as "conflicting interests" are simply inherent to people's actions and are inevitable. Financial conflicts of interest, by contrast, are identifiable and avoidable (Thompson 1993).

In the case of a pecuniary conflict, a decision maker will be disqualified if the first two (under common law) or all three (under American law) conditions are fulfilled: (1) The "decision maker must stand to gain or lose personally as a result of his decision" (Flick 1984). (2) The interest is not remote or does not arise upon a purely speculative series of events. Interestingly, some English and Commonwealth courts have argued that interest as a shareholder or ratepayer is sufficient to disqualify a person on the basis of bias (Flick 1984). (3) Under American law, the interest must also be substantial. The due process clause requires disqualification of a board member only if the interest is more than "*de minimis.*" In contrast, English and Commonwealth common law prescribe that a minimal interest is sufficient to disqualify a person on the basis of bias. The position of the common law courts is ably summarized by Justice Blackburn, who declared that the interest "may be less than a farthing [historical quarter of a penny], but still it is an interest" (Flick 1984).

In contrast to financial interest, personal involvement in a case only leads to disqualification if there is a real likelihood that a hearing will not be fair. A paradigmatic example of this is when there is a close kinship between one of the parties and one of the judges or adjudicators. This type of bias might pose greater risk in academic IRBs, where colleagues have to review protocols of persons with whom they are closely related. Such personal conflicts are less likely to occur in NIRBs.

Prejudgment is an even more flexible concept. Courts recognize that adjudicators, particularly those who serve on specialized boards and have experience in the field, have often formulated opinions on cases or situations similar to the ones they have in front of them. In fact, oftentimes the very motivation for selecting these persons as adjudicators is based on their having expressed opinions on certain issues. In the IRB context, one would hope that special expertise of IRB members would not be in and of itself grounds for disqualification. The opinion of expert members is often invaluable in assessing the validity of a given protocol. These experts will often have expressed authoritative opinions on particular issues in research. Similarly, community members' statements about the need for better protection of subjects should not constitute grounds for disqualification, and previous decisions by an IRB should not be invoked to challenge a later decision on a similar study. One could compare the situation to that of judges: their earlier decisions, and the unavoidable interpretations of the law expressed in them, do not disqualify them from ruling on a similar case in the future.

In conclusion, when reviewers or judges have financial interests, they are disqualified if there is a clear potential for personal loss and if the financial interest is not too remote. Financial interests are identified as creating conflicts, and are more clearly subject to regulation than other types of interest. Scrutiny of financial interests, rather than of personal involvement and prejudgment, seems appropriate for IRB review, in particular when we are dealing with research undertaken entirely within a commercial context. While some cases involving personal involvement and prejudgment may necessitate intervention, they do not require the same stringent regulations because they are often unavoidable and may be counterbalanced by the composition of the IRB. Personal involvement can only be decided on a case-by-case basis—for example, by looking at the specific relationship an IRB member has with a researcher who submits a protocol. We further believe that the public function of IRBs strengthens the need for stringent assessment of the impact of commercial interests on the review process. This public function emphasizes the need for a system that imposes public trust and thereby promotes participation in medical research.

The Role of Conflict-of-Interest Rules

We have argued that conflict-of-interest rules should provide an appropriate framework for review, and that they are essential to promote trust. Conflict-of-interest rules are particularly important when regulations allow much discretion and rely on the fairness and independence of individual decision makers. This is the case with research regulations. Two major types of rules are available for any type of regulation: procedural rules and substantive rules. Through procedural rules, legislators or regulatory agencies can establish a system of review and licensing. These procedural rules are ordinarily, if not always, accompanied by a set of substantive rules. Substantive rules specify what is allowed and what is forbidden. As applied to research ethics review, substantive rules specify *what* research is acceptable and procedural rules specify *how* one can decide and *who* can decide that a study is acceptable. Substantive rules describe the qualities the conduct of research itself needs to satisfy; procedural rules describe the qualities required of the decision-making process that validates the research project—including the ways in which substantive rules are applied and interpreted.

Research ethics codes and research regulations are characterized by the dominance of procedural rules. They typically provide details about the constitution and composition of IRBs, record keeping, and appeal procedures but are vague about how to weigh risks and benefits. IRB members are relied upon to make significant value judgments.

The FDA regulations, for example, contain concrete procedures but only general rules dealing with substantive issues. Issues such as IRB membership, the functioning of the IRB, the keeping of minutes, notification procedures, and so on, are specifically regulated (21 CFR 56). Yet, not so much direction is provided as to what criteria IRBs should use in rejecting or approving protocols. Research procedure, for example, must be consistent with "sound research design" and should not "unnecessarily" expose subjects to risks. Risks have to be "reasonable in relation to anticipated benefits." Selection of subjects has to be "equitable." FDA rules expand on subject selection, but only to create more room for IRB interpretation. In assessing the equitable nature of the selection, "the IRB should take into account the purposes of the research and the setting in which the research will be conducted." And while "coercion" or "undue influence" is to be avoided, what such avoidance in fact entails remains unspecified.

Research regulations, in other words, provide no absolute standards upon which IRBs can rely. Appropriate protocol review requires a fair exercise of intelligence and discretion on the part of IRB members. As Harold Edgar and David J. Rothman point out, "there are very few provisions in the regulations that protect against bodies [IRBs] that might be sloppy, venal, or subservient to the institution. Put another way, the quality of an IRB's work depends to an inordinate degree on the conscience and commitment of its volunteer members" (Edgar and Rothman 1995). Procedural rules dealing with the membership and composition of IRBs, including conflict-of-interest rules, are important in research ethics review precisely because there is so much reliance on the fairness of IRB members. Members should be sufficiently detached that they can be trusted to weigh risks and benefits fairly. There should be no suspicion that objectives other than the protection of research subjects will prevail. Unfortunately, current provisions on conflict of interest, particularly regarding the way they are to be interpreted, are too vague to be helpful.

Conflict-of-Interest Rules in Research Codes and Regulations

The recently revised World Medical Association Declaration of Helsinki states in its principle 13 that all protocols for medical research involving humans have to be submitted to an "especially appointed ethical review committee which has to be independent of the investigator, the sponsor or any other kind of undue influence" (World Medical Association 2000). It thus not only prohibits researchers from participating in the review of their own research, but also prescribes that reviewers should not be "dependent" on those who pay for the research. The reference to "any other kind of undue influence" was added under the last revisions to the Helsinki Declaration. It indicates that many potential sources of influence are recognized. While the notions of "dependence" and "undue influence" leave some room for interpretation, the provision clearly reflects the idea that reviewers should be kept at arm's length from investigators or sponsors.

Surprisingly, other research ethics codes and regulations totally fail to refer to this idea. The FDA rules point out that "No IRB may have a member . . . who has a conflicting interest," without providing further detail (21 CFR 56.107(e)). Data on FDA site visits to IRBs suggest that the FDA has identified conflicts of interest only when researchers participate in the review of their own research (Francis 1996). It is the duty of the local IRB to determine whether a situation gives rise to a conflict of interest. This seems to be a recipe for problems if the same rule applies to conflicts of interest within the IRB itself. If IRBs are supposed to decide what to do with conflicts of interest, what happens if its own members are in a conflict of interest?

The Office for the Protection from Research Risks' 1993 *Institutional Review Board Guidebook*, which provides further information on the rules of the federal policy, also avoids defining "conflict of interest" (Office for the Protection from Research Risks 1993). However, after stating that "[n]o IRB member may participate in the review of any project in which the member has a conflicting interest," the *Guidebook* mentions that a list of members must be kept by the IRB. This list must state "any employment or other relationship between each member and the institution (e.g., full-time employee, stockholder, unpaid consultant, or board member)." While both of these rules can be found under different sections of the federal policy (45 CFR 46.107(e); 45 CFR 46.103(b)(3)), the fact that they are lumped together in the *Guidebook* may indicate at least a recognition that these relationships can affect the functioning of the IRB.

Interestingly, while IRBs have to keep a list of the board members with the same details under the FDA Rules and Regulations as under the federal policy that applies to the funding agencies (21 CFR 56.115(a)(5)), the FDA does not itself keep records of the composition of these boards and does not require the boards to report any changes in membership or in the status of the members.

The absence of stringent central oversight, the lack of clear conflict-of-interest rules, and the reliance on the individual integrity of IRB members are reminiscent of the emphasis on the professional integrity of medical practitioners. The traditional approach to ethical problems in medicine in general, and in medical research in particular, has been to emphasize personal and professional responsibility. Research and its review take place in a context that is highly permeated by this Hippocratic model of personal integrity and professional responsibility of the trusted healer. Only after the ethical pitfalls in several high-profile cases were exposed in the sixties and seventies—such as Tuskegee, Brooklyn Jewish Chronic Disease Hospital, and Willowbrook—did the medical community fully realize that many research practices have an impact on patient care and that there is a need for stringent review (Beecher 1966; President's Advisory Commission on the Human Radiation Experiments 1996). However, the research community preempted attempts to establish a more publicly accountable national regulatory structure of protection in the sixties by adopting a system of flexible control through federal funding agencies (President's Advisory Commission on the Human Radiation Experiments 1996; Edgar and Rothman 1995). Under this system, funding agencies are key participants in the establishment and enforcement of general research ethics rules, which are interpreted and implemented by local IRBs in light of the local context in which they operate. It is worth noting that, to this day, both the funding agencies and the local committees remain characterized by a strong representation if not dominance of medical professionals (McNeill 1993; 1998). In other words, IRB review has remained very akin to professional self-regulation, in which reliance on individual integrity is a core value. This may explain why oversight of medical research has often been restricted and has not led to a very stringent control of the IRB system.

Another reason Edgar and Rothman invoke to explain the local character of IRBs is worth mentioning here. Local review was set up at a time when research was expected to take place within academic institutions and teaching hospitals. In these places, it was presumed, there was "a shared commitment to the ideals of good science [which] would far outweigh any tendency for persons to trade favors or elevate concerns for the financial viability of the institutions above their loyalty to the integrity of science or the well-being of subjects" (Edgar and Rothman 1995).

The emphasis on localism and context-sensitive review of individual research projects still has many supporters, including Edgar and Rothman. As Jonathan Moreno points out, "local review does allow for familiarity with local conditions that could be relevant for human subjects research, and it provides a convenient source of cheap labor in the form of professors who feel obliged to serve" (Moreno 1998). However, these and other observers do recognize that there are serious problems. The circumstances of research review have changed from the time of the inception of the IRB system. Recent research scandals support this view. If local factors warrant local variations in review, different temporal circumstances also warrant different remedies. For one reason, commercial involvement in medical research has clearly changed the academic landscape and has led to IRBs that are set up as profit-making ventures. The drafters of the IRB system did not anticipate for-profit IRB review or the increasing commercialization of medical research. They envisioned a system grounded in review by a balanced in-house committee, consisting of dedicated members of the academic community and some other volunteers, who participated in IRB review out of pure altruism. Without suggesting that this ideal vision was ever fully realized, we argue that the changed circumstances make it more necessary than ever to analyze what types of conflicts may undermine the independence of IRBs.

Conflict of Interest in Commercial IRBs

The English and Commonwealth decisions holding that an interest as a shareholder or ratepayer is sufficient to create a disqualifying bias are very interesting in the context of discussing financial conflicts of IRBs and IRB members. When individual IRB members are paid by a commercial IRB, they have an interest in keeping their contractual relationship with this IRB. NIRBs, in turn, have an interest in obtaining as many contracts as possible from CROs. When NIRBs are financially dependent on their clients, they surely have an interest that is less remote than that of a shareholder or ratepayer. An NIRB's decision to reject protocols submitted by a CRO may affect its client–service provider relationship. This, in turn, could have an impact on the earnings of individual IRB members. American law softens the rule on conflict of interest, by suggesting that an interest must be "substantial." This could imply that one has to look in more detail at the salaries IRB members receive, and what the percentage this amount is of their overall income. How do these rules apply to the two forms of commercial IRBs?

In the case of proprietary review, the company that establishes the IRB submits its own research protocols for review. Two situations are causes for concern here. First, individual IRB members may be recruited from among personnel of the company, which means they are employees of the institution submitting protocols for review. Consciously or inadvertently, directly or indirectly, pressure might exist to approve protocols or to be more flexible with respect to required modifications. While this situation also exists within academic IRBs, the pressure can be greater within private companies, whose practices are not subjected to the same level of public and academic scrutiny. Respect for superiors is part of the hierarchical corporate culture, and may be less prevalent in a university environment that values academic freedom. There might be fewer, or less reliable, means of protecting employee reviewers from corporate sanctions. In academic environments, where academic excellence and integrity should be core values, profit motives may be less likely to prevail. In a commercial context, profit is of the highest importance and the primary responsibility is to shareholders. By definition, CROs depend financially on the protocols that are submitted for review. Employees know very well that rejection of research protocols leads *de facto* to a loss for the company, since it means that lucrative research cannot be undertaken. They are also aware that when they insist on certain modifications to the protocol, research may be delayed or become more expensive. Moreover, systems of financial incentives within the company might increase the pecuniary consequences of rejecting protocols. Employees may receive shares in the company as part of their benefit package, in which case they have significant financial interests as shareholders in these companies. Every rejection of a protocol or any delay caused by the review process would have a negative impact on profit margins and thus on the value of the shares of the company.

Second, even if IRB members are attracted from outside the company, they are appointed by those in charge of the company. The latter have a primary interest in the profit margin of the company. They could easily terminate the appointments of IRB members whose decisions affect the profit margin of the company. Even if the board or president acts in good faith and respects the IRB's independence, the appearance of direct control over the IRB undermines the credibility of proprietary review. It is not unreasonable to expect that members may fear losing the financial advantages linked to membership and thus act accordingly. Certainly, this is also a possibility within a university environment, where deans or hospital and departmental directors may feel the pressure of corporate investments. But as we have argued, academic scrutiny might be higher and other values prevail, or should prevail, in this setting. Within a commercial context, financial profit is clearly the driving force essential to corporate survival. This situation should encourage us to be even more vigilant about financial pressures. This appearance of conflict makes it crucial to require public scrutiny and access to information on how IRB members are protected from corporate sanction, whether they have secure positions (e.g., by long-term contracts), and whether they have any other financial interests in research undertaken by the company.

According to the American rules on bias, it is important to look at how much money IRB members receive from their work, to determine whether payment for this work is a significant part of their regular income. If the remuneration for review work is marginal, compared to a member's overall income, conflict of interest may be less of a problem under the American approach. Discussing NIRBs, Erica Heath suggests in the same vein that "the remuneration is probably not enough to make any member wealthy" (Heath 1998). It is hard to obtain information about payment of members, but in a survey undertaken for the Canadian National Council of Ethics in Human Research, respondents reported numbers varying between $50 and $200 per meeting. Other commercial IRBs pay per protocol reviewed. If one assumes that an IRB meets once a week, this can easily amount to $10,000 per year, not an insignificant amount and likely to be more than "*de minimis.*" Some NIRBs meet even more frequently, up to twice a day (Kefalides 2000), which clearly means that IRB members can become financially dependent on their IRB work.

Presuming that some commercial IRBs pay their members less, which seems unlikely, IRB members who earn little income outside their work as reviewer may have a conflict of interest under the *de minimis* approach, while others who have another substantial source of income would have no conflict, even if they are paid more as members. The relatively small weight of the income they gain from participating in research review could be used to argue that external reviewers are more likely to be independent than, for example, a member of an academic IRB who is reviewing profit-oriented protocols submitted by the chair of her department.

Nevertheless, in the context of the commercial IRB structure, we feel more comfortable with the common law rules, which would see this as a situation in which conflicts of interest are inherent, regardless of the significance of IRB remuneration to a specific member. We have three reasons for holding this to be the case. First, it may not be practical to examine in detail how significant the remuneration is, with respect to the overall income of every individual IRB member. Second, the special role of IRBs within medical research demands that we err on the side of caution and develop policies that enhance public trust. This can only be done if rules on conflict of interest are clear and comprehensive. Third, IRB review requires, as we discussed, the exercise of much discretion. There is no clear standard to verify whether IRB members did perform their work without undue influence from their financial interests. Because of their particular work, strict detachment is required.

In the case of NIRBs, the financial interests are more remote. Much depends on the attitudes of the companies submitting the protocols for review. In an ideal world, NIRBs should not see their workload diminished by a thorough review of protocols. Serious review should be a marketable item. But CROs could cease to employ a NIRB that frequently rejects its protocols or requests substantial modifications if other IRBs, known to be more lenient, are also available. "Consistently unfriendly reviews," Leslie Francis points out, "might be thought to threaten ongoing relationships between IRBs and the institutions for which the studies are being reviewed" (Francis 1996). NIRBs may suffer if they frequently reject protocols, or request significant changes to protocols, which may result in delays for their clients. They may be dependent on a few very lucrative contracts with large CROs. In that case, their financial gains may be directly affected by performing a thorough, critical review. Outside the field of medical research, it is a general principle that reviewers or judges should not be directly paid by only one of the parties involved in the review. If this is such a fundamental rule elsewhere, why not in medical research?

Heath suggests that there is little difference between paying people to sit as professionals on IRBs or paying them to give their expert opinions as doctors or lawyers. They also "must occasionally deliver bad news to a client who seeks good news but also must pay regardless of the outcome" (Heath 1998). However, when doctors or lawyers give their expert opinion, the beneficiary of their opinion is the patient or client who is confronted with a medical problem or legal quandary. In the case of IRBs, the primary responsibility of the reviewers is not toward the investigators or sponsor of a trial, but toward research subjects and the public. Moreover, when doctors or lawyers feel they must give bad news, it is not so much based on a somewhat discretionary weighing of risks and benefits, but results from an empirically based diagnosis or an appraisal of the current state of the law. The reason for their decision is their realistic assessment of what will happen to their clients, who remain free to follow or ignore their advice. The basis underlying their recommendation is measurable and more precise. Doctors or lawyers who give unprofessional advice are easily held liable for doing so. They have a professional duty to try to prevent harm to their individual clients. IRBs, however, can hinder a research project from going ahead, even if it would not necessarily have caused major problems to their clients. On the contrary, when IRBs give a negative review, their clients are stopped from conducting research and may be financially hampered by doing so. For example, when an IRB rejects a research protocol with a biased design, it may very well be that there was no likelihood of serious and immediate harm to subjects and thus no risk of liability or financial hardship to the company conducting the research. The positive results of a scientifically flawed study may boost the sale of a particular drug without identifiable physical harm to patients or research subjects that could result in legal liability.

Remedies against Conflict of Interest

Can these conflicts of interest be avoided? Several procedural remedies have been suggested to solve them. The most common suggestions are disclosure, removal of voting right, and prohibition from participating in the review.

The disclosure remedy is based on the idea that people can make truly informed decisions if they are aware of all factors that could influence their physicians' enthusiasm for the trial. If those who could be harmed by a conflict of interest are informed, the argument goes, they can then freely decide whether to take the risk. While this rings true in some circumstances, it ignores the fact that people are often in situations which make them vulnerable, and dependent upon others to protect them. When people or institutions offer special expertise to protect people against harm, "[t]hey must act in good faith to avoid conflict *per se*, since resolution through disclosure may, in many cases, leave dependent parties without means of achieving further protection of independent aid" (Dickens 1995). Furthermore, the mere existence of a protective regime in the area of research, based on control by regulatory agencies and IRB review, indicates that reliance on informed consent is not sufficient. Mildred K. Cho and Paul Billings argue in favor of public disclosure rules because "research or review of review board activities may be facilitated by public disclosure of financial or other ties between review board members and investigators, or between funding sources and review board members or investigators" (Cho and Billings 1997). They thereby fail to distinguish between conflicts of interest of investigators and of IRB members. IRBs are themselves supposed to control conflict of interest among researchers. According to the latest revision to the Helsinki Declaration, for example, the IRB has an explicit duty to review financial relations between researchers and sponsors. It has to assess how financial interests could impact on the research process and on the recruitment of patients. Principle 13 states that "[t]he researcher should also submit to the committee, for review, information regarding funding, sponsors, institutional affiliations, other potential conflicts of interest and incentives for subjects" (World Medical Association 2000). A similar duty to scrutinize the research budgets for conflicts of interest is provided for by the Canadian Tri-Council Policy Statement (Medical Research Council, Social Sciences and Humanities Research Council, and Natural Sciences and Engineering Council 1998). When analyzing the potential conflicts, IRBs might consider that direct disclosure of a researcher's interest in a study is an appropriate remedy. But it seems odd to explain to research subjects that the committee protecting them against the negative impact of conflicts of interest is itself affected by such a conflict.

This is not to say that disclosure of financial conflicts is not a core requirement of conflict-of-interest policies. We support efforts by journals and academic centers to require disclosure of any financial ties with research sponsors. Disclosure of the financial interests of IRB members also seems appropriate to enhance public accountability if it is connected to a system of overview and authorization. It can be considered a minimum requirement and part of a larger system of public control to be exercised by other institutional authorities, funding agencies, or federal regulatory agencies. Disclosure of conflicts of interest to those within institutions and to regulators can be essential components of a third-party assessment of the seriousness of the conflicts. This information could then allow decision makers to disqualify reviewers who have conflicts of interest. However, disclosure on its own, particularly the mere disclosure of institutional conflicts of interest to research participants, is insufficient as a remedy.

Would all problems be solved if those who are in an employment relationship with the IRB abstain from participation? We argue that even in that case, there is an inherent conflict of interest in the way commercial IRB review is currently organized. Depending on the payment IRB members receive, they may rely financially on these earnings, and may have a significant interest in keeping their status as a member. More important, conflict-of-interest rules are as much about perception of influence as they are about real influence, since they focus on establishing trust. Is there any way, then, to remedy conflicts of interest in NIRBs and proprietary IRBs?

First, it seems very difficult to avoid or correct conflicts of interest in proprietary IRBs or NIRBs when employees or full-time paid administrators of the IRB are involved. The perception that secondary interests (financial gain, promotion, employment) may affect the duty of IRB members to protect research subjects is serious. One way to decrease conflicts of interest in proprietary review would be to establish a system of accredited reviewers who would have to follow clear substantive guidelines and who would be held accountable for violations of their professional code. The paradigm for such a system is the accredited accountant, who is paid by the company but adheres to professional rules. Presently, neither the procedural rules nor the substantive rules of IRB review are appropriate for such a system of review. There are no real restrictions on membership of IRBs, and educational programs are very diverse and in need of improvement (Mastroianni and Kahn 1998). Above all, there is no single clear and reliable research code containing substantive rules that must be respected. In this context, it becomes very difficult to establish procedures for oversight and accountability in research review. One route would be to establish a professional code for research review.

In the absence of a professional code for IRB members, one could argue that when IRB review becomes a core aspect of professional practice, reviewers who participate as members of their profession can be held accountable according to their professional code. When they approve research protocols that contradict standard research and clinical practice, they could be charged with professional misconduct. We are aware of one precedent of an IRB member being held accountable as reviewer by his professional organization. The New Zealand Medical Council found the chairman of an ethics committee, which approved a study in which women with cervical cancer died, guilty of professional misconduct for his role in inadequate review and monitoring of the trial (McNeill 1998). However, it may not be easy to establish whether those reviewers are participating as members of a profession, and what constitutes a violation of one's professional code in reviewing research, particularly in light of the vagueness of the rules of IRB review. Many members are clearly not bound by professional codes. Bioethicists, for example, who often play an important role in IRB review, have no professional code, and often have no training in research ethics when they start participating in the review of protocols. There is no agreement as to who qualifies as bioethicist and no generally recognized educational program and certification. Under the new Canadian Tri-Council Policy Statement, an IRB must have, among others, "at least one member knowledgeable in ethics" (Medical Research Council, Social Sciences and Humanities Research Council, and Natural Sciences and Engineering Research Council 1998). However, what "knowledgeable in ethics" means is undefined, and no specific training in research ethics is required. Consequently, it is naive to trust blindly in the appropriateness of the membership of IRBs and in their ability to always withstand secondary interests.

NIRBs differ in at least one interesting respect: they are, in theory, independent contractors. If they could be financially independent from large CROs, one would not necessarily fear conflicts of interest. But the only way to guarantee fully that they are not pressured to provide client-friendly review is to implement a system where forum shopping is avoided. In its report on independent boards, the Office of Inspector General stresses this concern. It mentions that several members of these boards support the idea of a federal requirement, obliging sponsors to inform the IRB of any prior review (Office of Inspector General 1998d). However, mere reporting seems insufficient to us, since it does not prevent an NIRB from approving a study that was rejected by a more exacting IRB.

If we want to have a credible system of research review, the possibility of forum shopping for friendly review should clearly be banned, with respect to not only NIRBs but also other IRBs. Forum shopping can be avoided by creating an administrative structure that involves exclusive, mandatory jurisdiction, accreditation, and control. Under such a system, CROs and others involved in medical research would have to pay a licensing fee for submitting protocols. CROs should have no direct financial or other link with the IRB members and should not be able to exercise pressure—directly or indirectly—on decisions made by the IRB.

The disadvantage of separating reviewers from the research sponsor or from the research community where the research takes place is that it becomes even more difficult for the IRB to follow up and monitor research. The National Commission for the Protection of Human Subjects of Biomedical and Behavioral Research recommended in 1978 against a system of regional or national review. It suggested that local review has "the advantage of greater familiarity with the actual conditions surrounding the conduct of research" and allows the IRBs to "work closely with investigators to assure that the rights and welfare of human subjects are protected" (National Commission for the Protection of Human Subjects of Biomedical and Behavioral Research 1978). Influenced by this policy option, federal agencies involved in human subjects research consider the distance between the NIRBs and the place where research is undertaken as already problematic (Office of Inspector General 1998d). This is why the Department of Health and Human Services has problems recognizing research review by nonlocal or noninstitutional review boards. This concern will have to be addressed if our recommendations are accepted. However, off-site IRBs seem now to be widely accepted, by the Food and Drug Administration and by many other national regulatory agencies, without proper regulation to safeguard their independence. It is time to review this choice of local review and to think about a more structured review system.

The idea of a system of official authorization and exclusive jurisdiction is not new. In Canada, the province of Alberta has introduced a system of provincial board review through the College of Physicians and Surgeons, requiring approval from the College's IRB for studies undertaken by independent physicians who engage in research. In France, the Code of Public Health prescribes that any research on human subjects must be submitted to one of the regional committees set up under the authority of the Minister of Health. The Minister of Health has the power to issue permits for regional "advisory committees for the protection of humans in biomedical research" (Code de la Santé Public (France) 1994, article L.209-11, 12). These committees have exclusive and mandatory jurisdiction in their territory, and the law specifies which committee has jurisdiction in case of multiregional trials. They are financed through statutory fees that are paid by research promoters for every protocol they submit. Members, who are selected from a list established by the regional authorities and appointed by the government, have to be fully independent and the minister may withdraw the committee's power if conditions of independence are no longer met (Hirtle, Lemmens, and Sprumont 2000; Mander 1996). In short, conflicts of interest are avoided while committees are assured of the financial means to do their work properly, without additional cost to the government.

In Denmark, research review is also undertaken by independent regional ethics committees in cooperation with a central committee. Members of the Danish regional scientific ethical committees are appointed by the Danish Medical Research Council, while the Minister of Education and Health appoints the members of the Central Scientific Ethical Committee (Law on the Scientific Ethics Committee System and the Examination of Biomedical Research Projects (Denmark) 1992). As under the French system, the financial independence of these committees is guaranteed through the levy of a fee and through governmental subsidies. Similar review committees with exclusive jurisdiction exist in other countries, including New Zealand and Sweden, and in several Swiss cantons (Hirtle, Lemmens, and Sprumont 2000).

In the absence of stringent rules on forum shopping, conflicts of interest can be reduced somewhat if the contractual relationships between the NIRBs and their clients, or the financing system of the proprietary IRBs, provide for long-term financial stability. For example, if an NIRB has a three-year contract with a CRO to review all its protocols, there is at least some financial guarantee. Similarly, if a proprietary IRB has received a guaranteed budget for several years, the IRB and its members cannot be put under constant pressure. However, this is not a guarantee of full independence. An NIRB can, as discussed earlier, be fully dependent on only a few large contracts. This dependence clearly constitutes a significant conflict of interest.

Under any system of IRB review, terms of appointment of IRB members should also be carefully determined. Short-term and contractual appointments place reviewers in a vulnerable position. In discussing administrative review, Geoffrey A. Flick points out: "[W]here the appointment of a staff employee is only for a short term of years or where there is a distinct flow of public officials into the industry they are supposed to be controlling, there may be a temptation on the part of the decision maker not to needlessly offend potential future employers by controversial decisions" (Flick 1984). Long-term appointments are preferable, and authority over appointments should be regulated, to decrease the likelihood of pressure on IRB members. The Danish law, for example, stipulates that members are appointed for a four-year renewable term (Law on the Scientific Ethics Committee System and the Examination of Biomedical Research Projects (Denmark) 1992). Also, appeal procedures should be established. External audits by regulatory agencies should be required when IRB members' mandates are terminated. Regulatory agencies should be able to verify whether terminations were sufficiently motivated.

Independence is not the only issue. As Deputy Inspector General of the Department of Health and Human Services George Grob points out, specialized training programs to educate IRB members are urgently needed (Grob 1998). In a 1998 report, the Office of Inspector General recommends that all federally funded institutions should have a program for educating its investigators on human subjects protection (Office of Inspector General 1998c). While training and continuous education are important for members of all IRBs, Grob asserts that "this would be especially relevant for noninstitutional and nonscientific members" (Grob 1998). Training and continuing education should be required of all IRB members, and should be part of a formal system of accreditation. Adequate protection of research subjects requires more than the goodwill of volunteers.

In fact, over the last three years, significant efforts have been undertaken to set up educational programs and to implement systems of accreditation of programs and of certification of IRB members. For example, the American organization Public Responsibility in Medicine and Research (PRIM&R; http://www.primr.org/index.html), founded in 1974, now also offers through affiliated organizations an accreditation system for human research protection programs and a certification program for IRB professionals. Two organizations have been set up to deal with the accreditation and the certification processes: the Association for the Accreditation of Human Research Protection Programs (AAHRPP; http://www.primr.org/aahrpp.html) and the Council for Certification of IRB Professionals (CCIP; http://www.primr.org/certification.html) and a first certification examination has taken place. The National Institutes of Health (NIH) also took a significant step by requiring since

October 1, 2000 that all investigators who want to obtain research funding must describe what educational program on the protection of human research participants they have followed (National Institutes of
Health 2000). The NIH also announced new programs to support research ethics education of researchers and to promote career development in research ethics. It remains to be seen whether these initiatives
and new requirements will lead to the implementation of an all-encompassing, transparent, and sufficiently controlled official accreditation
and certification system for IRBs and whether other countries will follow
suit.

Lessons for Institutional IRBs

How does this discussion relate to academic IRBs? As we pointed out,
some of the conflicts existing in academic review are very particular
to the institutional context. Academic IRB members may feel inclined
to accept studies of colleagues whom they trust, work with, and share
other research interests with (Glass and Lemmens 1999; Cho and Billings
1997; Francis 1996). Issues of promotion, future co-authorship, and simple collegiality of the working environment may also create pressure. As
Cho and Billings point out, scientist IRB members "rarely question their
own or colleagues' competence publicly" and nonscientist members may
be hesitant to enter the debate (Cho and Billings 1997). Comments of
nonscientist members are easily qualified by the professionals dominating the IRB meeting as being uninformed.

More important, although many academic IRBs do function in an
environment where profit motives are less immediate, IRBs and IRB
members increasingly feel the pressure of corporate sponsorship (Glass
and Lemmens 1999), particularly in light of the proportional decline
of governmental funding (Reed and Camargo 1999). Even if no direct
pressure is exercised on an IRB, most members are part of the institution
in which research is undertaken and are well aware of the importance
of attracting external funding. They may be tempted to accept studies
that come with needed research dollars, which will help significantly to
improve the research potential of their department or institute. When a
lucrative study is rejected, some IRB members may have to return the
department they just deprived of significant research funds. They may
be challenged directly by the "rejected" colleague and may have to face

researchers whose employment at the institution depends in part upon their role in obtaining commercial funding.

Academic research centers are increasingly entering into institutional relationships with some major pharmaceutical companies and may become partly dependent on them (Bodenheimer 2000). This exacerbates pressure within the research centers to actively pursue research proposed by those companies. In other words, the fundamental difference between academic research units and CROs is diminishing and so, too, the difference between academic and proprietary IRBs. Thus, it is essential to introduce institutional policies that address the appropriate independence of IRBs and the need to protect IRB members when developing commercial partnerships. One way would be to reinforce some of the core aspects and values of academic scholarship that are increasingly under stress: academic integrity and independence, the public role of academic researchers, and tenure. The first two are values that require education and persuasion by role models. These values may also be strengthened by more stringent conflict-of-interest guidelines and a stricter control of these guidelines by academic institutions. Tenure seems particularly important to reinforce public trust in the independence of IRB members operating within the context of a corporate health care and research environment. Unfortunately, tenure appointments for physicians are the exception rather than the rule. And, although physicians may sometimes lack appropriate protection, they are still less financially vulnerable in light of their employability. Other traditional IRB members, such as bioethicists, are often hired by institutions contractually, either on a yearly renewal basis or on a fee-for-service basis. Independence is clearly jeopardized in this context, and an academic label attached to the job does not guarantee meaningful academic freedom.

Thus, academic IRBs need stricter conflict-of-interest rules, education, and accreditation of IRB members and greater public accountability as well. The conflicts of interest created by the increasing commercial pressures in academia add to other problems the academic IRB system is encountering.

Overall, George Annas's severe assessment that "Institutional Review Boards should be radically overhauled" does not seem to be an exaggeration (Annas 1996). The loopholes in the system of commercial IRB review are only part of a much larger problem. While Annas does not detail his proposals for change, his suggestions also seem to support the creation of a more accountable review structure. He proposes to set up a national human research agency, that would "set the rules for research involving humans, monitor their enforcement, and punish those who fail to follow them" (Annas 1996). IRBs would be accountable to this agency, and no longer be supervised only by their own institution. We believe that an intermediary agency or institutional body, exercising a level of authority between that of a national or regional agency and the local IRB remains a valuable option. Greater local oversight of IRB function, combined with increased surveillance by federal agencies, seems a preferable model. However, this institutional supervision should be set up in a way that enhances the independence of IRBs and their public accountability.

One of us (Lemmens) was recently involved in the development of an ethics structure within a newly merged psychiatric institution. In order to strengthen the IRB's structural independence from commercial and other institutional interests, an umbrella ethics committee was set up at the level of the board of administrators. Members of this committee include members of the board of administrators, two bioethicists (one tenured), community representatives, chairs of the research and clinical ethics committees, and some members of senior management. The IRB's primary reporting relation is to this board committee, rather than to institutional players who may have a vested interest in attracting research funding. The function of this committee is to deal with organizational ethics issues, but it also serves to promote accountability of the IRB process and to strengthen its independence. IRB chairs and members, for example, are supposed to be formally appointed by this committee, which confirms their independence from hierarchical superiors. The central ethics committee also discusses issues that exceed the scope of IRB review, such as institutional conflicts of interest resulting from partnerships with industry. It remains to be seen whether this new type of structure will do the job and will strengthen the independence (real and perceived) of the IRB while also promoting open debate about issues of sponsorship and financial relations within the institution.

It should also be pointed out that new developments in research warrant the creation of specialized national review panels. Some novel types of genetic research, for instance, or research involving risks that transgress local boundaries or raise fundamental ethical concerns would benefit substantially from such national panels (Glass, Weijer, Cournoyer, et al. 1999; Edgar and Rothman 1995). A discussion of specialized review panels exceeds the scope of this paper, but it is notable that the recent controversies in gene therapy trials in the United States and Canada have highlighted that conflict of interest is only one of the problems of IRB review. The need for specialized national review panels, or the expansion of the mandate of existing ones, should be on the table when discussing needed reforms of the research review system.

Conclusion

We believe that the credibility and integrity of research review are affected by inherent problems of conflict of interest in IRBs. While conflicts of interest are also a significant problem in academic IRBs, we have focused on conflicts affecting commercial IRBs for a number of reasons. We have argued that commercial IRBs are currently affected by a structural problem that affects their independence and undermines their credibility. In the eyes of the public, these IRBs may qualify more easily as the industry's partner than as the public's guardian. Considering the public role of IRBs, more appropriate governmental control and clear regulations are urgently needed than the ones currently in place. The integrity of IRB members and administrators is not sufficient to remedy the problem. Suggesting stricter conflict-of-interest rules ought not to be seen as a reflection of distrust of individual IRB members (Kassirer and Angell 1993). Nor does it mean that many commercial IRBs are currently doing a bad job. However, conflict-of-interest rules are essential to safeguard public trust. They target the perception of bias as much as they target actual bias. The aim of our argument is, to use Thompson's words, "to minimize conditions that would cause reasonable persons to believe that professional judgment has been improperly influenced, whether or not it has" (Thompson 1993).

While the financial context in which commercial IRB review takes place is a reason for particular and urgent concern, conflict of interest in academic IRBs should also be addressed when developing appropriate regulations. The conflicts we have identified in proprietary IRBs are relevant for academic IRBs. With increasing commercial involvement in academic centers, the financial impact of any decision will become a more prominent cause for tension in the decision-making process. This increases the need for major wide-ranging reform of the research review system. Such reform should work toward reinforcing public trust in

580   *T. Lemmens and B. Freedman*

universities, in medical research, and in the institutions established to protect research participants.

References

Advisory Committee on Human Radiation Experiments. 1996. *Final Report*. New York: Oxford University Press.

Annas, G.J. 1996. Questing for Grails: Duplicity, Betrayal and Self-Deception in Postmodern Medical Research. *Journal of Contemporary Health Law and Policy* 12:297–324.

Beecher, H.K. 1966. Ethics and Clinical Research. *New England Journal of Medicine* 74:1354–60.

Bell, J., Associates. 1998. Final Report: Evaluation of NIH Implementation of Section 491 of the Public Health Service Act, Mandating a Program of Protection for Research Subjects. Prepared for the Office of Extramural Research, National Institutes of Health, June 15.

Bodenheimer, T. 2000. Uneasy Alliance—Clinical Investigators and the Pharmaceutical Industry. *New England Journal of Medicine* 342(20):1539–44.

Cho, M.K., and P. Billings. 1997. Conflict of Interest and Institutional Review Boards. *Journal of Investigative Medicine* 45(4):154–9.

Code de la Santé Publique (France). 1994. *International Digest of Health Legislation* 45(5):496.

Council for International Organizations of Medical Sciences. 1991. *International Guidelines for Ethical Review of Epidemiological Studies*. Geneva.

Council for International Organizations of Medical Sciences. 1993. *International Ethical Guidelines for Biomedical Research Involving Human Subjects*. Geneva.

Dickens, B. 1995. Conflicts of Interest in Canadian Health Care Law. *American Journal of Law and Medicine* 21(2–3):259–80.

Edgar, H., and D.J. Rothman. 1995. The Institutional Review Board and Beyond: Future Challenges to the Ethics of Human Experimentation. *Milbank Quarterly* 73(4):489–506.

Eichenwald, K., and G. Kolata. 1999a. Drug Trials Hide Conflicts for Doctors. *New York Times*, May 16.

Eichenwald, K., and G. Kolata. 1999b. A Doctor's Drug Studies Turn into Fraud. *New York Times*, May 17.

Erde, E.L. 1996. Conflicts of Interest in Medicine: A Philosophical and Ethical Morphology. In *Conflicts of Interest in Clinical Practice and Research*, eds. R.G. Spece, D.S. Shimm, and A.E. Buchanan, 12–41. New York: Oxford University Press.

Finn, P.D. 1987. Conflicts of Interest and Professionals. Paper presented at the Professional Responsibility Seminar, University of Auckland, May 29. Cited by Justice J. La Forest of the Canadian Supreme Court in *Hodgkinson* v. *Simms*, 117 D.L.R. (4th) 161 at 185 (September 30, 1994).

Flick, G.A. 1984. Natural Justice: Principles and Practical Applications. Sydney: Butterworths.

Francis, L. 1996. IRBs and Conflicts of Interest. In *Conflicts of Interest in Clinical Practice and Research*, eds. R.G. Spece et al., 418–36. New York: Oxford University Press.

Glass, K.C., and T. Lemmens. 1999. REBs, Conflict of Interest and Commercialization of Research: What Is the Role of Research Ethics Review? In *The Commercialization of Genetic Research: Ethical, Legal and Policy Issues*, eds. T. Caulfield and B. Williams-Jones, 79–99. New York: Plenum.

Glass K.C., C. Weijer, D. Cournoyer, et al. 1999. Structuring the Review of Human Genetic Protocols: Gene Therapy Studies. *IRB: A Review of Human Subjects Research* 21(2):1–9.

Grob, G. 1998. Institutional Review Boards: A Time for Reform. Testimony before the Committee on Government Reform and Oversight, Subcommittee on Human Resources, U.S. House of Representatives, June 11.

Halikas v. *University of Minnesota*. 1994. 856 F. Supp. 1331 (D. Minn.).

Health Industry Manufacturers Organization. 2000. *Commercial Institutional Review Board (IRB)* (online). http://www.himanet.com/irb.htm.

Heath, E.J. 1997. Personal communication via e-mail, April 24.

Heath, E. 1998. The Noninstitutional Review Board: What Distinguished Us from Them? *IRB: A Review of Human Subjects Research* 20(5):8–11.

Hewitt, D.J. 1972. *Natural Justice: An Inquiry Concerning Administrative and Domestic Tribunals and the Nature and Scope of the Rules as to Bias and the Right to a Hearing; with References to Great Britain, Canada, Australia and New Zealand.* Sydney: Butterworths.

Hirtle, M., T. Lemmens, and D. Sprumont. 2000. A Comparative Analysis of Research Ethics Review Mechanisms and the International Conference on Harmonisation Good Clinical Practice Guideline. *European Journal of Health Law* (forthcoming).

International Conference on Harmonisation. 1996. Tripartite Guideline for Good Clinical Practice.

Jones, D.J. 1995. Conflict of Interest in Human Research Ethics. *NCBHR Communiqué* 6(2):5–10.

Kassirer, J., and M. Angell. 1993. Financial Conflicts of Interest in Biomedical Research. *New England Journal of Medicine* 329:570–1.

Kefalides, P.T. 2000. Research on Humans Faces Scrutiny: New Policies Adopted. *Annals of Internal Medicine* 132:513–16.

Law on the Scientific Ethics Committee System and the Examination of Biomedical Research Projects (Denmark). 1992. Law No. 503 of June 24. *International Digest of Health Legislation* 43(4):758.

Lemmens, T., and P. Singer. 1998. Bioethics for Clinicians, 17: Conflict of Interest in Research, Education and Patient Care. *Canadian Medical Association Journal* 159:960–65.

Lemmens, T., and A. Thompson. 2000. Private Review Boards: How Do They Function, What Do They Do? *IRB: A Review of Human Subjects Research* (forthcoming).

Levine, R. 1988. *Ethics and Regulation of Clinical Research*, 2nd ed. New Haven: Yale University Press.

Maatz, T.C. 1992. Comment: University Physician-Researcher Conflicts of Interest: The Inadequacy of Current Controls and Proposed Reform. *High Technology Law Journal* 7(1):137–88.

Mander, T. 1996. The Legal Standing of Local Research Ethics Committees. *Medical Law International* 2:149–65.

Mastroianni, A.C., and J.P. Kahn. 1998. The Importance of Expanding Current Training in the Responsible Conduct of Research. *Academic Medicine* 73(12):1249–54.

McDonald, D.R. 1999. Administrative Law. (Fifth Circuit Survey: June 1997–May 1998). *Texas Tech Law Review* 30(2):333–61.

McNeill, P. 1993. *The Ethics and Politics of Human Experimentation*. New York: Cambridge University Press.

McNeill, P. 1998. International Trends in Research Regulation: Science as Negotiation. In *Research on Human Subjects: Ethics, Law and Social Policy*, ed. D.N. Weisstub, 234–63. Oxford: Pergamon.

Medical Research Council, Social Sciences and Humanities Research Council, and Natural Sciences and Engineering Council. 1998. *Tri-Council Policy Statement: Ethical Conduct for Research Involving Humans*. Ottawa: Public Works and Government Services Canada.

Mill, J.S. 1988. *Utilitarianism, On Liberty and Considerations on Representative Government*, ed. H.B. Acton. London: J.M. Dent.

Moreno, J.D. 1998. IRBs under the Microscope. *Kennedy Institute of Ethics Journal* 8(3):329–37.

National Commission for the Protection of Human Subjects of Biomedical and Behavioral Research. 1978. Institutional Review Boards:

Report and Recommendation of the National Commission for the Protection of Human Subjects of Biomedical and Behavioral Research. *Federal Register* 43 (30 November): 56186.

National Institutes of Health. 2000. Notice OD-00-039, Required Education in the Protection of Human Research Participants. http://grants.nih.gov/grants/guide/notice=files/NOT-OD-0.39.html.

Office for the Protection from Research Risks. 1993. *Protecting Human Subjects: Institutional Review Board Guidebook.* Washington: National Institutes of Health.

Office of Inspector General. 1998a. *Institutional Review Boards: Their Role in Reviewing Approved Research.* Washington, D.C.: U.S. Department of Health and Human Services.

Office of Inspector General. 1998b. *Institutional Review Boards: Promising Approaches.* Washington, D.C.: U.S. Department of Health and Human Services.

Office of Inspector General. 1998c. *Institutional Review Boards: A Time for Reform.* Washington, D.C.: U.S. Department of Health and Human Services.

Office of Inspector General. 1998d. *Institutional Review Boards: The Emergence of Independent Boards.* Washington, D.C.: U.S. Department of Health and Human Services.

Orlowski, R.P., and L. Wateska. 1992. The Effects of Pharmaceutical Firm Enticements on Physician Prescribing Patterns. *Chest* 102:270–3.

Pearlman v. *Manitoba Law Society Judicial Committee.* 1991. 2 S.C.R. 869.

Reed, C.R., and C.A. Camargo. 1999. Recent Trends and Controversies in Industry-sponsored Clinical Trials. *Academic Emergency Medicine* 6:833–9.

Schaad, B. 1999a. Cobayes humains: La Suisse importe des cobayes humains. *L'Hebdo*, no. 20. www.webdo.ch.

Schaad, B. 1999b. Cobayes humains: "Je me suis senti humilié." *L'Hebdo*, no. 20. www.webdo.ch.

Schaad, B. 1999c. Cobayes humains: La chimie bâloise paiera-t-elle le prix de la honte? *L'Hebdo*, no. 26. www.webdo.ch.

Schwartz, B. 1995. Bias in *Webster* and Bias in Administrative Law—The Recent Jurisprudence. *Tulsa Law Journal* 30:461–83.

Serjeant v. *Dale.* 1877. 2 Q.B.D. 558.

Shipp, A.C. 1992. How to Control Conflict of Interest. In *Biomedical Research: Collaboration and Conflict of Interest*, eds. R.J. Porter and T.E. Malone, 163–84. Baltimore: Johns Hopkins University Press.

584   *T. Lemmens and B. Freedman*

Stelfox, H.T., G. Chua, K. O'Rourke, and A.S. Detsky. 1998. Conflict of Interest in the Debate over Calcium-Channel Antagonists. *New England Journal of Medicine* 338(2):101–6.

Stolberg, S.G. 1997. "Unchecked" Research on People Raises Concern on Medical Ethics. *New York Times* (14 May):A1, A15.

Tendy, L.K. 1996. Independent Commercial IRBs (letter to the editor). *IRB: A Review of Human Subjects Research* 18(3):10–1.

Tennessee Cable Television Association v. *Tennessee Public Service Commission.* 1992. 844 S.W.2d 151.

Thompson, D. 1993. Understanding Financial Conflicts of Interest. *New England Journal of Medicine* 329:573–6.

Valley v. *Rapides Parish School Board.* 1997. 118 F.3d 1047 (5th Cir.).

Wadman, M. 1997. Ethics of Private Panels Comes under Scrutiny. *Nature* 387:445.

World Health Organization. 1995. *Guidelines for Good Clinical Practice (GCP) for Trials on Pharmaceutical Products.* Geneva: WHO Technical Reports Series, no. 850: 97–135.

World Medical Association. 1964, 1975, 1983, 1989, 1996, 2000. Declaration of Helsinki: Ethical Principles for Medical Research Involving Human Subjects. Adopted by the 18th World Medical Assembly, Helsinki, Finland, June 1964 and amended in Tokyo, 1975, in Venice, 1983, in Hong Kong, 1989, in Somerset West, 1996, and in Edinburgh, 2000. www.wma.net/e/policy/17-c_e.html.

Acknowledgments: Research for this paper was funded by a joint research grant of the Medical Research Council and the Social Sciences and Humanities Research Council of Canada and by the National Council on Ethics in Human Research. The authors thank Richard Devlin, Bernard Dickens, Carl Elliott, Paul Miller, Dominique Sprumont, and three anonymous reviewers for their constructive comments on earlier versions of this paper. Their former colleagues of the McGill Clinical Trials Research Group deserve recognition for providing the stimulating intellectual environment from which this paper benefited. This paper is dedicated to the memory of Benjamin Freedman, who died on March 20, 1997. A first version, of which he was a co-author, was presented on November 22, 1996, at the III World Congress of Bioethics in San Francisco. Although the paper has undergone some significant changes, his contributions to that first version, which contained the same core ideas, merits co-authorship. The first author is also confident that Freedman would be comfortable with any of the subsequent changes.

Address correspondence to: Trudo Lemmens, Faculty of Law, University of Toronto, 78 Queen's Park; Toronto, Ontario, Canada M5S 2C5 (e-mail: trudo. lemmens@utoronto.ca).

[34]

Dealing with Conflicts of Interest in Biomedical Research: IRB Oversight as the Next Best Solution to the Abolitionist Approach

Jesse A. Goldner

In the summer of 1995, Thomas W. Parham went to his physician, Peter Arcan, for an ordinary check up.[1] During his visit, Dr. Arcan suggested that Mr. Parham join a clinical trial studying a new drug to shrink enlarged prostates. Mr. Parham was confused because he never had prostate problems, but Dr. Arcan stated that the drug might prevent future difficulties. When asked why he joined the study, Mr. Parham stated, "I just followed his advice, just like if he said to take two aspirin instead of one. He's a doctor and I'm not."[2]

Mr. Parham should not have been entered into the study because he had been hospitalized a year earlier due to a chronic slow heart rate, a clear study-exclusion criterion that would disqualify him from being a subject in the protocol.[3] However, Dr. Arcan sought an exemption from the drug company stating that Mr. Parham's heart rate was only "mildly slow," failing to report the prior hospitalization.[4] After Mr. Parham began taking the study medication, he complained of fatigue, a symptom of a slow heart rate. Within weeks, after requesting to be taken off the study, he was hospitalized and a pacemaker was implanted for his slow heart rate.[5] The drug's manufacturer, SmithKline Beecham P.L.C., was paying Dr. Arcan $1,610 for each patient enrolled in the study. The fee covered study expenses, but was sufficient to give the recruiting physician a profit for each subject enrolled.[6]

In what has become one of the better known and more tragic stories involving problematic research, in 1999 an eighteen-year-old study subject, Jesse Gelsinger, died as a result of his participation in a gene therapy study at the University of Pennsylvania. Though suffering from a rare liver disorder, Gelsinger had been managing his illness on a

Journal of Law, Medicine & Ethics, 28 (2000): 379–404.
© 2000 by the American Society of Law, Medicine & Ethics.

combination of special drugs and diet.[7] After his death, Food and Drug Administration (FDA) investigators concluded that he was placed on the protocol and given an infusion of genetic material despite the fact that his liver was not functioning at the minimal level required under study criteria. Moreover, researchers had not notified the agency of severe side effects experienced by prior subjects that should have resulted in halting the study, nor was the agency told of the death of four monkeys who had undergone similar treatment. The consent form signed by Gelsinger did not inform him of those events.[8] Federal investigators determined that the University's Institute for Human Gene Therapy was unable to document that all patients had been informed of the risks and benefits of the procedures and that some patients should have been considered ineligible for the study because their illnesses were more serious that the protocols allowed.[9]

Ultimately, the FDA suspended all active or pending gene therapy studies at the Institute after finding numerous deficiencies in the way the trial was run,[10] and the University announced that the Institute would no longer experiment on people.[11] The director of the Institute that conducted the research, James M. Wilson, was identified as having a conflict of interest because he owned stock in Genovo, the company that financed research at the Institute.[12] Both Wilson and the former dean of Pennsylvania's medical school had patents on some aspects of the procedure.[13] Subsequently, Wilson admitted "he would gain stock worth $13.5-million from a biotechnology company in exchange for his shares of Genovo stock."[14] In addition, the University's contract with Genovo gave the company rights to gene research discoveries at the Institute in exchange for substantial financial support.[15] The University's equity interest in Genovo has been valued at $1.4 million dollars.[16]

Volume 28:4, Winter 2000

The Gelsinger family filed a lawsuit alleging negligence and fraud in recruiting their son for the research study.[17] The defendants in this lawsuit were the University of Pennsylvania, the research team, three other doctors, and two hospitals.[18] Part of the lawsuit claimed that the defendants intentionally failed to disclose their conflicts of interest.[19] The suit was recently settled but the terms of the settlement were undisclosed.[20]

Medical research on human subjects allows medical science to advance by the development of new medications, equipment, and procedures. Furthermore, it is a lucrative business. It is estimated that the average cost to develop a new medication can range from $300 million to $600 million.[21] More than half of the 6 billion dollars spent annually for clinical trials worldwide is paid by pharmaceutical companies to investigators in the United States.[22] Despite the fact that there has been a recent shift away from conducting research at academic centers, many research investigators are university faculty.[23] Researcher-physicians and others involved in the research enterprise, therefore, in the broadest sense have a financial interest in conducting research trials. Thus, a potential conflict of interest exists when a physician is conducting an objective research protocol while still receiving compensation or other forms of support for the research conducted.[24] The issue at hand is how best to protect research subjects from potentially unfortunate consequences of such conflicts of interest.

Given the government's recent flurry of activity in the area of human subject protections — largely focusing on the activities of institutional review boards (IRBs)[25] whose charge is to protect subjects' rights — it is ironic that, until very recently, relatively little official attention has been directed toward the conflicts of interest of individual investigators that might adversely impact subjects' rights. The *New York Times* and the *Chronicle of Higher Education* have published numerous articles identifying and discussing the financial conflicts of interest arising from investigators' ties with the pharmaceutical industry.[26] In addition, there has been increased recognition in the scientific community that financial conflicts of interest, of all types, can potentially bias the outcome of clinical trials, affect a subject's welfare, and diminish a subject's ability to provide fully informed consent.

Primary, secondary, and non-financial conflicts

Conflicts of interest in research can arise in two very different spheres: conflicts between different primary interests and those between primary and secondary interests. In their most general form, the primary interests of a physician-researcher are the health of his or her patients and the integrity of the research.[27] These primary interests should be the most important consideration in any professional decision.[28] In therapeutic encounters, for example, physicians

are expected to attend solely to the welfare of the individual patient.[29] More realistically, however, perhaps one ought to say they are expected to attend almost entirely to the patient's welfare. In research encounters, on the other hand, patient-subjects are being used for scientific ends.[30] Investigators, therefore, are committed both to their present patient-subjects and to abstract, future patients, thereby causing a conflict between competing primary interests. In such a situation, the investigator must educate the potential subject on the critical distinctions between clinical practice and research.[31] In addition, the investigator must correct the patient-subject's perception that an invitation to participate in research is a professional recommendation solely intended to serve the individual's treatment needs.[32]

The focus of this paper, however, is not so much on these competing primary interests, although in the ultimate analysis they may well come into play. Rather, it is on the conflicts that exist between the physician's primary or ethical interests and his or her secondary or personal interests. The conflict of interest here can be defined as a circumstance in which interests, such as career advancement or financial gain, have an influence on the researcher's judgment of a primary interest, such as a patient's welfare.[33] Such circumstances present the specter of altering physician-researcher judgments so that the risks to subjects participating in the research are increased.

A secondary interest is usually not illegitimate in itself — and may even be a necessary part of professional practice.[34] But, it is the relative weight of this secondary interest in professional decision-making that may be problematic and, consequently, serve as the source of both financial and non-financial conflicts of interest.

The desire to eliminate conflicts of interest arises from the natural belief that physicians and other researchers should not engage in endeavors that could endanger their ability to protect the interests of their patients.[35] Regardless of the treatment outcome, the determinative factors are the circumstances surrounding the physician's outside interests and the physician-patient relationship.

Conflicts of interest, of course, are by no means merely financial — at least in the narrowest sense of that word. The true issue may not necessarily be one of a physician's honesty or integrity but, rather, one of his or her unconscious biases and influences, which may be subtle and difficult to detect.[36] Some such conflicts, however, can be equally insidious. Motivation to conduct research is an enormously complex matter that no doubt differs among individuals. At one end of the spectrum may be the altruistic, unselfish incentive to improve the lives of others. At the other is the arguably crass, but surely comprehensible, human desire to improve one's financial situation and level of creature comforts by amassing and spending capital. Between these lies a range of potential sources of motivation: the simple joy that comes from successful efforts and progress, the satis-

The Journal of Law, Medicine & Ethics

faction felt when work is finally developed and completed, the desire to produce insights, and the quest for recognition through publications and professional advancement. Finally, institutional work environments themselves can generate immense pressures.

The prices we pay and the need for change

Concerns about the implications of unchecked conflicts of interest extend beyond the issue of the need to protect individual research subjects from inappropriate perils engendered by such conflicts. These conflicts, far too frequently, can lead to deficiencies in the validity of the data obtained and, thus, in the robustness of the analyses that result: that is, bad research. When this occurs, of course, the harm that transpires is not solely to the research subjects themselves — whose health and safety are put at risk — but also to individuals in the population at large who later may pass up more efficacious therapy in favor of intervention modalities that are seemingly effective, but only because the bad research supports them. The problem, however, extends even beyond members of this broader group that may be harmed. The result of conflicts of interest and bad research is that public confidence and trust in the entire research enterprise vanishes. This has implications for the willingness of individuals to participate as subjects in research, for the public to financially support research efforts, and ultimately for our very ability to continue to alleviate suffering, conquer disease, and treat painful medical conditions.

Finally, given what we know about human nature, we need to recognize that despite the existence of sound arguments that favor maximum efforts to prohibit conflicts of interest in biomedical research, the political reality is such that we simply may be unable to effectuate such a strategy. The abolitionist position, preferable though it is, may be impracticable in the current environment, where both institutions and individual investigators have so much at stake in maintaining some semblance of the status quo. Conflicts of interest may well be unavoidable. Consequently, the very most we can do is eliminate some, minimize those that remain, and provide adequate education to increase the likelihood that conflicts will be recognized and managed appropriately.

Section I of this paper focuses on the conflicts of interest facing individual investigators. It provides a taxonomy of the broad range of concerns that arise when an investigator conducts a clinical study in which he or she may have financial or other interests. These, in turn, may affect clinical judgment with individual research subjects as well as shape how the researcher spends his or her time. Section II briefly describes some of the conflicts of interest facing research institutions. Section III describes the current mechanisms that exist to regulate conflicts of interest, though primarily at the level of the relationship between investigators and the institutions in which research is conducted. These include regulatory requirements of federal agencies, such as the Food and Drug Administration (FDA), Public Health Service (PHS), and National Science Foundation (NSF). In addition, the section describes a small number of related efforts by research groups, professional societies, and individual institutions. In Section IV, attention will be directed to the potentially critical role of federally mandated institutional review boards in dealing with such conflicts, but at the very different level of the relationship between researchers and individual subjects. The final section of the paper makes specific recommendations for dealing with conflicts of interest in biomedical research.

The paper argues that efforts ought to be made to approximate the abolitionist position — to eliminate conflicts of interest — but recognizes that absent the political will to do so, conflicts need to be managed in a number of different ways. While existing mechanisms may well be necessary components of a management strategy, they are by no means sufficient. Largely designed to help protect the integrity of research data, they do little, if anything, to deal with the potential adverse impact of conflicts of interest on the autonomy rights of research subjects.

Admittedly, IRBs currently are justifiably under attack for attempting to do too much with too little in the way of resources. Thus, there should be a natural reluctance to burden boards with additional obligations, at least until such time as either additional resources are provided or federal authorities step back from what many perceive to be an unnecessary focus on minute regulatory concerns. At the same time, however, IRBs traditionally are charged with protecting the rights of research subjects in general and in mandating needed disclosures in particular. Given their historical experiences and expertise in doing so, they are uniquely qualified to assess the impact of conflicts of interest on the welfare of such research subjects.

IRBs should monitor the nature and extent of these conflicts. Upon identifying them, they must assiduously evaluate the need for remedial action and, when appropriate, prescribe methods to minimize their impact on the autonomy rights of subjects whose interests they are chartered to protect. To insure such IRB involvement, regulatory changes may be needed. In undertaking this responsibility, IRBs will not only further protect these autonomy rights, but, in addition, will aid in re-establishing and maintaining needed public trust in the biomedical research enterprise.

I. INDIVIDUAL CONFLICTS OF INTEREST

The issue of individual conflicts of interest ordinarily arises when an investigator conducts a clinical study in which he or she has a financial interest.[37] The investigator's financial

Volume 28:4, Winter 2000

interest in the research may manifest itself in a variety of ways.

In addition to the two instances described in the introduction to this paper, a further example of an individual conflict of interest is illustrated by the behavior of Dr. Joseph Oesterling, who was chief of urology at the University of Michigan Medical Center, editor of the journal *Urology*, and the main investigator of a clinical research trial for a medical procedure known as TUNA.[38] A credential that Dr. Oesterling failed to disclose, however, was that he was a member of the board of directors for ViaMed, a company for which he was conducting clinical research.[39] Dr. Oesterling had 13,334 shares of stock in the company and was paid to attend conferences promoting the medical procedure. It was estimated that ViaMed paid Dr. Oesterling tens of thousands of dollars in honoraria and travel expenses over, at minimum, a four-year period. Dr. Oesterling was also receiving honoraria and travel expenses from Abbott Laboratories, for whom he promoted the use of a test that the company had designed. In 1998, it was reported that Dr. Oesterling's peers accused him of misrepresenting the accuracy of test results in a conference presentation.[40] As a result, Dr. Oesterling was temporarily barred from the practice of medicine, resigned from his position as editor of *Urology*, and pled no contest to a felony charge.[41]

Although this is an extreme example of a physician's conflict of interest, it is not an isolated occurrence. In discussing conflicts of interest, one physician stated: "We have in our profession too many people who owe their jobs to the industry .... They get on a company's speakers' bureau list. They start out being objective, but they change over time."[42] Moreover, while much attention has been paid to conflicts of interest that arise in instances where investigators conduct research in institutional settings, the most significant challenges arise outside academia where there is little in the way of administrative oversight.[43]

A. Per capita payments and finder's fees

The first situation in which an investigator's conflict of interest may arise involves clinical trials sponsored by pharmaceutical manufacturers. It is a common practice in the pharmaceutical industry to pay investigators for their recruiting of subjects on a per capita basis.[44] To obtain a sufficient number of patient-subjects in an acceptable period of time, manufacturers offer investigators financial incentives to enter patients into studies.[45] One commentator estimates that remuneration levels are as high as $3,000 per subject.[46] Another indicates that such levels typically range from $2,000 to $5,000 per subject.[47] These payments purportedly are intended to offset medical expenses incurred by the subject's participation, as well as the data management costs incurred by the investigator,[48] but the amounts involved typically exceed these costs. In an academic setting,

the researcher commonly uses money in excess of that required for conducting the study to purchase supplies and equipment or to support travel to scientific meetings.[49] In addition, this money is often used to fund research efforts that may not have been judged sufficiently important or scientifically rigorous to warrant funding by government agencies via the standard peer review process.[50] But particularly outside of academic environments, the money left over after study-related expenses have been met will remain in the researcher-physician's pocket.

In addition to the per capita payments, pharmaceutical sponsors frequently offer investigators, or their staff, incentives to boost subject enrollment.[51] These incentives may be financial,[52] often in the form of bonus payments per subject enrolled; or they may be non-financial, such as granting the investigator authorship on a corresponding study paper, providing the research site with office or medical equipment, or offering gifts such as books.[53] There are several reasons, inherent in how the pharmaceutical industry operates, why sponsors offer these types of incentives.[54] First, sponsors are pushing tight enrollment deadlines. These shorter deadlines reflect the pharmaceutical companies' desire to be as profitable as possible.[55] The time for a drug patent starts running when the patent application is filed, which is prior to the clinical testing of the drug.[56] Sponsors seek to shorten the testing phase so that they may recoup research and development costs before similar drugs appear on the market.[57] Second, there is an intensified search for subjects. Sponsors need increasing numbers of subjects who meet particular eligibility criteria to fill more and larger clinical trials.[58] As a result of these pressures, pharmaceutical sponsors must offer researchers incentives to meet the sponsors' needs.

There is a concern that comes with the pressure to enroll large numbers of subjects quickly.[59] The fear is that investigators will encourage inappropriate or marginally appropriate subjects who do not meet the inclusion criteria to participate in the research. For example, it has been reported that patients have received drugs to treat conditions that they did not have, sometimes without being told that the drug was experimental.[60] In such an instance, the investigator is compromising patient care in exchange for monetary gain, in addition to compromising the results of the study.[61] A subject can also be considered inappropriate when other treatments or research protocols may be more beneficial for his or her particular condition. When an investigator enters a patient into a study when alternative treatments are known to be effective or thought to be superior, or when an investigator enrolls a patient who does not meet the study's inclusion or exclusion criteria, again he or she may be compromising patient care in exchange for monetary gain.[62]

Aside from per capita payments, physicians may also receive "finder's fees" for referring patients to participate

The Journal of Law, Medicine & Ethics

in clinical trials.[63] The category of finder's fees includes the practice of "paying bonuses to physician-investigators, research nurses, and others involved in a pharmaceutical industry-sponsored research study in order to speed up subject recruitment to meet industry-imposed study completion deadlines."[64] The practice of paying finder's fees has been pursued where there may not be an adequate patient population in a particular area where their research is being conducted.

Cynthia M. Dunn, a former drug industry executive who now directs the Clinical Research Institute at the University of Rochester, stated: "On one hand, many companies recognize it's [paying finder's fees] part of what we have to do to be competitive. On the other hand, they recognize they are setting up potential conflicts of interest for doctors."[65] Some commentators have noted that the payment of finder's fees may encourage the enrollment of patients who do not properly meet inclusion criteria.[66] Furthermore, finder's fees increase the total cost of clinical research, which is ultimately paid for by consumers.[67] Other scholars have noted that, in practice, offering finder's fees is similar to paying fees for the referral of patients, which is prohibited.[68] The underlying trust between the patient and the referring physician, researcher, and clinical research may be damaged when physicians are paid to refer the patient to a clinical study.[69]

B. Gifts from industry sponsors

Another conflict of interest stemming from links with the pharmaceutical industry is the research-related gift. Gifts from companies to academic and other investigators can be in the form of biomaterials, discretionary funds, and support for students, research equipment or trips to professional meetings. A study in the *Journal of the American Medical Association* found that 43 percent of researchers who responded to a survey had received a research-related gift in the last three years.[70] Of those researchers who had received a gift, 66 percent reported that the gift was important to their research.[71] The survey results also suggest that corporate gifts may have been associated with a variety of donor restrictions and expectations. For example, some donors expected pre-publication review of any articles or reports stemming from the use of the gift, while others expected ownership of all patentable results from research in which the gift was used.[72] In addition to difficulties stemming from the donor's expectations, research-related gifts are problematic in that they may cause an investigator to choose to develop or pursue one protocol over another out of a desire for future gifts. Alternatively, if an investigator is dependent on the gifts — similar to 13 percent of surveyed investigators who indicated that the gift was "essential" to their research[73] — he or she may be inclined to publish or emphasize favorable results or minimize unfavorable aspects

of a study, irrespective of the data, in order to help assure future gifts and support from a particular company.

Research indicates that, despite physician claims to the contrary, gifts have an effect on physicians. For example, a study published in the medical journal *Chest* examined the impact of an all-expense-paid trip to a resort hosting a seminar sponsored by a pharmaceutical company on physician prescribing patterns.[74] The majority of the physicians interviewed insisted that this elaborate gift would not influence their prescribing decisions.[75] The study demonstrated, however, that this promotional technique, used by some pharmaceutical companies, was associated with a significant increase in the prescribing of the promoted drugs at the institution studied.[76] Thus, such enticements clearly influenced the behavior of the physicians in clinical practice. If minor gifts influence the prescribing conduct of physicians, then more major gift incentives are likely to have a pernicious effect on the projects physician-researchers pursue and the way in which researchers report outcomes. This is why it is important for universities and other research institutions to control the existence of this type of conflict of interest by maintaining an appropriate policy regarding gifts from industry.

C. Stock ownership and similar financial interests

A financial conflict of interest in the research setting may also occur when an investigator holds stock in, or serves as a paid consultant to, the manufacturer whose drugs or devices are under investigation.[77] As noted earlier, a concern with these types of arrangements stems from the fear that the potential for profit may subtly affect an investigator's interpretation of his or her research or that the promise of large profits could affect the way the investigator presents his or her findings publicly.[78] The potential for monetary gain could also influence the investigator's view of ethical issues.[79] For example, if an investigator perceives the possible risk involved in the study to be great, he or she may attempt to offer the subjects higher levels of compensation as an inducement to enter the study.[80] If the investigator is still unsuccessful in enrolling subjects, he or she may target institutions with populations such as the mentally ill or mentally retarded as a source of subjects. Even in situations where the potential for profit does not affect the investigator's work product, the perception of bias may linger in the minds of other investigators and lay observers.[81]

In 1998, a comprehensive study of bias resulting from financial conflicts of interest was reported in an article published in the *New England Journal of Medicine*.[82] This study surveyed eighty-nine investigators who had published research on calcium channel antagonists and found that 96 percent of the supportive authors had financial ties to the manufacturers.[83] Only 60 percent of the authors of neutral papers and 37 percent of the authors of critical papers were

Volume 28:4, Winter 2000

found to have such ties.[84] In addition, only two of the seventy papers analyzed in the study included disclosures of the investigator's financial relationship with the manufacturer.[85] In part, as a result of this demonstration of the potential for bias, a relatively recent study indicated that some 15 percent of journals now require disclosure of stock ownership of companies the author is evaluating.[86]

Recently, the *New England Journal of Medicine* reviewed its own conflict-of-interest policy and procedures. This review was initiated by a finding that the *Journal* had published an analysis favorable to two popular hair-loss treatments written by an investigator who had been a paid consultant to the companies producing the products.[87] This investigator was also receiving research support from the companies.[88] The *Journal* editor who was overseeing the article, Alastair Wood, was aware of the investigator's ties to the companies when the investigator was invited to do the comparison of the hair-loss treatments.[89] The investigator was still a consultant at that time, but she assured Wood that she would cease those duties.[90] The editor was satisfied with this arrangement. Moreover, the editor determined that the companies' continuing support of the investigator's research should not preclude her from writing the article since the grant money was being paid directly to the university where the investigator worked and not to the investigator personally.[91]

When reports of the author's conflicts of interest were made public, the editor-in-chief of the *Journal* stated that the situation revealed inconsistencies between the *Journal*'s policy and practice, which needed to be assessed.[92] Sheldon Krimsky, a professor of urban and environmental policy, who studies the conflicts-of-interest policies of journals, stated that by publishing the review without the disclosure of the investigator's conflicts, readers may have been given a false sense of security about the reliability of the review.[93] In Krimsky's own study, he found that few scientific journals required the disclosure of financial interests, but even those that do rarely publish such disclosures.[94] The *New England Journal of Medicine* incident seems to confirm the results of Krimsky's study.

D. Conflicts of interest related to the academic research environment

All financial conflicts of interest facing individual investigators are not as overt as stock ownership, per capita payments, and gifts from pharmaceutical companies. There are, for example, conflicts of interest embedded in the highly competitive nature of academic research. Investigators often pursue clinical research in order to build their reputations and academic standing. In addition, investigators at different institutions may pursue the same clinical research simultaneously. Since recognition, future research grants, and job prospects generally go to those who publish first,[95]

and since criteria used to appoint, evaluate, and promote faculty emphasize publication output, investigators experience tremendous pressure to conduct and conclude research quickly.[96] This pressure to produce continues unremittingly throughout an investigator's career.[97] Therefore, an investigator's research may eventually fall prey to his or her desire for recognition.[98] Although the investigator's motivations may not necessarily be directly or even largely financial in these situations, conflicts may stem as much from the desire for recognition or advancement as from corresponding increases in compensation.

University researchers also face financial conflicts of interest as a result of the passage of the Bayh-Dole Act in 1980,[99] which "encourages academic institutions supported by federal grants to patent and license new products developed by their faculty members and to share royalties with the researchers."[100] The National Institutes of Health (NIH) has a standard process for determining who can take title to an invention and file a patent application.[101] After notifying the NIH of an invention, the awardee institution has two years to determine if it will do so, and the researcher himself will share in any profits.[102] If the institution does not elect to take title, then the NIH can choose to do so, in which case the individual inventor also is guaranteed a portion of any royalties received.[103] However, if the NIH does not take title, then the researcher-inventor himself may file for a patent.[104]

After the researcher files for a patent, he or she may form a biotechnology company or enter into a joint venture with these types of companies.[105] The stock options and directors' fees from these corporations may far exceed the salaries that the researchers receive from their universities.[106] The potential for commercialization may create incentives for academic researchers to pursue areas of research that are likely to result in patentable inventions. At the least, it is encouraging researchers to think from a business perspective instead of a purely scientific one.[107] Although this is an acceptable purpose, inadequate attention may have been given to conflicts of interest issues, which will always be a concern in an entrepreneurial environment.[108]

Distribution of faculty practice plan revenues and the role of research in such distribution may also create a financial conflict of interest for academic investigators. Faculty practice plans typically are organized along departmental or divisional lines and operate autonomously. Traditionally, each department has broad latitude regarding its priorities, the research grants that it solicits, and its business practices.[109] At many institutions, a portion of faculty practice plan revenues, ranging from 5 to 20 percent, is allocated to support general academic endeavors; this amount is commonly referred to as the "dean's tax."[110] Another portion of faculty practice plan revenues finances the central administration, and the balance accrues to the individual medical department or division. After the departments or

The Journal of Law, Medicine & Ethics

divisions cover administrative costs and invest appropriately in their practice, the remaining revenues typically are distributed to the clinical faculty.[111]

Distribution of faculty practice plan revenues to clinical faculty occurs through a variety of means. The method currently employed by many medical schools, however, is a tripartite "base, supplemental, incentive" salary formula.[112] The base salary is the guaranteed or "tenured" salary. The supplemental salary normally reflects the market value of the faculty member. This is negotiated on an annual basis and is usually contingent upon the availability of funds from faculty practice plan and other revenue sources.[113] The incentive or bonus, which is also generally contingent upon the availability of funds from these sources, usually is reflective of "productivity," either individually or departmentally or both.[114] In determining the amount of incentive salary, individual productivity may be measured on a point system in which the faculty member receives a designated number of points for contributions in areas including research, teaching, patient care, administration, and extracurricular activities.[115]

Incentives, and even supplemental salary, can be linked to productivity. Research endeavors provide an opportunity to increase a physician-researcher's overall compensation.[116] As a result, an investigator could feel pressure to complete as much research as possible in an effort to increase his level of compensation. Of course, under some other institutional incentive systems, such efforts may have a minimal effect on the investigators' overall compensation, particularly if the system places a heavy emphasis on production of clinical revenue through treating patients rather than through research projects. The changing world of institutional support, however, may radically alter this balance in the near future.

II. INSTITUTIONAL CONFLICTS OF INTEREST

Many academic medical centers are finding themselves squeezed for clinical revenue due to a combination of lower levels of government payments through Medicare and Medicaid and an increase in competition for managed care dollars from nonacademic medical centers.[117] As a result, the temptation to emphasize research dollars as a source of funding may well increase. Historically, federal and state governments provided funding for scientific research while the contributions from private industry were miniscule.[118] More recently, funds received from private industry have helped sustain many of these research budgets, which had previously declined.[119] Although, there is a strong incentive for universities to seek funding from private research companies, there is also a potential conflict of interest from the affiliation[120] because medical entrepreneurialism is not only a goal of individual researchers, but also of the universities themselves.[121] Conflict-of-interest issues arise as a result of

the tension between a desire to make contributions to improve medical treatment and the universities' financial interest in research.[122]

The passage of the Bayh-Dole Act has also compounded institutional conflicts of interest. Under the Act, sponsoring universities are given intellectual property rights in the inventions created with federal funding.[123] These rights are then freely transferable to private companies.[124] The purpose of the Bayh-Dole Act was to establish uniform vesting of patent rights in inventions resulting from federally funded research as well as to encourage the commercialization of such inventions.[125] The result, however, has been to give academic institutions and researchers intellectual-property rights.[126] Thus, the institution may potentially obtain valuable patent rights as a direct result of research conducted at the university. Furthermore, the passage of the Bayh-Dole Act has also strengthened the ties between academic institutions and for-profit industries because academic institutions need an avenue to facilitate the movement of new products, such as drugs or devices, from the institution to the marketplace.[127] Such ongoing relationships, however, may prove to be problematic in the long run as universities may become increasingly tempted to lose their objectivity.

One major risk of institutional conflicts of interest is adverse publicity.[128] The public, through the media, Congress, and other government entities, may question apparent profits from successful commercialization of discoveries made during research funded through government grants — although, ironically, it was Congress through Bayh-Dole that encouraged such commercialization.[129] The public may view the university's commercialism as incompatible with the institution's academic mission. Concerns "flow from an uneasy sense that programs to exploit technological development are likely to confuse the university's central commitment to the pursuit of knowledge and learning by introducing into the very heart of the academic enterprise a new and powerful motive — the search for commercial utility and financial gain."[130] A conflict of interest, therefore, develops when the institution's financial interest interferes, or even appears to interfere, with its primary mission.[131] This conflict becomes significant when it erodes public confidence in the university.

An example of a financial conflict of interest caused by a university's relationship with a start-up company occurred at the University of Florida. A researcher invented and patented a new drug delivery system, CDS (chemical delivery system).[132] In exchange for a patent license, a private company earmarked $1 million for university funding, and the physician who invented the system was named vice president of the start-up company that would develop the drugs to be used as carriers in the new chemical delivery system.[133] Prominent members of the university's faculty were also hired by the private company and compensated with company stock.

Volume 28:4, Winter 2000

Following these developments, another University of Florida researcher produced evidence that CDS was similar to a known neurotoxin and could cause symptoms similar to those found in patients suffering from Parkinson's disease.[134] This researcher's attempts to make his suspicions known were hampered by faculty members involved in the start-up company. After his findings did become public, the researcher received a negative review, resulting in a smaller salary increase than his professional accomplishments might otherwise have warranted.[135] Throughout the controversy, university officials refused to investigate the matter formally or conduct toxicity testing.[136] Moreover, the university continued to endorse the safety of CDS. Some commentators have suggested that the university was afraid of jeopardizing its relationship with the start-up company.[137] A university's failure to fully investigate potentially hazardous technologies due to financial interests could result in harm to both researchers and their subjects.[138] This type of conflict of interest also exists within pharmaceutical companies. It is arguable, however, that the public perception toward these companies is more skeptical, as opposed to the public's presumption that research within universities is legitimate and pure.

III. CURRENT REGULATORY REQUIREMENTS AT THE
       INSTITUTIONAL LEVEL

A. Existing federal conflict-of-interest mandates

As described in the next section, federal regulations addressing requirements for obtaining informed consent from human subjects prior to their inclusion as research subjects have not yet been interpreted to require the disclosure of an investigator's financial conflict of interest to research subjects. Nonetheless, the Food and Drug Administration (FDA) and Public Health Service (PHS) have promulgated regulations; and the National Science Foundation (NSF) has issued a policy addressing the issue of financial conflicts of interest.[139] These are to be assessed and dealt with at the level of the relationship between investigators on the one hand and either sponsors of their studies or institutions at which investigators conduct research on the other. The stated purpose of the FDA, NSF, and PHS rules is to minimize the potential for biased reporting of research results,[140] rather than to protect individual research subjects. Under certain circumstances, where conflicts of interest had not been appropriately disclosed or managed by the institution, the NSF and PHS regulations mandate disclosure of a conflicting interest during public presentations of the research.[141] Within the regulations, however, there is no discussion of — let alone requirement for — disclosure of final conflicts of interest to subjects participating in the research.

The FDA and PHS regulations and the NSF policy all mandate that the institutions conducting research obtain financial information from their investigators. The PHS and NSF documents, however, are broader in scope than the FDA document.[142] This can be seen as a reflection of the differences in the fundamental roles of the agencies. The FDA's concerns apply only to sponsors and investigators who submit clinical data in support of claims of "safety and effectiveness" of products regulated by the FDA.[143] The concerns of the PHS and NSF, on the other hand, include the stewardship of public research funds and the assurance of objectivity in research supported by these funds. PHS and NSF, therefore, are interested in protecting against bias in all research that they fund.[144] Other relevant differences between the FDA regulations and the PHS and NSF documents do exist. There are differences as to what is to be disclosed. Moreover, there are differences as to whether the agency requires a written conflict-of-interest policy to be in place.

Under the FDA's regulations, an applicant seeking FDA approval of a product must disclose to the agency each investigator conflict of interest enumerated by the regulations or certify that no investigator conflict exists.[145] Investigator financial interests that must be disclosed include:

- compensation tied to a favorable research outcome;
- compensation tied to product sales;
- equity interests in the sponsor corporations whose value is unascertainable through reference to public prices;
- equity interests in a publicly traded sponsor corporation whose value exceeds $50,000;
- proprietary interests, such as patent, trademark, copyright or licensing agreements, in the tested product; and
- payments from the sponsor that, less the costs of conducting the research, exceed $25,000.[146]

The FDA evaluates the financial information disclosed to determine the impact of any interests on the reliability of the study. If the FDA decides that the financial interests of any clinical investigator raise a serious question about the integrity of the data, the FDA will take any action it deems necessary to ensure the reliability of the data.[147] To verify the validity of the reported data, the FDA may initiate agency audits of the data derived from the clinical investigator in question, request further analyses of the data to evaluate the effect of the clinical investigator's data on the study's overall outcome, or request that the applicant conduct additional independent studies to confirm the results of the questioned study.[148] Moreover, if the sponsor fails to submit the required certification or disclosure, the FDA may refuse to file the product application.[149]

Under the PHS and NSF rules, the institution conduct-

The Journal of Law, Medicine & Ethics

ing the research must certify that it enforces a written institutional conflict-of-interest policy. The regulations require the institutional policy to include investigators' disclosure of known significant financial interests that would reasonably appear to be affected by the research to a representative of the institution.[150] Both agencies indicate that "significant financial interests" include salaries or other payments for services from the sponsor, equity interests, and intellectual property rights.[151] The term "significant financial interest" excludes salary, royalties, or other remuneration from the applicant institution, income from teaching engagements sponsored by public or non-profit entities, equity interests that do not exceed $10,000 in value or more than a 5 percent ownership interest in a single entity, or salary, royalties, or other payments that are not expected to exceed $10,000 during the twelve-month period.[152]

According to the NSF and PHS rules,[153] the institution itself need not further disclose any details regarding the conflict of interest unless they are unable to "manage, reduce or eliminate" the conflict.[154] Although the agencies do not define "manage, reduce or eliminate," the NSF and PHS rules do provide examples of conditions or restrictions that the institution may impose in order to "manage, reduce or eliminate" the conflict of interest.[155] These include modification of the research plan, public disclosure of significant financial interests, monitoring of the research by independent reviewers, disqualification from participation in all or a portion of the research funded by the agency, divestiture of significant financial interests, or severance of relationships that create the actual or potential conflicts.[156]

The PHS and NSF do have some mechanisms in place to respond to situations of biased design, conduct, or reporting of funded research. For example, if an institution determines that an investigator's failure to comply with the institution's conflict-of-interest policy has resulted in a biased design, conduct, or reporting of the funded research,[157] the institution is required to promptly notify the awarding component agency of the corrective action taken or to be taken.[158] The agency will consider the situation and, as necessary, either take appropriate action itself or refer the matter to the institution for further action.[159] This action may include directions to the institution on how to maintain appropriate objectivity in the funded project.[160]

Moreover, in any case in which the agency determines that a funded research project has been designed, conducted, or reported by an investigator with a conflicting interest that was not disclosed or managed, the institution must require the investigator to disclose the conflicting interest in each public presentation of the research.[161] In addition, the agency may at any time inquire into the institutional procedures and actions regarding conflicting financial interests in funded research, including a requirement for submission or on-site review of all pertinent records.[162] On the basis of its review of records and other information that

may be available, the agency may decide that a particular conflict will bias the objectivity of the funded research to such an extent that further corrective action is needed.[163] The agency may then determine whether suspension of funding is necessary until the matter is properly resolved.[164]

Although the PHS and NSF guidelines are useful in that they require institutions to implement a conflict-of-interest policy, they fail to offer specific standards to guide the institutions. For example, current PHS and NSF requirements do not prohibit any specific industry relationships. The requirements limit neither the amount of money researchers may receive as industry consultants nor the amount of stock or other equity interests a researcher can hold in a product he is investigating. In addition, the guidelines do not suggest a format for investigator disclosures nor do they suggest which office or official in the institution should be involved in administering the conflict-of-interest policy. The PHS and NSF regulations simply delegate the responsibility to individual research institutions without providing adequately specific guidelines. Moreover, as noted above, while they, as well as the FDA guidelines, direct their attention to disclosure between the investigator and his or her institution, or between the institution or sponsor and the federal agency, they do not contemplate disclosure of the financial conflict of interest to the research subject.

B. Institutionally imposed mandates

Due to the prevalence of conflict-of-interest issues that arise, some research groups, professional societies, and academic institutions have imposed conflict-of-interest guidelines on themselves. The purpose of this section is to review some notable examples of the guidelines imposed and how they function to reduce conflicts of interest.

1. Post-CABG clinical trial

Some clinical investigators have taken it upon themselves to reduce the risk and appearance of conflicts of interest. In the Post Coronary Artery Bypass Graft (Post-CABG) Surgery Clinical Trial,[165] for example, the participating investigators decided at the outset to develop a set of conflict-of-interest guidelines. These guidelines allowed the investigators to avoid situations that could have been perceived as involving a conflict.[166] The investigators explained that such guidelines were necessary because they "believe[d] that a defined conflict of interest policy [would] protect the integrity of the study and the credibility of the investigators as the trial [was] scrutinized by the scientific community and the public."[167]

The guidelines provided that investigators involved in the Post-CABG study would not buy, sell, or hold stock or stock options in any of the companies providing or distributing medication under the study.[168] Each investigator also

Volume 28:4, Winter 2000

agreed not to serve as a paid consultant to any of the companies.[169] The guidelines applied to the investigator as well as his spouse and dependents. Additional safeguards were imposed which required researchers to report activities not typically viewed as conflicts of interest. For example, any financial interests in the companies over which the investigator had no control, such as mutual funds, were reported annually to the trial's coordinating center.[170] The establishment of these guidelines by the Post-CABG investigators suggests that researchers are aware of the potential bias that may result from financial conflicts of interest. A *New England Journal of Medicine* editor praised the Post-CABG guidelines as "laudable voluntary guidelines, which for the time being other clinical investigators would do well to adopt."[171] The editor went on to add that "[a] broader and more institutionalized approach is needed, however."[172]

2. American Society of Gene Therapy

This past April, the American Society of Gene Therapy developed and implemented a conflict-of-interest policy imposed on all principal investigators researching gene therapy.[173] The policy begins by noting that the primary interest in all clinical trials must be the interest of the patient and that the standard-of-care guidelines must be strictly followed. In addition to following institutional and federal regulations on conflicts of interest, no investigator may have "equity, stock options or comparable arrangement in companies sponsoring the trial."[174] Since members of the American Society of Gene Therapy can be suspended "for actions deleterious to the purposes of the Society," the policy may help ensure that all members follow the guidelines it has instituted.[175]

3. Harvard Medical School

Harvard Medical School adopted conflict-of-interest guidelines after a keratoconjunctivitis sicca[176] study was performed at the university. In the late 1980s, an investigator conducting a trial of an ointment for the treatment of keratoconjunctivitis sicca published promising reports of its efficacy.[177] The individual failed to disclose his ownership of over $500,000 worth of stock in the company that manufactured the ointment.[178] As a result of this conflict of interest, a second multi-institutional, randomized, double blind study was conducted by investigators without links to the company.[179] These investigators concluded that the ointment was no more effective than a placebo.[180]

In response to concerns arising from this incident, Harvard Medical School adopted guidelines that addressed the issue of faculty members' potential conflicts of interest in clinical research.[181] Under these guidelines, faculty members are required to disclose annually all potential conflicts, and a standing committee of the faculty must approve most

financial connections between faculty and for-profit companies.[182] Faculty members must obtain approval from the Standing Committee of Harvard Medical Center[183] to conduct research sponsored by and for the benefit of a company in which they or their immediate family have an interest.[184] Other activities that require approval are serving as an executive for a biomedical company or having a financial interest in a product that is in competition with a product being investigated by researchers at the university.[185] In addition, disclosure and express approval is required before a faculty member conducting clinical trials may hold stock in or receive consulting fees from a company whose technology he or she is investigating.[186]

In an effort to prevent the loss of faculty members, Harvard had recently considered softening its guidelines.[187] Ultimately, the university decided not to amend them after ethicists published concerns about the implications of weaker guidelines.[188] As one commentator noted, if Harvard had decided to make its conflict-of-interest guidelines more lax, it would have been the wrong step for the prestigious university to take.[189] Instead, it has been argued, there should be an agreement among academic medical centers, whether self-imposed by universities or by governmental agencies, to have rigorous and uniform rules on managing conflicts of interest.[190] If such an agreement existed, there would be no concern about losing faculty[191] (except, of course, to the private sector). Thus, Harvard should encourage other centers to adopt stronger guidelines instead of softening its own.[192]

Commentators suggest that the financial conflict-of-interest rules adopted by Harvard are among the strictest of all American universities.[193] Certainly they do not entirely eliminate conflicts. It is possible, however, that if all institutions were to establish and enforce guidelines which are as detailed and as strict as Harvard's, the conflict-of-interest problem might well be brought under control, at least with respect to research conducted under institutional auspices. While requirements for disclosing any remaining conflicts of the investigator or the institution to subjects may be warranted, the pernicious effects of the conflicts may be minimized. Realistically, however, due to financial incentives and pressures, the likelihood that all universities will voluntarily implement such a policy is very small.

IV. THE ROLE OF THE INSTITUTIONAL REVIEW BOARD

A. Regulatory and historical perspectives

Federally mandated IRBs historically have been charged with playing a significant role in the protection of human research subjects.[194] IRBs are required to determine that the risks of research are reasonable in relation to its anticipated benefits and that informed consent will be sought from each

The Journal of Law, Medicine & Ethics

prospective subject.[195]

The past two-and-a-half years have been marked by an extraordinary amount of governmental and media attention directed toward oversight of regulatory and ethical policies affecting the conduct of biomedical research generally and the role of IRBs in evaluating and monitoring the conduct of research in particular. The history of the role of IRBs has been recounted elsewhere,[196] but three parallel, but related, series of events have taken place marking this renewed attention.

1. OIG reports

The recent highly publicized criticism of institutional review boards began in June 1998 with the release of a series of reports assessing the effectiveness of IRBs by the Office of Inspector General (OIG) at the Department of Health and Human Services.[197] According to the OIG, IRBs were providing inadequate oversight.[198] One reason for this inadequacy was that IRBs were being overwhelmed with an increasing numbers of research proposals. It was claimed that the review boards were assessing too many research proposals too quickly and with too little expertise.[199] Within five years, the workload of IRBs had increased an average of 42 percent, while the size of these boards and their budgets had remained the same.[200]

A follow-up report issued in April 2000 by the OIG concluded that only "minimal progress" had been made in improving the IRB situation during the interim period.[201] It also criticized the failure to streamline federal regulatory provisions so as to decrease the workload on IRBs.[202]

2. Institutional suspensions

The second series of events, beginning in October 1998, has been a number of suspensions or significant restrictions by federal regulators of institutional research programs involving human subjects. These actions have been taken either by the Food and Drug Administration (FDA) or by what was then called the Office of Protection from Research Risks (OPRR), the agency responsible for oversight of IRBs. The suspensions and restrictions have been due to findings that the institutions were not following regulations designed to protect the safety and dignity of research subjects. Among the institutions involved were Veterans Affairs Medical Center in West Lost Angeles, Duke University Medical Center, University of Illinois at Chicago, St. Jude's Children's Research Hospital, Virginia Commonwealth University, University of Alabama at Birmingham, University of Colorado Health Sciences Center, Institute for Human Gene Therapy of the University of Pennsylvania,[203] Rush Presbyterian-St. Luke's Medical Center,[204] University of Oklahoma College of Medicine in Tulsa,[205] University of Texas Medical Branch at Galveston, and the University of Miami.[206]

The reasons for the federal agencies' finding non-compliance varied from one institution to another. A summary of common reasons included, among other items:

- concerns regarding IRBs acting improperly by approving protocols or informed-consent documents that were inadequate;
- an absence of sufficient information regarding plans for subject recruitment and enrollment prior to approval;
- questions about the equitable selection of subjects;
- protocol deficiencies in protecting subject privacy and confidentiality;
- lack of quorums at IRB meetings;
- an inappropriate granting of exemptions from IRB review;
- omissions of required elements in informed-consent documents and failure to provide adequate detail regarding certain elements;
- inappropriately complex consent documents;
- inadequate IRB resources; and
- overburdened IRBs.[207]

In addition to the situation at the University of Pennsylvania discussed at the beginning of this paper,[208] a physician's conflict of interest may have also contributed to the research suspension at the University of Oklahoma after the Office for Human Research Protections, the OPRR replacement, determined that cancer patients were being placed at risk.[209] Dr. Michael McGee, the principal investigator of a research trial for patients with melanoma, a deadly form of skin cancer, was also the developer and manufacturer of the vaccine being tested.[210] The alleged violations included changing the protocol without IRB approval, misinforming patients of the potential benefits of participation in the research study, and not informing patients of the risk of suspending treatment while participating in the study.[211] It is unclear to what degree the investigator's interest in the vaccine he developed may have led to the reduction in patient protection.

Reaction to these enforcement efforts, as expected, has been very mixed. Some bioethicists, university officials, and researchers clearly applauded these regulatory actions as a necessary means of providing wake-up calls both to IRBs that were doing hardly more than rubber-stamping research proposals and to institutions that did little to support their IRBs.[212] Others, however, viewed them as unreasonable and overly focused on deficiencies in documentation and the like, rather than at situations where subjects were actually put at risk.[213] The concern voiced here has been that boards would now spend inordinate amounts of time attending to procedural requirements, thus diluting efforts at substantive review of research protocols.[214]

Volume 28:4, Winter 2000

3. Creation of the Office of Human Research Protections

The third significant action raising public awareness concerning failures in the system for protecting human subjects was the recent decision to relocate the OPRR from the NIH to the Office of the Secretary of Health and Human Services.[215] The name of the office has also been changed to the Office of Human Research Protections, and the position of director was upgraded.[216] The move was made as a result of recommendations by a panel appointed to review growing public concern about the adequacy of protections for human research subjects and was designed to enhance the OPRR's stature.[217] OPRR had been portrayed during congressional hearings as being "bureaucratically impotent" and questions had been raised about whether the OPRR's position within the NIH, which sponsors much research regulated by OPRR, might have created "the appearance and actuality of a conflict of interest."[218]

Dr. E. Greg Koski, an anesthesiologist with both a medical degree and a doctorate in physiology, who directed the human subject protection program at three teaching hospitals affiliated with Harvard Medical School, has replaced the former director, Gary Ellis.[219] While some commentators have questioned whether the change in personnel was a sign that enforcement would be far less strict,[220] others have suggested that Dr. Koski would be seeking an appropriate middle ground.[221]

Dr. Koski himself has stated that it may be necessary to bar both institutions and scientists from conducting research if they fail to fulfill their responsibilities to subjects and has suggested that IRBs ought to be strengthened.[222] Since his appointment, he has been quoted as saying that the entire system for protecting human research subjects was "dysfunctional" and in need of significant change.[223] He supports the development of more uniform national standards to guide IRBs as well as the inclusion of more nonscientists and members of the public on the boards.[224] On the issue of conflicts of interest, he has noted that they are "very real. They are very serious and they are a threat to our entire endeavor. These conflicts have certainly intensified over the last two decades and certainly during the last five years the system may have gotten entirely out of control."[225]

There also are indications of a change in emphasis in the activities of the OHRP and, hence, in the entire enterprise of protecting human research subjects. Dr. Koski's past writings indicate that he will be trying to promote less adversarial and more cooperative relationships among researchers, institutions, and the federal government.[226] A model he has suggested is that of the nation's system for airline safety, in which the early identification and correction of deficiencies before problems arise[227] is preferred to a punitive regulatory approach. Undoubtedly, there will be increased emphasis on education for all those involved in the research enterprise, including IRB members and researchers,[228] so as to develop "greater awareness of and sensitivity to ethical and regulatory matters."[229] The need to develop more uniform national standards to guide IRBs so that federal regulations are easier to interpret has also been noted by Dr. Koski.[230] It is possible that he will recommend steps to moderate the workload of IRBs so as to reduce administrative burdens and improve efficiency, encourage adequate provision of institutional resources devoted to the protection of subjects, increase assistance to institutions in order to optimize utilization of these resources, develop guidelines for staffing and workload levels, and accredit the review boards.[231]

B. IRB regulation of conflicts of interest

1. Current regulatory provisions

Presently the federal regulations, which IRBs are directed to enforce, do not specifically require boards to consider the issue of conflicts of interest prior to approving research.[232] Similarly, they do not require that informed-consent documents address the issue of what, if anything, investigators should disclose concerning conflicts of interest.[233]

One element within these regulations that might be interpreted as requiring disclosure of an investigator's apparent conflict of interest states that subjects should receive "[a] description of any benefits to the subject *or to others* which may reasonably be expected from the research."[234] There has been little official interpretation of this language. In commenting on this statement in the final rule appearing in the Federal Register, the FDA stated, "even if subjects receive no personal benefit from the study, others may receive some benefit, and, where it may reasonably be expected that others may benefit, that information should be disclosed."[235]

From this comment, it seems that the FDA considers the section directed solely toward the disclosure of benefits to future patients. Nonetheless, if an investigator initiates a clinical study with the expectation of either economical or professional gain, it could be argued that this section requires him or her to disclose such information to the subject.

Another element within the informed-consent regulations that could be interpreted to require disclosure of an investigator's apparent conflict of interest provides that an investigator should seek "consent only under circumstances that provide the prospective subject or the representative sufficient opportunity to consider whether or not to participate and that minimize the possibility of coercion or undue influence."[236] While it may be unlikely that potential or actual investigator conflicts of interest will be viewed as engendering truly coercive stratagems by investigators to encourage potential subjects to enroll, it is more likely they could result in less harsh, but still cognizable "undue influence" by investigators.

2. Recent initiatives

Presently, attention is being paid to the possibility that IRBs should consider the issue of financial conflicts of interest. In early June 2000, in the course of announcing a forum that would be held in August 2000 to discuss the sharing of information between IRBs and compliance offices responsible for institutional policies and procedures regarding conflicts of interest in the conduct of clinical trials, the National Institutes of Health noted the "recent highly publicized instances of apparent financial conflicts of interest [that] have generated concern within the research and lay communities."[237] In doing so, the NIH observed that objectivity in research is essential to public trust and researchers must pursue research based on scientific data, not other self-serving interests.[238]

While the NIH noted that there was no regulatory requirement for IRBs to consider investigators' financial conflicts of interest, it estimated that 25 percent of IRBs routinely dealt with this concern, incorporating conflict-of-interest issues in board deliberations.[239] It would appear that existing IRB review of conflicts of interest might be of recent vintage.

Subsequently, in a more detailed announcement regarding the August 2000 "Conference on Human Subject Protection and Financial Conflict of Interest," Secretary Donna Shalala of the Department of Health and Human Services again recognized that financial conflicts of interest in clinical trials are an area of concern. The secretary noted that there was little guidance available to IRBs to assist in handling such conflicts[240] and suggested, perhaps for the first time in an official document, the possibility that "information about the financial interests of investigators and research institutions should be disclosed to research subjects and others."[241]

As one part of her initiative to strengthen human-subject protections, Shalala announced that there would be "extensive public consultation to identify new or improved means to manage financial conflicts of interest that could threaten the safety of research subjects or the objectivity of the research itself."[242] She posed a series of questions to be addressed at the conference, including: (1) what types of financial interest were associated with human subjects research; (2) whether there was empirical evidence concerning the effects of informing research participants about financial relationships or conflicts of interest between the investigator, the institution, or the IRB; and (3) if information about financial interest were to be disclosed, what information should be provided, with what detail, and when and how should it be offered?[243]

3. Options for resolving or mitigating conflicts at the investigator-subject level

a. Mandating disclosure as part of the informed-consent process

i. Alternative standards of disclosure

In large part, the current view of appropriate standards of disclosure for informed consent have developed from medical malpractice litigation, which has arisen largely in a purely clinical, as opposed to research, setting. Three standards have been identified. The first standard, which is the least stringent of the three, often is described as the medical custom or medical professional practice standard. In the research context, this standard would require that subjects receive the quantity and quality of information that a reasonable medical researcher would provide.[244]

The second standard is the reasonable-person standard; it requires researchers to give subjects the kind of "objective" information that a similarly situated prudent person would desire.[245] Under this approach, "[t]he scope of the physician's communications to the patient ... must be measured by the patient's need, and that need is the information material to the decision."[246]

The third standard is the subjective or individual standard; it requires researchers to provide information that is tailored, whenever possible, to the subjective preferences of the particular research participants.[247] Presumably, this would be in addition to whatever information ought to be provided to the subject under the second objective, or reasonably prudent person, standard. This subjective standard is the most burdensome,[248] especially in the research setting where researchers often have limited knowledge about the preferences of individuals participating in the study. Arguably, it would require that the researcher engage the prospective subject in a discussion about the subjects' values and interests.

Slightly more than half of the jurisdictions within the United States follow the professional custom standard in therapeutic settings.[249] The unique circumstances surrounding most clinical research, however, supports the use of the reasonable-person standard, if not the subjective standard.

First, clinical research poses a higher degree of unascertainable risks than standard-of-care clinical therapy.[250] This uncertainty alone provides a strong argument for utilizing the reasonable-person standard in the clinical research environment. The uncertain risks, coupled with the concept of patient autonomy, strengthens the argument that "[t]he subject of medical experimentation is entitled to a full and frank disclosure of *all* the facts, probabilities and opinions which a reasonable man *might* be expected to consider before giving his consent" (emphasis added).[251]

Volume 28:4, Winter 2000

Second, the reasonable-person standard for clinical research is warranted because experimentation often provides little or no likely benefit to the subject. This is in contrast to traditional therapeutic treatments that invariably attempt to provide the subject with some physical or psychiatric benefit.[252] Investigators may argue that the standard for disclosure should vary depending on whether the research is beneficial or non-beneficial to the subject. If the treatment received by the subject is likely to benefit him or her, an investigator might conclude that the less stringent custom standard is appropriate. If the subject will not benefit from his or her participation in the study, however, investigators may be more willing to employ the reasonable-person standard. As the National Commission for the Protection of Human Subjects of Biomedical and Behavioral Research determined, the custom standard is inappropriate in clinical research because the voluntary subject may desire more information about his or her gratuitously taken risk[253] than a patient who seeks therapeutic treatment.[254] The Commission's report states:

> The extent and nature of information [provided] should be such that persons knowing that the procedure is neither necessary for their care nor perhaps fully understood can decide whether they wish to participate in the furthering of knowledge. Even when some direct benefit to them is anticipated, the subjects should understand clearly the range of risk and the voluntary nature of participation.[255]

Third, the reasonable-person standard should be adopted in the research setting because the interests of subject and investigator often conflict.[256] For example, the investigator's interests in the advancement of science conflict with the subject's desire to receive the newest treatment or the best care. Since investigators are often subject to these types of competing loyalties,[257] it is important to hold them to a stricter standard of disclosure, thereby reducing the likelihood that the investigator will receive less than fully informed consent.

ii. Arguments against disclosure

To some degree, disclosure of an investigator's apparent conflict of interest might be viewed as straining traditional notions of informed consent. Conventional informed-consent requirements allow patients to weigh a combination of likely risks against possible benefits.[258] In the case of an investigator's disclosure of a conflict of interest, however, the informed consent deals more with the investigator's expected benefits than any potential harm or benefit to the subject.[259] Therefore, even though one might expect information about the investigator's conflict of interest to im-

prove the value of the consent process, questions remain as to whether such information truly assists the subject in his or her decision-making.[260]

Disclosure may also be insufficient in that it "only reveals a problem, without providing any guidance for resolving it."[261] The subjects who receive the information may not know how to evaluate it.[262] Subjects who are considering the research for therapeutic reasons may feel only more anxious during an already stressful period at the investigator's disclosure of financial information.[263] On the other hand, some subjects may not comprehend the subsequent implications of the information;[264] they may not understand that a financial interest in the research could cause an investigator to encourage the subject to enter the study when it is not in his or her best interest.

Psychological studies demonstrate that despite accurate disclosure, subjects may not comprehend the information provided.[265] Detailed informed-consent forms may in fact obscure a subject's understanding.[266] In addition, the complete faith and trust many subjects place in the investigator may create a cavalier attitude towards informed-consent forms. Full disclosure, therefore, does not always give the subject understanding or control.[267] Despite existing disclosure requirements, many patients will continue to place complete confidence in their physicians and will, unhesitatingly, consent to participate in clinical research.

Moreover, ideally, disclosure is thought to promote communication and foster trust between physicians and patients.[268] One commentator suggests, however, that rather than increasing communication and trust, disclosure of a physician's financial interest is likely to provoke doubts about the value of the medical advice offered.[269] Disclosing financial ties is unlike revealing risks and benefits in that it warns not of the risks of the procedure, but of the limits of the physician as a loyal agent or fiduciary.[270] In applying this to the research setting, disclosure of an investigator's financial interest — it is said — is likely to cause the subject to question the investigator's motivations in suggesting the research. This may, in turn, cause a decrease in the number of subjects willing to participate in clinical studies.[271]

The fact that the patient's trust in his physician is a crucial factor in the patient's willingness to participate in the clinical study cannot be refuted.[272] As one physician-researcher noted:

> I could get most of my patients to participate in almost any kind of clinical study. They would swallow new drugs, receive infusions of calcium or glucagon, or even embrace esophageal or rectal catheters because they had faith in my goodwill or, I now fear, because they wanted to please me.[273]

iii. Why disclose financial conflicts?

It is this great trust in the physician-researcher, however, that makes it imperative that subjects participating in clinical research be alerted to any significant financial conflict of interest of the investigator and/or the institution, irrespective of whether it is likely to affect the subject's ultimate decision. Despite the obvious problems that arise when a disclosure is made, it remains one of the most effective tools available to the research community to protect a subject's autonomy. It would be nonsensical to abandon a tool simply because it cannot fix all potential problems. A better solution would be to maintain this tool and develop others to address the problems arising from disclosure.

In the one judicial opinion that explores the issue, the state court considered the question of a physician's obligation to disclose personal economic interests to the patient. In *Moore v. Regents of University of California*,[274] the California Supreme Court addressed the issue of whether a physician had a fiduciary duty to disclose such interests. John Moore was diagnosed as having hairy cell leukemia, and Dr. David Golde of the University of California at Los Angeles (UCLA) Medical Center recommended that Moore have his spleen removed. Before the operation, Golde made arrangements to obtain portions of Moore's spleen after it was removed and to take them to a separate research unit.[275] This was not intended to be for any purpose relating to Moore's medical care. At the time, Golde was aware that certain blood products were commercially valuable and that access to a patient whose blood contained these substances could be profitable. Golde did not inform Moore of his plan to conduct this research or request his permission to do so.[276]

Moore returned to UCLA numerous times over the next seven years for follow-up visits, and on each of these occasions, Golde withdrew additional samples of blood, skin, bone marrow, and other bodily fluids. Unknown to Moore, Golde was actually developing a cell line from the spleen and tissue samples. This "Mo-cell" line had an estimated worth of three billion dollars.[277]

The California Supreme Court held that "a physician who is seeking a patient's consent for a medical procedure must, in order to satisfy his fiduciary duty and to obtain the patient's informed consent, disclose personal interests unrelated to the patient's health, whether research or economic, that may affect his medical judgment."[278] The court stated that failure to disclose these unrelated personal interests might give rise to a cause of action for performing medical procedures without informed consent or for breach of fiduciary duty. Thus, from the *Moore* case, it appears that in at least one state there is a duty of the physician to disclose any preexisting or concurrent research interest in a patient. Therefore, the patient ought to be made aware of any conflicts so that he or she has sufficient information to

either consent to treatment or look for another source of medical care.[279] From this holding, it seems as if simply disclosing the conflict of interest would have fulfilled Dr. Golde's fiduciary duty.

Requiring that study subjects be provided with information concerning an investigator's potential conflict of interest could be viewed as a necessary and appropriate disclosure of an additional risk, in the sense that such a conflict might result in an investigator's conducting the study in a manner that would serve his own best interests rather than that of the subject. This requirement would thus further the goal of subject autonomy in the decision-making process regarding whether or not to participate in the study. In addition, disclosure inherently involves the investigator's identifying his or her motivations, and this, in and of itself, might result in the investigator's changing behavior to avoid embarrassment and to conduct the study more carefully and in a manner that is more protective of the subject's welfare.

iv. The reasonable-person standard

Although there is general agreement that the reasonable-person standard should be adopted in the research setting, the determination of what a reasonable person needs to make an informed decision is subject to debate. In formulating the appropriate disclosure, the investigator should begin by differentiating between significant and trivial information. Under this formula, the investigator must correct a subject's erroneous expectations, but he need not belabor the obvious.[280] To some commentators, an investigator's financial conflicts of interest fall into the "obvious" category.[281] These commentators contend that reasonably prudent subjects understand that investigators will seek both payments as well as recognition for their services.[282] If, on the other hand, the subject believes his or her participation in the clinical research will solely benefit the subject's and/or the public's good, the investigator may be duty-bound to clarify the misunderstanding.[283]

One could develop a standard disclosure format for some of the various types of conflicts of interest. For example, consider the situation in which a salaried clinical investigator employed by a not-for-profit institution, such as an academic medical center, is conducting a study and neither the investigator nor the institution has any equity or similar interest in the outcome of the research. In such a case, where the payment by a study sponsor merely covers the actual cost of conducting the research plus a modest amount that covers the institution's indirect costs or overhead, it may well be sufficient simply to tell prospective subjects that the institution is receiving financial support from the sponsor to aid in conducting the study. Certainly, however, applying such boilerplate language in all cases could defeat the purpose of informed consent. If the goal is

Volume 28:4, Winter 2000

to provide the potential subject with enough information about the investigator's financial interest to make an informed decision about participating in the study, then in situations other than our example the specific financial arrangements of each clinical study should receive consideration by the IRB. Where appropriate, the IRB would mandate the disclosure of additional information.

Given the variety of different conflicts of interest described above, numerous difficulties arise in developing a standard format for making disclosures. In fact, when asked if there was a suggested format for investigator disclosures at the *institutional* level (as opposed to disclosure to subjects), the National Science Foundation and the Public Health Service specifically declined to propose such a format for disclosure.[284] Rather than attempt to develop a standard disclosure for the numerous types of financial conflicts of interest, the agencies explicitly stated that "[t]he rules are designed to defer to the expertise of grantee institutions in developing policies and supporting documentation."[285] A similarly flexible approach is warranted for IRBs as they formulate formats for appropriate disclosure to subjects.

v. How should disclosure occur?

Disclosure during the informed-consent process may serve more to protect the investigator than to inform the subject. Consequently, the manner of disclosure may be critical. Some investigators may disclose their financial conflicts of interest in a way that induces passive capitulation rather than increases the subjects' understanding of the conflict. Investigators may seek to bury the information concerning the conflict within pages of technical or scientific terminology that the average subject is incapable of comprehending. Frustration with the complexity of the consent form may cause the subject to treat the form as "meaningless paperwork."[286] The investigator may then point to the subject's "informed consent" as the moral justification for a bad result that occurred during the research.[287]

Presented in this manner, disclosure will do little to mitigate the investigator's conflict of interest. Consequently, the IRB must see to it that if disclosure of financial conflicts of interest is warranted, it is done in a reasonable way, such that subjects can give the information the appropriate degree of weight according to the circumstance.

Given the problems associated with placing complete reliance on the disclosure of financial conflicts of interest in what presumably would be a very rare case, a monitoring system, coupled with disclosure, may be an appropriately effective means of protecting a subject's autonomy. The use of monitors or auditors is not unknown to health-care institutions generally or to some IRBs as they pursue vehicles for ensuring appropriate subject protections. Many health-care providers employ the services of

health-care consultants to ensure compliance with federal fraud and abuse rules. Similarly, IRBs have used auditors on occasion as an appropriate vehicle for insuring both (1) that subjects understand the risks and benefits of the research in which they are being asked or have agreed to participate, and (2) that they are willing to participate or to continue to participate in the research project.

With respect to the disclosure of financial conflicts of interest and the need to ensure that subjects understand both the nature and implication of any conflict of interest that the research presents, boards could utilize the same internal staff, IRB members, or independent auditors. While the use of auditors obviously could not occur without some costs, it may be viewed as a sound investment and is very much in line with current indications from the Office of Human Research Protections of the direction in which it would like to see IRBs move.

b. Mandating the sharing of profits

The reasons behind a subject's participation in clinical research may range from a desire to help his or her fellow man to a desire to obtain the latest treatment when all other traditional therapies have failed.[288] Due to these non-financial motivations, subjects generally receive, at best, only minimal compensation for their time, effort, and discomfort.[289] Similarly, at least when a patient consents to the use of removed tissue for research, typically the patient is not paid for his or her time, although there may be a modest payment for the discomfort or for the actual tissue or fluid itself.[290] Most patients feel comfortable with the idea that the donation is a gift.[291] This may change, however, when the possibility arises that a researcher, university, or corporation will receive substantial financial benefit as a result of the donated tissue or fluid.[292] When the terms of the gift are dramatically altered, the subject-donor may view the researcher-recipient in a different light.[293] The subject's best interest may no longer appear to be the researcher's priority; therefore, the subject's and the researcher's interests may no longer be congruent. This would be particularly true when it is clear, from the outset, that one of the obvious purposes of conducting the research is the development of commercially viable products from the blood or tissue samples.

Some commentators believe that, at least with respect to databanking DNA and developing cell lines from stored blood and tissue samples, sharing the profits with the subject is appropriate and would adequately resolve the investigator's conflict of interest.[294] The suggestion has been that subjects should receive anywhere between 10 and 25 percent of any profits for their role in providing the blood and tissue samples that become the foundation for a commercially viable product.[295] This percentage range is based on what would seem fair to "reasonable persons inside and outside of biomedical science."[296] This theory of sharing profits revolves around the idea that once a reasonable person understands that his or her cells may become commercially profitable, that person would expect to receive a portion of the profits as compensation.[297]

Investigators may argue that sharing profits with the subject will induce some to participate in the research for the wrong reasons. Subjects may not comprehend that the possibility of realizing the financial gain is no greater than their chances of winning a multistate lottery.[298] The desire for financial gain may cloud the subject's judgment and cause him or her to minimize the potential risks of the research. In addition, this proposed solution does not guarantee that the investigator will act in a manner that is not biased by personal interest. That is, clearly, the investigator's stake in the research will continue to subject him or her to subtle biases. This may result, for example, in removing more tissue than is therapeutically necessary or, when obtaining consent from the subject, in minimizing potential risks. Finally, although sharing profits with the subject will provide both subject and investigator with similar interests, it does not resolve the issue of whether the subject truly understands the nature of his or her participation — the essence of informed consent.

Investigators may also argue that the subject should not receive a percentage of the profits because the level of compensation otherwise received by the subject for his or her participation in the research is adequate. This may be especially true in situations where the subject's tissue is transformed in making the final commercially viable product. The subject merely supplied the original tissue sample, a sample that probably could have been provided by other subjects.[299] It is the researcher who is responsible for the transformation and it was his or her knowledge and skill that facilitated the development of the commercially viable product from the tissue sample. Therefore, it would be posited that it is only the study sponsor and perhaps the investigator who are entitled to any profits from the tissue's commercialization, and the subject ought not be entitled to a percentage of the proceeds.

An argument could also be made that the purpose of much research not involving the use of blood and tissues samples is to develop commercially viable products such as pharmaceuticals and medical devices. Thus, the question will arise concerning whether subjects in those studies ought to be entitled to a share of resulting profits, if any, should financial success ensue. Of course, in these situations, there are typically a large number of subjects involved and the role that any one subject plays may be viewed as marginal or incidental. But this would not be the case when a particular person's blood or tissue is utilized.

While various IRBs, no doubt, have handled this situation differently, not infrequently investigators and study sponsors have requested that consent forms contain statements to the effect that the subject understands that by participating in the research and signing the consent form the subject waives any rights he or she may have to proceeds from commercially viable products that may result from the development of blood or tissue samples.

As a result of concerns arising from *Moore*, several IRBs have added language to informed-consent documents in situations where commercialization may occur. One IRB, for example, voted to add the following language for a particular protocol:

> Tissues taken from you, including blood and other fluid samples, may be used in the making of new medical products. The persons conducting this research do/do not have a financial interest in any such product. You may or may not be entitled to receive profits from this product.[300]

In another situation, the consent form stated:

> I understand that cell lines containing material from the blood sample I supply will be established in laboratory culture. All rights to and title in these cell lines will reside with the institution conducting this study.[301]

Robert Levine has indicated that the Yale IRB would approve a consent form that included the following statement of purpose and benefits:

> The purpose of this research is to learn more than we know about cancer of the cervix. In particular, we wish to learn whether cells like yours can be used to make antibodies to cancer cells .... This research is not designed to bring benefits to you. Rather, we hope that the knowledge developed in the course of this research will form the basis for developing improved treatments for future patients with cancer of the cervix.[302]

He went on to conclude that it would be appropriate to add the following statement to the informed-consent document:

> If we are successful we may be able to develop a cure for cancer, which, of course, would have enormous market value.[303]

Levine then stated that in research that may yield a commercially viable product, the investigator should add a statement to the following effect:

> In the event this research project results in the development of a marketable product, you will

Volume 28:4, Winter 2000

have no rights to share in any profits from its sale and no obligations to share in any losses.[304]

The difficulty here is that such a statement may well violate the explicit provision in federal regulations that prohibits statements in consent documents that "include any exculpatory language through which the subject ... is made to waive or appear to waive any of the subject's legal rights, ..."[305] It would seem appropriate, however, to include a statement to the effect that should commercially viable products result from blood or tissue samples that researchers obtain from the research, there are no present plans to share the proceeds with research subjects. Such a statement, of course, would not preclude subsequent efforts by subjects to share any proceeds. Property law, as determined by the relevant state court, would control the question. While the California courts in the *Moore* case held that the physician and his research associates were entitled to sole ownership of the cell line created from Moore's tissue,[306] other states might make different determinations. Moreover, *Moore* was decided in the context of a situation where the issue of ownership had not been addressed by the patient and physician prior to the procedures involved. The result might well be different where ownership interests are so addressed.

Although some investigators may argue that contracting to pay the subject a percentage of the profits is potentially unfair and raises more problems than it solves, the advantages of profit-sharing, at least in some circumstances, may outweigh the risks. This is particularly true in those instances in which the development of commercially viable products is a clear goal of the research. Sharing profits with the subject has a number of potential benefits. It promotes the investigator's own awareness of his or her potential financial interest. While informing the subject of the potential commercial use of the tissue, the investigator is also disclosing his or her potential interest if the tissue has commercial value. The subject is then given an opportunity to make a conscious decision, with full knowledge of the investigator's interest, regarding the use of his or her tissue. Finally, if the subject's tissue turns out to be commercially valuable, the subject will receive compensation for the contributed tissue, thereby lessening the sense of injustice that may be felt by the public toward the financial benefits received by the investigator or institution.

Consequently, it would be sensible in appropriate situations for IRBs to consider the propriety of requiring investigators to share profits with subjects, to inform subjects of such a possibility, and to supervise the manner in which such information is provided and actual profits shared. For IRBs to make such a judgment in particular situations and on a case-by-case basis would not take them far afield from their traditional roles. IRBs are already involved in reviewing levels of compensation paid to subjects. The conventional concern here is that overly high amounts of compensation might well serve to encourage — inappropriately — higher than average rates of participation in research by poorer members of society. This would violate the bioethical principle of justice in the selection of subjects. This principle mandates that both the benefits and burdens of research fall on all segments of society equally.[307] By following this line of thought, one could conclude that sharing profits with the subject mitigates the investigator's conflict of interest because the subject's and researcher's interests are aligned more closely.

4. Existing financial disclosure experiences

Over twelve years ago, at least one IRB insisted on disclosing a financial conflict of interest to potential subjects. In that situation, the IRB required that the investigator disclose the fact that he or she would receive a per capita payment for each subject enrolled in the clinical trial. The disclosure read as follows:

> The investigator will be reimbursed a fixed amount by (company name) for each appropriate subject enrolled in the trial. Please feel free to ask about funding arrangements and amounts if you desire.[308]

At the Conference on Human Subject Protection and Financial Conflict of Interest last August, a number of institutions reported how they had handled disclosure of financial conflicts of interest to subjects. Typically, these were presented as part of the institution's broader program regarding such conflicts. The programs involved investigators' reporting conflicts to the institution as well as possibly to subjects after IRB review.

a. Children's Hospital in Boston

Children's Hospital in Boston has a multistep process for identifying and managing investigator conflicts of interest.[309] All investigators must complete a form and disclose any financial interests they have in a research protocol. The department chair reviews the form and determines whether there is an actual or potential conflict of interest. If a conflict of interest is identified, the chairman must present this to the president of the research administration, the trustee conflict-of-interest committee, or general counsel. Thus, the responsibility for reviewing the form and determining whether there is a conflict of interest is vested in the department chair, not the IRB.

The next step requires that clinical agreements be finalized before the IRB approves the protocol. The purpose of this requirement is to ensure that all funds received are justified and to guarantee that issues such as publication rights and ownership of data are resolved prior to begin-

The Journal of Law, Medicine & Ethics

ning the research. Another policy includes the prohibition of finder's fees.

To address potential institutional conflicts of interest, the informed consent must disclose whether the hospital holds stock as a result of a licensing agreement in the company owning the intellectual property invented at the hospital. If the hospital has equity in the licensing agreement, there must be an independent data safety monitoring board and the inventor may not supervise the clinical trial. Moreover, multicenter studies are required.

b. Washington University

At Washington University in St. Louis, the conflict-of-interest policy takes a different approach, according to Ted Cicero, the University's vice chancellor for research.[310] Similar to Children's Hospital in Boston, the investigator is required to disclose any conflict of interest. The department chair reviews this form to determine whether there is a conflict of interest and then a separate faculty disclosure review committee reviews the form. If an investigator holds equity in a company, the University may require either that the equity be placed in an escrow account held by a third party or that the investigator divest himself of the equity. The IRB asks for information about conflicts of interest, but largely relies on departmental chairs and the faculty disclosure review committee to deal with the situation.

Mr. Cicero noted, however, that there are two problems with the University's conflict-of-interest policy. The reporting system is essentially voluntary, trusting that the investigator will be honest in his disclosure. Additionally, due to the number of faculty members, there are no audits to ensure that the disclosure is adequate and complete.

c. Recent empirical studies of policies

Two recent articles appearing in the *New England Journal of Medicine* surveyed conflict-of-interest policies and policies on disclosure of conflicts of interest. The first article, which analyzed policies on conflict of interest from the ten medical schools receiving the largest amount of funding from the NIH, reported that six required disclosure of conflicts of interest to the institutional review board and two required disclosure to research subjects.[311] The second article was a broader national survey of policies on the disclosure of conflicts of interest at all 127 medical schools, 170 other research institutions receiving substantial grants from federal sources, journals, and federal agencies. Only 1 percent of those institutions having such policies required that disclosure of conflicts be made to the IRB; none indicated that the disclosure should either be managed by the IRB or by providing information to research subjects.[312] Neither article discussed what IRBs did with the information provided or how disclosure to subjects was handled.

V. RECOMMENDATIONS AND CONCLUSION

If we had a broadly effective "culture of conscience and responsibility," such that those engaged in research did "the right things for the right reason,"[313] there would be no need for regulations concerning conflicts of interest. This would, in effect, result in ubiquitous adherence to the abolitionist position. In the current climate, however, this hypothetical seems utopian. Certainly, if research groups, institutions, and professional societies were to voluntarily prohibit conflicts of interest, this would be ideal.

Federal authorities such as the FDA, OHRP, and the various research funding agencies should give strong consideration to imposing total bans on conflicts of interest to the extent they are able to do so. At the very least, the proscription should apply in those situations where a clinical investigator has a financial interest in the result of a clinical trial while also being responsible for the safety of subjects.[314]

Recently, the abolitionist argument in favor of prohibiting conflicts was posited most forcefully by Marcia Angell, the former editor of the *New England Journal of Medicine*, both in an editorial in that publication[315] and in a presentation at the August 2000 conference discussed above.[316] She asserts that institutional oversight is inadequate and that efforts at disclosure of conflicts to subjects "simply passes the buck to the patient subject, who is left to wonder how the investigator will balance his competing interest"; it "does nothing to remove the conflict of interest."[317] Nonetheless, she admits "not disclosing a conflict of interest is even worse because it is fundamentally deceptive."[318] She would prohibit researchers from having any financial ties to companies from which they receive grant support; prohibit payments for writing and speaking; bar industry payment for travel to industry-sponsored symposiums; and require that any payments for consulting go to pools earmarked to support research or other medical center missions.[319] She further argues that no strings should be attached to research; she would require investigators to design, analyze, and publish their own studies, and bar both institutions and their senior officials from investing in the health-care industry.[320]

There is little doubt that an outright prohibition is the preferable way to proceed. Were that to occur and be effective, requirements for disclosure at the levels of investigator/sponsor, investigator/institution, and investigator/subject would become unnecessary.

But even those such as Dr. Koski, the new OHRP director, who essentially seems to agree with Dr. Angell and believes that certain conflicts of interest can and probably should be avoided, have taken the position that such conflicts are "inherent .... intrinsic and unavoidable to the research process."[321] Practically speaking, many of Dr. Angell's suggestions may be impossible to achieve. The political will to effectuate her proposals does not seem to exist. The question then becomes how conflicts of interest can best be managed. One necessary, albeit not sufficient, way of man-

Volume 28:4, Winter 2000

aging them would be to prescribe institutional review board oversight of such conflicts for the reasons described in and in a manner detailed in the previous section of this paper.

If this is the approach to be taken, federal regulations should be amended in two respects. First, they should explicitly require among the criteria for IRB approval of research a determination that any conflicts of interest that exist be reasonable in relation to the nature of the study. Second, the provisions regarding general requirements for informed consent should include, as an additional element of informed consent when appropriate, a statement describing the conflict of interest.

As noted above, some IRBs are already reviewing conflicts of interest in the protocols before them. Moreover, the suggested approach is not dissimilar to other determinations they are asked to make. For example, IRBs are currently required to determine that the risks to subjects are reasonable in relation to the anticipated benefits. As part of their determination that the selection of subjects is equitable, IRBs typically review levels of compensation being offered to subjects and implicitly utilize prior determinations as a guide to each new case. In appropriate, though undoubtedly rare, cases as described above, IRBs might require that investigators agree to share profits from the development of blood or tissue samples should any profits result.

There is no reason to believe that investigators would be unable to provide good-faith estimates of financial arrangements involved in the conduct of the study, and these can be reviewed in the same manner as is information regarding scientific background, risks and their minimization, subject selection, and the like. Protocols should include information concerning the source and amount of funding for the research and how that funding will occur. Relevant excerpts from proposed contracts should be reviewed in the same manner as boards typically review scientific material that appears, for example, in pharmaceutical company-sponsored protocols. Investigators should identify any ownership or other financial interests that they or the institution may have in any sponsoring organizations.

No doubt, boards will have to develop some expertise in evaluating financial arrangements. Thus, for example, they will need to detect situations where a study budget attempts to hide profit through payments of overly excessive amounts for particular tests, such as endoscopies, that the investigator will be required to perform as part of the protocol. Still, this is not significantly different, in kind, from the expertise that is developed in identifying and assessing physical, emotional, or social risks.

With respect to disclosure requirements, in many cases boards will determine that no statement need be made. In other instances, a simple statement indicating that financial support is being provided to the institution conducting the study will suffice. Certainly, however, if a finder's fee is involved or if the investigator himself will receive any significant per-subject payment above and beyond the actual costs to conduct the study, more detailed disclosure would be necessary.

It is true that many, if not most, institutional review boards find themselves overwhelmed by current responsibilities. Consequently, any decision to add to their burdens must be made with some trepidation. But, in the absence of a wholesale prohibition on conflicts of interest, such as propounded by Dr. Angell, attention must be paid to the need to better ensure the protection of patient autonomy. Currently that is the task with which IRBs are most familiar. Should some of the directions suggested by Dr. Koski, the new OHRP director, be effectuated, IRBs will find themselves both more adequately supported and less concerned with unnecessary documentation and other procedural minutiae. They should then be in a position to better attend to substantive issues such as those presented by conflicts of interest.

ACKNOWLEDGMENTS

The research assistance of Martin M. Clay, Jr., Esq., Rebecca L. McCarty, and Lisa M. Re is gratefully acknowledged. I would also like to thank Ellen Wright Clayton, M.D., J.D., for her helpful comments. A summer grant from the Saint Louis University School of Law Faculty Research Program partially supported the writing of this paper.

REFERENCES

1. K. Eichenwald and G. Kolata, "Drug Trials Hide Conflicts for Doctors," *New York Times*, May 16, 1999, at A1.
2. *Id.*
3. *Id.*
4. *Id.*
5. *Id.*
6. *Id.*
7. D. Nelson and R. Weiss, "Penn Researchers Sued in Gene Therapy Death," *Washington Post*, Sept. 19, 2000, at A3 [hereinafter cited as Nelson and Weiss, "Penn Researchers Sued"].
8. R. Weiss and D. Nelson, "Methods Faulted in Gene Test Death, Teen Too Ill for Therapy, Probe Finds," *Washington Post*, Dec. 8, 1999, at A1.
9. J. Brainard and D.W. Miller, "U.S. Regulators Suspend Medical Studies at 2 Universities," *Chronicle of Higher Education*, Feb. 4, 2000, at A30.
10. R. Weiss, "FDA Halts Experiences on Genes at University: Probe of Teen's Death Uncovers Deficiencies," *Washington Post*, Jan. 22, 2000, at A1.
11. D. Nelson and R. Weiss, "Penn Ends Gene Trials on Humans," *Washington Post*, May 25, 2000, at A1 [hereinafter cited as Nelson and Weiss, "Penn Ends Gene Trial"].
12. B. Gose, "U. of Pennsylvania, Doctors, and Ethicist are Named in Suit Over Gene-Therapy Death," *Chronicle of Higher Education*, Sept. 29, 2000, at A34.
13. Nelson and Weiss, "Penn Researchers Sued," *supra* note 7.
14. *Id.*

The Journal of Law, Medicine & Ethics

15. Nelson and Weiss, "Penn Ends Gene Trial," *supra* note 11.

16. S. Hensley, "Targeted Genetics' Genovo Deal Leads to Windfall for Researcher," *Wall Street Journal*, Aug. 10, 2000 at B12.

17. Nelson and Weiss, "Penn Ends Gene Trial," *supra* note 11.

18. *Id.*

19. Gose, *supra* note 12.

20. A. Schneider, "U. of Pennsylvania Settles Lawsuit Over Gene-Therapy Death," *Chronicle of Higher Education*, Nov. 6, 2000.

21. T. Bodenheimer, "Uneasy Alliance- Clinical Investigator's and the Pharmaceutical Industry" (Health Policy Report), *N. Engl. J. Med.*, 342 (2000): 1539–44, at 1539.

22. *Id.*

23. *Id.*

24. M. Angell, "Is Academic Medicine for Sale?" (Editorial), *N. Engl. J. Med.*, 342 (2000): 1516–18, at 1517.

25. See text at notes 197–217 *infra*.

26. See, for example, Eichenwald and Kolata, *supra* note 1; K. Eichenwald and G. Kolata, "A Doctor's Drug Studies Turn Into Fraud," *New York Times*, May 17, 1999, at A1; V. Kiernan, "Financial Ties May Taint Researchers' Judgment," *Chronicle of Higher Education*, Jan. 23, 1998, at A18.

27. D.F. Thompson, "Understanding Financial Conflicts of Interest" (Sounding Board), *N. Engl. J. Med.*, 329 (1993): 573–76, at 573.

28. *Id.*

29. J. Katz, "Human Experimentation and Human Rights," *Saint Louis University Law Journal*, 38 (1993): 7–54, at 14.

30. *Id.* at 15.

31. *Id.* See also J.A. Goldner, "An Overview of Legal Controls on Human Experimentation and the Regulatory Implications of Taking Professor Katz Seriously," *Saint Louis University Law Journal*, 38 (1993): 64–134, at 120 [hereinafter cited as Goldner, "Legal Controls on Human Experimentation"].

32. *Id.*

33. Thompson, *supra* note 27, at 573.

34. *Id.*

35. R. Delgado and H. Leskovac, "Informed Consent in Human Experimentation: Bridging the Gap Between Ethical Thought and Current Practice," *UCLA Law Review*, 34 (1986): 67–130, at 91.

36. J.P. Kassirer and M. Angell, "Financial Conflicts of Interest in Biomedical Research," *N. Engl. J. Med.*, 329 (1993): 570–71.

37. E.J. Emanuel and D. Steiner, "Institutional Conflict of Interest" (Sounding Board), *N. Engl. J. Med.*, 332 (1995): 262–67, at 263.

38. TUNA is a procedure used to treat prostate disorders. T.M. Burton, "Urodollars: A Prostate Researcher Tested Firm's Product and Sat on Its Board," *Wall Street Journal*, Mar. 19, 1998, at A1.

39. *Id.*

40. *Id.*

41. Dr. Oesterling pled no contest to a felony charge of fraud after it was discovered that he had been double and triple billing for his trips and had not reported research money to the university. *Id.*

42. *Id.*

43. D. Vergano, "Drug Trials vex Medical Ethics American Experts put Testing by Private Companies Under a Microscope," *USA Today*, Aug. 8, 2000, at 9D; see also Eichenwald and Kolata,

supra note 1.

44. M.J. Finkel, "Should Informed Consent Include Information on How Research is Funded?," *IRB*, 13, no. 5 (1991): 1–3, at 1. Currently, the Department of Health and Human Services provides little guidance on recruitment. However, a recent OIG report recommended the development of such recruitment guidelines. See Office of Inspector General, "Recruiting Human Subjects: Pressures in Industry Sponsored Clinical Research" (June 2000): 1–79, at 33 [hereinafter cited as OIG Report, "Pressures in Industry Sponsored Clinical Research"].

45. D.S. Shimm and R.G. Spece, "Conflict of Interest and Informed Consent in Industry-Sponsored Clinical Trials," *Journal of Legal Medicine*, 12 (1991): 477–513, at 482.

46. R. Roizen, "Why I Oppose Drug Company Payment of Physician/Investigators on a Per Patient/Subject Basis," *IRB*, 10, no. 1 (1988): 9–10, at 9.

47. Shimm and Spece, *supra* note 45, at 482. Still another source states that pharmaceutical companies sometimes pay doctors as much as $6,000 per patient. See also S. Kaplan and S. Brownlee, "Dying for a Cure: Why Cancer Patients Often Turn to Risky Experimental Treatments — And Wind Up Paying With Their Lives," *U.S. News & World Report*, Oct. 11, 1999, at 34. It is not clear whether remuneration levels cited by commentators are in net or gross.

48. Shimm and Spece, *supra* note 45, at 482.

49. *Id.* See Roizen, *supra* note 46, at 9. See also OIG Report, "Pressures in Industry Sponsored Clinical Research," *supra* note 44, at 25.

50. Shimm and Spece, *supra* note 45, at 482.

51. Office of Inspector General, "Recruiting Human Subjects: Sample Guidelines for Practice" (June 2000): 1–23, at 8 [hereinafter cited as OIG Report, "Sample Guidelines for Practice"].

52. Some investigators indicate that sponsors continually cut initial study budgets, so bonuses help sites recoup the costs of conducting the trials. See OIG Report, "Pressures in Industry Sponsored Clinical Research," *supra* note 44, at 17.

53. See OIG Report, "Sample Guidelines for Practice," *supra* note 51, at 8.

54. OIG Report, "Pressures in Industry Sponsored Clinical Research," *supra* note 44, at 12–14.

55. *Id.* at 13.

56. *Id.*

57. *Id.*

58. *Id.*

59. See OIG Report, "Pressures in Industry Sponsored Clinical Research," *supra* note 44, at 25–26.

60. L.B. Andrews, "Money Is Putting People at Risk in Biomedical Research," *Chronicle of Higher Education*, Mar. 10, 2000, at B4.

61. Shimm and Spece, *supra* note 45, at 482.

62. *Id.*

63. E.A. Maher, "An Analysis of Finder's Fees in Clinical Research," *Canadian Medical Association Journal*, 150 (1994): 252–56, at 252.

64. E.G. DeRenzo, "Coercion in the Recruitment and Retention of Human Research Subjects, Pharmaceutical Industry Payments to Physician-Investigators, and the Moral Courage of the IRB," *IRB*, 22, no. 2 (2000): 1–5, at 2.

65. Eichenwald and Kolata, *supra* note 1.

66. Maher, *supra* note 63, at 255.

67. *Id.* at 255–56.

68. S.L. Lind, "Finder's Fees for Research Subjects," *N. Engl. J. Med.*, 323 (1990): 192–95, at 193.

Volume 28:4, Winter 2000

69. *Id.*

70. E.G. Campbell, K.S. Louis, and D. Blumenthal, "Looking a Gift Horse in the Mouth: Corporate Gifts Supporting Life Sciences Research," *JAMA*, 279 (1998): 995–99, at 995.

71. The study surveyed 2,167 faculty who conducted research. The survey asked the researchers to rate research-gifts as "essential," "very important," "important," "not very important," or "not at all important" to the progress of their research. *Id.* at 997.

72. *Id.* at 998.

73. *Id.* at 997.

74. J.P. Orlowski and L. Wateska, "The Effects of Pharmaceutical Firm Enticements on Physician Prescribing Patterns: There's no Such Thing as a Free Lunch," *Chest*, 102 (1992): 270–73.

75. *Id.*

76. *Id.* at 273.

77. B. Healy et al., "Conflict- of- Interest Guidelines for a Multicenter Clinical Trial of Treatment After Coronary Artery Bypass-Graft Surgery" (Special Report), *N. Engl. J. Med.*, 320 (1989): 949–51, at 950.

78. S. Hilgartner, "Research Fraud, Misconduct and the IRB," *IRB*, 12, no. 1 (1990): 1–4, at 4.

79. *Id.*

80. R. Macklin, "'Due' and 'Undue' Inducements: On Paying Money to Research Subjects," *IRB*, 3, no. 5 (1981): 1–6, at 1, 4. The risk-to-benefit ratio must be balanced or shown to be "in a favorable ratio. See National Commission for the Protection of Human Subjects of Biomedical and Behavioral Research, *The Belmont Report: Ethical Principles and Guidelines for the Protection of Human Subjects of Research*, DHEW Pub. No. (OS) 78–0012, (Washington, D.C.: U.S. Gov't Printing Office, 1978) [hereinafter cited as *The Belmont Report*]. Thus, offering patients money, as an inducement to participation in a study with high levels of risk, would violate principles of justice and accepted norms regarding the risk-benefit analysis.

81. Hilgartner, *supra* note 78, at 4.

82. H. Stelfox et. al., "Conflict of Interest in the Debate over Calcium-Channel Antagonists," *N. Engl. J. Med.* 338 (1998): 101–06. For a discussion of other studies demonstrating that financial conflicts of interest have an impact on the conclusions reached by researchers in published articles, see National Institutes of Health, "Conference on Human Subject Protection and Financial Conflicts of Interest," Transcript at 13–14 (August 15, 2000) [hereinafter cited as National Institutes of Health, "Transcript, Aug. 15, 2000"].

83. V. Kiernan, *supra* note 26.

84. *Id.*

85. *Id.*

86. "Scientific Journals Rarely Acknowledge Authors' Potential Conflicts, Study Finds," *Chronicle of Higher Education*, Feb. 5, 1999, at A39.

87. See G. Blumenstyk, "Medical Journal Reviews Its Policies After Author's Potential Conflict is Reported," *Chronicle of Higher Education*, Oct. 8, 1999, at A24. See also D. Orentlicher and M.K. Hehir, II, "Advertising Policies of Medical Journals: Conflicts of Interest for Journal Editors and Professional Societies," *Journal of Law, Medicine & Ethics*, 27 (1999): 113–118.

88. Blumenstyk, *supra* note 87.

89. *Id.*

90. *Id.*

91. *Id.*

92. *Id.*

93. *Id.*

94. "Scientific Journals Rarely Acknowledge Authors' Potential Conflicts, Study Finds," *supra* note 86.

95. Katz, *supra* note 29, at 37. See also Delgado and Leskovac, *supra* note 35, at 104.

96. B.A. Goldrick, E. Larson, and D. Lyons, "Conflict of Interest in Academia," *Image: Journal of Nursing Scholarship*, 27 (1995): 65–69, at 66.

97. Delgado and Leskovac, *supra*, note 35, at 104.

98. J.A. Goldner, "The Unending Saga of Legal Controls Over Scientific Misconduct: A Clash of Cultures Needing Resolution," *American Journal of Law & Medicine*, 24 (1998): 293–343, at 343.

99. See 35 U.S.C. §§ 200 et. seq. (1980). See also National Institutes of Health, "Transcript, Aug. 15, 2000," *supra* note 82, at 49. See also text at notes 123–127 *infra*.

100. Angell, *supra* note 24.

101. National Institutes of Health, "A '20-20' View of Invention Reporting to the National Institutes of Health" (visited Oct. 30, 2000) <http://grants.nih.gov/grants/guide/notice-files/not95-003.html>.

102. *Id.*

103. *Id.*

104. *Id.*

105. Andrews, *supra* note 60, at 2.

106. *Id.*

107. *Id.* at 3.

108. In fact, there is no mention of conflicts of interest in the legislative history of the Act.

109. J.K. Inglehart, "Rapid Changes for Academic Medical Centers," *N. Engl. J. Med.*, 332 (1995): 407–11, at 408.

110. *Id.* See also P.D. Fox and J. Wasserman, "Academic Medical Centers and Managed Care: Uneasy Partners," *Health Affairs*, (Spring 1993): 85–93, at 89.

111. *Id.*

112. A. Johnson, "Current Trends in Faculty Personnel Policies: Appointment, Evaluation and Termination," *Saint Louis University Law Journal*, 44 (2000): 81–112, at 88.

113. *Id.*

114. *Id.*

115. Taken from materials presented by Annette Johnson, Saint Louis University Health Law Symposium, April 1999. Materials on file with author.

116. See, for example, C. Hilton et al., "A Relative-value-Based System for Calculating Faculty Productivity in Teaching, Research, Administration, and Patient Care," *Academic Medicine* (1997): 787–93, at 792–93. For example, at Louisiana State University School of Medicine in New Orleans, physicians receive points for writing grants and publishing an abstract or manuscript. *Id.* Under the university's scheme, a physician has the opportunity to receive 4,150 points based on research projects, out of a total 14,612 possible points. *Id.* Thus, almost one-third of the total points may be obtained by participating in research; salary levels, in turn, reflect the total number of points awarded. *Id.*

117. Angell, *supra* note 24, at 1517.

118. H. Leskovac, "Ties that Bind: Conflicts of Interest in University-Industry Links," *U.C. Davis Law Review*, 17 (1984): 895–923, at 895.

119. *Id.* at 899.

120. H. Edgar and D.J. Rothman, "The Institutional Review Board and Beyond: Future Challenges to the Ethics of Human Experimentation," *Milbank Quarterly*, 73, no. 4 (1995): 489–506, at 500.

121. *Id.* at 499–500.

122. *Id.* at 500.

123. W.L. Geary, "Protecting the Patent Rights of Small Businesses — Does the Bayh-Dole Act Live Up to its Promise?" *AIPLA Quarterly Journal*, 20 (1992): 10–34, at 18. See also R.K. Yoshinaka, "Too Much of a Good Thing? Public Access to Medical Research in Washington After *Paws v. U.W.*," *Washington Law Review*, 70 (1995): 929–52, at 939. See text at notes 99–104 *supra*.

124. *Id.*

125. *Id.*

126. Andrews, *supra* note 60, at 2.

127. Angell, *supra* note 24.

128. D.A. Blake, "The Opportunities and Problems of Commercial Ventures: The University View, in Biomedical Research," in R.J. Porter and T.E. Malone, eds., *Biomedical Research: Collaboration and Conflict of Interest* (Baltimore: John Hopkins University Press, 1992): 88–92, at 88–89.

129. *Id.* This is true even though the Bayh-Dole Act gives sponsoring universities intellectual property rights to inventions stemming from federally funded research.

130. D. Bok, "Business and the Academy," *Harvard Magazine*, 83 (1981): 23–35, at 26.

131. Emanuel and Steiner, *supra* note 37, at 263.

132. C.T. Maatz, "University Physician-Researcher Conflicts of Interest: The Inadequacy of Current Controls and Proposed Reform," *High Technology Law Journal*, 7 (1992): 137–88, at 155.

133. *Id.*

134. *Id.*

135. *Id.*

136. *Id.* at 156.

137. *Id.* at 156.

138. *Id.*

139. See "Financial Disclosure by Clinical Investigators," 63 Fed. Reg. 5,233 (1998); "Objectivity in Research," 60 Fed. Reg. 35,810 (1995); and "Investigator Financial Disclosure Policy," 59 Fed. Reg. 33,308 (1994).

140. See "Financial Disclosure by Clinical Investigators," 21 C.F.R. § 54.1(a) (1998) and "Responsibility of Applicants for Promoting Objectivity in Research for Which PHS Funding is Sought," 42 C.F.R. § 50.601 (1996).

141. See "Responsibility of Applicants for Promoting Objectivity in Research for Which PHS Funding is Sought," 42 C.F.R. § 50.606 (1996).

142. "Financial Disclosure by Clinical Investigators," 59 Fed. Reg. 48,708 (1994).

143. *Id.* Federal support is not necessary for the FDA regulations to be applicable. The FDA regulations apply to any FDA-regulated article. See "NIH Regulatory Burden v. Human Subjects Protection — Workgroups Report" (visited at December 6, 2000) < http://grants.nih.gov/grants/policy/regulatoryburden/humansubjectsprotection.htm >.

144. *Id.*

145. "Financial Disclosure by Clinical Investigators," 21 C.F.R. § 54.4 (1998).

146. *Id.*

147. *Id.*

148. *Id.*

149. *Id.* at § 54.4(c).

150. "Responsibility of Applicants for Promoting Objectivity in Research for Which PHS Funding is Sought," 42 C.F.R. § 50.604 (1996).

151. *Id.* See also "Investigator Financial Disclosure Policy," 59 Fed. Reg. 33,311–12 (1994); F-D-C Reports, "Final PHS Conflict-of-Interest Rule Sets $10,000/5% Disclosure Threshold, Harmonizes With NSF Reg," *The Blue Sheet*, July 12, 1995.

152. "Responsibility of Applicants for Promoting Objectivity in Research for Which PHS Funding is Sought," 42 C.F.R. § 50.604 (1996). See also "Investigator Financial Disclosure Policy," 59 Fed. Reg. 33,311–12 (1994); F-D-C Reports, "Final PHS Conflict-of-Interest Rule Sets $10,000/5% Disclosure Threshold, Harmonizes With NSF Reg," *The Blue Sheet*, July 12, 1995.

153. The NSF and PHS guidelines are virtually identical. The main difference between the two is that, while all research funded by PHS is subject to the PHS guidelines, the NSF policy only applies to institutions accepting NSF grant funds that have more than 50 employees. See M. Barnes and S. Krauss, "Conflicts of Interest in Human Research: Risks and Pitfalls of 'Easy Money' in Research Funding," *BNA's Health Law Reporter*, 9, no. 35 (2000): at 1385.

154. "Responsibility of Applicants for Promoting Objectivity in Research for Which PHS Funding is Sought," 42 C.F.R. § 50.604 (1996). See also "Investigator Financial Disclosure Policy," 59 Fed. Reg. 33,311–12 (1994); F-D-C Reports, "Final PHS Conflict-of-Interest Rule Sets $10,000/5% Disclosure Threshold, Harmonizes With NSF Reg," *The Blue Sheet*, July 12, 1995.

155. *Id.*

156. *Id.*

157. The PHS and NSF rules do not specify what type of mechanisms an institution should have in place in order to detect an investigator's failure to comply with the institution's conflict-of-interest policy.

158. 42 C.F.R. § 50.606(a).

159. *Id.*

160. *Id.*

161. 42 C.F.R. § 50.606(c). The disclosure of financial conflicts of interest is required of all individuals presenting at Continuing Medical Education (CME) seminars.

162. 42 C.F.R. § 50.606(b).

163. *Id.*

164. *Id.*

165. The Post-CABG Clinical Trial was a multicenter, randomized, double blind study sponsored by the National Institutes of Health. Healy, *supra* note 77. See also Shimm and Spece, *supra* note 45, at 508.

166. Shimm and Spece, *supra* note 45, at 508.

167. F-D-C Reports, "Conflict-of-Interest Guidelines Established By Researchers Conducting NHLBI-Sponsored Trial," *The Blue Sheet*, April 12, 1989.

168. Shimm and Spece, *supra* note 45, at 508.

169. *Id.*

170. *Id.*

171. A.S. Relman, "Economic Incentives In Clinical Investigation," *N. Engl. J. Med.*, 320 (1989): 933–34, at 933.

172. *Id.*

173. See American Society of Gene Therapy, "Policy of The American Society of Gene Therapy on Financial Conflict of Interest in Clinical Research" (visited Oct. 30, 2000) < http://www.asgt.org/policy/index.html >.

174. *Id.*

175. See American Society of Gene Therapy, "American Society of Gene Therapy Bylaws" (visited Oct. 30, 2000) < http://www.asgt.org/bylaws.html >.

176. "Keratoconjunctivitis sicca" is defined as "inflammation of the cornea and conjunctiva [the membrane lining the eyelids]; a condition marked by hyperemia [an excess of blood] of the conjunctiva, thickening and drying of the corneal epithelium, and itching and burning of the eye." M. O'Toole et al., eds., *Miller-Keane Encyclopedia and Dictionary of Medicine, Nursing, and*

Allied Health, 5th ed. (Philadelphia: W.B. Saunders, 1992): at 811.

177. Shimm and Spece, supra note 45, at 507.

178. Id. See also F-D-C Reports, "Vitamin A Ophthalmic Ointment Studies By Tseng, et al., Violated Human Subject Protection Rules, NIH Finds," The Blue Sheet, March 8, 1989.

179. Id. at 507–08.

180. Id. at 508.

181. M. Witt and L.O. Gostin, "Conflict of Interest Dilemmas in Biomedical Research," JAMA, 271 (1994): 547–51.

182. Id. See also Shimm and Spece, supra note 45, at 508, n. 92.

183. See President and Fellows of Harvard College, "Guidelines for Conflicts of Interest" (visited Oct. 30, 2000) <http://www.hms.harvard.edu/integrity/guide.html>.

184. Witt and Gostin, supra note 181, at 549.

185. Id.

186. Id.

187. Angell, supra note 24, at 1516.

188. K.S. Mangan, "Harvard Medical School Will Keep Its Conflict-Of-Interest Policies," Chronicle of Higher Education, June 9, 2000, at A36.

189. Angell, supra note 24, at 1518.

190. Id.

191. Id.

192. Id.

193. Id.

194. See Goldner, "Legal Controls on Human Experimentation," supra note 31.

195. Id. at 101–103. Institutional review boards also conduct continuing review of approved research to ensure that human-subject protections remain in place. See also R.J. Levine, Ethics & Regulation of Clinical Research (Baltimore : Urban & Schwarzenberg, 1981): 326. See also 21 C.F.R. § 56.111(a)(2) and (4); 45 C.F.R. § 46.111(a)(2) and (4).

196. See Goldner, "Legal Controls on Human Experimentation," supra note 31, at 63, 90–103.

197. See generally Office of Inspector General, "Institutional Review Boards: Their Role in Reviewing Approved Research" (June 1998): i–15.

198. Id.

199. Id. at 9–11.

200. Id.

201. Office of Inspector General, "Protecting Human Subjects: Status of Recommendations" (April 2000): 1–25 [hereinafter cited as OIG Report, "Status of Recommendations"]. See also J. Brainard, "NIH, FDA Should Do More to Protect Human Subjects in Research, Report Says," Chronicle of Higher Education, April 21, 2000, at A38.

202. OIG Report, "Status of Recommendations," supra note 201, at 2–3.

203 "IRBs: Facing a Crackdown," Center Watch, 7 (April 2000).

204 J. Manier, "Rush is told why studies were halted," Chicago Tribune, Nov. 19, 1998, at A1.

205. P.J. Hilts, "Safety Concerns Halt Oklahoma Research," New York Times, July 11, 2000, at F12.

206. J. Brainard, "U.S. Regulators Call on 2 Universities to Suspend Studies Involving Prisoners," Chronicle of Higher Education, Sept. 15, 2000, at A26.

207. Office for Human Research Protections, "OHRP Compliance Activities: Common Findings and Guidance" (visited Oct. 30, 2000) <http://ohrp.osophs.dhhs.gov/references/findings.pdf>.

208. See text at notes 7–20 supra.

209. E.T. Pound, "Clinical trials halted Feds: Cancer study endangered patients," USA Today, July 10, 2000, at 1A.

210. E.T. Pound, "A case study in how not to conduct a clinical trial," USA Today, July 10, 2000, at 15A.

211. R. Weiss and D. Nelson, "U.S. Halts Cancer Tests in Oklahoma; Patient Protections Ignored, Agency Say," Washington Post, July 11, 2000, at A1.

212. J. Brainard, "Spate of Suspensions of Academic Research Spurs Questions About Federal Strategy," Chronicle of Higher Education, Feb. 4, 2000, at A29 [hereinafter cited as Brainard, "Spate of Suspensions"]. See also J. Brainard, "Agency Reassigns Head of Office That Oversees Human-Subjects Research," Chronicle of Higher Education, June 9, 2000, at A31 [hereinafter cited as Brainard, "Agency Reassigns Head of Office"].

213. Brainard, "Spate of Suspensions," supra note 212.

214. Id.

215. J. Brainard, "Physician May Lead New Human-Research Office," Chronicle of Higher Education, May 26, 2000, at A41. See also P. Healy, "Government to Upgrade Power of Watchdog on Human-Subject Research," Chronicle of Higher Education, July 30, 1999, at A28.

216. Healy, supra note 215; Brainard, supra note 215.

217. R. Weiss, "Panel Urges Major Upgrade for Medical Research Safety Office," Washington Post, June 4, 1999, at A16; Brainard, supra note 215.

218. Weiss, supra note 217.

219. Healy, supra note 215. See also J. Brainard, "Director Named for New Office to Protect Human Research Subjects," Chronicle of Higher Education, June 16, 2000, at A30.

220. Brainard, "Agency Reassigns Head of Office," supra note 212; J. Brainard, "Will 'Fresh Face' Bring a New Approach to Federal Protection of Human Subjects?" Chronicle of Higher Education, July 21, 2000, at A21 [hereinafter cited as Brainard, "Fresh Face"].

221. Brainard, "Fresh Face," supra note 220.

222. Id.

223. J. Brainard, "Top Official Criticizes Protection of Humans in Research," Chronicle of Higher Education, Oct. 6, 2000, at A34.

224. Id.

225. National Institutes of Health, "Conference on Human Subject Protection and Financial Conflicts of Interest," Transcript (August 16, 2000) [hereinafter cited as National Institutes of Health, "Transcript, Aug. 16, 2000"] (Statement of Greg Koski).

226. Brainard, "Fresh Face," supra note 220.

227. Id.

228. Office for Human Research Protections, "Statement of Greg Koski, Ph.D., M.D., Director, Office for Human Research Protections, Office of the Secretary, Department of Health and Human Services, for the Hearing on Human Subjects Protections in VA Medical Research Before The Subcommittee on Oversight and Investigations Committee on Veterans Affairs U.S. House of Representatives," Transcript (Sep. 28, 2000) (visited December 6, 2000) <http://ohrp.osophs.dhhs.gov/references/tkoski.htm> [hereinafter cited as OHRP, "Statement of Greg Koski"].

229. Brainard, supra note 215.

230. J. Brainard, "Top Official Criticizes Protection on Humans in Research," Chronicle of Higher Education, Oct. 6, 2000, at A34.

231. OHRP, "Statement of Greg Koski," supra note 228.

232. 45 C.F.R. § 46.111 (1991); 21 C.F.R. § 56.111 (1991).

233. 21 C.F.R. § 50.25 (1981); 45 C.F.R. § 46.116(c) (1991); 45 C.F.R. § 690.116(c) (1991).

The Journal of Law, Medicine & Ethics

234. *Id.* (emphasis added).
235. "Protection of Human Subjects; Informed Consent," 46 C.F.R. §§ 8942, 8947 (1981).
236. 21 C.F.R. § 50.20 (1981); 45 C.F.R. § 46.116 (1991); 45 C.F.R. § 690.116 (1991).
237. National Institutes of Health, "Financial Conflicts of Interest and Research Objectivity: Issues for Investigators and Institutional Review Boards" (June 5, 2000) (visited December 6, 2000) <http://grants.nih.gov/grants/guide/notice-files/NOT-OD-00-040.html>.
238. *Id.*
239. *Id.*
240. Department of Health and Human Services, "Human Subject Protection and Financial Conflicts of Interest: Conference," 65 Fed. Reg. 41,073–02 (2000).
241. *Id.*
242. *Id.*
243. *Id.*
244. R.F. Weir and J.R. Horton, "DNA Banking and Informed Consent — Part 1," *IRB*, 17, no. 4 (1995): 1–4, at 3 [hereinafter cited as Weir and Horton, Part 1].
245. *Id.*
246. *Canterbury v. Spence*, 464 F.2d 772, 786 (D.C. Cir. 1972).
247. Weir and Horton, Part 1, *supra* note 244, at 3.
248. *Id.*
249. B.R. Furrow et. al., *Liability and Quality Issues in Health Care*, 3rd ed. (St. Paul, Minnesota: West Publishing Co., 1997): at 381.
250. Delgado and Leskovac, *supra* note 35, at 88.
251. *Halushka v. University of Saskatchewan*, 53 D.L.R. 2d 436, 444 (Sask. 1965).
252. Delgado and Leskovac, *supra* note 35, at 90.
253. Of course, the subject's risk is not gratuitous if he or she is being compensated for time spent, or if he or she has contracted to receive a percentage of the profits if the research produces a commercially viable product. A subject, however, cannot be compensated for risk.
254. Goldner, "Legal Controls on Human Experimentation," *supra* note 31, at 114.
255. *Id.*, citing the National Commission for the Protection of Human Subjects of Biomedical and Behavioral Research, *The Belmont Report: Ethical Principles and Guidelines for the Protection of Human Subjects of Research*, DHEW Pub. No. (OS) 78-0012 (Washington, D.C.: U.S. Gov't Printing Office, 1978).
256. Delgado and Leskovac, *supra* note 35, at 92.
257. *Id.* at 91.
258. T.H. Murray, "Who Owns the Body? On the Ethics of Using Human Tissues for Commercial Purposes," *IRB*, 8, no. 1 (1986): 1–5, at 4.
259. *Id.*
260. M.A. Rodwin, "Physicians' Conflicts of Interest: The Limitations of Disclosure (Sounding Board)," *N. Engl. J. Med.*, 321, (1989): 1405–1409, at 1407 [hereinafter cited as Rodwin, "Limitations of Disclosure"]. See generally C.E. Schneider, *The Practice of Autonomy: Patients, Doctors and Medical Decisions* (New York: Oxford University Press, 1998).
261. Emanuel and Steiner, *supra* note 37, at 265.
262. *Id.*
263. *Id.*
264. Rodwin, "Limitations of Disclosure," *supra* note 260, at 1405.
265. *Id.*
266. *Id.*

267. *Id.*
268. *Id.*
269. M.A. Rodwin, *Medicine, Money and Morals: Physicians' Conflicts of Interest* (New York: Oxford Press, 1993): at 215.
270. *Id.* at 216.
271. *Id.* at 5; Murray, *supra* note 258, at 5.
272. Roizen, *supra* note 46, at 9.
273. *Id.* at 9, citing H.M. Spiro, "Mammon and Medicine: The Rewards of Clinical Trials," *JAMA*, 255 (1986): 1174–1175.
274. *Moore v. Regents of University of California*, 793 P.2d 479 (Cal. 1990).
275. *Id.* at 481.
276. *Id.*
277. *Id.* at 482.
278. *Id.* at 485.
279. A.T. Corrigan, "A Paper Tiger: Lawsuits Against Doctors for Non-Disclosure of Economic Interest in Patient's Cells, Tissues and Organs," *Case Western Reserve Law Review*, 42 (1991): 565–97, at 584.
280. Murray, *supra* note 258, at 4.
281. Finkel, *supra* note 44, at 2.
282. *Id.*
283. Murray, *supra* note 258, at 4.
284. "Frequently Asked Questions Concerning the Department of Health and Human Services Objectivity in Research Regulations and the National Science Foundation Investigator Financial Disclosure Policy," 61 Fed. Reg. 34,839 (1996).
285. *Id.*
286. Rodwin, "Limitations of Disclosure," *supra* note 260, at 1405.
287. R.W. Garnett, "Why Informed Consent? Human Experimentation and the Ethics of Autonomy," *The Catholic Lawyer*, 36 (1996): 455–511, at 458.
288. Delgado and Leskovac, *supra* note 35, at 102.
289. See Office for Protection from Research Risks, "Protecting Human Research Subjects: Institutional Review Board Guidebook" (1993): at 3-44–3-45.
290. Tissue is generally removed during a medically necessary procedure. Very few protocols call for tissue removal in excess of what is medically necessary for the subject's particular malady.
291. A "gift" is defined as a voluntary transfer of property to another made gratuitously and without consideration. *Bradley v. Bradley*, 540 S.W.2d 504, 511 (Tex. Civ. App. 1976).
292. Murray, *supra* note 258, at 1, 3.
293. *Id.*
294. R.F. Weir and J.R. Horton, "DNA Banking and Informed Consent — Part 2," *IRB*, 17, nos. 5–6 (1995): 1–8, at 8 [hereinafter cited as Weir and Horton, Part 2].
295. *Id.*
296. *Id.*
297. *Id.* at 2.
298. *Id.* at 8.
299. R. Levine, "Research that Could Yield Marketable Products from Human Materials: The Problem of Informed Consent," *IRB*, 8, no. 1 (1986): 6–7, at 7.
300. Bartolo, "Tales of Informed Consent: Four Years on an Institutional Review Board," *Health Matrix*, 2 (1992): 193–245, at 233.
301. Weir and Horton, Part 2, *supra* note 294, at 3.
302. Levine, *supra* note 299, at 6.
303. *Id.*
304. *Id.* at 7.
305. 45 C.F.R. § 46.116 (1991); 21 C.F.R. § 50.20 (1981).

306. *Id.* at 7.

307. 7 C.F.R. § 1.111 (2000). *The Belmont Report* states, "it can be seen how conceptions of justice are relevant to research involving human subjects. For example, the selection of research subjects needs to be scrutinized in order to determine whether some classes (e.g., welfare patients, particular racial and ethnic minorities, or persons confined to institutions) are being systematically selected simply because of their easy availability, their compromised position, or their manipulability, rather than for reasons directly related to the problem being studied." *The Belmont Report, supra* note 80, at 5.

308. Roizen, *supra* note 46, at 10.

309. See National Institutes of Health, "Conference on Human Subject Protection and Financial Conflicts of Interest," Transcript (August 15, 2000) [hereinafter cited as National Institutes of Health, "Transcript, Aug. 15, 2000"] (Statement of Susan Kornetsky).

310. *Id.* (Statement of Theodore J. Cicero).

311. B. Lo et al., "Conflict of Interest Policies for Investigators in Clinical Trials," *N. Engl. J. Med.*, 343 (2000): 1616–1620, at 1617.

312. S. Van McCrary et. al., "A National Survey of Policies on Disclosure of Conflicts of Interest in Biomedical Research," *N. Engl. J. Med.*, 343 (2000): 1621–1625, at 1623.

313. National Institutes of Health, "Transcript, Aug. 16, 2000," *supra* note 225 (Statement of Greg Koski).

314. See J.M. Drazen and G. Koski, "To Protect Those Who Serve" (Editorial), *N. Engl. J. Med.*, 343, (2000): 1643–1645, at 1644.

315. See Angell, *supra* note 24.

316. National Institutes of Health, "Transcript, August 16, 2000," *supra* note 225 (Statement of Marcia Angell).

317. *Id.*

318. *Id.*

319. *Id.* See also Angell, *supra* note 24.

320. National Institutes of Health, "Transcript, August 16, 2000," *supra* note 225 (Statement of Marcia Angell).

321. *Id.* (Statement of Greg Koski).

[35]

Restoring and Preserving Trust in Biomedical Research

Mark Yarborough, PhD, and Richard R. Sharp, PhD

ABSTRACT

Recent media depictions of the dangers of biomedical research have fueled public and regulatory scrutiny of academic research institutions. The authors argue that if these institutions are to preserve the trust that the public has historically bestowed upon them, they must go beyond mere compliance with regulatory mandates. Several steps are suggested that institutions can take to strengthen and supplement ongoing compliance efforts, steps the authors believe will bolster the public's confidence in the integrity of academic research institutions. These steps grow out of the authors' analysis of three key components of institutional trustworthiness: (1) shared goals between research institutions and the communities they serve, (2) robust institutional oversight of research

activities, and (3) training programs that build professional character. The authors' recommendations include the use of research advisory councils to assure the public that research goals reflect community interests, more collaborative relationships between institutional review boards and members of investigative teams, and educational programs that emphasize the importance of professional integrity in biomedical research. These efforts will help preserve public confidence that an institution's research priorities are appropriate and that the research it conducts is ethical. Preserving this public trust is central to the long-term success of biomedical research and the institutions in which such research takes place.
Acad. Med. 2002;77:8–14.

hese are important times for institutions involved in biomedical research. Compelling financial and professional incentives to conduct research with human subjects have increased public scrutiny of academic institutions and placed tremendous strain on the ever-fragile consensus regarding the ethics of research.[1] Recently, these concerns have been fueled by media coverage of the tragic deaths of two participants in research, a young man participating in a gene-modification study at the University of Pennsylvania and a young woman involved in an asthma study at Johns Hopkins University. These two incidents have drawn attention to a number of systemic problems reported in recent government reviews of the regulatory system for research involving human subjects.[2,3] In light of these developments, it is not surprising that federal regulatory agencies have toughened their stance with research institutions regarding compliance with existing regulations governing human-subjects research.[4,5] Gone is the time when government and the public unhesitatingly trusted research institutions to serve as responsible advocates of the public welfare. Research institutions are now searching for ways to restore and preserve public confidence in biomedical research.

Given the reality of increased government oversight and greater scrutiny by the public, it behooves research institutions to search for ways to preserve and build public trust that biomedical research is conducted responsibly and that the academic institutions wherein much of this research is conducted are responsible advocates of the public welfare. Despite the recent developments leading to greater regulation and scrutiny of research, the scientific community continues to occupy a position of tremendous influence and authority. The perspectives of this community, its ways of knowing, its goals and values, all predominate in medicine

Dr. Yarborough *is director, Center for Bioethics and Humanities, University of Colorado Health Sciences Center, Denver, Colorado; Dr. Sharp is biomedical ethicist, Office of the Scientific Director, National Institute of Environmental Health Sciences, Research Triangle Park, North Carolina, and an associate, Center for the Study of Medical Ethics and Humanities, Duke University, Durham, North Carolina.*

The views expressed in this paper represent the opinions of the authors alone and may not represent the positions of either the National Institute of Environmental Health Sciences or the National Institutes of Health.

Correspondence and requests for reprints should be addressed to Dr. Sharp, National Institutes of Health, National Institute of Environmental Health Sciences, P.O. Box 12233, 79 Alexander Drive, Bldg 4401, Room 108 (courier), Research Triangle Park, NC 27709-2233; telephone: (919) 541-3489; fax: (919) 541-4397; e-mail: ⟨sharp@niehs.nih.gov⟩.

and biomedical research. This extraordinary influence is emblematic of the trust that historically has been bestowed by the public on the research community and the institutions where its members work. But do investigators and the institutions where they work deserve this trust? What are research institutions doing to promote and reinforce that trust?

Many institutions' answers to these questions consist of little more than references to compliance with federal regulations. In this article, we explain why mere compliance with federal regulations reflects a minimal concern on the part of an institution with matters of ethical research. We argue that if institutions hope to inspire public trust and confidence, additional actions are required. If such efforts are not made by institutions to preserve and foster the public's trust and confidence, investigators may find it more difficult to recruit participants for their studies, and federal oversight of research may become more burdensome. Such developments would result in the delay or loss of the benefits of research. Consequently, how research institutions respond to public and government concerns about the conduct of research is critical. As stated above, we believe that the common institutional response to this decline of public confidence, namely, greater compliance with federal regulations pertaining to the conduct of research, while important, is of limited value in preserving and building public trust. With their heavy focus on informed consent and risk minimization,[6] these federal regulations are limited in scope and thus do too little to inspire the public's trust. The degree of public support for and confidence in the research enterprise is a direct reflection of other considerations, high among them being the degree of trust the public has that research priorities are correct and that research practices are ethical. Thus, it behooves research institutions to search for additional ways to bolster the public's trust in their research mission and activities.

We illustrate how this can be accomplished by discussing three distinct but complementary components of institutional trustworthiness: (1) how research institutions and their investigators determine what should be studied, (2) how oversight mechanisms ensure that research is conducted in a morally appropriate manner, and (3) how investigators are trained to conduct responsible research. These three components of trustworthiness merit attention from research institutions because whether people trust physician investigators and the institutions where they work largely determines whether they will volunteer to participate in research.[7] We argue that a broad institutional focus on the three elements of institutional trustworthiness described above more fully reflects the moral landscape of contemporary biomedical research than do institutional efforts that are limited to compliance with federal regulations. If we are correct, then institutions need to begin to view the restoration

and preservation of trust as comparable in importance to regulatory compliance.

THE COMPONENTS OF INSTITUTIONAL TRUSTWORTHINESS

As we discuss each of the three components of institutional trustworthiness, we avoid review of specific institutional policies, such as those designed to identify and address conflicts of interest or obligation.[8,9] We focus instead on delineating several broader institutional reforms that promote trustworthiness by creating mutually respectful relationships between research institutions and their constituents, relationships based upon shared goals and ongoing collaboration. Institutions may implement a variety of activities at the local level to establish these institution–constituent relationships that inspire trust. Since our suggested reforms involve institutional efforts, they differ from other proposals, which rely primarily on individual actions, external accrediting organizations,[10] or professional societies.[11]

Shared Research Goals: Setting Research Priorities

The goals of biomedical research—the relief of suffering, the advancement of knowledge, the preservation of life, and the promotion of human well-being—are goals that research institutions share with the supporting community. Since these shared goals justify the social resources dedicated to research, it is important to include community perspectives in deliberations about research priorities. This is especially so since a basic tenet of medical professionalism is that health care professionals "engage with the public in negotiating social priorities that balance medical values with other societal values."[12] According to this tenet, responsible research advocacy implies that the prioritization of research areas within an institution should not be chosen at the sole discretion of the institution or its individual investigators. Rather, in working to serve the public welfare, institutions should regularly consult members of the broader community regarding their research.

One way for institutions to assure regular community consultation is to establish a research advisory council whose members are drawn from both inside and outside the institution. Key leaders in the institution who are responsible for and knowledgeable about the organization's research should be among those who represent the institution on such an advisory council. Community council members should be selected from among the institution's various constituencies. Research sponsors, both public and private, should also be represented on such councils. Members of an advisory council can be selected according to a variety of criteria, but minimally these criteria should include the following. All members should care about the public welfare and the role of biomedical research in promoting that end. No member should be so closely wedded to any one particular research need or problem that he or she would be unwilling to negotiate the values that frame research priorities or the numerous potential research initiatives competing for resources. Finally, all members should be deeply committed to the notion that research ought to be conducted in a responsible manner.

If community advisory councils are to be effective, institutional administrators and institutional council members should not view community members as cheerleaders or uncritical champions of the institution and the research conducted there. Rather, because of their shared vision regarding the value and conduct of research, institutions must encourage and permit the active participation of community council members in discussing and shaping research goals and activities. This will require the institution to adopt a degree of humility and to believe there is something useful to be learned about the research enterprise by soliciting input from its constituents. If council members do not find within the institution a spirit of openness and a commitment to be held accountable for institutional research activities, convening an advisory council or some similar collaborative process will prove to be little more than window dressing gained at the expense of the participants' time, efforts, and commitment to serve the public welfare.

We recognize that institutions face difficulties implementing a meaningful collaborative process and making the transition from institutional insularity to active community collaboration. There are many powerful forces at work that influence what specific research gets done at an institution. Research advisory councils will have limited capabilities to counteract these influences. The most powerful of these, of course, is funding. Industry, private foundations, and government sponsors fund most biomedical research done today, and they typically work directly with individual investigators rather than institutions to conduct their research. Nevertheless, sponsors and investigators still require compliant institutions as well as a compliant public in order to conduct their research. So, institutions and the communities they serve are not powerless to shape research practices unless they choose to be so.

We further recognize that if an institution is to fully embrace a research advisory council or some similar collaborative process, risks are involved. Where industry-sponsored human-subjects research establishes financially lucrative ties between an institution and a corporate sponsor, but does little to serve the public welfare, community advisory councils will likely wrestle with the appropriateness of using human and institutional capital to serve corporate goals.[13] While not all industry-sponsored research is of this sort, the investigative community ought not underestimate the threat that industry-sponsored research can pose to its integrity.[14,15] Research advisory councils will likely be very sensitive to this threat, especially since all research expends the good will, trust, and resources of the supporting community. In its worst form, using public trust and resources to advance private interests borders on exploitation[16] and erodes rather than builds trust. Consequently, councils may determine that some industry-sponsored research exacts a high cost to the institution that exceeds the revenue that the research generates.

The presence of an active research advisory council will invite rather than deflect greater scrutiny of industry ties, and institutions must be willing to permit such scrutiny and heed the advice that results from it if a collaborative process between the institution and its community is to thrive. Such a process can serve as a counter, even if it might be a modest one, to the financial clout of research sponsors. That is why we believe it is worth it in the long run for institutions to accept these challenges and fully embrace research advisory councils or some similar collaborative process. The partnership that will result will ensure that no one loses sight of the fundamental fact that all biomedical research uses other people's time, money, and bodies. Those who offer their bodies as clinical laboratories for research do so because they believe that the sacrifices they make on behalf of the common good will in fact serve the common good. A successful partnership will promote public confidence in the research enterprise by reassuring laypersons that the public welfare, not institutional prestige or financial gain, is the principal beneficiary of the institution's research efforts. This assurance is essential to building trust between the institution and its constituents.

Robust Research Oversight

It is also essential that the public trust that they will not be treated like guinea pigs in clinical investigations; this reminds us that in every aspect of biomedical research there is a fundamental duty to treat research subjects with dignity and respect. Informed consent has emerged as the accepted sign of respectful treatment of research subjects, with investigators and institutional review boards (IRBs) having acquired the primary institutional responsibility to ensure that informed consent to research occurs. Institutional consent practices have their limits, however. Numerous studies question whether the obtaining of permission to conduct research by having subjects or their surrogates read and sign informed consent forms truly signifies that individuals have volunteered, based upon the information with which they have been presented, to be research subjects in investigational studies.[17–19] These findings suggest that while current informed consent practices may be useful in *gathering* information relevant to informed decision making, they frequently are ineffective at *conveying* that information to prospective research participants and thus assuring voluntary consent. Hence, neither IRBs nor research institutions should presume that signed consent forms guarantee that research subjects are true volunteers. Instead, IRBs need to pay more attention to the capacity of members of investigative teams to inform research subjects about the nature of their research and alternatives to participating in it as well as their capacity to assess subjects' understanding and consent.[20] IRBs might routinely require study recruiters to assess subjects' understanding by having those who want to enroll in a study verbally explain the purpose, risks, and benefits of the study as well as their options besides that of enrolling in the study. They might also encourage the use of educational strategies that have proved effective at conveying information to patients and research subjects, such as the use of video recordings and computer programs.[21,22]

Despite the limitations of informed consent documents, scrutiny of such forms, along with consideration of risk minimization and risk–benefit assessment, occupies the bulk of IRB deliberations. Yet there are other equally important requirements for the ethical conduct of research. Seven essential ethical requirements, adapted from major codes and declarations relevant to medical research, recently have been set forth in a framework for evaluating the ethics of clinical research.[23] In addition to matters related to risks and informed consent, these requirements address social value, scientific validity, subject selection, independent review, and respect for subjects of research trials. Some of these, such as the scientific validity of proposed studies, fall beyond the scope of most IRBs' deliberations. For others, such as subject selection and respectful treatment of participants, IRBs are often poorly positioned to oversee their practical application and implementation. Consequently, if each of these requirements of ethical research is to be met, IRB members and others within the institution must put forth additional efforts to assure the public that research subjects are treated with the full measure of respect they are due.

With the increasing number of government mandates being placed on investigators and IRBs, this change will be difficult to achieve, but the mandates themselves accentuate the need for the change. Anyone familiar with the transformation of IRBs over the last several months as well as with much of the literature about IRBs is aware of the primary emphasis on protecting research subjects from risks.[24] This emphasis on protectionist concerns obscures other salient ethical dimensions of research and in the process creates an inappropriately narrow focus of IRBs, a focus at odds with a more robust understanding of the fundamental ethical dimensions of research: respect for persons, beneficence, and

justice.[25] A primary concern for protection from risks creates a tendency to reduce the demands of respect for persons to an obligation to disclose risks, to reduce the demands of beneficence to an obligation to minimize risks, and to reduce the demands of justice to an obligation to fairly distribute research risks.

While IRBs are institutionally positioned to prompt a broader emphasis on the ethics of research if they are provided with adequate financing and expertise, they cannot do it in isolation from those who conduct the research. This is especially true when one considers that IRB members, compared with members of investigative teams, may have limited understanding of the most ethically salient aspects of many clinical investigations if they lack adequate familiarity with unique clinical and other characteristics of a given research project. Although IRB members by and large are very familiar with the general ethical framework for the responsible conduct of research, ethical deliberation and decision making requires bringing these general considerations to bear on specific questions that arise in specific settings. No IRB has comprehensive scientific and clinical representation. Astute investigators, on the other hand, can be very knowledgeable about the ethical challenges embedded in a particular study. Hence the need for strong collaboration between investigative teams and their IRBs.

Such collaboration can be difficult to achieve, since the IRB is viewed by many investigators as an entity whose approval is an obstacle to be overcome rather than a group of research colleagues whose counsel is valuable. Consequently, until there is a climate of regular communication and collaboration about specific investigations among members of the investigative team and the IRB, neither the IRB nor the investigators can fully discharge their obligations to complete a thorough ethical review of research activities. This is true even when institutional educational programs about the ethics and regulation of research with human subjects are in place and comply with existing federal mandates. In order to foster this collaboration, IRBs need to have members with research ethics expertise that goes beyond an understanding of research regulation, and they need to make these members available for consultation with investigative teams. In this way, IRBs can play an institutional role similar to that currently played by clinical ethics committees when they conduct ethics consultations.[26]

When ethically challenging research issues arise, expert IRB members can foster moral deliberation and provide "hands on" ethical counsel. This consulting role is critical because when IRBs work closely with individual investigative teams, they promote the public's trust by establishing a climate of moral deliberation within the institution regarding its research enterprise. Joining moral circumspection with the intellectual curiosity of research scientists assures the public that the institution is interested not just in doing good things, but in doing them in the right way. Thus, these activities promote public confidence in research in a much stronger way than is possible when institutional efforts are limited to mere compliance with federal mandates.

Training Responsible Investigators

Most institutions that conduct biomedical research simultaneously train the next generation of investigators. To continue to warrant the public's trust, new researchers must be trained as responsible investigators, i.e., researchers who conduct investigations with both scientific and ethical rigor. Recognizing this, the NIH has recently augmented its longstanding requirement that its trainees have access to education in research ethics.[27] While we are in agreement with this development, we believe that compliance with this new mandate is insufficient to ensure that the next generation of researchers will be adequately trained in the ethics of research. If research ethics education is to be effective, it is important that this educational focus be experienced by students as an integral part of their professional training. Stand-alone courses or lectures, while they may satisfy sponsor-mandated training requirements, are insufficient for building and maintaining professional commitments to the integrity of research. To assure the public's trust, it is essential that junior investigators learn why research with human subjects must be conducted ethically and how this is done. This requires training programs to mentor students to acquire the virtues of self-effacement and self-sacrifice[28] so that they will learn to habitually set aside personal interests in professional advancement for the sake of their research subjects. Such training will not stifle development of the predominant professional characteristic of wanting to investigate hypotheses so as to generate new knowledge. Instead, it will join with this characteristic a willingness to discontinue research investigations when their continuation would require compromising the ethical tenets that assure trustworthy science. Such willingness reflects the acquisition of the requisite virtues and characteristics. These are acquired over time through education, through careful mentoring, and with experience; hence the need for a longitudinal, multifaceted emphasis on professionalism and ethics throughout biomedical training programs.[29]

Changes that have occurred over the last few decades in the way science is conducted also support the need for this emphasis.[30] Biomedical research today is highly sophisticated, requiring a variety of discipline-specific skills and creating a division of labor for the successful completion of research. The consequence of this division of labor is that most research is conducted by teams of researchers, frequently at different geographic locations. As a result, no single team member is intimately familiar with all the evidence in support of the findings of the team. Rather, team members believe what is reported to them from colleagues, illustrating how important trust is in gathering, reporting, and interpreting data.[31,32] In the absence of such trust, it is impossible to derive any conclusions. Thus, trustworthiness is not only an ethical requirement of research; it is an epistemologic requirement of modern science.[9]

FROM INSTITUTIONAL COMPLIANCE TO INFORMED TRUST

Responsible research is best described as a joint partnership that seeks to improve the public welfare through a better understanding of human health and disease and that treats those who participate in the enterprise with the full measure of respect and dignity they are due.[33] This partnership is characterized by notable asymmetries of knowledge and power as well as of privilege and vulnerability. Often joined with these asymmetries are tempting and pervasive conflicts of interest, all existing in institutional settings frequently characterized by the decentralization of institutional power and oversight. The many disparate elements of this partnership are held together by trust. Hence our contention that the creation of institutional processes that promote and preserve trust ought to be a central focus of research institutions.

Investigators and others who work for biomedical research institutions can take pride in being part of an enormously valuable effort that has enhanced human well-being by mitigating the effects of human disease. It is the public that is the beneficiary of the ever-growing capacity of medicine to extend the duration and quality of human life. It is important to remember, however, that the public has also been an essential contributor to this success. Without volunteers, this research would never have occurred. And the funds for much research are public ones. We believe the public should and will continue its support of research, provided institutions create opportunities to promote the public's informed trust.

We are not the only commentators to recognize the importance of trust for the future of biomedical research. Many organizations have recently signed a "reaffirmation of trust between medical science and the public."[34] We think researchers and institutional officials should take care in signing such declarations until they have established institutional processes along the lines of those we have described. Although these kinds of statements are intended as a signal to the community that biomedical institutions consider themselves trustworthy, such declarations may prove counterproductive. More than anything else, they may lull institutional leadership into believing a declaration alone signifies that they are already deserving of the very trust they need to actively seek.

Affirmations and declarations mean nothing if they are not backed up by a meaningful institutional commitment to promoting public confidence in research. Trustworthiness is an accomplishment, not a pronouncement. If it exists, it is embodied in the daily actions of the institution and its members. This in turn requires that an organization take time to deliberate about whether it is in fact trustworthy and whether it is doing what it ought to promote and preserve that trustworthiness.

CONCLUSION

The public must trust that research priorities sufficiently reflect social priorities if they are to be expected to support research. Research participation is based on the assumption that the goals of the investigator (and supporting research institutions) coincide with those of the subject and the public at large. This trust is also based in part upon public confidence that appropriate oversight of research occurs, that researchers are accountable to their colleagues and their research subjects, that safeguards are in place to prevent unnecessary harm from befalling research participants, and that there are oversight mechanisms in place to reduce and address mistakes of judgment if they should occur.[35] Additionally, trust is founded upon reassurance that investigators are persons of exemplary professional character who inspire confidence and respect. Since the findings of research are only as reliable as the trustworthiness of scientific investigators,[36] the development of virtuous researchers is a critical part of an institution's commitment to bolstering public trust in biomedical research.

The adoption of institutional processes such as those we have described will reflect a broad and deep interest in promoting the informed trust of the public in research. Strong and consistent advocacy for research that promotes the public welfare, the use of oversight mechanisms to create a culture of moral deliberation regarding biomedical research, and the training of new investigators with a keen sense of professionalism all demonstrate to the institution's partners in research that the institution has an abiding commitment to advance the public good in an ethically responsible fashion. These activities serve not only to secure but also to promote the trust essential to the research enterprise. Conversely, institutions that limit their efforts to mere regulatory compliance, with a narrow focus on protecting the public from harm rather than a broader focus on promoting public welfare, place the future of the research enterprise at risk.

The research undertaken to create this document was supported in part by the Division of Intramural Research at the National Institute of Environmental Health Sciences (RS). The authors thank Phil Candilis, Therese Jones, John Penta, Bob Truog, and several anonymous reviewers for their thoughtful comments on earlier versions of the paper.

REFERENCES

1. Woodward B. Challenges to human subject protections in U.S. medical research. JAMA. 1999;282:1947–52.
2. Inspector General, Department of Health and Human Services. Institutional Review Boards: A Time for Reform. Publication OEI-01-97-00193. Washington, DC: U.S. Department of Health and Human Services, 1998.
3. U.S. General Accounting Office. Scientific Research: Continued Vigilance Critical to Protecting Human Subjects. Publication GAO/HEHS-96-72. Washington, DC: U.S. General Accounting Office, 1996.
4. Ellis GB. Protecting the rights and welfare of human research subjects. Acad Med. 1999;74:1008–9.
5. Russell-Einhorn M, Vaitukaitis J, Snyderman R, et al. Far beyond informed consent: U.S. research institutions keep close watch on OPRR's suspensions. J Investig Med. 1999;47:259–66.
6. Federal policy for the protection of human subjects; notices and rules. Fed Reg. 1991;56, June 18:28002–32.
7. Kass NE, Sugarman J, Faden R, Schoch-Spana M. Trust: the fragile foundation of contemporary biomedical research. Hastings Center Rep. 1996;26:25–9.
8. Lo B, Wolf LE, Berkeley A. Conflict-of-interest policies for investigators in clinical trials. N Engl J Med. 2000;343:1616–20.
9. McCrary SV, Anderson CB, Jakovljevic J, et al. A national survey of policies on disclosure of conflicts of interest in biomedical research. N Engl J Med. 2000;343:1621–6.
10. Committee on Assessing the System for Protecting Human Research Subjects, Institute of Medicine. Preserving Public Trust: Accreditation and Human Research Participant Protection Programs. Washington, DC: National Academy Press, 2001.
11. Rhodes R, Strain JJ. Trust and transforming medical institutions. Cambridge Quarterly of Healthcare Ethics. 2000;9:205–17.
12. Wynia MK, Latham SR, Kao AC, et al. Medical professionalism in society. N Engl J Med. 1999;341:1612–6.
13. Angell M. Is academic medicine for sale? N Engl J Med. 2000;342:1516–8.
14. Rothman DJ. Medical professionalism—focusing on the real issues. N Engl J Med. 2000;342:1284–6.
15. Bodenheimer T. Uneasy alliance: clinical investigators and the pharmaceutical industry. N Engl J Med. 2000;342:1539–44.
16. Benatar SR. Avoiding exploitation in clinical research. Cambridge Quarterly of Healthcare Ethics. 2000;9:562–5.
17. Appelbaum PS, Roth LH, Lidz CW, et al. False hopes and best data: consent to research and the therapeutic misconception. Hastings Center Rep. 1987;17:20–4.
18. Sugarman J, McCrory DC, Hubal RC. Getting meaningful informed consent from older adults: a structured literature review of empirical studies. J Am Geriatr Soc. 1998;46:517–24.
19. Sugarman J, McCrory DC, Powell D, et al. Empirical research on informed consent: an annotated bibliography. Hastings Center Rep. 1999; 29(Jan–Feb):S1–S42.
20. Handelsman M, Department of Psychology, University of Colorado, Denver, CO. Personal communication, June 2001.
21. Green MJ, Fost N. Who should provide genetic education prior to gene testing? Computers and other methods for improving patient understanding. Genetic Testing. 1997;1:131–6.
22. Green MJ, Biesecker BB, McInerney AM, Mauger DT, Fost N. An interactive computer program can effectively educate patients about

genetic testing for breast cancer susceptibility. Am J Med Genet. 2001; 103:16–23.

23. Emanuel EJ, Wendler D, Grady C: What makes clinical research ethical? JAMA. 2000;283:2701–11.

24. National Institutes of Health Office for Protection from Research Risks. Protecting Human Research Subjects: Institutional Review Board Guidebook. Washington, DC: U.S. Government Printing Office, 1993.

25. The Belmont Report. Fed Reg. 1979;44, 18 Apr:23192–7.

26. Kuczewski M, Pinkus G, Rosa LB. An Ethics Casebook for Hospitals: Practical Approaches to Everyday Cases. Washington, DC: Georgetown University Press, 1999.

27. National Institutes of Health. Required education in the protection of human research participants. Notice OD-00-039, ⟨http://grants.nih.gov/grants/guide/notice-files/NOT-OD-00-039.html⟩, June 5, 2000; accessed 10/01/01.

28. McCullough LB, Chervenak FA, Coverdale JH. Ethically justified guidelines for defining sexual boundaries between obstetrician–gynecologists and their patients. Am J Obstet Gynecol. 1996;175:496–500.

29. Wear D, Castellani B. The development of professionalism: curriculum matters. Acad Med. 2000;75:602–11.

30. Reiser SJ. The ethics movement in the biological sciences: a new voyage of discovery. In: Bulger RE, Heitman E, Reiser SJ (eds). The Ethical Dimensions of the Biological Sciences. New York: Cambridge University Press, 1993;1–15.

31. Grinnell F. Ambiguity, trust, and the responsible conduct of research. Science and Engineering Ethics. 1999;5:204–14.

32. Whitbeck C. Trust and trustworthiness in research. Science and Engineering Ethics. 1995;1:403–16.

33. Ramsey P. The Patient as Person: Explorations in Medical Ethics. New Haven, CT: Yale University Press, 1970.

34. Association of American Medical Colleges. Clinical Research: A Reaffirmation of Trust Between Medical Science and the Public. Proclamation and Pledge of Academic, Scientific, and Patient Health Organizations. Washington, DC: Association of American Medical Colleges, 2000. ⟨http://www.aamc.org/newsroom/pressrel/000608b.htm⟩; accessed 10/8/01.

35. Shalala D. Protecting research subjects—what must be done. N Engl J Med. 2000;343:808–10.

36. Hardwig J. The role of trust in knowledge. Journal of Philosophy. 1991; 88:693–708.

[36]

Privatized Biomedical Research, Public Fears, and the Hazards of Government Regulation: Lessons from Stem Cell Research

DAVID B. RESNIK

2S-17 Brody Medical Sciences Building, East Carolina University, School of Medicine, Greenville NC 27858-4354, USA (Phone: 252 816 2492; Fax: 252 816 2319; E-mail: dresnik@brody.med.ecu.edu)

Abstract. This paper discusses the hazards of regulating controversial biomedical research in light of the emergence of powerful, multi-national biotechnology corporations. Prohibitions on the use of government funds can simply force controversial research into the private sphere, and unilateral or multilateral research bans can simply encourage multi-national companies to conduct research in countries that lack restrictive laws. Thus, a net effect of government regulation is that research migrates from the public to the private sphere. Because private research receives less oversight and external scrutiny than public research, it can threaten the welfare and rights of human subjects, scientific progress and openness, and the quality of the approval process for new biomedical technologies. In order to avoid the harmful effects of government regulation of biotechnology, society should promote meaningful discussion and dialogue among scientists, industry leaders, and the public before resorting to regulatory solutions. Legislative or executive initiatives should be applied with great discretion and care, and should be crafted in such a way that they protect public health and safety, promote scientific progress, and avoid the hazards of privatized research and polarized debates.

Key words: biomedical research, government regulation, biotechnology industry, privatization, scientific progress, public debates

Introduction

In the November 6, 1998 issue of the journal *Science*, James Thomson et al. published potentially one of the most important biomedical discoveries in the 1990s (Thomson, 1998). In their paper, the authors reported that they had isolated and cultured pluripotent stem cells derived from human embryos, a landmark study which helps to open the door to the engineering of human tissues and organs. Since the United States (US) government has a law forbidding the use of federal funds for research on human embryos, Thomson et al. conducted their work using private funds from Geron Corporation and the Wisconsin Alumni Research Foundation. In order to insure that this

274

work did not violate National Institutes of Health (NIH) regulations, they set up a separate lab on the University of Wisconsin campus to conduct the privately funded, stem cell research (Marshall, 1998). When Thomson et al. announced their important results, John Gearhart announced that he and his colleagues had obtained similar results. The Gearhart team published their work four days later in the *Proceedings of the National Academy of Sciences* (Gearhart, 1998). Gearhart's work was also funded by private funds from Geron Corporation.

Shortly after the publication of this cutting-edge research, a panel of biologists led by NIH Director Harold Varmus testified before Congress on the importance of stem cell research and the need to provide federal funding for this kind of work. The panel urged Congress to rethink the ban on the funding of embryo research in light of these dramatic discoveries (Bagla, 1998). A few weeks after this meeting, Harriet Raab, General Counsel of the Department of Health and Human Services (DHHS), which oversees the NIH, ruled that current laws allow federal funds to be used for research on embryonic stem cells (Marshall, 1999). However, 77 anti-abortion congressmen wrote a letter to the DHHS criticizing this ruling and they vowed to block stem cell research (Wadman, 1999). Currently, the National Bioethics Advisory Commission (NBAC) is studying this issue and the debate about the legal and ethical aspects of human stem cell research continues (Andrews, 1999).

This is not the first time that controversial research has been conducted in the private sector due to restrictions on the use of public funds. It seems like only yesterday that Ian Wilmut stunned the scientific world by cloning 'Dolly' from adult sheep cells (Campbell, 1997). Wilmut, who lost government funding after his work was published in the journal *Nature*, now receives private funds to conduct research on the genetic engineering of livestock at the Roslin Institute, near Edinburgh, U.K. (Wilmut, 1998). When President Clinton took office in 1993, he modified the ban on fetal tissue research to allow government funds to be used to conduct medical research with fetal tissue. During this four-year funding restriction, private corporations and individuals sponsored studies on Parkinson's disease that used fetal tissue transplants (Kolata, 1994). The controversial 'abortion' pill, RU486, was tested and developed in Europe long before clinical trials began in the US. Since the US government's ban on fetal tissue research has prevented the NIH from funding research on RU486, clinical trials conducted in the US have used private funds (Pence, 1995).

Although the NIH will probably find a way to fund stem cell research, this episode in the recent history of science represents a disturbing and potentially hazardous development in the sponsorship of science. While private industry should continue to play a key role in the funding of research, there are potential risks to science and society when important discoveries and inventions occur only within this part of the economy. In his testimony before Congress, Varmus expressed his concerns about research that is conducted *exclusively* in the private sector using private funds. Some of the concerns voiced by Varmus' and others can be summarized as follows.

Protecting Human Subjects

First, research conducted in private laboratories has less institutional oversight than research conducted at public institutions (Andrews, 1999). In the US, the Food and Drug Administration (FDA) requires that all research on human subjects, whether conducted in private or public institutions, be reviewed by independent committees known as Institutional Review Boards (IRBs). IRBs are charged with reviewing new research proposals in order to insure that study designs and protocols are scientifically rigorous and ethically legitimate. IRBs attempt to protect the welfare and rights of human subjects while promoting sound research methods. In order to obtain FDA approval for a new item (food, drug or medical device), a company must conduct preliminary studies that are approved by an IRB. These studies must also pass muster with the FDA, which will then sponsor its own studies before approving a new item (Brody, 1995). To accelerate review and approval of research protocols, many biotechnology and pharmaceutical companies have established their own, private IRBs.

Although all human subjects research must be reviewed by an IRB, private IRBs do not have to meet all of the oversight requirements mandated by the DHHS. The FDA and DHHS requirements are similar, but the DHHS has more stringent safety, informed consent, record keeping, and data monitoring standards (Brody, 1995). Additionally, the deliberations and records of private IRBs are not subject to the same types of openness rules that apply to public IRBs. Although the FDA can obtain access to the deliberations and records of private IRBs when it reviews a drug or device for potential approval, these IRBs do not normally operate under the threat of potential public scrutiny. Furthermore, private studies of new drugs that are not submitted for FDA approval may never be brought out in the open. One need look no further than the Department of Energy's human radiation experiments to see how ethical and scientific problems can proliferate when research is shielded from public scrutiny (*PACHRE*, 1996). A Bill was introduced in Congress in 1997 that would have extended stringent human subjects regulations to the private sector, but this proposed legislation failed (Walker, 1997).

276

In addition to being concerned about secrecy, one should also be concerned about financial and institutional stresses that can affect the quality of the review process. A 1998 DHHS report on institutional review boards concluded that all IRBs (public and private) have been strained by the 42% increase in the number of primary reviews that has occurred in the last five years. The report also noted that private IRBs are under intense pressure to accelerate or streamline the review process, and that financial interests may encourage all IRBs (public or private) to compromise their standard of oversight and review in order to process a high volume of research proposals (DHHS, 1998). One might argue that any IRB has a potential conflict of interest when the financial interests of the institution interfere with the objectivity and thoroughness of review (Francis, 1998). However, this conflict can become more egregious in the private sector due to increased financial pressures.

Although we do not have strong empirical evidence that private IRBs pose dire threats to human subjects, we should be concerned about the risks to human subjects and scientific quality posed by private research under the authority of private IRBs. Decreased openness and increased pressure for accelerated or streamlined review make the private IRB a less than ideal method for promoting scientific and ethical standards in research on human subjects. Additionally, we should be wary of any general trend toward an increase in private IRB review. It is not hard to understand how a privately-funded clinical researcher working at a university could be tempted to move his research to a private lab, in order to avoid the hassles and delays of the university's IRB. If this scenario repeats itself many times, then we would have good reasons to be concerned about the increased risks of private human subjects research.

Threat to the Quality of FDA Approval

A second reason why we should be concerned about the increased privatization of biomedical research is that it poses a potential threat to the quality of the approval process. The problem may arise if the shift from public to private research leads to an over-reliance on industry-generated data in making approval decisions. As mentioned previously, the FDA relies on previous experiments, which may include privately funded and publicly funded studies (Brody, 1995). Obtaining data from studies *other than* those conducted by a company seeking FDA approval helps to improve the quality of the approval process. Since private companies have strong financial interests in obtaining FDA approval, the FDA cannot rely solely on industry-generated results, since these results may be biased or incomplete. Private companies have a 'conflict of interest' because their financial interests conflict with their duties to conduct objective research (Huth, 1998). To compensate for this conflict of interest, the FDA needs to rely on independent sources of information (Korn, 1997). When these independent sources of information, e.g. FDA studies or other non-industry studies, are scarce, then the objectivity and completeness of the approval process can be at risk. If the FDA had no limits on time or money, then it could compensate for a lack of non-industry studies by conducting its own studies. However, the FDA has a limited budget and it is under great pressure to approve new items as quickly as possible. Thus, when research is conducted only in the private sector and public funds are scarce, the quality of the approval process and public safety are at risk (ibid.). Death, injury, and unnecessary suffering are possible long-term effects of the privatization of biomedical research when we depend too much on industry-generated studies in approving new items. For example, more thorough non-industry studies of sildenafil (trade name: Viagra) before it was approved for clinical use could have given us more information about the risks of mycardial infarction associated with this drug, which would have saved human lives (Martinez, 1998).

Threat to Scientific Openness

A third reason why we should be concerned about the privatization of biomedical research is that private companies often have strict rules and policies designed to prevent funded researchers from sharing data or results. Many companies require scientists to sign contracts transferring intellectual property rights to the organization, including the right to publish data or results (McCain, 1996; Marshall, 1998). In some cases, companies have suppressed scientific research in order to promote their own economic interests (Wadman, 1996). In other cases, companies have delayed publication (Marshall, 1998). Finally, many biotechnology companies now pursue patents with the primary goal of preventing competitors from exploiting particular areas of research. Companies may seek to obtain a patent on a particular gene, for example, even when they do not know how that gene functions or how they can transform the gene into a useful application. The use of these 'blocking' patents can stifle scientific progress by restricting the dissemination of scientific information. (Sagoff, 1999). In any case, the failure to share data and results in a timely fashion threatens the progress of science and medicine (Altman, 1996). Because openness plays such an important role in scientific collaboration, cooperation, criticism, and confirmation, the free and open exchange of information is widely recognized as one of the most

278

important principles of research (Resnik, 1998a). Thus, the privatization of research, in and of itself, represents a potential threat to scientific progress.

However, as long as we recognize and desire the benefits of industry-sponsored research, this trade-off between openness and private funding cannot be avoided (Resnik, 1998b). In order to obtain returns on their research investments, companies need to be able to use scientific information to their advantage. To insure that research has public benefits, companies should be given incentives to disclose data, results, materials, and methods. The key is to strike a balance between public and private control of research that promotes the advancement of science and medicine while allowing corporations to profit from their research investments. The current patent system, which grants corporations or individuals specific rights in return for public disclosure, is designed to strike a balance between public and private control of research (Foster, 1993).

We also should seek a balance between public and private when it comes to sponsoring and conducting research. Although a great deal of research can and should be sponsored and conducted by private industry, a substantial amount of research, especially *important research*, should be conducted in public laboratories using public funds. The privately funded stem cell research is troubling, in large part, because this work has great scientific and medical value. Very few eyebrows would be raised by this research if it were a study to develop a baldness cure or a new deodorant. Thus, government regulation can threaten the delicate balance between public and private research by encouraging scientists to conduct their work in the private sector in order to obtain funding or to avoid the inconvenient delays and paperwork created by the government rules and procedures. It is likely that these concerns played some role in the decision to conduct stem cell research in the private sector.

Privatized Biomedical Research

These issues concerning the relationship between government regulation and the privatization of research transcend this particular episode in the recent history of science. To think about these broader concerns, we need to understand the changing role of private industry in the funding of science and the role of public opinion in science policy. Several trends in the funding of science need to be comprehended. First, privately funded research and development (R&D) in the US doubled between 1980 and 1995. In 1980, industry funded $50 billion worth of R&D (measured in 1994 dollars) in the US; by 1995, that total increased to $100 billion (Jaffe, 1996). Second, even though government-sponsored research also increased between 1980 and 1995, it did not keep pace with industry-sponsored R&D. Industry-sponsored research amounted to about 48% of all R&D spending in the US in 1980, but that figure climbed to 60% by 1995. Government-sponsored research, on the other hand, totaled about 48% of all US R&D in 1980, but dropped to 35% by 1995 (ibid.). Third, privately funded basic research in the US nearly tripled between 1980 and 1995. In 1980, industry funded $3 billion worth of basic research; by 1995 that amount jumped to $8 billion (ibid.). Fourth, more research in now conducted in private laboratories. In 1980, about 62% of all R&D in the US was conducted in private laboratories; by 1995, this total increased to 71%. (ibid.). Fifth, private industry's contribution to biomedical R&D has risen dramatically since 1980. In 1980, the private sector contributed $2 billion to biomedical R&D; by 1990 that number rose to $16 billion (Beardsley, 1994) (Overall, biomedical R&D funds represents roughly half of all R&D funding) (Jaffe, 1996). Sixth, other Western nations also increased their private and public funding of R&D during the 1980s, although these funding increases have leveled off since then (ibid.). However, since many of the US-based pharmaceutical and biotech companies are multi-national, it is difficult to make international comparisons concerning R&D funding, since funds can travel from one country to another through a large corporation (Beardsley, 1994).

These statistics all indicate a trend toward the privatization of biomedical research and development, including basic research (ibid.). Although the government remains an important factor in the sponsorship of research, its overall influence on biomedical R&D has decreased relative to industry's influence. Given the world's current economic trends, we should expect private industry to continue to increase its influence on biomedical R&D in the US and around the world. In the last two decades, biotechnology has emerged as a new force in the global economy (Enriquez, 1998). Biotech and pharmaceutical companies are now some of the most powerful corporations in the world. Biomedical science now plays a key role in some of these new technologies, such as the genetic engineering of plants and animals, genetic diagnosis and therapy, drug and vaccine design and production, and tissue engineering (Shenk, 1997; Marshall, 1999). Since it provides the foundation for a great deal of work in biomedicine, the discipline of genomics has emerged as a vanguard in this economic revolution (Enriquez, 1998). Efforts to identify, isolate, sequence and patent genes have much in common with the gold and silver 'rushes' of the 19th century. Private companies now compete with each other and with government-funded researchers in the 'race' to decipher the human genome (Wade, 1998; Cohen, 1997). Privately funded gene hunters have also begun 'prospecting' for useful human and non-human genes in countries around the globe (Carey, 1997). As the global economy evolves, it is likely that this biotechnology revolution will continue. Just as

280

the 19th century witnessed the industrial revolution, the 21st century may witness a biotech revolution (Carey, 1997; Sheldon, 1991). This forecast means that we cannot and should not ignore or underestimate the role that private industry will play in biomedical research and development.

Public Opposition to Biotechnology

The other trend we should not ignore is a growing public opposition to biotechnology. Although some members of the public have always opposed the development of science and technology, since the late 1960s a new kind of technophobia has emerged. These new Luddites, which I will dub 'biotechno-phobes,' are opposed to new developments in biomedicine and biotechnology. Biotechnophobes are a diverse group, consisting of religious conservatives, environmentalists, and pro-government liberals. The most vocal and contro-versial biotechnophobe is Jeremy Rifkin, a man who has made a career out of opposing developments in biotechnology (Stix, 1997).

When scientists developed recombinant DNA techniques, biotechno-phobes, feared that genetic accidents would escape the laboratory and cause human and environmental degradation (Ramsey, 1970). When in vitro fertil-ization methods produced the first 'test tube' baby, biotechnophones worried that this technology would demean human reproduction and create harmful mutations (Kass, 1985). When agricultural engineers developed genetically modified crops, biotechnophobes warned that these new crops could be dangerous to humans and the environment (Rifkin, 1983). When cloning techniques were developed in the 1990s, biotechnophones speculated that this technology might be used to create beings for 'spare parts,' carbon copies of existing people, or a race of Hitlers (Annas, 1998).

Every step of the way, the media has fed public fears of biomedicine and biotechnology through sensationalized coverage of landmark events, such as the birth of Louise Brown and the unveiling of 'Dolly' (Priest, 1999; Pence, 1998). This powerful combination of biotechnophobia and a fear-mongering press has energized popular movements aimed at convincing political leaders of the need to impose additional regulations on biomed-ical research. In Europe, grassroots movements have opposed agricultural biotechnology, gene patenting, genetic engineering, embryo research, and human cloning (Williams, 1998; Schatz, 1998). The US, which has a ban on federally-funded human embryo research, narrowly defeated a Bill to ban human cloning (Marshall, 1998). Other regulations in other countries are pending (Butler, 1998; Williams, 1997).

From Fear to Paradox

Many of these fears and concerns about biotechnology may be justified, and we need to consider pro-biotech and anti-biotech perspectives in assessing the risks and benefits of new developments in biotechnology, I recognize the importance of the objections made by the critics. What concerns me most is the growing public opposition to biotechnology combined with the increased privatization of research. These two trends can reinforce each other and make our worst fears come true. How might his happen? Let's start with public opposition to biotechnology. This opposition often leads to more government regulation and control. Case in point, the cloning debate. After the press spread the news of Dolly around the globe, interest groups, grassroots campaigns, and other political forces voiced their concerns about the possible cloning of human beings. This public turmoil triggered a response from world leaders, including the Clinton administration, which issued an executive order banning the use of federal funds for human cloning research (Clinton, 1997). The administration also ordered the NBAC to study the issues and to make some policy recommendations. After several months, the NBAC concluded that there should be a ban on the use federal funds to study human cloning, although the NBAC did not go so far as to say that cloning should be illegal. The NBAC hoped that private industry would cooperate with the government in controlling human cloning (*NBAC*, 1997). Shortly after the NBAC report, Congress began to consider legislation to ban human cloning. Public fears played a key role in prompting the administration to choose the regulatory path: polls taken at the time showed nearly unanimous opposition to cloning human beings (Pence, 1998).

Although lobbying from a group of scientists stopped the anti-cloning steamroller from destroying this new area of research, a great deal of damage had been done. Scientists who had witnessed the effects of public opposition to biotechnology, such as Wilmut and Thomson, decided to conduct their work in the safer confines of the private sector. As the debate over cloning continued, other scientists working in the private sector revealed that they had succeeded in cloning mice, cows and pigs. A physicist announced that for a fee he would clone a human being, and a team of Korean scientists announced that they had repeated the 'Dolly' procedure (somatic cell nuclear transfer) on humans (Pennisi, 1997, 1998; Kestendbaum, 1998). In a bizarre turn of events, a private company, Advanced Cell Technologies, announced in November 1998 that it had used some of the nuclear transfer techniques used by Wilmut to fuse human DNA with a cow's egg to create a new type of human cell (Marshall, 1998).

Most people, including scientists, would rather avoid excessive regulation and controversy. As scientists seek to avoid government control and regu-

282

lation or the perceived threat of regulation, they look for private sources of funding and private venues. In the cloning controversy, public opposition to cloning did not stop this new technology; it merely forced it into the private sector. Since there is a ban on the use of federal funds for research on human embryos, stem cell researchers knew that they would need to do their work in the private sector. Hence, public opposition has also forced this important research into the private sector. However, the saga does not end here, since the public's fear of biotechnology is based, at least in part, on its concerns about a growing and uncontrollable biotechnology industry (Rifkin, 1998; Shenk, 1997). Taken together, these anxieties complete an ironic feedback loop: fears of biotechnology lead to increased governmental regulation and control, which encourages the further privatization of biotechnology, which exacerbates the fear of biotechnology.

If biotechnology migrates from the public to the private sector, this will not be the first time that an important industry became privatized after getting its start in the public sector. History reminds us that not very long ago most computers were clumsy machines that took up a lot of space on university campuses or government laboratories. Other recent examples of technologies that have migrated to the private sector after getting their start in the public sphere include lasers, radar, jet airplanes, and antibiotics (Volti, 1995). Indeed, the economic argument for government funding of research is premised on the transfer of information and technology from the public to the private sphere. Public investments in R&D are justified, according to many, because they will pay economic dividends by generating technologies to be developed by private industry (Resnik, 1998a). However, since biotechnology can have such profound and far-reaching social consequences, we should be concerned about trends toward privatization. Some industries are simply too important to be placed *solely* in the hands of the private sector.

Taking Stock: Regulation or Dialogue?

An important lesson to be learned from stem cell research is that we should be concerned about the trend toward the privatization of biomedical research in the light of governmental regulation of biotechnology. Scenarios like this one may be repeated many times as companies seek to make a profit in the rapidly evolving world of biotechnology. There are two distinct ways to respond to this trend, the way of regulation and the way of dialogue. Those who follow the regulatory path react to scientific and technical developments by urging society to enact new laws and rules in order to reign in the biotechnology industry and biomedical researchers (Rifkin, 1998). These proposed rules might take the form of restrictions on the use of federal funds or bans on particular kinds of research. The motto of the regulatory route is to 'regulate first and ask serious questions later.' The Clinton administration followed the regulatory approach in response to the public uproar over cloning (The White House, 1997; NBAC, 1997).

Those who seek to promote dialogue, on the other hand, react to scientific and technical developments by attempting to foster genuine and well-informed public discussion about social and ethical issues. The motto of the dialogic route is to 'to educate and talk first and regulate only when necessary.' Although there are not many good examples of the dialogic model at work, I suggest our current debates about information technology fit this approach. In the US, political leaders have taken a very restrained approach toward regulating the World Wide Web and the Internet, and the courts have not shown great sympathy for legislation designed to regulate information technology (Berghel, 1997). Citizens, industry leaders, and scholars have also engaged in a sincere and well-informed debate about the benefits and risks of the computer revolution. For the most part, this discussion has focused on social, ethical, and cultural responses to the computer revolution instead of regulatory ones. Indeed, many scholars argue that the legal and regulatory approaches will not be very effective in controlling computing technology, given its global dimension (Connolly, 1996). So far, this approach has promoted the responsible use of a very powerful, intractable, and potentially hazardous technology.

Which approach should we take in response to the biotech revolution? Several points made in this essay suggest that the regulatory approach is likely to be ineffective or even self-defeating. Prohibitions on the use of federal funds are likely to be self-defeating because they will force biomedical R&D into the private sector. If research is useful and profitable, then companies will pay for it, regardless of whether government funding is also available. Before the biotech revolution, prohibitions on the use of government funds would have stifled biomedical R&D. Since private industry is now more than willing to fund biomedical R&D, these responses are only likely to contribute to the further privatization of research, a result that we should be careful to avoid. The ban on the use of federal funds to conduct research on human embryos did not stop stem cell research; it merely drove it into the private sphere.

All-encompassing research bans are also likely to be ineffective. First, prohibitions on certain types of research are likely to be difficult to enforce, especially in a world where large, multi-national corporations conduct research across the globe. It would take an incredible amount of human resources to police biomedical research in the US, and a great deal of inter-national cooperation to develop and enforce global research regulations that

284

apply to private industry. Before the biotech revolution, it would also have been easier to police biomedical research, but the situation has changed dramatically in the last decade or so as the biotech industry has become more global (Beardsley, 1994; Enriquez, 1998). Unilateral or multilateral bans on research may do nothing more than drive that research out of the countries that forbid it. A ban on human cloning or stem cell research in the US will not stop human cloning or stem cell research in other countries. While the US and Europe were debating possible bans on human cloning, a South Korean team cloned a human adult cell by fusing a somatic cell nuclei with an unfertilized egg (Pennisi, 1997). A large multinational corporation interested in conducting cloning or stem cell research could simply seek science-friendly venues, much in the same way that large corporations often decide to conduct manufacturing processes in countries with lax employment laws in order to avoid restrictive employment regulations.

Finally, an added drawback of the regulatory approach is that it can stifle genuine debate and prevent people from reaching compromises and pragmatic solutions. For example, consider the abortion debate in the US. In the last three decades America has debated, proposed, and adopted a variety of abortion laws and policies, yet the abortion controversy continues and genuine public discourse has been sorely lacking. Instead of partaking in meaningful dialogue, pro-life and pro-choice sides of the issue have chosen to use other means of engagement, such as protests, political slogans and litmus tests, lobbying, harassment, and violence. Although it is impossible to know whether regulation has had a beneficial or harmful effect on this debate, some writers have argued that the focus on regulation has hampered meaningful discourse and that it has polarized the debate (Weston, 1997).

Thus, a second important lesson to be learned from stem cell research is that we should be wary of regulatory responses to new and controversial sciences, since these responses can be self-defeating or ineffective, especially when large multi-national corporations have strong economic interests in funding biotech R&D.

The most useful response to the biotechnology revolution, I believe, is to promote an ongoing dialogue among researchers, industry leaders, and the public about the benefits and risks of new discoveries and inventions. We should have a serious, informed, and sincere debate about the social, ethical, cultural, and scientific issues associated with biomedicine and biotechnology before enacting more rules and regulations. Since fear and distrust are usually based on ignorance, education will play a key role in any meaningful debate. Parties on all sides of the debate need to learn from each other. Scientists need to provide the public with information about new developments in biomedicine and biotechnology, industry leaders need to articulate and defend their

285

economic strategies and goals, and the public needs to be able to express its ethical and social concerns. Ideally, this debate would eventually lead to ethical guidelines that would be acceptable to researchers, industry leaders, and the public. Without a doubt, society will still need to adopt some laws and government policies to promote public health and safety. However, in order to avoid the harmful effects of regulation, legislative or executive initiatives should be applied with great discretion and care. They should be crafted in such a way that they protect public health and safety, promote scientific progress, and avoid the hazards of privatized research and polarized debates.

References

Altman, K. (1996) Secrecy is Hurting Medical Research, a U.S. Official Says. *New York Times* (10 February), 11.

Andrews, L. (1999) Legal, Ethical, and Social Concerns in the Debate Over Stem-cell Research. *The Chronicle of Higher Education* (Jan 29) **45**(21), B4.

Annas, G. (1998) Why We Should Ban Human Cloning. *New England Journal of Medicine* **339**, 122–125.

Bagla, P. (1998) Use of Stem Cells Still Legally Murky, But Hearing Offers Hope. *Science* **282**, 1962–1963.

Beardsley, T. (1994) Big-Time Biology. *Scientific American* **271**(5), 90–94.

Berghel, H. (1997) Post Mortem for the Communications Decency Act. *Computers and Society* **27**(4), 8–11.

Brody, B. (1995) *Ethical Issues in Drug Testing, Approval, and Pricing*. New York: Oxford University Press.

Butler, D. (1998) Human Genome Declaration Looks Set for United Nations Approval. *Nature* **396**, 297.

Campbell, K., McWhire, J., Ritchie, W. and Wilmut, I. (1997) Sheep Cloned by Nuclear Transfer From a Cultured Cell Line. *Nature* **385**, 810–813.

Carey, J., Freudlich, N., Flynn, J. and Gross, N. (1997) The Biotech Century. *Business Week* (10 March), 79–88.

Clinton, W. (1997) *Prohibition on Federal Funding For Cloning Human Beings: Memorandum for the Heads of Executive Departments and Agencies*. The White House: Office of the Press Secretary, 4 March.

Cohen, J. (1997) The Genomics Gamble. *Science* **275**, 767–772.

Connolly, F. (1996) A Call For a Statement of Expectations for the Global Information Infrastructure. *Science and Engineering Ethics* **2**, 167–176.

Department of Health and Human Services (1998) *Institutional Review Boards: a System in Jeopardy?* Washington, DC: DHHS, June.

Enriquez, J. (1998) Genomics and the World's Economy. *Science* **281**, 925–926.

Foster, F. and Shook, R. (1993) *Patents, Copyrights, and Trademarks*. New York: John Wiley and Sons.

Francis, L. (1998) IRBs and Conflicts of Interest. In R. Spece, D. Shimm and A. Buchanan (Eds.), *Conflicts of Interest in Clinical Practice and Research* (pp. 418–436). New York: Oxford University Press.

286

Gearhart, J. (1998) New Potential For Human Embryonic Stem Cells. *Science* **282**, 1061–1062.

Huth, E. (1998) Conflicts of Interest in Industry-Funded Clinical Research. In R. Spece, D. Shimm and A. Buchanan (Eds.), *Conflicts of Interest in Clinical Practice and Research* (pp. 407–417). New York: Oxford University Press.

Jaffe, A. (1996) Trends and Patterns in Research and Development Expenditures in the United States. *Proceedings of the National Academy of Sciences* **93**, 12658–12663.

Kass, L. (1985) *Toward a More Natural Science: Biology and Human Affairs.* New York: Free Press.

Kestendbaum, D. (1998) Cloning Plan Spawns Ethics Debate. *Science* **279**, 315.

Kolata, G. (1994) Parkinson Patients Set for First Rigorous Test of Fetal Cell Implants. *New York Times* (8 February), C3.

Korn, D. (1997) FDA Under Siege: The Public at Risk. *Science* **276**, 1627.

Marshall, E. A. (1998) Versatile Cell Line Raises Scientific Hopes, Legal Questions. *Science* **282**, 1014–1015.

Marshall, E. (1998) Disclosing Data Can Get You in Trouble. *Science* **276**, 671–672.

Marshal, E. (1998) Claim of Human-Cow Embryo Greeting with Skepticism. *Science* **282**, 1390–1391.

Marshall, E. (1998) Biomedical Groups Derail Fast-tack Anticloning Bill. *Science* **279**, 1123–1124.

Marshall, E. (1999) Ruling May Free NIH to Fund Stem Cell Studies. *Science* **283**, 465–467.

Marshall, E. and Pennisi, E. (1999) Hubris and the Human Genome. *Science* **280**, 994–995.

Martinez, F., Maillet, R., Legendre, C. and Buisson, C. (1998) Acute Myocardial Infarction Associated with Sildenafil. *Lancet* **352**, 1937.

McCain, K. (1996) Communication, Competition and Secrecy: The Production and Dissemination of Research-Related Information in Genetics. *Science, Technology and Human Values* **16**, 492.

National Bioethics Advisory Commission (1997) *(NBAC) Cloning Human Beings: Report and Recommendations.* Rockville, MD: National Bioethics Advisory Commission, June.

NBAC (1997) *Cloning Human Beings: Report and Recommendations.* Rockville, MD: NBAC.

Pence, G. (1995) *Classic Cases in Medical Ethics*, 2nd ed. New York: McGraw Hill.

Pence, G. (1998) *Who's Afraid of Human Cloning?* Lanham, MD: Rowman and Littlefield.

Pennisi, E. (1997) The Lamb That Roared. *Science* **278**, 2038–2039.

Pennisi, E. (1998) After Dolly, a Pharming Frenzy. *Science* **279**, 646–649.

Presidential Advisory Committed on Human Radiation Experiments (PACHRE). (1996) *The Human Radiation Experiments.* New York: Oxford University Press.

Priest, S. (1999) Popular Beliefs, Media, and Biotechnology. In S. Friedman, S. Dunwoody and C. Rogers (Eds.), *Communicating Uncertainty* (pp. 95–112). Mahwah, NJ: Lawrence Earlbaum, 1999.

Ramsey, P. (1970) *Fabricated Man: The Ethics of Genetic Control.* New Haven: Yale University Press.

Resnik, D. (1998a) *The Ethics of Science.* New York: Routledge.

Resnik, D. (1998b) Industry-Sponsored Research: Secrecy versus Corporate Responsibility. *Business and Society Review* **99**, 31–34.

Rifkin, J. (1983) *Algeny.* New York: Viking Press.

Rifkin, J. (1998) *The Biotech Century.* New York: Putnam.

Sagoff, M. (1999) DNA Patents: Marking Ends Meet. In A. Chapman (Ed.), *Perspectives on Genetic Patenting* (pp. 245–267). New York: American Association for the Advancement of Science.

Schatz, G. (1998) The Swiss Vote on Gene Technology. *Science* **281**, 1810–1811.

Sheldon, K. (1991) *Biotechnics and Society: The Rise of Industrial Genetics*. New York: Praeger.

Shenk, D. (1997) Biocapitalism. *Harper's Magazine* (December), 37–45.

Stix, G. (1997) Profile: Jeremy Rifkin. *Scientific American* **277**(2), 28–32.

The White House, Office of Communications (1997) *Directive on Cloning* (March 3).

Thomson et al. (1998) Embryonic Stem Cells Derived From Human Blastocysts. *Science* **282**, 1145–1147.

Volti, R. (1995) *Society and Technological Change*, 3rd edn. New York: St. Martin's Press.

Wade, N. (1998) It's a Three-Legged Race to Decipher the Human Genome. *New York Times* (23 June), 3.

Wadman, M. (1996) Drug Company Suppressed Publication of Research. *Nature* (2 May) **381**, 4.

Wadman, M. (1999) Congress May Block Stem-cell Research. *Nature* **397**, 639.

Walker, P. (1997) Bill Would Stiffen Rules for Informed Consent. *The Chronicle of Higher Education* **43**(22), A38.

Weston, A. (1997) *A Practical Companion to Ethics*. New York: Oxford University Press.

Williams, N. (1997) Cloning Sparks Calls for New Laws. *Science* **275**, 1415.

Williams, N. (1998) Agricultural Biotech Faces Backlash in Europe. *Science* **281**, 768–771.

Wilmut, I (1998) Cloning for Medicine. *Scientific American* (December) **279**, 58–63.

Name Index